MANUAL OF
CRITICAL CARE

MANUAL OF
CRITICAL CARE

Applying Nursing Diagnoses to Adult Critical Illness

Edited by

PAMELA L. SWEARINGEN, R.N.
Special Project Editor

MARILYN SAWYER SOMMERS, R.N., M.A., C.C.R.N.
Director of Critical Care Nursing,
University of Cincinnati

KENNETH MILLER, R.N., M.S., Ph.D.
Assistant Professor, University of California,
San Francisco

THE C. V. MOSBY COMPANY

St. Louis • Washington, D.C. • Toronto   1988

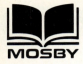

A TRADITION OF PUBLISHING EXCELLENCE

Editor: Don E. Ladig
Assistant Editor: Robin Carter
Production: Editing, Design & Production, Inc.
Design: Liz Fett

Printed in the United States of America

The C.V. Mosby Company
11830 Westline Industrial Drive, St. Louis, Missouri 63146

Library of Congress Cataloging-in-Publication Data

Manual of critical care.

  Includes bibliographies and indexes.
  1. Intensive care nursing.   2. Diagnosis.
I. Swearingen, Pamela L.   II. Sommers, Marilyn Sawyer.
III. Miller, Kenneth, 1948-   [DNLM: 1. Critical Care—
nurses' instruction.   2. Nursing Assessment.   WY 154 M294]
RT120.I5M364   1988   616'.028   87-28253
ISBN 0-8016-5028-3

C/D/D   9   8   7   6   5   4   3   2   1   01-A-047

CONTRIBUTORS

LINDA S. BAAS, R.N., M.S.N., C.C.R.N.
Cardiac Clinical Nurse Specialist
Consultation Department
University Hospital, University of Cincinnati
  Medical Center
Cincinnati, Ohio

MIMI CALLANAN, R.N., M.S.N.
Epilepsy Clinical Specialist
Mid-Atlantic Regional Epilepsy Center
Medical College of Pennsylvania
Philadelphia, Pennsylvania

**URSULA J. EASTERDAY, R.N., M.S.N.,
C.C.R.N.**
Clinical Nurse Specialist—Care of the Adult
Community Hospital North
Indianapolis, Indiana

**ANNA GAWLINSKI, R.N., M.S.N.,
C.C.R.N.**
Cardiovascular Clinical Nurse Specialist
UCLA Medical Center;
Assistant Clinical Professor
UCLA School of Nursing
Los Angeles, California

MIMA M. HORNE, R.N., M.S.N.
Staff Nurse, Dialysis Services
El Camino Hospital
Mountain View, California;
Instructor, Nursing Continuing Education
De Anza College
Cupertino, California

CHERI A. HOWARD, R.N., M.S.N.
Unit Director
Indiana University Hospital
Indianapolis, Indiana

**JANET HICKS KEEN, R.N., M.S.,
C.C.R.N., C.E.N.**
Trauma Clinical Nurse Specialist
Georgia Baptist Medical Center
Atlanta, Georgia

LESLIE S. KERN, R.N., M.N., C.C.R.N.
Cardiothoracic Surgery Clinical Nurse
  Specialist
UCLA Medical Center;
Assistant Clinical Professor
UCLA School of Nursing
Los Angeles, California

DONNA KERSHNER, R.N., B.S.N.
M.S.N. candidate
University of California, San Francisco
San Francisco, California

CAROL E. LANG, R.D., M.S.
Assistant Director, Clinical Nutrition Services
Department of Dietary Services
University of Cincinnati Medical Center
Cincinnati, Ohio

KENNETH MILLER, R.N., M.S., Ph.D.
Assistant Professor, Department of
  Physiological Nursing,
University of California, San Francisco;
Project Coordinator, Transfusion Safety Study
UCSF Department of Laboratory Medicine
San Francisco, California

**NANCY MUNRO, R.N., M.S.N.,
C.C.R.N.**
Critical Care Clinical Nurse Specialist
Georgia Baptist Medical Center
Atlanta, Georgia

**DENNIS G. ROSS, R.N., M.S.N.,
M.A.E., C.N.O.R.**
Associate Professor of Nursing
Castleton State College
Castleton, Vermont

**MARILYN SAWYER SOMMERS, R.N.,
M.A., C.C.R.N.**
Director, Critical Care Nursing
University Hospital, University of Cincinnati
  Medical Center
Cincinnati, Ohio

SUSAN KLAUSEN STONE, R.N., M.S., C.N.S.
Clinical Nurse Researcher
Northeast Georgia Medical Center
Gainesville, Georgia

ANN COGHLAN STOWE, R.N., M.S.N.
Instructor
West Chester University, Department of Nursing
West Chester, Pennsylvania

BARBARA L. TUELLER, R.N., M.S., C.C.R.N., C.E.N.
Assistant Professor
Samuel Merritt College of Nursing
Oakland, California

DAVID UNKLE, R.N., B.S.N., C.C.R.N., C.E.N.
Clinical Research Coordinator
Division of Trauma and Emergency Medical Services
Robert Wood Johnson Medical School at Camden
Cooper Hospital/University Hospital
Camden, New Jersey

PATRICIA D. WEISKITTEL, R.N., M.S.N.
Renal Clinical Nurse Specialist
University Hospital, University of Cincinnati Medical Center
Cincinnati, Ohio

MARIBETH WOOLDRIDGE-KING, R.N., M.S.
Associate Director, Nursing Education
Long Island College Hospital
Brooklyn, New York

CONSULTANT BOARD

PREFACE

Manual of Critical Care: Applying Nursing Diagnoses to Critical Illness was developed to provide nurses with a portable compendium of more than 70 of the clinical phenomena seen in critical care. Focusing on nursing diagnoses and interventions that are specific to each critical disorder, the book also provides a brief review of pathophysiology and discusses assessment data, diagnostic tests, medical management, and surgical interventions. The order of presentation provides a hierarchy of information that enables the nurse to make nursing diagnoses and determine interventions specific to the individual patient. Most critical illness discussions also provide rehabilitation and patient-family teaching concepts, a section that enumerates the data patients and their significant others need to ensure patients' optimal recovery and rehabilitation. While patient teaching in critical care may, by necessity, be concentrated on immediate learning needs (for example, coughing, deep breathing, leg exercises), ideally the information provided in this section will be incorporated before discharge, orally or *via* written instructions.

For the sake of clarity and consistency throughout the book, normal values are provided for hemodynamic monitoring and other measurements. However, all values should be individualized to correspond to the patient's normal range of measurements. Although the book offers a host of interventions for each critical disorder, not all interventions are appropriate for every patient. It is our intent that interventions that do apply to the individual patient be used in the development of a personalized care plan. Further, if the patient has needs that are not listed under the discussion at hand, the reader is invited to find appropriate nursing diagnoses by reviewing the section "Index of Nursing Diagnoses Used in this Manual," p. 543. In addition, nursing diagnoses common to most critically ill patients are found in the appendixes "Providing Nutritional Support," p. 490, "Caring for the Critically Ill on Prolonged Bed Rest," p. 506, "Caring for the Critically Ill with Life-Threatening Disorders," p. 511, and "Caring for the Family of the Critically Ill," p. 522. The last two sections discuss psychosocial nursing diagnoses that are appropriate for critically ill patients.

Manual of Critical Care was written to supplement critical care textbooks and assumes that the reader already has a background in critical care pathophysiology and assessment parameters. The book can serve as a resource not only for clinicians but also for academicians and students. The text and numerous tables will stimulate recall of previously learned concepts for the clinician. Academicians can use the book in teaching students how to apply theoretical concepts to clinical practice. Students will find the book an excellent tool in assessing the patient systematically, as well as setting priorities for nursing interventions. Our primary goal is to help staff and students in critical care locate clinical information quickly and easily and apply nursing diagnoses in the critical care environment. Reviewers indicate that we have achieved this objective. We welcome comments from nurses who use the book on a daily basis so that we can enhance its usefulness in future editions.

P.L.S
M.S.S.
K.M.

CONTENTS

3   RENAL-URINARY DYSFUNCTIONS

4   NEUROLOGIC DYSFUNCTIONS

5   ENDOCRINOLOGIC DYSFUNCTIONS: Donna Kershner

6   GASTROINTESTINAL DYSFUNCTIONS: Janet Keen

1
RESPIRATORY DYSFUNCTIONS

Status asthmaticus

Acute pneumonia

Pulmonary hypertension

Adult respiratory distress syndrome

Perfusion disorders

Pneumothorax

Chest trauma

Near drowning

Acid-base imbalances

Acute respiratory failure and management of the adult
on mechanical ventilation

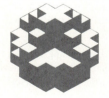

Status asthmaticus

Hyperreactive airways disease is an obstructive lung process more commonly known as asthma. The hyperreactive bronchial airways respond to a variety of irritants with diffuse narrowing due to bronchospasm, mucosal edema, increased mucus production, and plugging. If these problems are not controlled, status asthmaticus (SA) can occur. SA can be defined as a severe, unrelenting asthma attack that is not reversed after 24 hours by maximum doses of traditional therapy. Precipitating factors include allergens (airborne or ingested), respiratory infection, chemical irritants (e.g., smoke, air pollution), physical irritants (e.g., cold air, exercise), and emotional stress in some individuals. Although the attack can happen suddenly, there usually is a more gradual onset, with symptoms of increased sputum production, coughing, wheezing, and dyspnea occurring over several days. The patient experiences increased work of breathing, which increases insensible water loss through exhaled water vapor and diaphoresis. Oral intake may be decreased, which contributes further to the hypovolemia. Mucus becomes thick and begins to plug the airways. Terminal bronchioles become occluded completely from mucosal edema and tenacious secretions. Ventilation-perfusion mismatch occurs as the alveoli, which are not being ventilated, continue to be perfused. Shunting of blood from nonventilated alveoli to other alveoli cannot compensate for the diminished ventilation, and hypoxia occurs. Tachypnea and tachycardia evolve as compensatory mechanisms. As a result, oxygen requirements and work of breathing increase. If the patient is not treated promptly, respiratory collapse can occur and death by asphyxiation becomes possible.

ASSESSMENT

Signs and symptoms: Coughing, chest tightness, increased sputum production, increased RR (>20 breaths/min), labored breathing, dyspnea, fatigue, insomnia, anorexia, restlessness, and confusion.

Physical assessment: Agitation, use of accessory muscles of respiration, chest retractions, nasal flaring, diaphoresis, decreased tactile fremitus and hyperresonance over lung areas in which there is air trapping; dullness over areas of atelectasis. Expiratory wheezing, prolonged expiratory phase, and coarse rhonchi may be auscultated. In addition, the patient may have hypotension, pulsus paradoxus >10 mm Hg, and apical tachycardia (HR >100 bpm). Cyanosis of the lips and nailbeds is a late sign.

< N O T E : An absence of wheezing in the presence of other signs and symptoms of respiratory distress may be a result of severe bronchial constriction, which dangerously narrows airways during both inspiratory and expiratory phases. The volume of air moved through the airways is so minimal that it does not cause a sound. If this occurs, respiratory collapse may be imminent.

DIAGNOSTIC TESTS

1. *ABGs:* Determine status of oxygenation and acid-base balance. Initially, Pa_{O_2} is normal and then decreases as the ventilation-perfusion mismatch described earlier becomes more severe. Usually, Pa_{CO_2} is decreased in early stages of status asthmaticus due to hyperventilation. When Pa_{CO_2} is normal or greater than normal, respiratory failure may be imminent due to relative hypoventilation.

2. *Pulmonary function testing:* Forced expiratory volume (FEV) is decreased during acute episodes because of severely narrowed airways that prevent forceful exhalation of inspired volume. See Table 1-1.

3. *Chest x-ray:* Useful in ruling out other causes of respiratory failure (e.g., foreign body aspiration, pulmonary edema, pulmonary embolism, pneumonia). The x-ray usually shows lung hyperinflation due to air trapping and a flat diaphragm related to increased intrathoracic volume.

4. *Sputum:* Gross exam may show viscosity or actual mucous plugs. Culture and sensitivity may show microorganisms if infection was the precipitating event.

5. *CBC:* Differential will show increased eosinophiles, which are indicative of allergic response, in patients not on corticosteroids. The hematocrit may be increased due to hypovolemia.

6. *Serum theophylline level:* Important baseline indicator for patients who are on this therapy. Acceptable therapeutic range is 10-20 µg/ml. The therapeutic level is close to the toxic level and the patient must be monitored for toxic side effects (e.g., nausea, CNS stimulation, dysrhythmias). Serial levels are drawn at frequent intervals.

7. *EKG:* Presence of sinus tachycardia is an important baseline indicator because the use of some bronchodilators (e.g., metaproterenol) may produce cardiac stimulant effects and dysrhythmias.

TABLE 1-1

Pulmonary function tests in status asthmaticus (SA)

Test	Description	Normal values	Parameters in SA
Forced vital capacity (FVC)	Total amount of gas exhaled as forcefully and as rapidly as possible after maximal inspiration	≥80% of predicted normal	Normal or slightly decreased due to air trapping
Forced expiratory volume in one second (FEV_1)	Volume of gas exhaled over first second of FVC. (FEV_2 and FEV_3 also may be measured at two and three seconds, respectively.)	≥75% of predicted normal	Decreased due to airway obstruction. It may return to normal after administration of aerosolized bronchodilator.
Forced mid-expiratory flow (FEF). Formerly this was called maximal mid-expiratory flow (MMF).	Average rate of flow during middle half of FEV. It is an accurate estimate of airway resistance.	≥80% of predicted normal	Decreased due to small airways obstruction. It may return to normal after administration of aerosolized bronchodilator.

8. *Urine specific gravity:* An important indicator of hydration. Values higher than normal (1.010-1.030) occur with dehydration.

MEDICAL MANAGEMENT

Primarily, management is directed toward decreasing bronchospasm and increasing pulmonary ventilation. Other interventions are directed toward treatment of sequelae resulting from SA.

1. **Oxygen therapy:** Generally, these patients suffer from profound hypoxia and can tolerate high doses of oxygen (4-8 L). However, if the patient has chronic CO_2 retention, he or she will not tolerate >2-3 L oxygen, as doses higher than this might impair the drive to breathe, which is a hypoxic drive. Oxygen therapy is begun immediately to correct hypoxemia and the Pao_2 is kept above normal to compensate for the increased oxygen demands imposed by the increased work of breathing. The oxygen is humidified to help liquefy secretions. A nasal cannula is preferred because most patients cannot tolerate a mask due to feelings of suffocation. The degree of hypoxemia and patient response determines the method of oxygen delivery.

2. **Pharmacotherapy:** Vigorous therapy is initiated to improve bronchospasm. Treatment is continued until wheezing is eliminated and pulmonary function tests return to baseline.
   - *Bronchodilators:* Dilate smooth muscles of the airways (see Table 1-2).
   - *Corticosteroids:* Given IV during the acute phase of SA to decrease the inflammatory response. Dosage varies according to severity of episode and whether patient is currently taking steroids.

< N O T E : Acute adrenal insufficiency can develop in patients who take steroids routinely at home if these drugs are not given to the patient during hospitalization.

   - *Sedatives and tranquilizers:* Generally avoided unless patient is extremely agitated and unable to cooperate with therapy, as these agents depress the CNS response to hypoxia, hypercapnea, and airway obstruction.
   - *Buffers:* Metabolic acidosis may develop as a compensatory mechanism for early respiratory alkalosis during which patient is hyperventilating and exhaling greater than normal amounts of CO_2. Sodium bicarbonate may be given to correct severe metabolic acidosis. The physiologic response to bronchodilators improves with correction of metabolic acidosis.
   - *Antibiotics:* Given if infectious pulmonary process is present, as evidenced by fever, purulent sputum, or leukocytosis.

3. **Fluid replacement:** To liquefy secretions and replace insensible losses. Generally, crystalloid fluids (i.e., D_5W or D_5NS) are used.

4. **Intubation and mechanical ventilation:** Elected if $Paco_2$ continues to rise or if patient has deterioration in LOC. Therapy ensures adequate alveolar ventilation and provides a pathway for clearing airway secretions *via* suctioning.

5. **Chest physiotherapy:** Generally contraindicated in acute phases of SA owing to acute respiratory embarrassment and hyperreactive state of airways. Once the crisis is over, the patient may benefit from percussion and postural drainage q2-4h to help mobilize secretions.

TABLE 1-2
Bronchodilators used in status asthmaticus

Medication	Usual dosage	Action	Side effects
Epinephrine	0.2-0.5 ml of a 1:1000 solution given SC q15-30min	Immediate adrenergic effects; activates adrenergic sympathomimetic receptors; acts on alpha, beta-one, and beta-two receptors; relieves bronchospasm	Cardiac stimulation, palpitations, anxiety
Terbutaline	0.2-0.3 ml given SC q30min × 3 doses	Selective beta-adrenergic; relaxes bronchial smooth muscle	Fewer than with epinephrine and usually transient; increased HR (>20 bpm), nervousness, tremor, palpitations, nausea, vomiting, headache.
Methylxanthine	*Loading dose:* 6 mg/kg given IV bolus. *Maintenance dose:* 0.1-0.5 μg/kg/hr given *via* continuous IV infusion.	Short-acting nonadrenergic; directly relaxes smooth muscle of bronchial airways and pulmonary vasculature	Nausea, vomiting, GI bleeding, gastric distress, HR >20 bpm, decreased BP, restlessness. NOTE: Because toxic levels are close to therapeutic loads, serum levels should be monitored to ensure correct dosage adjustment. Dysrhythmias may result from toxic levels of theophylline.
Isoproterenol/ Isoetharine	Inhalants usually avoided during acute SA as gas flow may be too minimal to provide adequate distribution of medication.		

NURSING DIAGNOSES AND INTERVENTIONS

Impaired gas exchange related to decreased alveolar ventilation secondary to narrowed airways

---

Desired outcome: Patient has adequate gas exchange as evidenced by $Pao_2 \geq 60$ mm Hg, $Paco_2 \leq 45$ mm Hg, pH 7.35-7.45, and RR 12-20 breaths/min (or values consistent with patient's baseline).

---

1. Observe for signs and symptoms of hypoxia (e.g., restlessness, agitation, changes in LOC). Remember that cyanosis of the lips and nailbeds is a late indicator of hypoxia.
2. Position patient for comfort and to promote optimal gas exchange. Usually this is accomplished using high-Fowler's position, with the patient leaning forward and elbows propped on the over-the-bed table to promote maximal chest excursion. Record patient's response to positioning.
3. Auscultate breath sounds at frequent intervals. Monitor for decreased or adventitious sounds (e.g., crackles or wheezes).
4. Monitor ABG results. Be alert to decreasing Pao_2 and increasing $Paco_2$, which are signals of respiratory failure.
5. Deliver oxygen as prescribed; monitor Fio_2 to ensure that oxygen is within prescribed concentrations.
6. Encourage patient to breathe slowly and deeply. Utilize pursed-lip breathing technique to assist patient with controlling his or her respirations:
   - Inhale through the nose.
   - Form lips in an "O" shape as if whistling.
   - Exhale slowly through pursed lips.
   Record patient's response to breathing technique.

Ineffective airway clearance related to presence of viscous secretions

---

Desired outcome: Patient's airway remains free of adventitious breath sounds.

---

1. At frequent intervals, assess patient's ability to clear tracheobronchial secretions. Keep emergency suction equipment at the bedside.
2. Encourage oral fluid intake within patient's prescribed limits to help decrease viscosity of the secretions.
3. After crisis phase of SA has been resolved, ensure that patient receives chest physiotherapy as prescribed; document patient's response to treatment.
4. Ensure that oxygen is humidified to aid in liquefying tracheobronchial secretions.
5. Encourage patient to cough effectively at frequent intervals to clear secretions.
   - Instruct patient to take several deep breaths.
   - After the last inhalation, teach patient to perform a succession of coughs (usually three or four) on the same exhalation until most of the air has been expelled.
   - Explain that patient may need to repeat this technique several times before the cough becomes productive.

Activity intolerance related to fatigue secondary to increased work of breathing and inability to meet metabolic demands for oxygen

---

Desired outcome: Patient verbalizes a decrease in fatigue and associated symptoms.

---

1. Organize and group assessment procedures and activities to provide patient with frequent rest periods (optimally, of at least 90-120 minutes).
2. Assess temperature q2h. Inform MD of increases and provide treatment as prescribed to decrease temperature and, hence, oxygen demands.
3. If patient is restless, which increases oxygen demand, ascertain etiology of the restlessness. For example, if restlessness is related to anxiety, help reduce anxiety by providing reassurance, enabling family members to stay with patient, and offering distractions (e.g., soft music, television).

See "Acute Pneumonia" for the following: **Potential for infection** (nosocomial pneumonia), p. 13. For other nursing diagnoses and interventions, see "Caring for the Critically Ill with Life-Threatening Disorders," pp. 511-522; and "Caring for the Family of the Critically Ill," pp. 522-526.

REHABILITATION AND PATIENT-FAMILY TEACHING CONCEPTS

Give patient and significant others verbal and written instructions for the following:
1. Irritants that can precipitate an attack and the importance of removing these irritants from patient's environment.
2. Importance of adequate hydration to decrease airway irritation and minimize viscosity of tracheobronchial secretions. Teach patient to limit intake of tea, coffee, and alcoholic beverages, as they may have a diuretic effect, which in turn can precipitate hypovolemia.
3. Signs and symptoms of pulmonary infection (e.g., increased cough, increasing sputum production, change in color of sputum from clear-white to yellow-green, fever) or bronchial irritation (e.g., dry, hacking cough).
4. Medications, including name, route, purpose, dose, precautions, and potential side effects. In addition, teach patient the proper use of metered-dose inhalers, documenting accurate return of demonstration before hospital discharge. Remind patient that OTC inhalers contain medications that can interfere with the prescribed therapy. Instruct patient to contact MD before taking any OTC medications.

Acute pneumonia

Pneumonia is an acute infection that causes inflammation of the parenchyma (alveolar spaces and interstitial tissue) of the lung. As a result of the inflammation, the involved lung tissue becomes swollen and the air spaces fill with liquid. Pneumonias can be classified into two groups: community-acquired and hospital-associated (nosocomial). A third type that occurs is pneumonia in the immunocompromised host.

Community-acquired pneumonias: Individuals with this type of pneumonia seldom require hospitalization and are seen in intensive care areas only when an underlying medical condition such as COPD, cardiac disease, diabetes mellitus, or an immunocompromised state necessitates special care.

Hospital-associated (nosocomial) pneumonias: These pneumonias usually occur following aspiration of oropharyngeal flora in an individual whose resistance is altered or whose coughing mechanisms are impaired, for example, a patient who has undergone thoracoabdominal surgery. Bacteria invade the lower respiratory tract *via* three routes: aspiration of oropharyngeal organisms (most common route), inhalation of aerosols that contain bacteria, or hematogenous spread to the lung from another site of infection (rare). Gram-negative pneumonias have a high mortality rate, even with appropriate antibiotic therapy. *Aspiration pneumonia* is a nonbacterial cause of hospital-associated pneumonia that occurs when gastric contents are aspirated. If the alveolar-capillary membrane is affected, ARDS may be seen.

Pneumonias in the immunocompromised patient: Immunosuppression and neutropenia are predisposing factors in the development of nosocomial pneumonias, both from common and unusual pathogens. The patient's underlying disease state is a determining factor in susceptibility to specific pathogens. Usually, patients with neutropenia resulting from acute leukemia or cytotoxic agents have gram-negative bacilli as the source of pneumonia. Severely immunocompromised patients are affected not only by bacteria, but by fungi *(Candida, Aspergillus)*, viruses (Cytomegalovirus), and protozoa *(Pneumocystis carinii)* as well. Most commonly, *Pneumocystis carinii* is seen in patients with AIDS or in those who have received organ transplants.

ASSESSMENT

Findings are influenced by the patient's age, extent of the disease process, underlying medical condition, and pathogen involved.

General signs and symptoms: Cough (productive and nonproductive); sputum (rust-colored, purulent, bloody, or mucoid); fever; pleuritic chest pain (more common in community-acquired bacterial pneumonias); dyspnea; chills; headache; myalgia. Elderly individuals may be confused or disoriented and run low-grade fevers, but may present with few other signs and symptoms.

General physical assessment findings: Presence of nasal flaring and expiratory grunt; use of accessory muscles of respiration (scalene, sternocleidomastoid, external intercostals); decreased chest expansion caused by pleuritic pain; dullness on percussion over affected areas; tachypnea (RR $>$20 breaths/min), tachycardia (HR $>$100 bpm), high-pitched inspiratory crackles (increased by or heard only after coughing), and low-pitched inspiratory crackles caused by airway secretions.

$<$ N O T E :   Findings may be normal, even with an abnormal chest x-ray.

Risk factors: In addition to the risk factors listed in Table 1-3, any factor that alters the integrity of the lower airways, thereby inhibiting ciliary activity, increases the likelihood of pneumonia. These factors may include hypoventilation, hyperoxia (increaed FIO_2), hypoxia, chemical irritants, and viral pneumonia.

DIAGNOSTIC TESTS

1. *ABG levels:* Hypoxemia (Pao_2 $<$80 mm Hg) and hypocarbia ($Paco_2$ $<$35 mm Hg), with a resultant respiratory alkalosis (pH $>$7.45), will be seen in the absence of an underlying pulmonary disease.
2. *CBC:* WBC count will be increased ($>$11,000 μl) in the presence of bacterial pneumonias. Normal or low WBC will be seen with viral or mycoplasma pneumonias.

TABLE 1-3

Assessment guidelines by pneumonia type

Type/Pathogen	Risk groups	Onset	Defining characteristics	Complications/Comments
Community acquired				
Pneumococcal (*pneumococcus pneumoniae, Streptococcus pneumoniae*)	Aged people with debilitating diseases (e.g., diabetes mellitus, CHF)	Abrupt	Single shaking chill, fever, pleuritic chest pain, severe cough, SOB, rust-colored sputum	Herpes labialis, abdominal distention, meningitis, empyema, pericarditis, impaired liver function, septicemia. Mortality rate increases if more than one lobe is involved.
Mycoplasma (*Mycoplasma pneumoniae*)	School-aged children to young adult (5–30 yrs). Intrafamilial spread is common.	Gradual	Cough, sore throat, fever, lower lobe involvement, ear involvement (usually in children)	Rare. Persistent cough and sinusitis are possible.
Legionnaires' (*Legionella pneumophilia*)	Middle-aged, elderly (males at increased risk) populations; cigarette smokers; individuals with malignancy, immunosuppression, chronic renal failure	Abrupt	Malaise, headache within 24 hrs, fever with normal HR, shaking chills, nonproductive cough progressing to cough with purulent sputum. GI symptoms	Respiratory failure, hypotension, shock, acute renal failure
Viral Influenza A	Elderly people with chronic diseases (e.g., COPD, diabetes mellitus, CHF); pregnancy	One week after onset of influenza symptoms	Severe dyspnea, cyanosis, scant sputum with gross blood	Rapid course leading frequently to acute respiratory failure; secondary bacterial pneumonia

Continued.

T A B L E 1 - 3 cont'd.
Assessment guidelines by pneumonia type

Type/Pathogen	Risk groups	Onset	Defining characteristics	Complications/Comments
Nosocomial Klebsiella (*Klebsiella pneumoniae*)	Males >40 yrs; alcoholics; patients with diabetes mellitus or COPD	Abrupt	Chills, fever, productive cough (copious gray-green, brick-red sputum). Severe pleuritic chest pain, delirium, tenacious dark-brown or red-currant jelly sputum. Cyanosis and dyspnea, jaundice, vomiting, and diarrhea	Lung abscess and empyema, necrotizing pneumonitis with cavitation, acute respiratory failure. High mortality rate.
Pseudomonas	Patients receiving sedatives, endotracheal intubation, IPPB, numerous courses of antibiotic therapy	Gradual	Fever, shaking, chills, hyperventilation, confusion, delerium, bradycardia, sputum (green, foul-smelling)	Primary *Pseudomonas* is rare. Bacteremic *Pseudomonas* can result in circulatory collapse and has a high mortality rate.
Proteus	Patients receiving antibiotics or who have undergone urinary tract instrumentation	Abrupt	High fever, chills, pleuritic chest pain	Rare. Localizes to areas that already are damaged. Presents as a mixed infection. Has four pathogenic species with differing antibiotic susceptibilities.

Staphylococcus aureus	Patients with debilitating diseases (e.g., diabetes mellitus, renal failure, liver disease, malnutrition, influenza, measles, COPD)	Abrupt with community-acquired pneumonia; insidious with hospital-associated pneumonia	Cough, early peripheral vascular collapse, chills, high fever, progressive dyspnea, cyanosis, pleuritic pain, bloody sputum	Pulmonary abscesses or empyema. Response to antibiotics is slow.
Aspiration of gastric contents	Patients with impaired gag/cough reflexes; general anesthesia; presence of NG/ET tube.	Gradual: latent period between aspiration and onset of symptoms.	Fever, wheezes, crackles (rales), rhonchi, dyspnea, cyanosis	Physiologic response depends on pH of material aspirated: ≥ 2.5, little necrosis occurs; <2.5, atelectasis, pulmonary edema, hemorrhage, and necrosis can occur.

N O T E : *Enterobacter* and *Serratia* are enteric organisms that cause pneumonia with the same clinical pattern as *Klebsiella*.

Immunocompromised patient

Pneumocystis (*Pneumocystis carinii*)	Patients with AIDS or organ transplants	Insidious	Severe dyspnea and tachypnea. Nonproductive cough, progressive hypoxemia, few auscultatory signs, minimal or absent fever. Cyanosis is a late sign.	Open lung biopsy is most reliable method of diagnosis. High mortality rate.
Aspergillosis (*Aspergillus*)	Patients with AIDS, transplants, COPD; those receiving cytotoxic agents or steroids	Abrupt with immunosuppression; insidious with COPD	Hemoptysis; fungal ball within lung cyst or cavity	Biopsy necessary for definitive diagnosis. Hematogenous spread common in immunocompromised patient.

3. *Sputum for Gram stain and culture and sensitivity tests:* Sputum must be obtained from lower respiratory tract before initiation of antibiotic therapy. It can be obtained *via* expectoration, suctioning, transtracheal aspiration, bronchoscopy, or open-lung biopsy.

4. *Blood culture and sensitivity:* To determine presence of bacteremia and aid in the identification of the causative organism.

5. *Culture and sensitivity of pleural effusion fluid:* Especially useful in identifying pathogen involved in nosocomial pneumonias.

6. *Serologic studies:* Acute and convalescent titers are drawn to diagnose viral pneumonia. Rises in antibody titers are positive for viral infection.

7. *Acid-fast stains and cultures:* To rule out tuberculosis.

8. *Chest x-ray:* To identify anatomic involvement; extent of disease; and presence of consolidation, pleural effusions, and cavitation.
   - *Lobar:* Entire lobe involved.
   - *Segmental* (lobular): Only parts of a lobe involved.
   - *Bronchopneumonia:* Affects alveoli contiguous to the involved bronchi.

MEDICAL MANAGEMENT

1. **Oxygen therapy:** Administered when ABGs demonstrate presence of hypoxemia. Special care must be taken not to abolish the drive to breathe if patient has a chronic lung disorder and is known to retain CO_2. (Normally, the drive to breathe occurs with increased Pa_{CO_2} levels; in patients with CO_2 retention, the drive to breathe occurs with decreased Pa_{O_2} levels.) Initially, oxygen is delivered in low concentrations, with a close watch of ABG levels. If Pa_{O_2} does not rise to acceptable levels ($\geq$60 mm Hg), FI_{O_2} is increased in small increments, with concomitant ABG checks.

2. **Intubation and mechanical ventilation:** Intubation may be necessary if patient is unable to maintain a patent airway because of tenacious or copious secretions, ineffective cough, or fatigue. Mechanical ventilation is required if patient is unable to maintain adequate ABGs ($Pa_{O_2} \geq$60 mm Hg) with supplemental oxygen. High concentrations of oxygen and positive end expiratory pressure (PEEP) may be necessary in severe cases of pneumonia leading to acute respiratory failure.

3. **Antibiotic agents:** Prescribed empirically, based on presenting signs and symptoms, clinical findings, and chest x-ray results until sputum or blood culture results are available. Erythromycin is the most commonly used antibiotic in community-acquired pneumonia. Many of the organisms responsible for nosocomial pneumonias are resistant to multiple antibiotics. Proper identification of the organism and determination of sensitivity to specific antibiotics are critical for appropriate therapy.

4. **Antipyretics and analgesics:** To reduce temperature and provide relief for pleuritic pain.

5. **Hydration:** IV fluids may be necessary to replace fluids lost from insensible sources (e.g., tachypnea, diaphoresis with fevers).

6. **Isolation:** Some patients with pneumonia may require isolation. If the hospital follows the 1983 Centers for Disease Control (CDC) guidelines for *disease-specific* isolation precautions, the procedures are tailored to the specific pathogen involved. If the hospital follows the 1983 CDC guidelines for *category-specific* isolation precautions, the following procedures may be followed:
   - *Contact isolation:* Multiply-resistant bacteria, infection, or colonization with

Staphylococcus aureus or group A *Streptococcus*. This type of isolation requires masks, gowns if soiling is likely, and gloves if touching infective material (e.g., respiratory secretions) is anticipated. Hands must be washed after touching patient or potentially contaminated articles and before taking care of another patient. Articles contaminated with infective material are discarded or bagged and labeled before being sent for decontamination and reprocessing. A private room is indicated but patients with same organism may share the room.

- *Respiratory isolation:* Meningococcal; *Haemophilus influenzae* in infants and children. Hands must be washed after touching patient or potentially contaminated articles and before taking care of another patient. Masks are required for those in close contact with patient, but gowns and gloves are not. Articles contaminated with infective material should be discarded or bagged and labeled before being sent for decontamination and reprocessing.
- *Acid-fast bacilli (AFB) isolation:* Required if patient has current (active) tuberculosis (TB), a positive sputum smear, or a chest x-ray suggestive of active TB. A mask is required if the patient is coughing and doesn't cover his or her mouth reliably. A gown is indicated only if soiling of clothing is anticipated.

Body substance isolation: A relatively new concept in infection control, this procedure advocates treating *all* patients in an identical manner. Gloves are worn when contact with body substances, nonintact skin, or mucous membranes is anticipated, regardless of the patient's diagnosis. A mask may be required if the suspected or diagnosed disease is transmitted by an airborne route. Mask and eye protection are necessary if splashing of body substances into the eyes or mucous membranes is likely to occur (e.g., with suctioning). A gown is required only if soiling of clothing is anticipated.

7. **Percussion and postural drainage:** Indicated if deep breathing, coughing, and moving about in bed or ambulation are ineffective in raising and expectorating sputum.

NURSING DIAGNOSES AND INTERVENTIONS

Potential for infection (nosocomial pneumonia) related to high risk secondary to recent thoracoabdominal surgery, aspiration, exposure to contaminated respiratory equipment, respiratory instrumentation, colonization of oropharynx with aerobic gram-negative bacilli, or immunosuppression

---

Desired outcome: Patient is free of infection as evidenced by body temperature ≤37.5° C, WBC count ≤11,000 μl, and sputum clear to whitish in color.

---

1. Perform good handwashing after contact with respiratory secretions (even though gloves were worn) and before and after contact with patient who has a tracheostomy or is intubated.
2. Identify presurgical candidate who is at increased risk for nosocomial pneumonia: individuals who are >70 years old or obese; who have COPD or history of smoking, abnormal pulmonary function tests (especially decreased forced expiratory flow rate), tracheostomy; who will be intubated for a prolonged period of time; or who will have upper abdominal or thoracic operations.
   - Before surgery, provide patient with verbal and written instructions and dem-

onstrations of exercises to perform after surgery to prevent respiratory tract infection. Make sure that patient verbalizes knowledge of the exercises and their rationale and *returns* the demonstrations appropriately. Encourage smokers to discontinue smoking, especially during preoperative and postoperative periods.

- Be aware that most patients can expand their lungs effectively after surgery but won't do so unless they are encouraged. At frequent intervals, enforce the following regimens that expand the lungs: deep-breathing exercises, coughing, turning in bed, and walking (not as likely in critical care). In addition, use of incentive spirometry promotes periodic, voluntary lung expansion greater than tidal volume.
- If pain interferes with lung expansion, control it by administering medications ½ hour before deep-breathing exercises and providing support of wound areas with hands or pillows placed firmly across site of incision.
- In the high-risk patient who is too weak to deep-breathe independently, confer with MD regarding use of intermittent positive pressure breathing (IPPB). However, the role of IPPB in preventing pneumonia following surgery has not been determined.
- For patient who cannot remove secretions effectively by coughing, perform procedures that stimulate coughing such as chest physiotherapy, which includes breathing exercises, postural drainage, and percussion.

3. Identify patients who are at high risk for aspiration: individuals with a depressed LOC, those with dysphagia, or those who have an NG tube in place.
- For patient with depressed LOC, confer with MD regarding need for a method of feeding in which risk of aspiration is minimal, for example, small-bore weighted feeding tube that migrates to the duodenum, IV hyperalimentation, or gastrostomy.
- For patient with NG tube in place, turn onto side rather than back during feeding and provide small, frequent feedings rather than large ones. Elevate HOB to at least 30 degrees at all times.

4. Recognize the following ways in which nebulizer reservoirs can contaminate patient: introduction of nonsterile fluids or air, manipulation of nebulizer cup, or backflow of condensate from delivery tubing into reservoir or into patient when tubing is manipulated.
- Use only sterile fluids and dispense them aseptically.
- Replace (rather than replenish) solutions and equipment at frequent intervals. For example, empty reservoir completely and refill with sterile solution q8-24 hours, according to agency protocol.
- Change breathing circuits q48h; if used for the multiple patients, replace breathing circuit with sterilized or disinfected breathing circuit between patients.
- Fill fluid reservoirs immediately before use (not far in advance).
- Discard any fluid that has condensed in tubing; do not allow it to drain back into reservoir or into patient.

5. Recognize risk factors for patients with tracheostomy or endotracheal tubes: presence of underlying lung disease or other serious illness, increased colonization of oropharynx or trachea by aerobic gram-negative bacteria, greater access of bacteria to lower respiratory tract, and cross-contamination due to manipulation of these tubes.

- Employ "no-touch" technique or use of sterile gloves on both hands until tracheostomy wound has healed or formed granulation tissue around the tube.
- Suction on an "as needed" rather than routine basis, as frequent suctioning increases risk of trauma and cross-contamination.
- Use sterile catheter for each suctioning procedure, along with sterile solutions, if secretions are tenacious and catheter flushing is necessary.
- Always wear gloves on both hands to suction.

See "Status Asthmaticus" for the following: **Ineffective airway clearance** related to presence of viscous secretions, p. 6; and **Activity intolerance** related to fatigue, p. 6. See "Near Drowning" for the following: **Impaired gas exchange** related to decreased diffusion of oxygen secondary to alveolar capillary membrane changes and fluid accumulation in the lung, p. 39. As appropriate, see nursing diagnoses and interventions in "Management of the Adult on Mechanical Ventilation," pp. 66-70; "Providing Nutritional Support," pp. 490-505; "Caring for the Critically Ill on Prolonged Bed Rest," pp. 506-511; "Caring for the Critically Ill with Life-Threatening Disorders," pp. 511-522; and "Caring for the Family of the Critically Ill," pp. 522-526.

REHABILITATION AND PATIENT-FAMILY TEACHING CONCEPTS

Give patient and significant others verbal and written instructions for the following:
1. Techniques that promote gas exchange and minimize stasis of secretions, for example, deep breathing, coughing, use of incentive spirometry, increasing activity level as much as possible for patient's medical condition, and percussion and postural drainage, as necessary.
2. Medications, including drug name, purpose, dosage, frequency, precautions, and potential side effects, particularly of antibiotics.
3. Signs and symptoms of pneumonia and importance of reporting them promptly to health professional should they recur. Teach patient's significant others that changes in sensorium may be the only indicator of pneumonia if patient is elderly.

Pulmonary hypertension

Pulmonary hypertension is defined as a mean pulmonary artery pressure (MPAP) greater than 20 mm Hg. Primary pulmonary hypertension, which is rare, is a process for which a cause cannot be diagnosed. With secondary pulmonary hypertension, the cause can be identified. See Table 1-4 for a discussion of etiologic factors.

Rising pulmonary artery pressure (PAP) increases pulmonary vascular resistance (PVR), which in turn causes two responses in the vasculature: stand-by vessels open to increase the surface area available for perfusion and the capillaries distend to accommodate the increased blood flow. Although these responses reduce PVR initially, the system eventually fails if the increased pressure becomes chronic due to vasoconstriction that occurs in response to chronic hypoxia. While most of the vascular system responds to hypoxia by dilating in an effort to increase blood flow to vital organs, the pulmonary vasculature responds with vasoconstriction. Generally, Pao_2 decreases to ≤ 60 mm Hg before vasoconstriction occurs; the lower the Pao_2, the more severe the vasoconstriction.

T A B L E 1 - 4

Etiologic factors in the development of pulmonary hypertension

Cause	Clinical examples
Congenital heart disease with left-to-right shunt	Ventricular septal defect Atrial septal defect Patent ductus arteriosis
Congenital heart disease with diminished pulmonary blood flow	Tetralogy of Fallot Transposition of the great vessels
Obstruction to pulmonary venous outflow (congenital and acquired)	Mitral valve disease Left ventricular failure Stenosis of large pulmonary veins Portal hypertension
Pulmonary embolism and thrombosis	
Chronic alveolar hypoxia	High-altitude hypoxia Chronic obstructive pulmonary disease Obstructive sleep apnea Obesity-hypoventilation syndrome Neuromuscular disease processes
Diffuse pulmonary fibrosis	Lupus erythematosus Systemic sclerosis Sarcoidosis Idiopathic interstitial fibrosis

The rise in PAP and the resulting increase in PVR from acute hypoxia are completely reversible after the hypoxia has been resolved. However, in the presence of chronic hypoxia, pulmonary vasculature undergoes permanent changes (i.e., hypertrophy and hyperplasia), causing thickening of the vessel and narrowing of the lumen. In addition, polycythemia develops as a compensatory mechanism for increasing oxygen transport; this condition increases blood viscosity, which in turn increases PVR.

The functions of the heart and lungs are interdependent—factors that affect one may dramatically affect the other. The heart's first response to increased PVR is to increase the pumping force of the right ventricle to maintain adequate cardiac output. The right ventricle dilates and hypertrophies under the constant strain and workload. Eventually, the right side of the heart becomes weakened and is unable to accommodate venous blood returning to the heart. As a result, the circulatory system backs up and pressure in the systemic venous circulation increases, causing cor pulmonale or right-sided heart failure. See "Congestive Heart Failure/Pulmonary Edema," p. 85, for further discussion of right-sided heart failure.

ASSESSMENT

Because the low-resistance pulmonary vascular bed is clinically silent until late in the disease process, onset is insidious.

Signs and symptoms

- *Early:* Hyperventilation, vague chest discomfort.
- *Late:* Tachypnea, dyspnea, orthopnea, chest congestion.

Physical assessment: Cyanosis of the lips and nailbeds, edema of the hands and feet, anasarca (generalized, massive edema), distended jugular veins, right ventricular heave (visible left parasternal systolic lift), accentuated pulmonary component of the second heart sound, right ventricular diastolic gallop, pulmonary ejection click, distant breath sounds, basilar crackles (rales).

Hemodynamic measurements: MPAP will be >20 mm Hg. Normally, pulmonary artery pressures (PAP) range from 8-15 mm Hg during diastole to 20-30 mm Hg during systole, with a MPAP of 15 mm Hg.

DIAGNOSTIC TESTS

1. *ABG values:* Will vary but are important to the differential diagnosis of the cause of pulmonary hypertension. Generally, Pao_2 will be <60 mm Hg, while $Paco_2$ will be within normal limits (35-45 mm Hg), unless COPD is the cause of the pulmonary hypertension.
2. *Chest x-ray:* Will confirm anatomic abnormalities associated with chronic right ventricular failure (right ventricular dilatation or hypertrophy), enlarged pulmonary artery secondary to increased pressure, and diminished diaphragmatic excursion.
3. *EKG:* May show right-axis deviation, right bundle-branch block, and enlarged P waves.
4. *Echocardiogram:* May reveal enlarged right atrium and right ventricle, diminished wall motion, pulmonic valve malfunction (mid-systolic closure or delayed opening).
5. *Pulmonary function tests:* Also important for the differential diagnosis of the underlying pathology and will vary according to cause.
6. *Pulmonary angiography and perfusion scans:* To rule out an embolic event as the underlying cause.
7. *Hemodynamic monitoring:* Pressures in the pulmonary vasculature are measured by way of the flow-directed pulmonary artery (e.g., Swan-Ganz) catheter. Data will differentiate or quantify the contribution of the left or right ventricular failure and measure the response to pharmacotherapy.
8. *Open lung biopsy:* Usually avoided unless the cause of pulmonary hypertension cannot be diagnosed using less invasive studies. Data obtained from biopsy may establish the type of pulmonary vascular disease and assess extent of the disease process.
9. *RBC/Hct values:* Assess extent of polycythemia.

MEDICAL MANAGEMENT

The goal of medical management is to diagnose and treat the underlying disorder or process causing the pulmonary hypertension. Treatment is directed primarily toward increasing myocardial contractility or reducing right ventricular afterload caused by the high pulmonary vascular resistance.

1. **Oxygen therapy:** By eliminating hypoxia, pulmonary vascular vasoconstriction is reduced, which in turn may reduce ventricular overload.
2. **Diuretics:** Reduce circulating volume *via* loss of sodium and water, which will decrease PAP and right ventricular workload. In turn, this reduces leftward septal bulging seen with right ventricular overload.
3. **Digitalis:** Generally used only in cor pulmonale with biventricular failure. Otherwise, the inotropic effects of digitalis can increase cardiac output and increase

pulmonary resistance, which are deleterious in the presence of right ventricular failure.

4. **Bronchodilators** (e.g., methylxanthine, isoproterenol, terbutaline): Act as afterload reducers by decreasing pulmonary vascular resistance and increasing right ventricular ejection fraction. By improving gas exchange, bronchodilators may decrease hypoxic vasoconstriction of the pulmonary vascular bed.

5. **Vasodilators** (e.g., nitrates, hydralazine, calcium-channel blockers): Reverse pulmonary vasoconstriction, which will reduce right ventricular afterload and enhance pulmonary blood flow.

NURSING DIAGNOSES AND INTERVENTIONS

See "Near Drowning" for the following: **Impaired gas exchange** related to decreased diffusion of oxygen secondary to alveolar capillary membrane changes and fluid accumulation in the lung, p. 39. Refer to "Congestive Heart Failure/Pulmonary Edema," pp. 86-89 for nursing diagnoses and interventions related to the care of patients with heart failure. As appropriate, see nursing diagnoses and interventions in the following: "Providing Nutritional Support," pp. 490-505; "Caring for the Critically Ill on Prolonged Bed Rest," pp. 506-511; "Caring for the Critically Ill with Life-Threatening Disorders," pp. 511-522; and "Caring for the Family of the Critically Ill," pp. 522-526.

REHABILITATION AND PATIENT-FAMILY TEACHING CONCEPTS

Refer to this section in Congestive Heart Failure/Pulmonary Edema, p. 89.

Adult respiratory distress syndrome

Adult respiratory distress syndrome (ARDS) can be defined as pulmonary edema that exists in the presence of normal cardiac output. Although the cause of ARDS is not understood completely, the site of injury is the alveolar-capillary membrane. Normally this membrane is permeable only to smaller molecules, such as water and electrolytes. The balance of the forces of hydrostatic pressure (pushing) and osmotic pressure (pulling) keeps fluids in their proper place and maintains the interstitium and alveoli in a relatively dry state. All of the etiologic factors leading to the development of ARDS (see "History and risk factors," on p. 19) cause an increase in the permeability of the alveolar-capillary membrane, either by altering hydrostatic or osmotic pressure or by injuring the alveolar epithelium or capillary endothelium. This enables the passing of larger molecules (e.g., albumin and globulin) through the membrane. Essentially, this altered permeability leads to a leaky membrane and an accumulation of protein-rich fluid in the interstitial and intraalveolar spaces, interfering with gas exchange at this critical level. In addition, surfactant activity is reduced, either because the cell producing the surfactant is destroyed or because the surfactant is inactivated. The alveoli tend to collapse in the absence of surfactant unless they are filled with fluid. In either case, gas exchange no longer can occur and these areas become a mass of interstitial and alveolar edema, hemorrhage, and focal atelectasis. As the leak grows larger, the interstitium, alveoli, and terminal airways become filled with fluid, blood, and protein. Ventilation is wasted on these areas because they no longer participate in gas exchange. As a result, ventilation-perfusion mismatching with resultant hypoxia occurs. The patient becomes fatigued as the work of breathing increases in response to ever-stiffening lungs and respiratory failure becomes possible. Mortality rate for ARDS exceeds 50%.

ASSESSMENT

Signs and symptoms: Will vary, depending on the pathophysiology contributing to the ARDS. The following are general early and late indicators. The goal is to diagnose ARDS in the early stages when treatment is much less complex and the patient is less critically ill.

- *Early indicators:* Dyspnea, restlessness, cough, increased work of breathing, chest clear to auscultation.
- *Late indicators:* Cyanosis, pallor, grunting respirations, adventitious breath sounds, intercostal-suprasternal retractions, tachypnea, tachycardia, diaphoresis, mental obtundation.

History and risk factors: Trauma, hemorrhagic shock, gram-negative sepsis, sepsis with disseminated intravascular coagulation (DIC), inhalation of toxic substances, severe pneumonitis, aspiration of gastric contents, near drowning, air or fat embolus, hemorrhagic pancreatitis, postperfusion cardiopulmonary bypass, oxygen toxicity, drug overdose, neurologic injury, and massive blood transfusion.

DIAGNOSTIC TESTS

1. *ABG analysis:* Essential to the diagnosis of ARDS. Refractory hypoxemia (decreasing PaO_2 that is unresponsive to increasing FIO_2) is a key indicator. Initially, the pH is above normal (>7.45) because the patient hyperventilates and exhales greater-than-normal levels of CO_2. As ARDS worsens, the pH falls below 7.35 due to respiratory acidosis, which may be further complicated by metabolic acidosis resulting from the anaerobic metabolism induced by hypoxia.

2. *Serial chest x-rays:* May be normal in the early stages. As ARDS progresses, the lung shows bilateral diffuse infiltrates. In later stages, there may be few air spaces left in the lung, a condition that gives the lung a completely white appearance on x-ray.

3. *Pulmonary function tests:* Static and dynamic lung compliance will be decreased. Lung volumes, particularly functional residual capacity (FRC) also will be decreased.

4. *Hemodynamic monitoring:* Measurements of PAWP are important to the differential diagnosis. PAWP is normal in ARDS, whereas it is high (>12 mm Hg) in cardiogenic pulmonary edema. PAWP is a more sensitive indicator of fluid balance than CVP and will be obtained at frequent intervals in conjunction with fluid therapy.

5. *Tracheal protein/plasma protein ratio:* A relatively new diagnostic tool used to differentiate between cardiogenic and noncardiogenic pulmonary edema (ARDS). It compares total protein in tracheal aspirate with total protein in plasma. Ratio in cardiogenic pulmonary edema is <0.5; whereas the ratio in ARDS generally is >0.7.

6. *Lactic acid level:* Lactic acid is a by-product of anaerobic metabolism and will accumulate in the serum in the presence of hypoxemia. The presence of arterial lactate contributes to acidosis.

7. *P(A-a)O_2:* Alveolar-arterial oxygen tension difference. Normally, it increases

approximately 4 mm Hg with each decade of life. The value increases above normal in ARDS to reflect the difficulty with which oxygen diffuses across the alveolar-capillary membrane.

8. *QS/QT:* Ratio of shunt to cardiac output. Measures intrapulmonary shunting. Normal physiologic shunt is 3-4%; may increase to 15-20% with ARDS.

MEDICAL MANAGEMENT

The goals for medical management are twofold: first, maintenance of adequate arterial oxygenation and pulmonary ventilation; and second, treatment of underlying pathophysiology that caused the ARDS.

1. **Oxygen therapy:** To provide acceptable Pao_2 levels ($\geq$60 mm Hg) with FIo_2 $\leq$0.50.

2. **Mechanical ventilation:** Indicated if patient cannot be oxygenated adequately with acceptable concentrations of FIo_2 ($\leq$0.50). Nearly all patients with ARDS require intubation and mechanical ventilation, owing to decreased lung compliance, increased physiologic pressures, and increased work of breathing.

3. **Positive end expiratory pressure (PEEP):** Increases functional residual capacity and is used in conjunction with mechanical ventilation. High doses of PEEP often are required to maintain acceptable levels of Pao_2 with FIo_2 $\leq$0.50. Generally, 5-20 cm H_2O pressure is maintained at the end of the expiratory cycle (sometimes even higher levels are required). This pressure allows alveoli to remain open and participate in gas exchange. It will assist in maintaining adequate Pao_2 with lower concentrations of FIo_2. For a more complete discussion of PEEP, see p. 62 in "Management of the Adult on Mechanical Ventilation."

4. **Corticosteroids:** While use of steroids is controversial and their efficacy is not well established, short-term, high-dose corticosteroids are believed to be useful in stabilizing the alveolar-capillary membrane to prevent further deterioration.

5. **Fluid therapy:** Primary goal is to maintain a minimum PAWP to provide adequate cardiac output. Usually, the patient is kept slightly volume depleted due to leakage of excess fluids into the interstitium through damaged capillary membrane. The use of crystalloid versus colloid fluids is controversial. Both types of fluid have been shown to leak across the alveolar-capillary membrane. Currently, colloids are reserved for those patients who are hypoalbuminemic and crystalloids are used for all other patients.

6. **Sedation:** Extremely agitated patients may be medicated with morphine sulfate. Those patients too combative to cooperate with mechanical ventilation may be paralyzed with a neuroblocking agent, such as pancuronium bromide (Pavulon). It is imperative that the caregiver recognize that while the paralyzed patient may appear comatose, he or she may be wide awake and extremely anxious due to the total lack of control. These patients should receive some type of sedation to alleviate anxiety and will require expert psychosocial nursing interventions.

7. **Nutritional support:** Energy outlay with respiratory failure is high, due in part to the increased work of breathing. If the patient is unable to consume enough calories with enteral feedings, total parenteral nutrition *via* peripheral or central access is instituted.

NURSING DIAGNOSES AND INTERVENTIONS

Impaired gas exchange related to decreased diffusion of oxygen secondary to atelectasis and fluid accumulation in the alveoli

Desired outcome: Patient has adequate gas exchange as evidenced by $PaO_2 \geq 60$ mm Hg, $PaCO_2 \leq 45$ mm Hg, pH 7.35-7.45, RR 12-20 breaths/min with a normal pattern and depth (eupnea); and absence of restlessness, use of accessory muscles of respiration, and adventitious breath sounds.

1. Assess and document character of respiratory effort: rate, depth, rhythm, and use of accessory muscles of respiration.
2. Assess patient for signs and symptoms of respiratory distress: restlessness, anxiety, confusion, tachypnea (RR >20 breaths/min).
3. Assess breath sounds with each VS check to ascertain their presence and character. Adventitious sounds usually are present in the later stages of ARDS, but not as likely during the early stage.
4. Monitor serial ABG values and report significant changes (i.e., variances of 10-20 mm Hg in PaO_2 and $PaCO_2$).
5. Administer oxygen and monitor FIO_2 as prescribed.
6. Monitor and record pulmonary function tests as prescribed, especially tidal volume and minute ventilation. Expect decreased tidal volume and increased minute ventilation with respiratory distress.
7. Encourage patient to slow the rate of respirations and use pursed-lip breathing, which may help to hold airways open and improve gas exchange.
8. Position patient for comfort and to promote adequate gas exchange. Usually, semi- to high-Fowler's position is therapeutic.
9. Keep oral airway and self-inflating manual ventilating bag at the bedside for emergency use. Keep emergency intubation equipment at the bedside for use should patient's condition deteriorate.

As indicated, see nursing diagnoses and interventions in "Management of the Adult on Mechanical Ventilation," pp. 66-70; "Providing Nutritional Support," pp. 490-505; "Caring for the Critically Ill on Prolonged Bed Rest," pp. 506-511; "Caring for the Critically Ill with Life-Threatening Disorders," pp. 511-522; and "Caring for the Family of the Critically Ill," pp. 522-526.

REHABILITATION AND PATIENT-FAMILY TEACHING CONCEPTS

Give patient and significant others verbal and written instructions for the following:
1. Importance of assessment, including ABG analysis, which will be performed at frequent intervals. Explain the purpose of ABG analysis.
2. Precipitating factors specific to patient's development of ARDS.
3. Cause of changes in mental status, should they occur: increase in arterial carbon dioxide and decrease in arterial oxygen. Reassure patient and significant others that changes in sensorium might be temporary and may be resolved with treatment.
4. If patient is on mechanical ventilation, the reason for and location of the alarms, and explanation of their purpose. For other information, see "Management of the Adult on Mechanical Ventilation," p. 65.

5. Potential for grave consequences related to development of ARDS. Overall mortality rates exceed 50%. Significant others need to be prepared for this outcome.

Perfusion disorders

Pulmonary perfusion disorders are the result of any obstruction of blood flow in the pulmonary vasculature. The two most common abnormalities of pulmonary perfusion are pulmonary emboli and fat emboli. Other less common causes include thrombi from the right atrium, thrombi released from septic foci, tumors, and amniotic fluid emboli.

Pulmonary emboli (PE): The most common pulmonary perfusion abnormality, a pulmonary embolus is caused by a blood clot dislodged from the systemic circulation, typically the deep veins of the legs or pelvis. Most often, the ileofemoral venous system is implicated. Thrombus formation is the result of one or more of the following factors: blood stasis, alterations in clotting factors, and injury to vessel walls. Many patients with PE do not exhibit signs and symptoms of deep vein thrombosis (DVT). The formed thrombus becomes dislodged and travels to the pulmonary circulation, where it obstructs one or both branches of the pulmonary artery or a subdivision. Total obstruction leading to pulmonary infarction is rare because the pulmonary circulation has multiple sources of blood supply. Early diagnosis and appropriate treatment reduce mortality to under 10%. Although most pulmonary emboli resolve completely, leaving no residual deficits, some patients may be left with chronic pulmonary hypertension.

Fat emboli: The most common nonthrombotic cause of pulmonary perfusion disorders, fat emboli are the result of two events: the release of free fatty acids causing a toxic vasculitis, followed by thrombosis and obstruction of small pulmonary arteries by fat.

ASSESSMENT

Signs and symptoms of pulmonary emboli: Often are nonspecific but may involve sudden onset of dyspnea, tachypnea, restlessness, and anxiety. The patient also may have a nonproductive cough, palpitations, nausea, and syncope. With a large embolism, oppressive substernal chest discomfort will be present. Fever, pleuritic chest pain, and hemoptysis are present with pulmonary infarction.

Physical assessment: RR >20 breaths/min, HR >100 bpm, crackles (rales), decreased chest wall excursion secondary to splinting, S_3 and S_4 gallop rhythms, diaphoresis, edema, and cyanosis. Temperature may be elevated if infarction has occurred, and transient friction rub may be present.

History and risk factors
1. *Prolonged immobolization:* Especially significant when it co-exists with surgical or nonsurgical trauma, carcinoma, or cardiopulmonary disease. Risk increases as length of immobilization increases.
2. *Cardiac disorders:* Atrial fibrillation, congestive heart failure, myocardial infarction, rheumatic heart disease.
3. *Surgical intervention:* Risk increases in postoperative period, especially for patients with pelvic, thoracic, and abdominal surgery and for those with extensive burns or musculoskeletal injuries of the hip or knee.
4. *Pregnancy:* Especially during the postpartum period.
5. *Chronic pulmonary disease*

6. *Trauma:* Especially fractures of the lower extremities and burns. The degree of risk is related to the severity, site, and extent of trauma.
7. *Carcinoma:* Particularly neoplasms involving the breast, lung, pancreas, and genitourinary and alimentary tracts.
8. *Obesity:* A 20% increase in ideal body weight is associated with an increased incidence of PE.
9. *Varicose veins or prior thromboembolic disease*
10. *Age:* Risk of thromboembolism is greatest between 55-65 years of age.

Signs and symptoms of fat emboli: Typically, patient is asymptomatic for a period lasting 12-24 hours following embolization; this period ends with sudden cardiopulmonary and neurologic deterioration: restlessness, confusion, delirium, coma, and dyspnea.

Physical assessment: RR >20 breaths/min; HR >100 bpm; increased BP; elevated temperature; petechiae, especially of the upper torso and axillae; inspiratory crowing; and expiratory wheezes.

History and risk factors
1. *Multiple long bone fractures:* Especially fractures of the femur and pelvis.
2. *Trauma to adipose tissue or liver*
3. *Burns*
4. *Osteomyelitis*
5. *Sickle cell crisis*

DIAGNOSTIC TESTS

Pulmonary emboli
1. *ABG values:* Hypoxemia (PaO_2 <80 mm Hg), hypocarbia ($PaCO_2$ <35 mm Hg), and respiratory alkalosis (pH >7.45) usually are present. A normal PaO_2 does not rule out the presence of pulmonary emboli.
2. *Chest x-ray:* Initially, the chest x-ray is normal or an elevated hemidiaphragm will be present. After 24 hours, the x-ray may reveal small infiltrates secondary to atelectasis from decrease in surfactant. More specific findings are abnormal blood vessel diameters (i.e., obstruction of right pulmonary artery would cause dilation of left pulmonary artery) and shapes (i.e., the affected blood vessel may taper to a sharp point and disappear). If pulmonary infarction is present, infiltrates and pleural effusions may be seen within 12-36 hours.
3. *EKG:* If PE are extensive, signs of acute pulmonary hypertension may be present: right-shift QRS axes, tall and peaked P waves, ST-segment changes, and T-wave inversion in leads V_1-V_4.
4. *Pulmonary ventilation-perfusion scan:* A scan is used to detect presence of abnormalities of ventilation or perfusion in the pulmonary system. The patient inhales radioactive-tagged gases and radioactive particles are injected peripherally. If there is a mismatch of ventilation and perfusion (e.g., normal ventilation with decreased perfusion), vascular obstruction is likely.
5. *Pulmonary angiography:* This is the definitive study for pulmonary emboli. It is an invasive procedure involving right heart catheterization and injection of dye into the pulmonary artery (PA) to visualize pulmonary vessels. An abrupt vessel ''cut off'' may be seen at the site of embolization. Usually, filling defects are seen.
6. *Hemodynamic studies:* If PE lead to increased pulmonary vascular resistance,

PA pressure will be elevated. PA pressure increases significantly (>20 mm Hg) if 30-50% of the pulmonary arterial tree is affected. If massive PE are present and PA pressure increases to ≥40 mm Hg, right ventricular failure can develop, leading to a decrease in cardiac output and hypotension.

Fat emboli

1. *ABG values:* Hypoxemia ($Paco_2$ <80 mm Hg) and hypercarbia ($Paco_2$ >45 mm Hg) will be present with a respiratory acidosis (pH <7.35).
2. *Chest x-ray:* A pattern similar to adult respiratory distress syndrome is seen: diffuse, extensive bilateral interstitial and alveolar infiltrates.
3. *CBC:* May reveal decreased hemoglobin and hematocrit secondary to hemorrhage into the lung, in addition to thrombocytopenia.

MEDICAL MANAGEMENT

Management of pulmonary emboli

1. **Oxygen therapy:** Delivered at appropriate concentration to maintain a Pao_2 of ≥60 mm Hg.
2. **IV heparin therapy:** Treatment of choice; it is started immediately in patients without bleeding or clotting disorders and in whom PE are strongly suspected.
   - *Initial dose:* IV bolus of 5,000-10,000 units.
   - *Maintenance dose:* Two to four hours after initial dose, either a continuous infusion of 1000 units/hour or 5000-7500 units IV q4h. Maintenance continues for 7-14 days, during which time the patient is on bed rest, to ensure that the thrombus is firmly attached to the vessel wall before ambulation is attempted.

< N O T E : If IV route is unavailable, 7500 units can be given SC q6h or 10,000 units q8h.

   - *Goals of therapy:* To inhibit thrombus growth, promote resolution of the formed thrombus, and prevent further embolus formation. These goals are achieved by keeping partial thromboplastin time (PTT) at 1.5-2.5 times normal. This test should be done just prior to the next intermittent dose of heparin. In addition, platelet counts should be done q3days because thrombocytopenia and paradoxical arterial thrombosis can occur secondary to heparin therapy.
   - *Protamine sulfate:* Heparin antidote, which should be readily available during heparin therapy. Fatal hemorrhage occurs in 1-2% of patients undergoing heparin therapy. Risk of bleeding is greatest in women who are >60 years of age.
3. **Oral anticoagulants (warfarin sodium):** Started 48-72 hours after initiation of heparin therapy. The two are given simultaneously for 6-7 days to allow time for warfarin to inhibit vitamin K-dependent clotting factors before heparin is discontinued.
   - *Prothrombin time (PT):* Monitored daily, with the goal that of 1¼-1½ times normal. Once the patient has stabilized and the heparin is discontinued, weekly monitoring of PT is acceptable. After hospital discharge, the PT should be monitored q2weeks for as long as the patient continues to take warfarin.
   - *Maintenance:* Usually 10 mg/day, continued for 3-6 months based on the

continued presence of risk factors. Certain tumors (e.g., Trousseau syndrome) necessitate lifetime therapy.

< N O T E : Subcutaneous heparin therapy is an effective alternative to warfarin, with less risk of bleeding. The dose of heparin must be adjusted while the patient is hospitalized to ensure a PTT of 1½ times normal. No further monitoring is required after hospital discharge.

- *Vitamin K:* Reverses the effects of warfarin in 24-36 hours. Fresh frozen plasma may be required in cases of serious bleeding.
- **Caution.** Warfarin crosses the placental barrier and can cause spontaneous abortion and birth defects.

4. **Thrombolytic therapy (i.e., streptokinase and urokinase):** These drugs lyse clots *via* conversion of plasminogen to plasma and may be given in the first 24-72 hours after PE to speed the process of clot lysis. After the first 24-72 hours of thrombolytic therapy, heparin therapy is initiated. Thrombolytic therapy may be preferred for initial treatment of PE in patients with hemodynamic compromise (>30% occlusion of pulmonary vasculature) and in whom therapy has been initiated no later than 3 days after onset of PE.

- *Streptokinase:* Loading dose of 250,000 IU in normal saline or D_5W given IV over a 30-minute period. Maintenance dose is 100,000 IU/hr given IV for 24-72 hours.
- *Urokinase:* Loading dose of 4400 IU/kg of body weight in 5 ml of solution given IV over 10 minutes. Maintenance dose is 4400 IU/kg/hr for 12 hours.
- *Thrombin time:* Monitors therapy for both drugs. The test is repeated q4h during therapy to ensure adequate response, which should be between 2-5 times normal. A PTT can be used instead of thrombin time and should be 2-5 times control. Once thrombolytic therapy is stopped, thrombin time or PTT should be checked frequently until values fall below 2 times normal. When the values are below 2 times normal, heparin is started and continued as described above under "heparin therapy."
- *Contraindications:* Active internal bleeding, cerebrovascular accident, or intracranial bleeding within 2 months of PE. Other contraindications include trauma or surgery within 15 days of PE, diastolic hypertension >100 mm Hg, recent cardiopulmonary resuscitation, pregnancy, and <10 days postpartum.

< N O T E : Up to 33% of patients receiving thrombolytic therapy have hemorrhagic complications. Discontinuing the drug and administering fresh frozen plasma are the appropriate treatments.

5. **Surgical interventions:** Vena caval interruption and pulmonary embolectomy are surgical treatments used only in select cases owing to the success rate of anticoagulant therapy.

Management of fat emboli

1. **Oxygen:** Concentration of oxygen is based on clinical picture, ABG results, and patient's prior respiratory status. Intubation and mechanical ventilation may be required.
2. **Steroids:** Cortisone 100 mg or methylprednisone 30 mg/kg is used to decrease local injury to pulmonary tissue and pulmonary edema.

3. **Diuretics:** Approximately 30% of patients with fat emboli develop pulmonary edema necessitating use of diuretics.

NURSING DIAGNOSES AND INTERVENTIONS

Impaired gas exchange related to ventilation-perfusion mismatch secondary to pulmonary or fat emboli

---

Desired outcome: Patient exhibits adequate gas exchange and ventilatory function as evidenced by RR 12-20 breaths/min with normal pattern and depth (eupnea), $Pao_2 \geq 60$ mm Hg, $Paco_2 \geq 35$ mm Hg, and pH ≤ 7.45 (or values consistent with acceptable baseline parameters).

---

1. Monitor serial ABG values, assessing for the desired response to treatment: increased Pao_2 and correction of respiratory alkalosis. Report lack of response to treatment or worsening ABG values.
2. Monitor patient for signs and symptoms of increasing respiratory distress: respiratory rate increased from baseline, increasing dyspnea, anxiety, and cyanosis.
3. Ensure delivery of prescribed concentrations of oxygen.
4. Position patient for comfort and optimal gas exchange. Ensure that the area of the lung affected by the emboli is not dependent when patient is in the lateral decubitus position, and elevate HOB 30 degrees. This will ensure a better ventilation-perfusion match, thereby improving Pao_2.
5. Avoid positioning patient with knees bent (i.e., gatching the bed) as this impedes venous return from the legs and can increase the risk of pulmonary emboli.
6. Decrease metabolic demands for oxygen by limiting or pacing patient's activities and procedures.
7. Ensure that patient performs deep-breathing and coughing exercises 3-5 times q2h.

Potential for injury related to risk of bleeding or hemorrhage secondary to anticoagulation or thrombolytic therapy

---

Desired outcomes: Patient does not exhibit evidence of frank or occult bleeding, and body secretions test free of blood. PTT is 1¼-1½ times control and thrombin time is 2-5 times normal.

---

1. Monitor serial PTT or thrombin times. Report values outside the desired therapeutic ranges.
2. Ensure easy access to antidotes for prescribed treatment.
   - *Protamine sulfate:* 1 mg counteracts 100 units of heparin. Usually, the initial dose is 50 mg.
   - *Vitamin K:* 20 mg given SC.
   - *E-aminocaproic acid* (e.g., Amicar): Reverses the fibrinolytic condition related to thrombolytic therapy. < N O T E : Use of this drug as an antidote has not been documented in humans. It may, however, be used in emergency situations.

3. Inspect the following sites for evidence of bleeding: any entry site of an invasive procedure, oral mucous membranes, wounds, nares, torso, or extremities for evidence of petechiae or ecchymoses. Also check stool, urine, sputum, and vomitus for occult blood, using agency-approved method for testing.

4. Apply pressure over puncture sites until bleeding stops; apply pressure dressing over arterial puncture sites to stop oozing of blood.

5. To prevent hematoma formation, avoid giving IM injections.

6. Monitor hemoglobin and hematocrit. Report significant findings to MD, including decreases in values or failure to see appropriate increases after transfusion.

7. To avoid negative interactions with anticoagulants or thrombolytic therapy, establish compatability of all drugs before administering them.
   - *Heparin:* Digitalis, tetracyclines, nicotine, and antihistamines decrease the effect of heparin therapy. Consult with pharmacist regarding compatability before infusing other IV drugs through heparin IV line.
   - *Warfarin sodium:* Numerous drugs result in a decrease or increase in response to treatment with warfarin. Consult with pharamacist to obtain specific information about patient's medication profile.
   - *Thrombolytic therapy:* No specific drug interactions are noted. However, consult with pharmacist before infusing any other medication through the same IV line.

8. Because aspirin and nonsteroidal anti-inflammatory drugs (e.g., ibuprofen) are platelet aggregation inhibitors and can prolong episodes of bleeding, avoid use of *any* drug that contains these medications.

9. Discuss with patient and significant others the importance of reporting promptly the presence of bleeding from any source.

10. Teach patient the necessity of using cotton swabs and mouthwash for oral care to minimize the risk of gum bleeding during hospitalization when anticoagulant therapy is most intensive. Instruct patient to shave with an electric rather than straight razor.

11. If patient is restless and combative, provide a safe environment: pad the side rails, restrain patient as necessary to prevent falls, and use extreme care when moving patient to avoid bumping of extremities into side rails.

Knowledge deficit: Oral anticoagulant therapy, potential side effects, and foods and medications to avoid during therapy

---

Desired outcome: Patient verbalizes knowledge of his or her prescribed anticoagulant drug, the potental side effects, and foods and medications to avoid while on oral anticoagulant therapy.

---

1. Determine patient's knowledge of oral anticoagulant therapy. As appropriate, discuss the drug name, purpose, dosage, and schedule.

2. Inform patient of the potential side effects of anticoagulant therapy: easy bruising, prolonged bleeding from cuts, spontaneous nose bleeds, black and tarry stools, and blood in urine and sputum.

3. Discuss with patient the importance of laboratory testing and follow-up visits with MD.

4. Explain the importance of informing all health-care providers (e.g., dentists and other physicians) that patient is on anticoagulant therapy. Suggest that patient wear a Medic-Alert tag or other method of informing health-care providers about the anticoagulant therapy.

5. Teach patient about foods high in vitamin K (e.g., fish, bananas, dark green vegetables, tomatoes, and cauliflower), which can interfere with anticoagulation.

6. Caution patient that a soft-bristled, rather than hard-bristled, toothbrush and an electric, rather than straight, razor should be used during anticoagulant therapy.

7. Instruct patient to consult with physician before taking OTC or prescribed drugs that were used prior to initiation of anticoagulants. The following are among many drugs that enhance the response to warfarin: aspirin, cimetidine, and trimethoprem. Drugs that decrease the response include antacids, diuretics, oral contraceptives, and barbiturates, among others.

REHABILITATION AND PATIENT-FAMILY TEACHING CONCEPTS

Give patient and significant others verbal and written instructions for the following:
For pulmonary emboli

1. Risk factors related to the development of thrombi and embolization and preventive measures to reduce the risk.

2. Signs and symptoms of *thrombophlebitis:* swelling of the calf, tenderness or warmth in the involved area, possible presence of pain in affected calf when ankle is flexed, slight fever, distention of veins in affected leg; and *pulmonary embolism:* sudden onset of dyspnea and anxiety, nonproductive cough, palpitations, nausea, syncope.

3. Rationale and application procedure for antiembolism hose. Explain that patient should put them on in the morning before getting out of bed.

4. Importance of preventing impairment of venous return from the lower extremities by avoiding prolonged sitting, crossing legs, and constrictive clothing.

< N O T E :   Rehabilitation and family teaching concepts for fat emboli are nonspecific.

Pneumothorax

Pneumothorax is an accumulation of air between the parietal and visceral pleura. There are three types:

Spontaneous: Also referred to as closed pneumothorax because the chest wall remains intact with no leak to the atmosphere. It results from the rupture of a bleb or bulla on the visceral pleural surface, usually near the apex. Generally, the cause of the rupture is unknown, although it may result from a weakness related to a respiratory infection or from an underlying pulmonary disease (e.g., COPD, tuberculosis, malignant neoplasm). The affected individual is usually young (20-40 years), previously healthy, and male. Generally, onset of symptoms occurs at rest, rather than with vigorous exercise or coughing. Potential for recurrence is great, with the second pneumothorax occurring an average of 2-3 years after the first.

Traumatic: Can be open or closed. An open pneumothorax occurs when air enters the pleural space from the atmosphere through an opening in the chest wall, such as with a gunshot wound, stab wound, or invasive medical procedure (e.g., lung biopsy, thoracentesis, or placement of a central line into a subclavian vein).

A closed pneumothorax occurs when the visceral pleura is penetrated, but the chest wall remains intact with no atmospheric leak. This usually occurs with blunt trauma that results in a fracture and dislocation of the ribs. It also may occur from the use of positive end expiratory pressure (PEEP) or after CPR. For more information about blunt chest injuries, see ''Chest Trauma,'' p. 32.

Tension: Occurs when air enters the pleural space through a pleural tear when the individual inspires. Air continues to accumulate but cannot escape during expiration because of intrapleural pressure, which is greater than alveolar pressure. This leads to a one-way or flap-valve effect. As the pressure increases, it is transmitted to the mediastinum. This results in a mediastinal shift toward the unaffected side, which further impairs ventilatory efforts. The increase in pressure also compresses the vena cava, which impedes venous return, leading to a decrease in cardiac output and ultimately, to circulatory collapse if it is not diagnosed and treated quickly. Tension pneumothorax is a life-threatening medical emergency. Although it can occur with a spontaneous pneumothorax, it is most often associated with trauma or infection, or it can occur in patients with ARDS who require mechanical ventilation.

ASSESSMENT

Clinical presentation will vary in degree, depending on the type and size of pneumothorax.

Spontaneous or traumatic: Sudden onset of sharp, stabbing chest pain on the affected side, which may radiate to the shoulder; moderate to severe dyspnea; anxiety.

- *Inspection:* Decreased chest wall movement on affected side.
- *Palpation:* Tracheal shift toward unaffected side, subcutaneous emphysema (crepitus), tactile and vocal fremitus decreased or absent on affected side.
- *Percussion:* Hyperresonance on affected side.
- *Auscultation:* Absent or decreased breath sounds on affected side; increased RR.

Tension: Severe dyspnea; chest pain on affected side; cool, clammy, mottled skin; anxiety and restlessness.

- *Inspection:* Decreased chest wall movement on affected side, expansion of affected side throughout respiratory cycle, jugular vein distention.
- *Palpation:* Tracheal shift toward unaffected side, subcutaneous emphysema in neck and chest.
- *Percussion:* Hyperresonance on affected side.
- *Auscultation:* Absent or decreased breath sounds on affected side, distant heart sounds, increased RR (>20 breaths/min), decreased BP, increased HR (>100 bpm).

< C A U T I O N : Tension pneumothorax is life-threatening. Immediate medical intervention is critical.

DIAGNOSTIC TESTS

1. *Chest x-ray:* Will show size of the pneumothorax and any tracheal shift. The affected side will show air in the pleural space, expansion of the chest wall, lowering of the diaphragm, and partial to total collapse of the lung.
2. *ABG values:* Hypoxemia (Pao$_2$ <80 mm Hg) will be evident immediately after a large pneumothorax. Twenty-four hours following the pneumothorax, arterial

oxygen saturation returns to normal. Hypoxemia may be accompanied by respiratory acidosis (pH <7.35) and hypercarbia ($Paco_2$ >45 mm Hg).

MEDICAL MANAGEMENT AND SURGICAL INTERVENTIONS

1. **Oxygen therapy:** Administered when ABG values demonstrate the presence of hypoxemia, which usually occurs with a large pneumothorax.
2. **Analgesia:** Provides relief of pain of pneumothorax or its treatment.
3. **Thoracentesis:** Performed immediately in tension pneumothorax to remove air from the chest cavity. A large-bore needle is inserted in the second intercostal space, midclavicular line, which correlates to the superior portion of the anterior axillary lobe. A sudden rushing out of air confirms the diagnosis of tension pneumothorax. To decrease risk of further pleural laceration as the chest reexpands, a stylet introducer needle with a plastic sheath may be used. The needle is removed after penetration and the plastic catheter sheath is left in place to allow decompression of the chest cavity. Following air aspiration, chest tubes are inserted.
4. **Chest tube placement:** A chest tube is inserted in any patient who is symptomatic of a pneumothorax. Chest tubes produce inflammation and, ultimately, scarring of the pleura and may help prevent recurrent spontaneous pneumothoraces. Patients with recurrent pneumothoraces require chest tubes because their visceral pleurae do not seal promptly. Chest tubes (26-30F) are inserted in the second or third lateral intercostal space, midclavicular line. During insertion, the patient should be in an upright position so that the lung falls away from the chest wall. A small, 1-2 cm incision is made and the chest tube is placed, sutured in place, and connected to an underwater-seal drainage system. Usually simple underwater-seal drainage is all that is necessary for 6-24 hours. Suction may be used, depending on size of the pneumothorax, patient's condition, and amount of drainage. If drainage is minimal and no suction is required, a one-way flutter valve may be used instead of an underwater-seal drainage system. After chest tube insertion and removal of air from the pleural space, the lung begins to reexpand. A chest tube may produce inflammation of the pleura, causing pleuritic pain, slight temperature elevation, and pleuritic friction rub.
5. **Thoracotomy:** Often indicated if patient has had two or more spontaneous pneumothoraces on one side, owing to the risk of continuous recurrence, or if resolution of the pneumothorax does not occur within seven days. Thoracotomy may involve mechanical abrasion of the pleural surfaces with a dry sterile sponge or chemical abrasion *via* an agent such as tetracycline solution or talc, both of which result in pleural adhesions to prevent recurrence. A partial pleurectomy may be performed instead of mechanical or chemical abrasion.

NURSING DIAGNOSES AND INTERVENTIONS

Impaired gas exchange related to ventilation-perfusion mismatch secondary to diminished lung capacity

---

Desired outcome: Patient exhibits adequate gas exchange and ventilatory function as evidenced by Pao_2 ≥60 mm Hg and $Paco_2$ ≤45 mm Hg (or values within acceptable baseline parameters, which are dependent on underlying pathophysiology), RR ≤20 breaths/min with normal depth and pattern (eupnea), and orientation to person, place, and time.

1. Monitor serial ABG results to detect continued presence of hypercapnea or hypoxemia. Report significant findings to MD for treatment.
2. Observe for indicators of hypoxia, including increased restlessness, anxiety, and changes in mental status. Cyanosis is a late sign.
3. Assess patient for increasing respiratory distress: increased RR, diminished or absent movement of chest wall on affected side, complaints of increased dyspnea, and cyanosis. Evaluate HR and BP for indications of shock state.
4. Position patient to allow for full expansion of unaffected lung. Semi-Fowler's position usually provides comfort and allows adequate expansion of chest wall.
5. Change patient's position q2h to promote drainage and lung reexpansion and facilitate alveolar perfusion.
6. Encourage patient to take deep breaths, providing necessary analgesia to decrease discomfort during deep-breathing exercises. Deep breathing will promote full lung expansion and may decrease the risk of atelectasis. Coughing will facilitate mobilization of tracheobronchial secretions, if present.
7. Deliver oxygen and monitor oxygen delivery as indicated.
8. Assess and maintain closed chest-drainage system.
   * Tape all connections and secure chest tube to thorax with tape.
   * Avoid all kinks in the tubing, and ensure that the bed and equipment are not compressing any component of the system.
   * Maintain fluid in underwater-seal chamber and suction chamber at appropriate levels.
   * Be aware that the suction apparatus does not regulate the amount of suction applied to the closed drainage system. The amount of suction is determined by the water level in the suction control chamber. Minimal bubbling is acceptable.
   * **Note:** Suction aids in the reexpansion of the lung, but removing suction for short periods of time, such as for transporting, will not be detrimental or disrupt the closed drainage system.
   * Follow institution's policy regarding chest tube stripping. Be aware that this mechanism for maintaining chest tube patency is controversial and has been associated with creating high negative pressures in the pleural space, which can damage fragile lung tissue. Chest tube stripping may be indicated when bloody drainage or clots are visible in the tubing. Squeezing alternately hand-over-hand along the drainage tube may generate sufficient pressure to move fluid along the tube.
   * Be aware that fluctuations in the long tube of the underwater seal chamber are indicative of a patent chest tube. Fluctuations stop when either the lung has reexpanded or there is a kink or obstruction in the chest tube.
   * Bubbling in the underwater-seal chamber occurs on expiration and is a sign that air is leaving the pleural space.
   * Continuous bubbling on both inspiration and expiration in the underwater seal chamber is a signal that air is leaking into the drainage system. Locate and seal the system's air leak, if possible.
   * Keep necessary emergency supplies at the bedside: petrolatum gauze pad to

apply over insertion site if the chest tube becomes dislodged, and sterile water in which to submerge the chest tube if it becomes disconnected from the underwater seal system. *Never* clamp a chest tube without a specific directive from the MD, as clamping may lead to tension pneumothorax because the air can no longer escape.

Alteration in comfort: Acute pain related to alteration in pleural integrity and inflammation

---

Desired outcome: Patient expresses both verbally and behaviorally that a reduction in the level of discomfort has occurred.

---

1. At frequent intervals, assess patient's degree of discomfort, using patient's verbal and nonverbal cues. Medicate with analgesics as prescribed, evaluating and documenting effectiveness of medication.
2. Position patient on unaffected side to minimize discomfort from chest tube insertion site. Premedicate patient 30 minutes before initiating the move.
3. Teach patient to splint affected side when coughing, moving, or repositioning. Move patient as a unit to enhance stability and comfort.
4. Schedule activites to provide for periods of rest, which may increase patient's pain threshold.
5. Stabilize chest tube to reduce pull or drag on latex connector tubing. Tape chest tube securely to thorax and loop latex tubing on bed beside patient.

Also see appropriate nursing diagnoses and interventions in the following: "Caring for the Critically Ill with Life-Threatening Disorders," pp. 511-522; and "Caring for the Family of the Critically Ill," pp. 522-526.

REHABILITATION AND PATIENT-FAMILY TEACHING CONCEPTS

Give patient and significant others verbal and written instructions for the following:
1. Purpose for chest tube placement and maintenance.
2. Potential for recurrence of spontaneous pneumothorax. Average time between occurrences is 2-3 years. Explain the importance of seeking medical care immediately if the condition recurs.

Chest trauma

Chest trauma is a complex and multi-dimensional problem. It is usually categorized by etiology.

Blunt injury: Occurs as a result of a direct, forceful blow to the chest. Usually the injury is "closed" in that there is no communication of the chest cavity with outside atmospheric pressure. A typical occurrence is an automobile accident, during which there is impact of the thorax with the steering wheel. A crushing injury to the thorax is also considered blunt chest trauma.

Penetrating injury: Occurs as a result of stab or missile wounds to the thorax. This is an open chest injury because there is communication between the chest cavity and outside atmospheric pressure. Gunshots are the most common missile-type penetrating injuries, while knife wounds represent the most common stabbing chest injuries.

Both blunt and penetrating chest wounds can lead to pneumothorax (see "Pneumothorax," p. 28). In addition, thoracic injury may be severe enough to cause interference with the mechanical functions of the heart and lungs; therefore, in-depth physical assessment is critical during the early phase of the patient's injury.

ASSESSMENT

Subtle signs and symptoms and changes in the patient's condition can be clues to serious problems. Treat the patient as though a spinal cord injury has occurred until diagnostic tests have ruled it out. Be aware that subtle changes in mental status can signal a central nervous system insult.

Blunt injury: Dyspnea, SOB, severe chest pain during respirations that patient can localize, agitation, restlessness, anxiety.

- *Potential complications:* Pneumothorax, flail chest, hemothorax, pulmonary contusion, myocardial contusion, cardiac tamponade.
- *Inspection:* RR >20 breaths/min; hyperpnea; ventilatory distress; use of accessory muscles of respiration; nasal flaring; decreased tidal volume; hemoptysis; asymmetrical chest wall motion; paradoxical chest wall motion; inability to clear tracheobronchial secretions; splinting; jugular venous distention; cyanosis or pallor of the skin, lips, and nailbeds; and ecchymosis, which can signal injury to underlying organs.
- *Palpation:* Tracheal deviation; subcutaneous emphysema of the neck and upper chest; tenderness at fracture points; flail chest segment; weak pulse; cool, clammy skin; protrusion of bony fragments.
- *Percussion:* Dullness over lung fields, which can signal hemothorax or atelectasis; hyperresonance over lung fields, signalling pneumothorax.
- *Auscultation:* Diminished or absent breath sounds, respiratory stridor, bony crepitus over fracture sites, muffled heart tones, decreased BP, pericardial friction rub, paradoxical pulse, apical tachycardia. In addition, bowel sounds may be heard in the thorax due to rupture or tear of the diaphragm allowing herniation of abdominal contents into the thorax.

Penetrating injury: Dyspnea, SOB, moderate chest pain, restlessness, anxiety.

< N O T E : It is essential to perform a complete and rapid assessment with the clothing removed. Entry sites may be deceptive, as the skin has an elastic quality and tends to close behind the penetrating object, thereby masking the size and extent of injury.

- *Potential complications:* Hemothorax, pneumothorax, tension pneumothorax, hemorrhage, shock, and infection.
- *Inspection:* RR >20 breaths/min; hyperpnea; respiratory distress; use of accessory muscles of respiration; nasal flaring; decreased tidal volume; asymmetric chest-wall movement; inability to clear tracheobronchial secretions; splinting; cyanosis or pallor of the skin, lips, and nailbeds. During inspection, estimate blood loss on clothing and locate both entry and exit sites. Be alert to presence or severity of other wounds; and presence of ecchymosis, which can signal injury to underlying internal organs. Also, note presence or absence of pulsations of the penetrating object, which may be imbedded in a major organ or blood vessel. Do not remove any penetrating object, as the object

may have caused a sealing effect, and removing it could result in uncontrollable bleeding of the organ or vessel.

- *Palpation:* Tracheal deviation; subcutaneous emphysema; weak or irregular pulse; cool, clammy skin.
- *Percussion:* Dullness over lung fields secondary to hemothorax or atelectasis, hyperresonance over lung fields secondary to pneumothorax.
- *Auscultation:* Sucking sound over point of entry during inspiratory phase; diminished breath sounds; respiratory stridor; muffled heart tones; apical tachycardia or bradycardia, depending on stage of shock; bowel sounds in thorax.

Flail chest: A severe complication of blunt chest trauma, which occurs when three or more adjacent ribs fracture in two or more places (or the sternum is fractured, along with ribs adjacent to the sternum fracture). The fracture segment is free of the bony thorax and moves independently in response to intrathoracic pressure. Paradoxical chest-wall motion is the hallmark symptom in diagnosing flail chest. Normally the chest expands on inspiration, creating a negative intrathoracic pressure; and on expiration, the chest wall retracts in response to positive pressure inside the chest. Because a flail chest segment is no longer attached to the bony thorax, it follows the pressure and retracts on inspiration (negative pressure is a pulling pressure) and bulges on expiration (positive pressure is a pushing pressure).

DIAGNOSTIC TESTS

1. *Chest x-ray:* Confirms presence of air or fluid in the pleural space; assists in determining extent of hemo- or pneumothorax; and confirms presence or absence of fractures of the bony thorax, as well as mediastinal shift.
2. *ABG analysis:* Determines adequacy of oxygenation and presence or absence of acid-base abnormalities. Typical results will reflect hypoxemia (Pao_2 <80 mm Hg) and hypercapnia ($Paco_2$ >45 mm Hg) with concomitant respiratory acidosis (pH <7.35.)
3. *EKG:* Reveals presence or absence of life-threatening dysrhythmias and provides a more thorough analysis of the heart's electrical activity. Although dysrhythmias are a common complication following chest trauma, this important test is often overlooked.
4. *Hemoglobin/hematocrit:* Levels determine the need for blood transfusion or fluid volume replacement.
5. *WBC count:* A baseline indicator of infectious process.

MEDICAL MANAGEMENT AND SURGICAL INTERVENTIONS

Medical interventions are directed toward managing acute respiratory compromise while correcting the underlying pathophysiology or injuries that complicate or aggravate the patient's condition.

1. **Oxygen therapy:** Delivered by mask or cannula, depending on extent of hypoxemia.
2. **Intubation:** Maintains patent airway, decreases airway resistance and respiratory effort, provides route for easy removal of airway secretions, and allows for manual or mechanical ventilation, as necessary.
3. **Mechanical ventilation:** For cases of extreme respiratory distress or ventilatory collapse.

4. **Blood replacement:** A high priority in the trauma victim. Generally, blood loss is replaced with whole blood or packed red blood cells. Use of colloid versus crystalloid fluids for volume replacement remains controversial. Many factors specific to patient's condition and history dictate which fluid is the better volume expander. Volume usually is replaced with crystalloid fluids (e.g., normal saline, D_5W) rather than colloidal IV fluids (e.g., plasma, albumin) because colloids fail to provide significant benefits and carry with them the risk of development of ARDS and renal failure. Cost also is prohibitive. A large-bore venous line may be inserted so that large volumes of fluid can be replaced rapidly.

5. **Chest tube insertion:** To remove accumulation of fluid or air from the chest cavity. A large-bore (26-30F) thoracic catheter is inserted into the chest cavity through the second intercostal space, midclavicular line, or fifth lateral intercostal space, midaxillary line. Placement depends on the location and extent of the hemothorax or pneumothorax and principles of gravity drainage. The catheter is then connected to a one-way flutter valve or to a closed chest-drainage system.

6. **Analgesia:** Manages pain, which can interfere with work of breathing. Generally, narcotics are avoided because of their respiratory depressive side effects. Intercostal nerve block may be performed to provide local pain relief.

7. **Thoracentesis:** Relieves life-threatening tension pneumothorax. A 14-gauge needle is inserted into the second intercostal space at the midclavicular line to ventilate the pressurized chest cavity or, in an emergency situation, to remove a massive hemothorax.

8. **Stabilization and fixation of flail chest:** Most flail chest injuries stabilize within 10-14 days without surgical intervention. Internal fixation involves the use of a volume-cycled ventilator to stabilize the fracture(s). In some cases, the flail segment is fixated externally during a surgical procedure by wiring or otherwise attaching the segment to the intact bony structures.

9. **Thoracotomy:** Generally avoided unless patient develops complications after stabilization. Indications for thoracotomy include massive air leak in a functioning drainage system, continued or increased bleeding through a chest tube, refractory hypotension, acute deterioration, cardiac tamponade.

NURSING DIAGNOSES AND INTERVENTIONS

Potential fluid volume deficit related to decreased circulating volume secondary to risk of excessive bleeding occurring with chest trauma

---

Desired outcomes: Patient is asymptomatic of excessive bleeding as evidenced by stable weights, balanced I&O, urinary output ≥30 ml/hr, HR ≤100 bpm, BP >90/60 mm Hg (or within patient's normal range), chest drainage ≤100 ml/hr, and RR ≤20 breaths/min. Hemoglobin is ≥12 g/dl (female) or ≥14 g/dl (male).

---

1. Assess patient's hydration status by monitoring daily weight as well as amounts of fluid intake and urinary output.
2. Monitor patient's hemoglobin as an indicator of hemostasis. Be alert to a decrease in hemoglobin, which can occur with blood loss.

3. Assess VS at frequent intervals. Be alert to decreased BP, increased HR, and increased RR, which can signal an impending shock state.

4. Monitor drainage in closed chest drainage system. Report significant increase in bright red blood or excessive drainage. Amounts >100 ml/hour usually are considered excessive.

5. Note condition of dressings at frequent intervals. Be sure to check sheets underneath patient. Report excessive drainage or bleeding, for example, if dressings are saturated more frequently than q4h during the first 24-48 hours. After the first 48 hours, bleeding should subside and the dressing should not require changing more often than BID. At that time, drainage should be serosanguinous or serous; however, any bright red bleeding should be reported promptly.

See "Pneumothorax" for the following: **Impaired gas exchange** related to ventilation-perfusion mismatch secondary to diminished lung capacity, p. 30, and **Alteration in comfort:** Acute pain, p. 32. For other nursing diagnoses and interventions, see "Caring for the Critically Ill with Life-Threatening Disorders," pp. 511-522 ; and "Caring for the Family of the Critically Ill," pp. 522-526.

REHABILITATION AND PATIENT-FAMILY CONCEPTS

Give patient and significant others verbal and written instructions for the following:

1. Restriction of activities that might apply pressure or stress to ribs or thoracic musculature. Instruct patient to call for assistance when changing position. Teach patient to maintain active ROM on the operative side to prevent development of stiff shoulder from immobility.

2. Procedure for splinting area of injury with hand or pillow to decrease discomfort.

3. Importance of avoiding pulmonary infections and the necessary precautions to take, such as getting adequate amounts of rest, avoiding large crowds, and getting immunization against influenza during appropriate seasons.

Near drowning

Near drowning can be defined as survival longer than 24 hours following asphyxia related to submersion. Many adult drownings or near drownings are preceded by alcohol or drug ingestion, diving injuries, or medical catastrophies, such as seizures or myocardial infarctions. Hypoxia, hypotension, pulmonary edema, and respiratory and metabolic acidosis are the most common problems following near drowning. Potential complications include neurologic deficits from cerebral anoxia, acute renal failure secondary to acute tubular necrosis, and disseminated intravascular coagulation (DIC). Near drowning can be categorized as follows:

Near drowning with aspiration (wet): Occurs in 85-90% of near drowning victims. The aspirant is either the submersion fluid or gastric contents. Hypoxia results from a variety of mechanisms, including laryngospasm, bronchospasm, airway obstruction from aspirated contaminants, or pulmonary edema. *Freshwater* (hypotonic) *aspiration* results in loss of surfactant, caused by the presence of hypotonic solution in the lungs. This can lead to atelectasis because surface tension of the lung tissue increases, causing alveoli to collapse. A decrease in lung compliance also occurs. In turn, the atelectasis and pulmonary edema lead to a ventilation-perfusion mismatch, which adds to the hypoxia and acidosis. Fresh-water drowning is associated with hypervolemia, hemodilution, and occasionally hemoptysis. *Saltwater* (hypertonic) *aspiration* results in a rapid shift of water and plasma proteins from the circulation into the alveoli. These fluid-filled alveoli are not ventilated, and the continued perfusion leads to hypoxia and ventilation-perfusion mismatch. Saltwater drowning is associated with hypovolemic shock and hemoconcentration. In addition, aspirated contaminants (e.g., algae, chemicals, sand) can cause or contribute to obstruction and lead to asphyxiation. Bacterial pneumonia can develop, depending on the type of contaminant in the aspirant, and chemical pneumonitis can occur if gastric contents were aspirated.

Near drowning without aspiration (dry): Represents 10-15% of near drowning victims. Death, if it occurs, results from asphyxiation secondary to laryngospasm. Laryngospasm is usually caused by water entering the airway, although it can be triggered by fear or pain.

Many deaths that have been attributed to near drowning may, in fact, be the result of one of two separate phenomena that can lead to aspiration: (1) *immersion syndrome,* which occurs with sudden immersion in cold water, resulting in hyperventilation. This increases the risk of swallowing or inhaling large amounts of cold water, which can lead to a vagally stimulated bradycardia that results in loss of consciousness; and (2) *hyperventilation syndrome,* which occurs when divers hyperventilate in order to increase the duration time of breath holding underwater. The normal impetus to breath (increased $Paco_2$) is not present, and with exercise, oxygen stores continue to deplete. Because breath holding may not be terminated before oxygen supplies have reached dangerously low levels, dysrhythmias, seizure, or death from hypoxia can occur. *Hypothermia* also is significant in near drowning. It is defined as a drop in core temperature to 33° C (91.4° F), or below. Its progression can cause muscle activity and vital functions to cease and ventricular fibrillation to occur (this happens at 28° C [83° F]). In some instances hypothermia protects the brain from permanent damage, depending on the victim's age and the degree of hypothermia, because of the decrease in cerebral metabolism that occurs when core body temperature reaches 25° C (77° F). This helps protect the brain from the affects of anoxia. Resuscitation should be continued until the victim is rewarmed to at least 32° C (90° F), because the heart may start beating at that temperature. Resuscitation is possible, even after 30 minutes of submersion.

ASSESSMENT

The following parameters are based on post-resuscitation findings:

Signs and symptoms (depending on degree of CNS involvement): Unconsciousness, seizures, nonspecific alterations in mental status (e.g., confusion, irritability, lethargy), neurologic deficits (motor, speech, visual), mild coughing, coughing up of pink and frothy sputum, vomiting, substernal chest pain, mottled and cold skin, cyanosis, fixed and dilated pupils, abdominal distention.

Physical assessment: In the presence of pulmonary edema, there may be resonance over lung fields and normal tactile fremitus. Auscultation of lung fields may reveal apnea, tachypnea (RR >20 breaths/min), shallow or gasping respirations, crackles (rales), rhonchi, wheezes, supraventricular dysrhythmias, bradycardia (HR <60 bpm), tachycardia (HR >100 bpm), and ventricular fibrillation.

DIAGNOSTIC TESTS

1. *ABG values:* Initially may reflect hypoxemia (Pao_2 <80 mm Hg), hypercapnia ($Paco_2$ >45 mm Hg), and metabolic and respiratory acidosis (pH <7.35, serum bicarbonate <22 mEq/L).

< N O T E : Initial ABG values may be within acceptable range, but because respiratory status can deteriorate quickly, serial monitoring is essential.

2. *CBC:* To determine baseline hematologic status and presence of infection, hemodilutional anemia (from freshwater aspiration), or hemoconcentration (from saltwater aspiration), depending on tonicity of the fluid aspirated.

3. *Serum electrolytes:* Life-threatening changes in electrolytes are unusual following near drowning. Electrolyte disturbances are related to the quantity and tonicity of the water aspirated. Saltwater aspiration leads to hemoconcentration, while freshwater aspiration can cause hemodilution.

4. *BUN and creatinine:* To determine effects of hypoxia on renal tubular function. Creatinine is the most sensitive indicator of renal dysfunction. Acute tubular necrosis is a potential complication of near drowning.

5. *Chest x-ray:* Serial x-rays are necessary to determine presence or development of infiltrates, atelectasis, and pulmonary edema. Alveolar filling pattern is evaluated with pulmonary edema, and is evidenced on x-ray by a soft, fluffy appearance with poorly demarcated lesions, often referred to as a ground-glass appearance.

6. *Skull and spine x-rays:* If CNS trauma has not been ruled out as a precipitating event, these x-rays are crucial. Until x-ray results are known, the patient's neck and spine must be immobilized.

MEDICAL MANAGEMENT

1. **Oxygen therapy:** One hundred percent oxygen is initiated immediately to treat hypoxia. High concentrations of oxygen are continued, even in alert patients with spontaneous ventilation, because of the likelihood of hypoxia and acidosis. Warmed oxygen 40-43° C (104-110° F) may be used as part of the rewarming process for patients with hypothermia.

2. **Endotracheal intubation and positive end expiratory pressure (PEEP):** Required when pulmonary edema or hypoxia is present and unresponsive to increasing levels of oxygen (up to .40 FIo_2). Intubation also assists in the maintenance of clear airways in patients who are unable to manage secretions independently. PEEP improves oxygenation by preventing the collapse of alveoli during expiration. It is especially useful after freshwater aspiration, because it keeps alveoli open in the absence of adequate surfactant. PEEP should be removed cautiously because levels of surfactant can remain low for 48-72 hours after freshwater aspiration.

3. **Mechanical ventilation:** Utilized with respiratory failure, when lung compliance is decreased, or when the patient is unable to maintain effective respiratory effort. PEEP is continued with mechanical ventilation when indicated. Patients with freshwater aspiration require 1½-2 times normal tidal volume at slower rates to allow optimal lung expansion and ventilation of alveoli. If neurologic involvement is present, decreased levels of $Paco_2$ can be achieved *via* mechanical hyperventilation.

4. **Bronchoscopy:** To remove aspirated contaminants, if necessary.

5. **Rewarming for hypothermia:** Warm, moist oxygen 40-43° C (104-110° F)

may be used to elevate core temperature. Peritoneal lavage also is used for rewarming. Fluid for lavage is warmed to 37° C (98.6° F). The goal is quick rewarming to achieve a normal core temperature.

6. **Medications:** Metabolic acidosis is treated with sodium bicarbonate and careful monitoring of arterial pH. If bronchospasm is present, aerosol epinephrine or isoproterenol may be used. Use of steroids and prophylactic antibiotics is controversial. Temperature elevation up to 38° C (101° F) during the first 24 hours can be a normal response to injury. Antibiotics may be prescribed if fever ≥38° C (101° F) persists for longer than 24 hours after the submersion.

7. **Fluid and electrolyte management:** Although uncommon, fluid and electrolyte abnormalities may occur, especially with saltwater aspiration. Usually, no specific therapy is required for minor disturbances. Fluid volume may be replaced with volume expanders (plasmanate, Ringer's lactate, dextran). If anemia is present secondary to hemodilution or hemolysis from freshwater aspiration, a transfusion with packed red blood cells may be necessary.

8. **Neurologic support:** Depends on severity of the neurologic impairment. Severe impairment may necessitate intracranial pressure monitoring, steroids, hyperosmolar diuretics (e.g., mannitol), mechanical ventilation to maintain $Paco_2$ <30 mm Hg or to manage barbiturate coma (see discussion in "Head Injuries," p. ●●●) and deep hypothermia (core temperature <30° C).

9. **Management of event that precipitated the near drowning:** For example, alcohol or drug ingestion, seizure, myocardial infarction.

NURSING DIAGNOSES AND INTERVENTIONS

Impaired gas exchange related to decreased diffusion of oxygen secondary to alveolar capillary membrane changes and fluid accumulation in the lung

---

Desired outcome: Patient has adequate gas exchange as evidenced by Pao_2 ≥60 mm Hg and $Paco_2$ ≤45 mm Hg.

---

1. Auscultate lung fields at frequent intervals. Note the type and extent of adventitious breath sounds (e.g., crackles, rhonchi, friction rubs); document the findings. Notify MD of significant findings.

2. Monitor ABG values. Hypoxemia is common. Progressive hypoxemia may require increased concentrations of oxygen or mechanical ventilation. Alert MD accordingly.

3. Assess patient for indicators of increased respiratory effort: complaints of SOB, tachypnea (RR >20 breaths/min), change in the use of accessory muscles of respiration, nasal flaring, grunting, restlessness, and anxiety.

4. Place patient in semi-Fowler's position to optimize lung expansion and decrease work of breathing.

5. Assess patient's need for suctioning at frequent intervals. Document color, consistency, and amount of sputum; frequency of suctioning to maintain clear airway; and patient's response to the procedure.

6. If patient is on PEEP, be aware that alveoli collapse when PEEP is removed. Oxygenation levels achieved prior to suctioning will not be attained immediately after PEEP is reinstituted because the effect PEEP exerts on alveoli is not instantaneous. To prevent dramatic decreases in Pao_2 with suctioning, use of a PEEP adaptor on manual resuscitator is recommended for patients on high levels

of PEEP. See "Management of the Adult on Mechanical Ventilation," pp. 61-70.

7. Provide rest periods between activities to decrease oxygen demands.
8. Explain all procedures to patient and provide emotional support to decrease anxiety.

Hypothermia related to prolonged exposure to cold water during submersion

---

Desired outcome: Patient's core temperature will be ≥35-37° C (95-98.6° F), followed by a return of surface body temperature to ≥35-37° C within an acceptable period of time.

---

1. Use temperature probe to obtain a continuous measurement of patient's core temperature. If a pulmonary artery catheter is in place, the cardiac output thermodilution probe can be used to monitor core body temperature. The temperature of inspired gases may affect accuracy of this measurement. Other methods for measuring core temperature include bladder thermometry, rectal probe, or esophageal temperature probe, which is positioned in the lower third of the esophagus.
2. Monitor patient's response to rewarming. Assess temperature and humidity level of inspired oxygen. Monitor temperature of instilled peritoneal lavage fluid. Do not attempt surface or external warming until core temperature is within acceptable limits (i.e., 35-37° C [95-98.6° F]). Premature surface rewarming can lead to the return of cold blood to the heart and precipitate an "after drop" in core temperature.
3. After core temperature has reached acceptable limits, monitor patient's response to active rewarming of body surface. Rewarming can be achieved by warm baths, heating pads, or lights. Use of blankets alone is an inadequate method of rewarming surface areas except in cases of mild hypothermia.
4. Be aware of the likelihood of decreased drug metabolism during patient's hypothermic period.

Potential fluid volume deficit related to decrease in circulating volume secondary to fluid shift to pulmonary system occurring with saltwater aspiration

---

Desired outcome: Patient is normovolemic as evidenced by BP >90/60, HR ≤100 bpm, urine output ≥30 ml/hr, brisk capillary refill (<3 seconds), CVP ≥2 mm Hg (or ≥5 cm H_2O), BUN 10-20 mg/dl, and creatinine 0.7-1.5 mg/dl.

---

1. Assess patient for signs of hypovolemia: BP decreased from baseline, increased HR, urine output <30 ml/hour, increased capillary filling time, and decreased CVP. Document findings and notify MD of significant changes.
2. Monitor serum electrolyte values, BUN, and creatinine for evidence of hemoconcentration. With dehydration, BUN increases disproportionately to the rise in creatinine.
3. As appropriate, monitor patient's response to volume expanders. Be alert to crackles (rales) as a sign of pulmonary edema secondary to volume overload.

Potential for infection related to susceptibility secondary to aspiration of water, gastric contents, and contaminants present in water

---

Desired outcome: Patient is free of infection as evidenced by core temperature ≤37.5° C (99.6° F) after the first 24 hours, WBC ≤11,000 μl, and negative sputum culture.

---

1. Monitor temperature q2h. Increases in temperature up to 38° C (100.4° F) are common during the first 24 hours. After 24 hours, an increased temperature may be indicative of infection.
2. Monitor WBC count, being alert to increases from baseline values.
3. Inspect sputum for changes in color, consistency, and amount.
4. Use meticulous aseptic technique when suctioning patient.
5. Collect sputum specimen for Gram stain and culture and sensitivity as prescribed. These tests will identify the pathogen if infection is present.

See other nursing diagnoses and interventions in the following: "Caring for the Critically Ill with Life-Threatening Disorders," pp. 511-522; and "Caring for the Family of the Critically Ill," pp. 522-526.

Acid-base imbalances

For optimal functioning of the cells, metabolic processes maintain a steady balance between acids and bases. Arterial pH is an indirect measurement of hydrogen ion (H^+) concentration and is a reflection of the balance between carbon dioxide (CO_2), which is regulated by the lungs, and bicarbonate (HCO_3^-), a basic buffer regulated by the kidneys. Carbon dioxide, when dissolved in water, becomes carbonic acid (H_2CO_3). Because H_2CO_3 cannot be measured directly, the amount of H_2CO_3 in the blood is reflected by the $Paco_2$ (see p. 43). Normal acid-base ratio is 1:20, representing one part CO_2 (potential H_2CO_3) to twenty parts HCO_3^-. If this balance is altered, derangements in pH occur. If extra acids are present, acidosis exists. If extra base is present or there is loss of acid and the pH is higher than 7.40, alkalosis is present.

SECTION ONE: Evaluating acid-base balance

Several mechanisms regulate acid-base balance. These mechanisms are exceptionally sensitive to minute changes in pH. Usually, the body is able to maintain pH without outside intervention, if not at a normal level, at least in a life-sustaining range.

Buffer system responses

BUFFERS

Buffers are present in all body fluids and act immediately (within 1 second) after an abnormal pH occurs. They combine with excess acid or base to form substances that do not affect pH. Their effect, however, is limited.

1. **Bicarbonate:** The most important buffer, it is present in the largest quantity in body fluids. It aids in the excretion of H^+ and is generated in the kidneys.
2. **Phosphate:** Aids in the excretion of H^+ in the renal tubules.
3. **Ammonium:** The kidneys produce an acidic urine by adding H^+ to ammonia (NH_3) to form ammonium (NH_4^+).
4. **Protein:** Present in cells, blood, and plasma. Hemoglobin is the most important protein buffer.

RESPIRATORY SYSTEM

Hydrogen ions (H^+) exert direct action on the respiratory center in the brain. Acidemia increases alveolar ventilation to 4-5 times the normal level, while alkalemia decreases alveolar ventilation to 50-75% of the normal level. The response occurs quickly—within 1-2 minutes, during which time the lungs eliminate or retain carbon dioxide in direct relation to arterial pH. While the respiratory system cannot correct imbalances completely, it is 50-75% effective.

RENAL SYSTEM

This system regulates acid-base balance by increasing or decreasing bicarbonate concentration in body fluids. This is accomplished through a series of complex reactions that involve H^+ secretion, Na^+ reabsorption, HCO_3^- conservation, and ammonia synthesis for excretion in the urine. H^+ secretion is regulated by the amount of carbon dioxide in extracellular fluid: the greater the concentration of carbon dioxide, the greater the amount of H^+ secretion, resulting in an acidic urine. When H^+ is excreted, bicarbonate is generated by the kidneys, helping to maintain the 1:20 ratio of acids and bases. When extracellular fluid is alkalotic, the kidneys conserve H^+ and eliminate sodium bicarbonate, resulting in alkalotic urine. Although the kidneys' response to an abnormal pH is slow—several hours to days, they are able to adjust the imbalance to normal because of their ability to excrete large quantities of excess bicarbonate and H^+ from the body.

Blood gas values

Blood gas analysis usually is based on arterial sampling. Venous values are given as a reference.

Arterial Values	Venous Values
pH: 7.35-7.45	pH: 7.36
$Paco_2$*: 35-45 mm Hg	Pco_2: 46 mm Hg
Pao_2: 80-95 mm Hg	Po_2: 40 mm Hg
Saturation: 95-99%	Saturation: 75%
Base excess: + or − 1	
Serum bicarbonate (HCO_3^-)†: 22-26 mEq/L:	

*$Paco_2$ multiplied by 0.30 (solubility coefficient) equals the amount of carbonic acid.
†Although serum bicarbonate is a buffer, it usually is reported as "CO_2 content" or "total CO_2" and not as serum bicarbonate. The serum HCO_3^- concentration usually is obtained separately from ABG analysis and is critical in the determination of acid-base status, although this value may be calculated from $Paco_2$ and pH results *via* the ABG analysis. Values should be obtained with the initial assessment and daily thereafter.

ARTERIAL BLOOD GAS ANALYSIS

1. **pH:** Measures H^+ concentration to reflect acid-base status of the blood. Values reflect whether arterial pH is normal (7.40), acidic (<7.40), or alkalotic (>7.40). Because of the ability of compensatory mechanisms to "normalize" the pH, a near-normal value does not exclude the possibility of an acid-base disturbance.

2. **Paco₂:** Partial pressure of carbon dioxide in the arteries. It is the respiratory component of acid-base regulation and is adjusted by changes in the rate and depth of pulmonary ventilation. Hypercapnia ($Paco_2$ >45 mm Hg) signals alveolar hypoventilation and respiratory acidosis. Hyperventilation results in a $Paco_2$ <35 mm Hg and respiratory alkalosis. Respiratory compensation occurs rapidly in metabolic acid-base disturbances. If any abnormality in $Paco_2$ exists, it is important to analyze pH and HCO_3^- parameters to determine if the alteration in $Paco_2$ is the result of a primary respiratory disturbance or a compensatory response to a metabolic acid-base abnormality.

3. **Pao₂:** Partial pressure of oxygen in the arteries. It has no primary role in acid-base regulation if it is within normal limits. The presence of hypoxemia (Pao_2<80 mm Hg) can lead to anaerobic metabolism, resulting in lactic acid production and metabolic acidosis. There is a normal decline in Pao_2 in the aged.

4. **Saturation:** Measures the degree to which hemoglobin is saturated by oxygen. It can be affected by changes in temperature, pH, and $Paco_2$. When the Pao_2 falls below 60, there is a large drop in saturation.

5. **Base excess or deficit:** Indicates, in general terms, the amount of blood buffer (hemoglobin and plasma bicarbonate) present. Abnormally high values reflect alkalosis; low values reflect acidosis.

6. **HCO₃⁻:** Serum bicarbonate is the major renal component of acid-base regulation. It is excreted or regenerated by the kidneys to maintain a normal acid-base environment. Decreased bicarbonate levels (<22 mEq/L) are indicative of metabolic acidosis (seen infrequently as a compensatory mechanism for respiratory alkalosis); elevated bicarbonate levels (>26 mEq/L) reflect metabolic alkalosis—either as a primary metabolic disorder or as a compensatory alteration in response to respiratory acidosis.

STEP-BY-STEP GUIDE TO ABG ANALYSIS

A systemic step-by-step analysis is critical to the accurate interpretation of ABG values. For further information, see Table 1-5.

1. **Step one:** Determine if pH is normal. If abnormal, identify whether it is on the acidotic (<7.35) or alkalotic (>7.45) side of normal.

2. **Step two:** Check $Paco_2$ and HCO_3^- to determine which value corresponds to the pH value. For example, if the pH is acidotic, which value most closely reflects acidosis? This determines whether the primary problem is respiratory or metabolic in nature.

3. **Step three:** If both $Paco_2$ and HCO_3^- are abnormal, the value that deviates the most from normal points to the primary disturbance responsible for the altered pH. A mixed metabolic-respiratory disturbance or compensatory elements may be present.

4. **Step four:** Check Pao_2 and oxygen saturation to determine whether they are decreased, normal, or increased. Decreased Pao_2 and O_2 saturation can lead to

TABLE 1-5
ABG comparisons of acid-base disorders

		Alkalosis			Acidosis	
	$Paco_2$	pH	HCO_3^-	$Paco_2$	pH	HCO_3^-
Simple Respiratory	25	7.6	24	50	7.15	25
Metabolic	44	7.54	36	38	7.20	15
Compensated Respiratory	25	7.54	21	66	7.37	34
Metabolic	50	7.42	31	23	7.28	9
Mixed Disorder	40	7.56	38	50	7.2	20

lactic acidosis and may signal the need for increased concentrations of oxygen. Conversely, high Pao_2 may be indicative of the need to decrease delivered concentrations of oxygen.

ARTERIAL-VENOUS DIFFERENCE

The difference between arterial oxygen content and venous oxygen content (A-VO_2) reflects the tissue extraction of oxygen. This difference increases when ventricular performance is impaired. Simultaneous analysis of arterial and pulmonary artery blood sampling provides an accurate and reliable index of ventricular function.

SECTION TWO: Caring for adults with acid-base imbalances

Acute respiratory acidosis

Respiratory acidosis (hypercapnia) occurs secondary to alveolar hypoventilation and results in an elevated $Paco_2$. $Paco_2$ derangements are direct reflections of the degree of ventilatory function or dysfunction. The degree to which the increased $Paco_2$ alters the pH depends on the rapidity of onset and the body's ability to compensate through the blood buffer and renal systems. The acidemia may develop rapidly because of the delay (hours or days) before renal compensation occurs. Acute rises in $Paco_2$ do precipitate a rise in extracellular bicarbonate even before renal compensation occurs, but the extracellular rise is not sufficient to maintain a normal pH in the presence of an elevated $Paco_2$.

ASSESSMENT

Signs and symptoms: Dyspnea; asterixis; restlessness leading to lethargy, confusion, and coma.

Physical assessment: Increased heart and respiratory rates, diaphoresis, and cyanosis. Severe hypercapnia may cause cerebral vasodilatation, resulting in increased ICP with papilledema. Another finding may be dilated conjunctival and facial blood vessels.

Monitoring parameters: Presence of ventricular dysrhythmias; increased ICP.

History and risk factors

1. *Acute respiratory disease*
2. *Overdose of drugs:* Oversedation with drugs that cause respiratory center depression.
3. *Chest wall trauma:* Flail chest, pneumothorax.
4. *CNS trauma/lesions:* Can lead to depression of respiratory center.
5. *Asphyxiation:* Mechanical obstruction; anaphylaxis.
6. *Impaired respiratory muscles:* Can occur with hypokalemia, hyperkalemia, polio, Guillain-Barré syndrome.
7. *Iatrogenic:* Inappropriate mechanical ventilation (increased dead space, insufficient rate or volume); high FIo_2 in the presence of chronic CO_2 retention.

DIAGNOSTIC TESTS

1. *ABG analysis:* Aids in diagnosis and determination of severity of respiratory acidosis. Pa_{CO_2} will be >45 mm Hg and pH will be <7.35.
2. *Serum bicarbonate:* HCO_3^- reflects metabolic and base balance. Initially, HCO_3^- values will be normal (22-26 mEq/L) unless a mixed disorder is present.
3. *Serum electrolytes:* Usually not altered; depend on etiology of respiratory acidosis.
4. *Chest x-ray:* Determines presence of underlying respiratory disease.
5. *Drug screen:* Determines presence and quantity of drug if patient is suspected of taking an overdose.

MEDICAL MANAGEMENT

1. **Restoration of normal acid-base balance:** Accomplished by supporting respiratory function. If Pa_{CO_2} is >50-60 mm Hg and clinical signs such as cyanosis and lethargy are present, the patient usually requires intubation and mechanical ventilation. Generally, use of bicarbonate is avoided because of the risk of alkalosis when the respiratory disturbance has been corrected. Although a life-threatening pH must be corrected to an acceptable level promptly, a normal pH is not the immediate goal.
2. **Treatment of underlying disorder**

NURSING DIAGNOSES AND INTERVENTIONS

Nursing diagnoses and interventions are specific to the pathophysiologic process. See appropriate section(s) in this and other chapters for diagnoses such as **Impaired gas exchange, Ineffective airway clearance,** and **Activity intolerance.** A list of nursing diagnoses used in this manual begins on p. 543.

Chronic respiratory acidosis (compensated)

This disorder occurs in pulmonary diseases (e.g., chronic emphysema and bronchitis) in which effective alveolar ventilation is decreased and a ventilation-perfusion mismatch is present. Chronic hypercapnia also can occur with obesity. In patients with a chronic lung disease, a nearly normal pH can be seen if renal function is normal, even if the Pa_{CO_2} is as high as 60 mm Hg. Chronic compensatory metabolic alkalosis (serum HCO_3^- >26 mEq/L) occurs and maintains an acceptable acid-base environment, which results in compensated respiratory acidosis and a normal or near normal pH. Patients with chronic lung disease can experience acute rises in Pa_{CO_2} secondary to superimposed disease states such as pneumonia. If the chronic compensatory mechanisms in place (e.g., elevated HCO_3^-) are inadequate to meet the sudden increase in Pa_{CO_2}, decompensation may occur with a resultant decrease in pH.

ASSESSMENT

Signs and symptoms: If the Pa_{CO_2} does not exceed the body's ability to compensate, no specific findings will be noted. If Pa_{CO_2} rises rapidly, the following may occur: dyspnea, asterixis, agitation, and insomnia progressing to somnolence and coma.

Physical assessment: Tachypnea, cyanosis. Severe hypercapnia (Pa_{CO_2} >70 mm Hg) may cause cerebral vasodilatation resulting in increased ICP, papil-

T A B L E 1 - 6

Quick assessment guide to acid-base imbalances

Acid-base imbalance	pH	Paco₂	HCO₃⁻	Clinical signs and symptoms	Common causes
Acute respiratory acidosis	Decreased	Increased	No change	Tachycardia, tachypnea, diaphoresis, headache, restlessness leading to lethargy and coma, cyanosis, dysrhythmias, hypotension.	Acute respiratory failure, cardiopulmonary disease, drug overdose, chest wall trauma, asphyxiation, CNS trauma/lesions, impaired muscles of respiration.
Chronic respiratory acidosis (compensated)	Decreased	Increased	Increased	Dyspnea & tachypnea, with increase in CO_2 retention that exceeds compensatory ability; progression to lethargy, confusion, and coma.	COPD, extreme obesity (Pickwickian syndrome), superimposed infection on COPD.

Continued.

T A B L E 1 - 6 cont'd.
Quick assessment guide to acid-base imbalances

Acid-base imbalance	pH	$Paco_2$	HCO_3^-	Clinical signs and symptoms	Common causes
Acute respiratory alkalosis	Increased	Decreased	No change (a decrease will occur if condition has been present for hours, providing that renal function is adequate).	Paresthesias, especially of the fingers; dizziness.	Hyperventilation, salicylate poisoning, hypoxia (e.g., with pneumonia, pulmonary edema, pulmonary thromboembolism), gram-negative sepsis, CNS lesion, decreased lung compliance, inappropriate mechanical ventilation.
Chronic respiratory alkalosis	Increased	Decreased	Decreased	No symptoms	Hepatic failure; CNS lesion.
Acute metabolic acidosis	Decreased	Decreased	Decreased	Tachypnea leading to Kussmaul respirations, hypotension, cold and clammy skin, coma, and dysrhythmias.	Shock, cardiopulmonary arrest (secondary to lactic acid production), ketoacidosis (e.g., diabetes, starvation, alcohol abuse), acute renal failure, ingestion of acids (e.g., salicylates), diarrhea.

Chronic metabolic acidosis	Decreased	Decreased (not as much as acute type)	Decreased	Fatigue, anorexia, malaise. Symptoms may be related to chronic disease process as well as acidosis.	Chronic renal failure
Acute metabolic alkalosis	Increased	Increased (can be as great as 60)	Increased	Muscular weakness and hyporeflexia (due to severe hypokalemia), dysrhythmias, apathy, confusion, and stupor.	Volume depletion (Cl^- depletion) as a result of vomiting, gastric drainage, diuretic use, post-hypercapnea. Hyperadrenocorticism (e.g., Cushing's syndrome), aldosteronism, severe potassium depletion, excessive alkali intake.
Chronic metabolic alkalosis	Increased	Increased	Increased	Usually asymptomatic.	Upper GI losses through continuous drainage; correction of hypercapnia if Na^+ and K^+ depletion remains uncorrected.

ledema, and dilated conjunctival and facial blood vessels. Depending on underlying pathophysiology, edema may be present secondary to right ventricular failure.

History and risk factors

1. *COPD:* Predominantly emphysema and bronchitis.
2. *Extreme obesity:* Pickwickian syndrome.
3. *Development of superimposed acute respiratory infection in a patient with COPD.*
4. *Exposure to pulmonary toxins:* Occupational risk; pollution.

DIAGNOSTIC TESTS

1. *ABG values:* Provide data necessary for determining the diagnosis and severity of respiratory acidosis. Although the $Paco_2$ will be elevated, the pH will be on the acidic (low) side of normal in patients who are not experiencing acute pulmonary infection. If the $Paco_2$ has increased abruptly from baseline value, a pH lower than normal may be seen.
2. *Serum electrolytes:* Serum bicarbonate (HCO_3^-) is especially helpful in determining the level of metabolic compensation that has occurred (i.e., HCO_3^- increased with a near normal pH if fully compensated). This information is particularly useful in identifying "mixed" acid-base disturbances because the HCO_3^- is expected to be elevated in chronic respiratory acidosis. If the HCO_3^- is normal or low, this could be diagnostic of a second pathologic process concurrent with the first.
3. *Chest x-ray:* Determines extent of underlying pulmonary disease and identifies further pathologic changes that may be responsible for acute exacerbation, for example, pneumonia.
4. *EKG:* Identifies cardiac involvement from COPD. For example, right-sided heart failure is a complication of chronic bronchitis.
5. *Sputum culture:* Determines presence of pathogens causing an acute exacerbation of a chronic pulmonary disease (e.g., pneumonia) present in a patient with COPD.

MEDICAL MANAGEMENT

1. **Oxygen therapy:** Used cautiously in patients with chronic CO_2 retention for whom hypoxia, rather than hypercapnia, stimulates ventilation. Patient may require intubation and mechanical ventilation for stupor and coma precipitated by oxygen if drive to breathe is eliminated by high concentrations of oxygen.
2. **Pharmacotherapy:** Bronchodilators and antibiotics, as indicated. Narcotics and sedatives can depress the respiratory center and are avoided unless patient is intubated and mechanically ventilated.
3. **IV fluids:** Maintain adequate hydration for mobilizing pulmonary secretions.
4. **Chest physiotherapy:** Aids in expectoration of sputum. Includes postural drainage if hypersecretions are present. Assess patient closely during this procedure because it may be poorly tolerated, especially the postural drainage component.

NURSING DIAGNOSES AND INTERVENTIONS

Impaired gas exchange related to trapping of CO_2 secondary to pulmonary tissue destruction (appropriate for the patient with COPD)

Desired outcome: ABG values reflect a $Paco_2$ and pH within acceptable range, based on patient's underlying pulmonary disease.

1. Monitor serial ABG results to assess patient's response to therapy. Report significant findings to MD: an increasing $Paco_2$ and a decreasing pH.
2. Assess and document patient's respiratory status: respiratory rate and rhythm, exertional effort, and breath sounds. Compare pretreatment findings to posttreatment (e.g., oxygen therapy, physiotherapy, or medications) findings for evidence of improvement.
3. Assess and document patient's LOC. If $Paco_2$ increases, be alert to subtle, progressive changes in mental status. A common progression is agitation → insomnia → somnolence → coma. To avoid a comatose state secondary to rising CO_2 levels, always evaluate the "arousability" of a patient with elevated $Paco_2$ who appears to be sleeping. Notify MD if patient is difficult to arouse.
4. Ensure appropriate delivery of prescribed oxygen therapy. Assess patient's respiratory status after every change in FIo_2. Patients with chronic CO_2 retention may be very sensitive to increases in FIo_2, resulting in depressed ventilatory drive. If patient requires mechanical ventilation, be aware of the importance of maintaining the compensated acid-base environment. If the $Paco_2$ were rapidly decreased by a high respiratory rate per mechanical ventilation, a severe metabolic alkalosis could develop. The sudden onset of metabolic alkalosis may lead to hypocalcemia, which can result in tetany (see "Hypocalcemia," p. 232).
5. Assess for presence of bowel sounds and monitor for gastric distention, which can impede movement of the diaphragm and restrict ventilatory effort further.
6. If patient is not intubated, encourage use of pursed-lip breathing (inhalation through nose, with slow exhalation through pursed lips), which helps airways to remain open and allows for better air excursion. Optimally, this technique will diminish air entrapment in the lungs and make respiratory effort more efficient.

Acute respiratory alkalosis (hypocapnia)

Respiratory alkalosis occurs as a result of an increase in the rate of alveolar ventilation (alveolar hyperventilation). It is defined as $Paco_2$ <35 mm Hg. Acute alveolar hyperventilation most frequently results from anxiety and is commonly referred to as "hyperventilation syndrome." In addition, numerous physiologic disorders (see "History and risk factors," below) can cause acute hypocapnia, which results in increased pH. The rise in pH is modified to a small degree by intracellular buffering. To compensate for increased CO_2 loss and the resultant base excess, hydrogen ions are released from tissue buffers, which in turn lowers plasma bicarbonate concentration.

ASSESSMENT

Signs and symptoms: Lightheadedness, anxiety, paresthesias, circumoral numbness. In extreme alkalosis, confusion, tetany, syncope, and seizures may occur.

Physical assessment: Increased rate and depth of respirations.

EKG findings: Cardiac dysrhythmias.

History and risk factors

1. *Anxiety:* Patient is often unaware of hyperventilation.
2. *Acute hypoxia:* Pulmonary disorders (e.g., pneumonia, pulmonary edema, and pulmonary thromboembolism) cause hypoxia, which stimulates the ventilatory effort.
3. *Hypermetabolic states:* Fever; sepsis, especially gram-negative induced septicemia.
4. *Salicylate intoxication*
5. *Excessive mechanical ventilation*
6. *CNS trauma:* May result in damage to respiratory center.

DIAGNOSTIC TESTS

1. *ABG values:* $Paco_2$ <35 mm Hg and pH >7.45 will be present. A decreased Pao_2, along with the clinical picture (e.g., pneumonia, pulmonary edema, pulmonary embolism, and ARDS), may help diagnose etiology of the respiratory alkalosis.
2. *Serum electrolytes:* Determine presence of metabolic acid-base disorders.
3. *EKG:* Detects cardiac dysrhythmias, which may be present with alkalosis.

MEDICAL MANAGEMENT

1. **Treatment of underlyling disorder**
2. **Reassurance or sedation:** If anxiety is the cause of decreased $Paco_2$. If symptoms are severe, it may be necessary for patient to rebreathe CO_2 through an oxygen mask with an attached CO_2 reservoir.
3. **Oxygen therapy:** If hypoxia is the causative factor.
4. **Adjustments to mechanical ventilators:** Settings are checked and adjustments made to ventilatory parameters in response to ABG results that signal hypocapnia. Respiratory rate and/or volume are decreased and dead space is added, if necessary.
5. **Pharmacotherapy:** Sedatives and tranquilizers may be given for anxiety-induced respiratory alkalosis.

NURSING DIAGNOSES AND INTERVENTIONS

Nursing diagnoses and interventions are specific to the pathophysiologic process. See appropriate nursing diagnoses (e.g., **Ineffective breathing pattern** related to hyperventilation) in this and other chapters. A list of nursing diagnoses used in this manual begins on p. 543.

Chronic respiratory alkalosis

This is a state of chronic hypocapnia, which stimulates the renal compensatory response and results in a decrease in plasma bicarbonate. Maximal renal compensatory response requires several days to occur.

ASSESSMENT

Signs and symptoms: Individuals with chronic respiratory alkalosis usually are asymptomatic.

Physical assessment: Increased respiratory rate and depth.

History and risk factors

1. *Cerebral disease:* Tumor, encephalitis.
2. *Chronic hepatic insufficiency*
3. *Pregnancy*
4. *Chronic hypoxia:* Adaptation to high altitude; cyanotic heart disease; lung disease resulting in decreased compliance (e.g., fibrosis).

DIAGNOSTIC TESTS

1. *ABG values:* $PaCO_2$ will be <35 mm Hg, with a nearly normal pH; PaO_2 may be decreased if hypoxia is the causative factor.
2. *Serum electrolytes:* Probably will be normal, with the exception of plasma bicarbonate (HCO_3^-), which will decrease as renal compensation occurs.
3. *Phosphate levels:* Hypophosphatemia (as low as 0.5 mg/dl) may be seen with intense hyperventilation. Alkalosis causes increased uptake of phosphate by the cells.

MEDICAL MANAGEMENT

1. **Treatment of underlying cause**
2. **Oxygen therapy:** If hypoxia is present and identified as causative factor in respiratory alkalosis.

NURSING DIAGNOSES AND INTERVENTIONS

Nursing diagnoses and interventions are specific to the pathophysiologic process. See appropriate medical disorders and nursing diagnoses in this and other chapters. A list of nursing diagnoses used in this manual begins on p. 543 in the appendix.

Acute metabolic acidosis

Metabolic acidosis is caused by a primary decrease in plasma bicarbonate, as reflected by a serum bicarbonate of <22 mEq/L with a pH <7.40. The decrease in serum bicarbonate is caused by one of the following mechanisms: (1) increase in the concentration of hydrogen ions in the form of nonvolatile acids (e.g., ketoacidosis associated with diabetes and alcoholism; lactic acidosis); (2) loss of alkali (e.g., severe diarrhea, intestinal malabsorption); and (3) decreased acid excretion by the kidneys (e.g., acute and chronic renal failure). The decrease in pH stimulates respirations. Attempts to compensate occur rapidly, as manifested by lowering of the $PaCO_2$, which may be reduced by as much as 10-15 mm Hg. The most important mechanism for ridding the body of excess H^+ is the increase in acid excretion by the kidneys. However, nonvolatile acids may accumulate more rapidly than they can be neutralized by the body's buffers, compensated for by the respiratory system, or excreted by the kidneys.

ASSESSMENT

Signs and symptoms: Findings vary, depending on underlying disease states and severity of acid-base disturbance. There may be changes in LOC that range from fatigue and confusion to stupor and coma.

Physical assessment: Decreased BP, tachypnea leading to alveolar hyperventilation (Kussmaul's respirations), cold and clammy skin, presence of dysrhythmias and shock state.

History and risk factors

1. *Renal disease:* Acute renal failure, renal tubular acidosis.
2. *Ketoacidosis:* Diabetes mellitus, alcoholism, starvation.
3. *Lactic acidosis:* Respiratory or circulatory failure, drugs and toxins, hereditary disorders, septic shock. It can be associated with other disease states, such as leukemia, pancreatitis, bacterial infection, and uncontrolled diabetes mellitus.
4. *Poisonings and drug toxicity:* Salicylates, methanol, ethylene glycol, ammonium chloride.
5. *Loss of alkali:* Draining wounds (e.g., pancreatic fistulas), diarrhea, ureterostomy.

DIAGNOSTIC TESTS

1. *ABG values:* Determine pH (usually <7.35) and degree of respiratory compensation as reflected by $Paco_2$, which usually is <35 mm Hg.
2. *Serum bicarbonate:* Determines presence of metabolic acidosis (HCO_3^- <22 mEq/L).
3. *Serum electrolytes:* Elevated potassium may be present because of the exchange of intracellular potassium for hydrogen ions in the body's attempt to normalize acid-base environment.

   In attempt to identify cause of metabolic acidosis, an analysis of serum electrolytes to detect anion gap may be helpful. Anion gap reflects unmeasureable anions present in plasma and is calculated by subtracting the sum of chloride and sodium bicarbonate from plasma sodium concentration. Anion gap = Na^+ − (Cl^- + HCO_3^-). Normal anion gap is 12 (+ or − 2) mEq/L. Normal anion gap acidosis results from direct loss of HCO_3^- (e.g., diarrhea, renal tubular acidosis, pancreatic fistulas) or the addition of chloride-containing acids (e.g., ammonium chloride, hydrochloric acid), some hyperalimentation fluids, and oral calcium chloride). An increased anion gap acidosis >12-14 mEq/L results from accumulation of nonvolatile acids (acids from lactic acidosis, diabetes ketoacidosis, uremia, and salicylate and methanol toxicity).
4. *EKG:* Detects dysrhythmias, which may be caused by acidosis or hyperkalemia. Changes seen with hyperkalemia include peaked T waves, depressed ST-segment, decreased size of R waves, decrease or absence of P waves, widened QRS complex.

MEDICAL MANAGEMENT

1. **Sodium bicarbonate ($NaHCO_3^-$):** Indicated when arterial pH is ≤7.2. The usual mode of delivery is IV drip: 2-3 ampules (44.5 mEq/ampule) in 1000 ml D_5W, although $NaHCO_3$ frequently is given IV push in emergencies. Concentration depends on severity of the acidosis and presence of any serum sodium disorders. $NaHCO_3$ must be given cautiously to avoid metabolic alkalosis and pulmonary edema secondary to the sodium load.
2. **Potassium replacement:** Usually, hyperkalemia is present, but a potassium deficit can occur. If a potassium deficit exists (K^+ <3.5), it must be corrected before $NaHCO_3$ is administered because when the acidosis is corrected, the potassium shifts back to intracellular spaces. Therefore, this could result in serum hypokalemia with serious consequences, such as cardiac irritability with

fatal dysrhythmias and generalized muscle weakness. See "Hypokalemia," p. 226, for more information.

3. **Mechanical ventilation:** If necessary. However, it is important that the patient's compensatory hyperventilation be allowed to continue, to prevent acidosis from becoming more severe. Therefore, the respiratory rate on the ventilator should not be set lower than the rate at which patient has been breathing spontaneously, and the tidal volume should be large enough to maintain compensatory hyperventilation until the underlying disorder can be resolved.

4. **Treatment of underlying disorder**
   - *Diabetes ketoacidosis:* Insulin and fluids. If acidosis is severe (with a pH of <7.1 or HCO_3^- 6-8 mEq/L), sodium bicarbonate may be necessary.
   - *Alcoholism-related ketoacidosis:* Glucose and saline.
   - *Diarrhea:* Usually occurs in association with other fluid and electrolyte disturbances; correction addresses concurrent imbalances.
   - *Acute renal failure:* Hemodialysis or peritoneal dialysis to maintain an adequate level of plasma bicarbonate.
   - *Renal tubular acidosis:* May require modest amounts (<100 mEq/day) of bicarbonate.
   - *Poisoning and drug toxicity:* Treatment depends on the drug ingested or infused. Hemodialysis or peritoneal dialysis may be necessary.
   - *Lactic acidosis:* Correction of underlying disorder. Mortality associated with lactic acidosis is high. Treatment with $NaHCO_3$ is only transiently helpful.

NURSING DIAGNOSES AND INTERVENTIONS

Nursing diagnoses and interventions are specific to the pathophysiologic process. In addition to **Alterations in oral mucous membrane** related to mouth breathing (see appendix, p. 535, for this and other nursing diagnoses used in this manual), refer to nursing diagnoses and interventions in the following sections: "Management of the Adult on Mechanical Ventilation," pp. 66-70; "Acute Renal Failure," p. 173; "Diabetic Ketoacidosis," p. 330; "Caring for the Critically Ill with Life-Threatening Disorders," pp. 511-522; and "Caring for the Family of the Critically Ill," pp. 522-526.

Chronic metabolic acidosis

Most often, this condition is seen with chronic renal failure in which the kidneys' ability to excrete acids (endogenous and exogenous) is exceeded by acid production and ingestion. The acidosis usually is mild in the initial stage, with HCO_3^- 18-22 mEq/L and a pH of 7.35. Treatment is indicated when serum bicarbonate levels reach 15 mEq/L. Respiratory compensation does occur, but to a limited degree. A modest decrease in $Paco_2$ will be noted on ABG values.

ASSESSMENT

Signs and symptoms: Usually patient is asymptomatic, although fatigue, malaise, and anorexia may be present in relation to underlying disease.

History and risk factors: Chronic renal failure.

DIAGNOSTIC TESTS

1. *ABG values:* $Paco_2$ will be <35 mm Hg; pH will be <7.35.
2. *Serum bicarbonate:* Will be <22 mEq/L (usually 18-21 mEq/L). With severe acidosis, it will be ≤15 mEq/L.
3. *Serum electrolytes:* Serum calcium level is checked before treatment of acidosis is initiated to prevent tetany induced by hypocalcemia (caused by a decrease in ionized calcium). Serum phosphorus level is evaluated to determine presence of hyperphosphatemia, a common complication of chronic renal failure. Serum potassium level should be monitored after acidosis has been corrected to detect hypokalemia, as potassium shifts back into the cells.

MEDICAL MANAGEMENT

1. **Alkalizing agents:** For serum bicarbonate levels <15 mEq/L, oral alkali are administered (sodium bicarbonate tablets or sodium citrate—Shohl's solution). They are used cautiously to prevent fluid overload and tetany caused by hypocalcemia.

   < C A U T I O N : Be alert to the possibility of pulmonary edema if oliguria is present and bicarbonate is administered parenterally.

2. **Oral phosphates:** Given if hypophosphatemia is present (not common with chronic renal failure, but may result from overuse of phosphate binders given to treat hyperphosphatemia).
3. **Hemodialysis or peritoneal dialysis:** If indicated by chronic renal failure or other disease processes. See discussion, pp. 200-201.

NURSING DIAGNOSES AND INTERVENTIONS

Nursing diagnoses and interventions are specific to the underlying pathophysiologic process. See renal chapter, p. 173, in particular, and p. 543 for a list of nursing diagnoses used in this manual.

Acute metabolic alkalosis

This disorder results in an elevated serum bicarbonate (up to 45-50 mEq/L) as a result of hydrogen ion loss or excess alkali intake. A compensatory increase in $Paco_2$ (up to 50-60 mm Hg) will be seen. Respiratory compensation is limited because of hypoxia, which develops secondary to decreased alveolar ventilation. The major causes of this disturbance are loss of gastric acid from vomiting or NG suction, posthypercapneic alkalosis (which occurs when chronic CO_2 retention is corrected rapidly), excessive sodium bicarbonate administration (i.e., overcorrection of a metabolic acidosis), and diuretic therapy.

ASSESSMENT

Signs and symptoms: Muscular weakness, neuromuscular instability and hyporeflexia secondary to accompanying hypokalemia. Decrease in GI tract motility may result in an ileus. Severe alkalosis can result in apathy, confusion, and stupor.

EKG findings: Frequent PVCs as a result of cardiac irritability occurring secondary to hypokalemia; U waves.

History and risk factors

1. *Clinical circumstances associated with volume/chloride depletion:* Vomiting or gastric drainage.
2. *Posthypercapneic alkalosis*
3. *Excessive alkali intake:* May be iatrogenic from overcorrection of metabolic acidosis (frequently seen during CPR).

DIAGNOSTIC TESTS

1. *ABG values:* Determine severity of alkalosis and response to therapy.
2. *Serum bicarbonate:* Values will be elevated to >26 mEq/L.
3. *Serum electrolytes:* Usually, serum potassium will be low (<4.0 mEq/L) as will serum chloride (<95 mEq/L).
4. *EKG:* To assess for dysrhythmias, especially if profound hypokalemia or alkalosis is present.

MEDICAL MANAGEMENT

Management will depend on the underlying disorder. Mild or moderate metabolic alkalosis usually doesn't require specific therapeutic interventions.

1. **Saline infusion:** Normal saline infusion may correct volume (chloride) deficit in patients with gastric alkalosis secondary to gastric losses. Metabolic alkalosis is difficult to correct if hypovolemia and chloride deficit are not corrected.
2. **Potassium chloride (KCl):** Indicated for patients with low potassium levels. KCl is preferred over other potassium salts because chloride losses can be replaced simultaneously.
3. **Sodium and potassium chloride:** Effective for posthypercapneic alkalosis, which occurs when chronic CO_2 retention is corrected rapidly (e.g., *via* mechanical ventilation). If adequate amounts of chloride and potassium are not available, renal excretion of excess bicarbonate is impaired and metabolic alkalosis continues.
4. **Cautious IV administration of isotonic hydrochloride solution, ammonium chloride, or argenine hydrochloride:** May be warranted if severe metabolic alkalosis (ph >7.6 and HCO_3^- >40-45 mEq/L) exists, especially if chloride or potassium salts are contraindicated. The medication is delivered *via* continuous IV infusion at a slow rate, with frequent monitoring of IV insertion site for signs of infiltration. Ammonium chloride and argenine hydrochloride may be dangerous to patients in renal or hepatic failure.

NURSING DIAGNOSES AND INTERVENTIONS

Nursing diagnoses and interventions are specific to the underlying pathophysiologic process. See renal chapter, p. 173, in particular, and p. 543 for a list of nursing diagnoses used in this manual.

Chronic metabolic alkalosis

Chronic metabolic alkalosis results in a pH >7.45. $Paco_2$ will be elevated (>45 mm Hg) to compensate for the loss of H^+ or excess serum HCO_3^-. There are three clinical situations in which this can occur: (1) abnormalities in the kidneys' excretion of HCO_3^- related to a mineralocorticoid effect; (2) loss of H^+ through the GI tract; and (3) diuretic therapy.

ASSESSMENT

Signs and symptoms: Patient may be asymptomatic. With severe potassium depletion and profound alkalosis, patient may experience weakness, neuromuscular instability, and decrease in GI tract motility, which can result in ileus.

EKG findings: Frequent PVCs or U waves with hypokalemia and alkalosis.

History and risk factors

1. *Diuretic use:* Thiazide diuretics cause a loss of chloride, potassium, and hydrogen ions. Massive depletion of potassium stores with loss of up to 1000 mEq, which is 1/3 of total body potassium, may occur, causing profound hypokalemia (≤2.0).

2. *Hyperadrenocorticism:* Cushing's syndrome, primary aldosteronism. This is not a chloride deficit but a chronic loss of potassium, which can lead to total body depletion of potassium with profound hypokalemia (K ≤2.0 mEq/L).

3. *Chronic vomiting or chronic GI losses through GI suction*

4. *Milk alkali syndrome:* An infrequent cause of metabolic alkalosis. Hypercalcemic nephropathy and alkalosis develop secondary to excessive intake of absorbable alkali.

DIAGNOSTIC TESTS

1. *ABG values:* Determine severity of acid-base imbalance. $Paco_2$ will be increased (>45 mm Hg) and pH will be >7.40.

2. *Serum bicarbonate:* Will be >26 mEq/L.

3. *Serum electrolytes:* Usually, potassium will be profoundly low (may be ≤2.0 mEq/L). Chloride may be <95 mEq/L. Magnesium may be <1.5 mEq/L in both renal system abnormalities.

MEDICAL MANAGEMENT

The goal is to correct the underlying acid-base disorder *via* the following interventions:

1. **Fluid management:** If volume depletion exists, normal saline infusions are given.

2. **Potassium replacement:** If a chloride deficit also is present, potassium chloride is the drug of choice. If a chloride deficit does not exist, other potassium salts are acceptable.

   - *IV potassium:* If the patient is on a cardiac monitor, up to 20 mEq/hour of potassium chloride is given for serious hypokalemia. Concentrated doses of KCl (>40 mEq/L) require administration through a central venous line because of the risk of blood vessel irritation.

   - *Oral potassium:* Tastes *very* unpleasant. 15 mEq per glass is all most patients can tolerate, with a maximum daily dose of 60-80 mEq. Slow-release potassium tablets are an acceptable form of KCl. All forms of KCl may be irritating to gastric mucosa.

   - *Dietary:* Normal diet contains 3 grams or 75 mEq of potassium, but not in the form of potassium chloride. Dietary supplementation of potassium is not effective if a concurrent chloride deficit is also present.

3. **Potassium-sparing diuretics:** May be added to treatment if thiazide diuretics are the cause of hypokalemia and metabolic alkalosis.

4. **Identification and correction of the cause of hyperadrenocorticism**

NURSING DIAGNOSES AND INTERVENTIONS

Nursing diagnoses and interventions are specific to the underlying pathophysiologic process. See the renal chapter, p. 173, in particular, and p. 543 for a list of nursing diagnoses used in this manual.

Acute respiratory failure and management of the adult on mechanical ventilation

Acute respiratory failure is a disorder in which there is impairment of alveolar ventilation and pulmonary vascular perfusion. Clinically, respiratory failure exists when Pao_2 is <50 mm Hg with the patient at rest and breathing room air. $Paco_2$ ≥50 mm Hg or pH <7.35 is significant for respiratory acidemia. While a variety of disease processes can lead to respiratory failure, four basic mechanisms are involved:

Alveolar hypoventilation: Occurs secondary to reduction in alveolar minute ventilation. Because differential indicators (cyanosis and somnolence) occur late in the process, the condition may go unnoticed until hypoxia is severe.

Ventilation-perfusion mismatch: Considered the most common cause of hypoxia. Normal alveolar ventilation occurs at a rate of 4 L/min, with normal pulmonary vascular blood flow occurring at a rate of 5 L/min. Normal ventilation-perfusion ratio is 0.8. Any disease process that interferes with either side of the equation upsets the physiologic balance and can lead to respiratory failure as a result of reduction in arterial oxygen levels.

Diffusion disturbances: Processes that physically impair gas exchange across the alveolar-capillary membrane. Diffusion is impaired owing to the increase in anatomic distance the gas must travel from alveoli to capillary and capillary to alveoli.

Right-to-left shunt: Occurs when the above processes go untreated. Large amounts of blood pass from the right side of the heart to the left and out into the general circulation without adequate ventilation; therefore, blood is poorly oxygenated. This mechanism occurs when alveoli are atelectatic or fluid-filled, as these conditions interfere with gas exchange. Unlike the first three responses, hypoxia secondary to right-to-left shunting does not improve with the administration of oxygen because the additional FIo_2 is unable to cross the alveoloar-capillary membrane.

< N O T E: See Table 1-7 for a description of some of the disease processes that can lead to acute respiratory failure.

ASSESSMENT

Signs and symptoms: Clinical indicators of acute respiratory failure vary according to the underlying disease process and severity of the failure. Acute respiratory failure is one of the most common causes of impaired LOC. Often, it is misdiagnosed as CHF, pneumonia, or CVA. Sometimes the onset of acute respiratory failure is so insidious that it is missed because the staff does not want to disturb the patient who appears to be sleeping.

- *Early indicators:* Restlessness, anxiety, headache, fatigue, cool and dry skin, increased BP, tachycardia, and cardiac dysrhythmias.
- *Intermediate indicators:* Confusion, lethargy, tachypnea, hypotension caused by vasodilatation, cardiac dysrhythmias.
- *Late indicators:* Cyanosis, diaphoresis, coma, respiratory arrest.

TABLE 1-7
Disease processes leading to the development of respiratory failure

Impaired alveolar ventilation
A. COPD (emphysema, bronchitis, asthma, cystic fibrosis)
B. Restrictive pulmonary disease (interstitial fibrosis, pleural effusion, pneumothorax, kyphoscoliosis, obesity, diaphragmatic paralysis)
C. Neuromuscular defects (Guillain-Barré syndrome, myasthenia gravis, multiple sclerosis, muscular dystrophy)
D. Depression of respiratory control centers (drug-induced cerebral infarction, inappropriate use of high-dose oxygen therapy)

Diffusion disturbances
A. Pulmonary/interstitial fibrosis
B. Pulmonary edema
C. Adult respiratory distress syndrome
D. Anatomic loss of functioning lung tissue (tumor pneumonectomy)

Ventilation or perfusion disturbances
A. Pulmonary emboli
B. Atelectasis
C. Pneumonia
D. Emphysema
E. Chronic bronchitis
F. Bronchiolitis
G. Adult respiratory distress syndrome

Right-to-left shunting
A. Atelectasis
B. Pneumonia
C. Pulmonary edema
D. Pulmonary emboli
E. Oxygen toxicity

DIAGNOSTIC TESTS

1. *ABG analysis:* Assesses adequacy of oxygenation and effectiveness of ventilation. Typical results are $Pao_2 \leq 60$ mm Hg, $Paco_2 \geq 45$ mm Hg, and pH <7.35, which are consistent with severe respiratory acidosis.
2. *Chest x-ray:* Ascertains presence of underlying pathophysiology or disease process that may be contributing to the failure.

MEDICAL MANAGEMENT

1. **Correction of hypoxemia:** First treatment priority. Pao_2 levels <30 mm Hg for longer than a few minutes may cause permanent brain damage or death. Oxygen therapy and chest physiotherapy, in conjunction with pharmacotherapy (e.g., bronchodilators, steroids, antibiotics), often improve ABGs sufficiently to get the patient out of danger.
2. **Correction of abnormal pH:** Second treatment priority. Adequate cellular and metabolic functioning are hindered when pH remains outside the normal range of 7.35-7.45. A pH <7.25 may be treated with IV sodium bicarbonate; a pH >7.45 may be managed by placing the patient on a rebreathing mask or increasing dead space on mechanical ventilator circuitry.
3. **Intubation and mechanical ventilation:** Early intubation can prevent further airway collapse and tissue injury. In most cases the patient will require intubation and mechanical ventilation to provide adequate respiratory function and stabilize ABGs. Mechanical support is used until the underlying cause of the failure can be corrected and the patient can resume ventilatory efforts independently. Mechanical ventilation is discussed in greater depth in the following section.

Mechanical ventilation

To ensure optimal care of the patient requiring mechanical ventilation, the practitioner must have adequate knowledge of the equipment and processes involved in mechanical ventilation. An in-depth discussion of the entire process is beyond the scope of this book; it is therefore assumed that the reader has adequate baseline knowledge on which to build.

VENTILATORS

Three categories of ventilators are used to deliver oxygen and artificial respiration.

1. **Pressure-cycled:** Terminates inspiration once a preset pressure is reached, at which time the patient exhales passively. When airway resistance increases due to mucous secretions or bronchospasm, the inspiratory cycle may terminate before adequate tidal volume is delivered.

2. **Volume-cycled:** Most widely used ventilator. It is designed to deliver preset volume of gas (tidal volume). The machine continues to deliver the predetermined tidal volume independent of changes in airway resistance or lung compliance. The ventilator is equipped with safety valves that can be set to terminate inspiration when peak pressures are excessive. Generally, these pressure limits are set at 10-20 cm H_2O pressure over the patient's normal delivery pressure. Refer to agency policy regarding alarm limits.

3. **Negative pressure:** Intrapleural pressure ranges from -2 to -10 cm H_2O. The positive pressure ventilators discussed above generate 5-10 cm H_2O pressure to deliver a breath. Negative pressure ventilators generate sub-atmospheric pressure to the thorax and trunk to initiate respiration and do not require intubation for use. The iron lung, chest cuirass shell, and poncho chest shell are examples of such devices. While they rarely are used in today's modern hospitals, these devices are useful in long-term home therapy.

4. **Jet ventilation and oscillation:** An alternative mode of ventilation in which small tidal volumes are delivered at high rates. The resulting lower airway and intrathoracic pressures may reduce the risk of injury secondary to barotrauma, which is associated with the high peak airway pressures of conventional ventilatory modes. Tidal volume is low and minute ventilation is high, making this the ideal mode for ventilation of patients with major airway disruption. Jet ventilation requires the use of special ventilators and a specially designed endotracheal tube. Three basic mechanisms are used and are discussed in Table 1-8.

MODES OF MECHANICAL VENTILATION

1. **Controlled mechanical ventilation (CMV):** Delivers preset tidal volume at a preset rate, ignoring the patient's own ventilatory drive. Its use is restricted to patients with CNS dysfunction, drug-induced paralysis or sedation, or severe chest trauma for whom negative pressure driven respiratory effort is contraindicated. This is the least frequently used mode.

2. **Assist-control ventilation (ACV):** Delivers preset tidal volume when the patient initiates a negative pressure respiratory effort (inspiration). With adequate tidal volume delivery, work of breathing is decreased and alveolar ventilation improves. Machine sensitivity can be adjusted to prevent hyperventilation in patients whose respiratory rate increases due to mild anxiety or neurologic factors. If hyperventilation cannot be controlled, the patient may need to be changed to the IMV mode (see p. 62).

TABLE 1-8
High-frequency jet ventilation

Mode	Rate	Tidal volume	Mechanism
High-frequency positive pressure ventilation (HFPPV)	60–100 bpm	3–6 cc/kg	Pneumatically controlled valve connected to high pressure gas source pulses gas into airway, while additional gases are entrained into the airway *via* a humidification circuit.
High-frequency jet ventilation (HFJV)	100–200 bpm	50–400 cc/kg	Gas under pressure is propelled through a narrow cannula (inserted in endotracheal tube), while additional gases are entrained through a humidifier.
High-frequency oscillations (HFO)	>200 bpm (800–3000 vibrations/ min)	50–80 cc/kg	Gas is oscillated through endotracheal tube *via* a piston. Gas flows over the connection and PEEP is created *via* resistant tubing on the outflow port. Gas exchange occurs primarily by diffusion.

3. **Intermittent mandatory ventilation (IMV):** Delivers a preset tidal volume at a preset rate. In addition, the patient can breathe spontaneously (at his or her own rate and tidal volume) between ventilator breaths from an oxygen reservoir that is attached to the machine. This is considered the standard mode of ventilation.

4. **Synchronized intermittent mandatory ventilation (SIMV):** Identical to IMV, but with one additional sensitivity factor: the ventilator is synchronized to deliver the mandatory breath when the patient initiates inspiratory effort. Optimally, this mode prevents breath stacking caused by exhaling against machine-delivered inspirations.

5. **Peak end expiratory pressure (PEEP):** Frequently used as an adjunct to mechanical ventilation to improve ventilatory function of the lungs, thereby increasing Pao_2. PEEP increases functional residual capacity (FRC), the amount of air left in the lungs at end of expiration, by applying a given pressure at the end of expiration. This pressure counteracts small airway collapse and keeps

alveoli open so that gas exchange can occur across the alveolar-capillary membrane. Areas of the lungs that are poorly ventilated normally can participate in adequate gas exchange, thereby decreasing shunting. This mechanism is effective for atelectatic alveoli, as well as alveoli that are filled with fluid, but does not improve lung function if the problem is one of poor perfusion. Generally, PEEP pressures range from 2.5 to 10 cm H_2O. Higher pressures may be used if the patient can tolerate the increase and if the condition warrants. Application of this pressure increases intrathoracic pressure and can compromise the patient's hemodynamic status by decreasing venous return and cardiac output, potentially leading to hypotension and shock.

< N O T E : Continuous positive airway pressure (PAP) functions in the same manner as PEEP but is a mode used independently of the ventilator.

COMPLICATIONS RELATED TO MECHANICAL VENTILATION

1. **Barotrauma:** Can occur when ventilatory pressures increase intrathoracic pressure, causing damage to major vessels or organs in the thorax and referring damage to the abdomen.

2. **Tension pneumothorax:** Develops when pressurized air enters the thoracic cavity. The high pressure of positive pressure ventilation may blow a hole in diseased or fragile lung tissue, leading to this life-threatening complication. In addition to the usual indicators of pneumothorax, the patient on mechanical ventilation will develop sudden and sustained increases in peak inspiratory pressure.

< C A U T I O N : If it is suspected that the patient has developed a pneumothorax, disconnect the ventilator and ventilate the patient manually with 100% oxygen while an assistant notifies the physician. Prepare for immediate emergency chest tube placement.

3. **Gastrointestinal complications:** Peptic ulcers with profound hemorrhage may develop as a result of physiologic pressures and stress. Antacids, cimetidine, and ranitidine routinely are administered to prevent these ulcers from developing. In addition, gastric dilatation can occur due to the large amounts of air swallowed in the presence of an artificial airway. If left untreated, the patient may develop paralytic ileus, vomiting, and aspiration. Extreme dilatation can compromise respiratory effort because of the restriction of diaphragmatic movement. Treatment includes insertion of an NG tube and application of intermittent suction to the GI tract.

4. **Hypotension with decreased cardiac output:** Develops as a result of decreased venous return secondary to increased intrathoracic pressure. Generally, this phenomenon is transient and is seen immediately after the patient has been placed on mechanical ventilation. PEEP may increase the incidence and severity of this phenomenon because of the significant increase in intrathoracic pressure that occurs with its use. Monitor heart rate and BP qh, or more frequently if the patient is unstable. Monitor cardiac output as prescribed *via* flow-directed pulmonary artery (Swan-Ganz) catheter. Refer to "Management of the Adult with Hemodynamic Monitoring," p. 165, for details regarding cardiac output.

5. **Increased intracranial pressure:** Occurs as a result of decreased venous re-

turn, which causes pooling of blood in the head. See "Head Injury," pp. 270-281 for more information about increased intracranial pressure.

6. **Fluid imbalance:** Increased production of antidiuretic hormone (ADH) occurs as a result of increased pressure on baroreceptors in the thoracic aorta, which causes the system to react as if the body were volume depleted. ADH stimulates the renal system to retain water in the presence of hypovolemia. Patients may need diuretics if signs of hypervolemia are present. Be alert to new symptoms of dependent edema or adventitious breath sounds.

WEANING THE PATIENT FROM MECHANICAL VENTILATION

This can involve weaning from oxygen, PEEP, mechanical ventilation, and the artificial airway. Physiologic factors (cardiovascular, fluid and electrolyte, acid-base, and nutritional status, as well as comfort and sleep pattern) and emotional factors (fear, anxiety, coping skills, general emotional state, and ability to cooperate) are important and must be evaluated both before and during the weaning process. In addition, pulmonary function parameters must be met before the weaning process is begun (see Table 1-9 for discussion). Traditionally, two methods are employed for weaning the patient from mechanical ventilation:

1. **T-piece adaptor:** Patient is taken off the ventilator and initiates spontaneous respiratory effort for increasingly longer periods of time. In this manner, the patient builds strength and endurance for independent respiratory effort. CPAP may be added to prevent alveolar collapse, thus allowing for more efficient gas exchange.

TABLE 1-9

Pulmonary function parameters for the patient being weaned from mechanical ventilation

Pulmonary function	Optimal parameters	Definition
Minute ventilation	≤ 10 L/minute.	Tidal volume $\times$ respiratory rate. If adequate, means the patient is breathing at a stable rate with adequate tidal volume.
Negative inspiratory force	≥ -10 to -20 cm H_2O	The maximum negative pressure patient is able to generate to initiate spontaneous respirations. It is indicative of patient's ability to initiate inspiration independently.
Maximum voluntary ventilation	$\geq 2 \times$ resting minute ventilation	Indicates patient's ability to sustain maximal respiratory effort.
Tidal volume	5–10 ml/kg	Indicates patient's ability to ventilate lungs adequately.
Arterial blood gases	$Pao_2 \geq 60$ mm Hg $Paco_2 \leq 45$ mm Hg pH 7.35-7.45	
FIo_2	$\leq .40$	

TABLE 1 - 10

Processes contributing to high-pressure alarm situations

Increased airway resistance	Decreased lung compliance
Patient requires suctioning.	Pneumothorax.
Kinks in ventilator circuitry.	Pulmonary edema.
Water or expectorated secretions in circuitry.	Atelectasis.
Patient coughs or exhales against ventilator breaths.	Worsening of underlying disease process.
Patient biting endotracheal tube.	
Bronchospasm.	
Herniation of airway cuff over end of artificial airway.	
Change in patient position that restricts chest wall movement.	

2. **Intermittent mandatory ventilation (IMV):** Ventilator-generated breaths are decreased gradually while patient builds strength and endurance. This is the most widely accepted method for patients on long-term ventilatory support. If the patient has multiple failures at weaning, the T-piece method may be used, starting with 1-2 minutes off the ventilator, followed by 58-59 minutes on, with a gradual reversal of this ratio until the patient breathes independently.

TROUBLESHOOTING MECHANICAL VENTILATOR PROBLEMS

The most important assessment factor in troubleshooting a mechanical ventilator is the effect on the patient. Regardless of which alarm sounds, always assess the patient first to evaluate his or her physiologic response to the problem. See Tables 1-10 and 1-11 for processes that contribute to high-pressure and low-pressure alarm situations.

TABLE 1 - 11

Processes contributing to low-pressure alarm situations

Patient disconnected from machine.
Leak in airway cuff
  • Insufficient air in cuff
  • Hole or tear in cuff
  • Leak in one-way valve of inflation port
Leak in circuitry
  • Poor fittings on water reservoirs
  • Dislodged temperature-sensing device
  • Hole or tear in tubing
  • Poor seal in circuitry connections
Displacement of airway above vocal cords
Loss of compressed air source

NURSING DIAGNOSES AND INTERVENTIONS

Potential for impaired gas exchange related to inadequate ventilation secondary to malfunction or improper setting of mechanical ventilator

---

Desired outcome: Patient has adequate gas exchange as evidenced by $Pao_2 \geq 60$ mm Hg, $Paco_2$ 35-45 mm Hg, and RR 12-20 breaths/min.

---

1. Observe for, document, and report any changes in patient's condition consistent with increasing respiratory distress. See "Signs and symptoms," p. 59.
2. Monitor serial ABG results. Be alert for decreases in Pao_2 or increases in $Paco_2$ with concomitant decrease in pH (<7.35), which can signal inadequate gas exchange. Also observe for decreased $Paco_2$ (<35 mm Hg) with increased pH (>7.35), which may signal mechanical hyperventilation. Notify MD of dysrhythmias, which can occur even with modest alkalosis if the patient has heart disease or is receiving cardiotropic medications. Arrange for ABG analysis when change in patient's condition warrants.
3. Position patient to allow for maximal alveolar ventilation and comfort. Remember that in normal situations, the dependent lung receives more ventilation and more blood flow than the nondependent lung; however, when a patient is ventilated mechanically, the dependent portion of the lung receives less distribution of tidal volume than the nondependent areas. Follow body positioning protocol:
   - Analyze ABG results with patient in different positions to determine adequacy of ventilation.
   - Utilize postural drainage principles where appropriate.
   - In unilateral lung disease, position patient with healthy lung down.
   - In bilateral lung disease, position patient in the right lateral decubitus position, as the right lung has more surface area. If ABG results show that the patient tolerates left lateral decubitus position, alternate between the two positions.
   - Turn patient q2h or more frequently if signs of deteriorating pulmonary status occur.
4. Auscultate over artificial airway to assess for leaks.
5. Assess ventilator for proper functioning and parameter settings, including FIo_2, tidal volume, rate, mode, peak inspiratory pressure, sigh volume and rate, and temperature of inspired gases. In addition, ensure that circuits are tight and alarms are set.
6. Keep ventilator circuitry free of condensed water and expectorated secretions, as these fluids may obstruct the flow of gases to and from the patient.

Potential ineffective airway clearance related to interruption in normal respiratory mechanics secondary to intubation and mechanical ventilation

---

Desired outcome: Patient maintains a patent artificial airway as evidenced by auscultation of normal breath sounds over the lung fields and absence of adventitious breath sounds or signs of respiratory distress such as restlessness and anxiety.

---

1. Maintain the artificial airway in a secure and proper alignment.
2. Maintain correct temperature (32-36° C) of inspired gas. Cold air will irritate airways and hot air may burn fragile lung tissue.
3. Maintain humidification of inspired gas to prevent drying of tracheal mucosa. In addition, without humidification, tracheobronchial secretions may become thick and tenacious, creating mucous plugs that put patient at risk for development of atelectasis and infection.
4. Assess and document breath sounds in all lung fields at least qh. Note quality and presence or absence of adventitious sounds.
5. Monitor patient for restlessness and anxiety, which can signal early airway obstruction.
6. Using sterile technique, suction patient as needed to maintain patency of airway. Document amount, color, and consistency of tracheobronchial secretions. Report significant changes (e.g., increase in production of secretions, tenacious secretions, bloody sputum) to MD. In addition, document patient's tolerance to suctioning procedure.

Potential for ineffective breathing pattern related to hyperventilation secondary to anxiety due to use of mechanical ventilation

Desired outcome: Patient has effective breathing pattern as evidenced by stable RR of 12-20 breaths/min (synchronized with ventilator) and absence of restlessness, anxiety, lethargy, and/or sounding of high-pressure alarm.

1. Monitor respiratory rate and quality and monitor for signs of respiratory distress (e.g., tachypnea, hyperventilation, anxiety, restlessness, lethargy, and cyanosis, which is a late sign).
2. Monitor for evidence that patient is fighting ventilator: frequent sounding of high-pressure alarm when patient breathes against mechanical inspiration or mismatch of patient's respiratory rate and ventilator cycle.
3. Administer prescribed pain medication or sedation when indicated.
4. Teach patient the importance of relaxing and breathing in synchrony with the ventilator. Stay with the patient until the respirations are under control. Assure patient that he or she will be able to synchronize respirations with the ventilator once he or she relaxes.

Potential for infection related to compromise of normal defense mechanisms secondary to intubation, contamination of respiratory equipment, or immunosuppression

Desired outcome: Patient is free of infection as evidenced by normothermia, WBC count ≤11,000 μl, clear sputum, and negative sputum cultures.

1. Assess patient for signs and symptoms of infection, including temperature >38° C (100.4° F), tachycardia (HR >100 bpm) erythema of wound, and foul-smelling sputum. Document all significant findings.

2. Culture secretions or wound drainage; administer antibiotics as prescribed.

3. To minimize the risk of cross-contamination, wash hands before and after contact with the respiratory secretions of any patient (even though gloves were worn) and before and after contact with patient who is intubated.

4. Recognize that bacteria and spores can be introduced easily during suctioning; follow standard techniques:
   - Use aseptic technique when suctioning patient, including use of sterile catheter, gloves, and suctioning or lavage solutions.
   - Suction tracheobronchial tree before the oropharynx to avoid introducing oral pathogens into tracheobronchial tree.
   - Never store or reuse suction catheter.
   - Clean suction cannisters daily. Change cannisters and tubing between patients.
   - Tightly recap saline bottle used for suctioning. Be sure bottle is dated and timed; dispose of unused portion after 24 hours.

< C A U T I O N :   Wear gloves on both hands when handling secretions as a protection against Herpes whitlow virus.

5. To reduce the risk of infection caused by trauma or cross-contamination, suction patient on an ''as needed'' basis rather than routinely.

6. Use sterile gloves when performing tracheostomy care to prevent colonization of stoma with bacteria from practitioner's hands.

7. Provide good oral hygiene at least qshift to prevent overgrowth of normal flora and aerobic gram-negative bacilli.

8. Recognize ways that water reservoirs and ventilator equipment can be potential sources of contamination by following these precautions:
   - Use only sterile fluids in all humidifiers and nebulizers.
   - To prevent formation of mold or other pathogens, replace reservoir and the fluid in it with a sterilized unit q24h.
   - Change all ventilatory circuitry q24h or sooner if soiled with secretions. Disposable circuitry may be changed q48h if not soiled or contaminated during use.
   - Empty condensed water or expectorated secretions in tubes into attached traps—not back into patient.
   - Empty water traps on tubing during each ventilator check.
   - When disconnecting patient from ventilatory circuits, keep end of connectors sterile by placing them on opened sterile gauze pads.
   - Keep connectors on manual resuscitator bags clean and free of secretions between use. Although there are no data suggesting that bags be changed with any frequency when used for only one patient, they should not be used between patients without being sterilized.

9. Maintain appropriate seal on artificial airway cuff to prevent aspiration of oral secretions.

10. Keep cuff sealed and HOB elevated 30-45 degrees for patients receiving continuous NG feedings. Monitor patient for reflux of feedings, as well as signs of intolerance to feedings (absence of bowel sounds, abdominal distention, residual feedings >100 mL), which can precipitate vomiting and result in pulmonary aspiration of gastric contents.

11. Be aware of special risk factors for patients with tracheostomy tubes and intervene accordingly:
    • Maintain tracheostomy tube in a secure and proper alignment to avoid irritation of stoma from too much movement.
    • Change tracheostomy ties q24h or more frequently if heavily soiled with secretions or wound exudate.
    • Perform stoma care at least q8h, using aseptic technique until stoma is completely healed. Keep area around stoma dry at all times to prevent maceration and infection. Change stoma dressing as needed, to keep it dry and free of copious secretions.
    • Avoid use of cotton-filled gauze or other material that may shed small fibers. Patient may aspirate fibers, which in turn can lead to infection.
    • Use aseptic technique (including use of sterile gloves and drapes) when changing tracheostomy tube.
12. Isolate patient from others (other patients, staff, family members) who have active infectious processes. Exposure, even to common pathogens, is dangerous for the patient with a compromised immune system.

Anxiety related to actual or perceived threat to biologic integrity secondary to need for or presence of mechanical ventilation

---

Desired outcome: Patient relates the presence of emotional comfort and exhibits a decrease in irritability, with a HR within patient's normal range.

---

1. Because the general public equates being put on a ventilator with a hopelessly chronic, vegetative state, reassure patient and significant others that ventilatory support may be a temporary measure until the underlying pathophysiologic process is resolved. At that time, the patient may be weaned from the ventilator.
2. Reassure patient that he or she will not be left alone.
3. Explain all procedures to patient and significant others before they are initiated. Inform patient of his or her progress.
4. Describe and point out the alarm system, explaining that it will alert staff in the event of an accidental disconnection.

Potential for impaired gas exchange related to decreased diffusion of oxygen secondary to weaning from mechanical ventilation

---

Desired outcome: Patient has adequate gas exchange as evidenced by $Pao_2 \geq 60$ mm Hg, $Paco_2 \leq 45$ mm Hg, and pH 7.35-7.45.

---

1. Observe for indicators of hypoxia, including tachycardia, tachypnea, cardiac dysrhythmias, anxiety, and restlessness.
2. Assess and record VS q15min for the first hour of weaning, then hourly if patient is stable. Report significant findings to MD, such as increased respiratory effort, hyperventilation, anxiety, lethargy, cyanosis.
3. Check patient's tidal volume after the first 15 minutes of weaning, and as needed. Optimally, it will be within 5-10 ml/kg.

4. Obtain specimen for ABG analysis 20 minutes after weaning has been initiated, or as prescribed.
5. Maintain patient in a comfortable position to enhance ventilation. Many patients find that semi-Fowler's position promotes effective respirations.

Anxiety related to perceived threat to biologic integrity secondary to weaning process

Desired outcome: Patient expresses the attainment of emotional comfort and is asymptomatic of the signs of harmful anxiety as evidenced by HR $\leq$100 bpm, RR $\leq$20 breaths/min, and BP within patient's normal range.

1. Before weaning process is initiated, discuss plans for weaning with patient and significant others. Explain that patient will be assessed at frequent intervals during the weaning procedure. Provide time for questions and answers about the procedure.
2. Stay with patient during the initial phase of weaning, keeping patient informed of progress being made. Provide positive feedback for positive efforts.
3. Instruct patient to take deep breaths if he or she is capable of doing so. This may provide the confidence of knowing that he or she can initiate and sustain respirations independently.
4. Leave call light within patient's reach before leaving bedside. Reassure patient that help is nearby.

Also see nursing diagnoses and interventions in the following: "Caring for the Critically Ill on Prolonged Bed Rest," pp. 506-511; "Caring for the Critically Ill with Life-Threatening Disorders," pp. 511-522; and "Caring for the Family of the Critically Ill," pp. 522-526.

REHABILITATION AND PATIENT-FAMILY TEACHING CONCEPTS

Give patient and significant others verbal and written information about the following during the period of time patient is mechanically ventilated:
1. Assessment, including ABG analysis, which will be performed at frequent intervals. Explain the purpose of ABG analysis.
2. Basic operation of the mechanical ventilator, especially the alarms and safety devices.
3. Procedure and purpose of chest physiotherapy, which can be alarming to family members. Reassure them that although percussion is loud, it is not painful.
4. Suctioning procedure and purpose.
5. Patient's inability to communicate verbally while ventilated and the frustration this may cause to both patient and significant others. (See discussion in appendix under **Impaired verbal communication,** p. 513.)

SELECTED REFERENCES

Biddle C: Hypothermia: Implications for the critical care nurse. *Crit Care Nurs* 1985; 5(2): 34-37.

Burrel L, Burrell Z: *Critical Care,* 4th ed. Times Mirror/Mosby, 1982.

Burton G, Hodgkin J: *Respiratory Care: A*

Guide to Clinical Practice, 2nd ed. Lippincott, 1984.

Celentano L, Conforti C: The effects of body position on oxygenation. *Heart & Lung* 1985;14(1): 45-51.

Centers for Disease Control 1982: Guidelines for prevention of nosocomial pneumonia. US Department of Health and Human Services.

Centers for Disease Control 1983: Guidelines for isolation precautions in hospitals. US Department of Health and Human Services.

Chalikian J, Weaver T: Mechanical ventilation: Where it's at, where it's going. *Am J Nurs* Nov 1984; 11: 1373-1379.

Dantzker D: *Cardiopulmonary Critical Care.* Harcourt, Brace, Jovanovich, 1986.

Elguinda A, et al: Pulmonary embolism: Evaluation and management. *Hosp Formulary* 1986; 21: 688-693.

Emanuelson K, Densmore M: *Acute Respiratory Care.* Wiley, 1981.

Griffin J, Carlon G: Medical and nursing implications of high-frequency jet ventilation. *Heart & Lung* 1984; 13(3) 250-254.

Guenter C: *Pulmonary Medicine,* 2nd ed. Lippincott, 1982.

Kinney M, et al: AACN's *Clinical Reference for Critical Care Nursing.* McGraw-Hill, 1981.

Lederer JR: Respiratory Disorders. In: *Manual of Nursing Therapeutics: Applying Nursing Diagnoses to Medical Disorders.* Swearingen PL (editor). Addison-Wesley, 1986.

Lynch P, Jackson M: Isolation practices: How much is too much or not enough. *ASEPSIS: The Infection Control Forum* 1986 8(4): 2-5.

Mills J, et al, eds: *Current Emergency Diagnosis and Treatment,* 2nd ed. Lange, 1985.

Petersdorf A, et al: *Harrison's Principles of Internal Medicine,* 10th ed. McGraw-Hill, 1983.

Petty T: *Intensive and Rehabilitative Respiratory Care,* 3rd ed. Lea & Fabiger, 1982.

Smothers P: Drowning and near drowning: An update. *Jour Emerg Nurs* 1982; 8(4): 176-180.

Thompson, JM, et al: *Clinical Nursing.* Times Mirror/Mosby, 1986.

Traver GA: Ineffective airway clearance: Physiology and clinical application. *Dim Crit Care Nurs* July/Aug 1985; 4(4): 198-208.

Woodruff M: Pulmonary thromboembolism: Risk factors, pathophysiology, and management *Crit Care Nurs* 1984; 4(4): 52-63.

2
CARDIOVASCULAR DYSFUNCTIONS

Acute chest pain

Acute myocardial infarction

Congestive heart failure/pulmonary edema

Cardiomyopathy

Dysrhythmias and conduction disturbances

Cardiac arrest

Cardiac trauma

Acute cardiac tamponade

Acute infective endocarditis

Acute pericarditis

Hypertensive crisis

Aortic dissection

Cardiogenic shock

Percutaneous transluminal coronary angioplasty

Percutaenous balloon valvuloplasty

Intra-aortic balloon pump

Heart-assist device

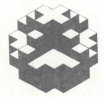

Coronary artery bypass graft

Valvular heart disease and valve surgery

Automatic implantable cardioverter-defibrillator

Coronary artery thrombolysis

Management of the adult with hemodynamic monitoring

Acute chest pain

Chest discomfort or pain associated with myocardial ischemia is called angina pectoris. It can occur at rest or with exercise and may result from a sudden decrease in coronary blood flow due to coronary thrombosis or spasm or from the inability to increase coronary blood flow sufficiently to meet myocardial oxygen demands (e.g., during exercise). Acute chest pain due to ischemia may occur when coronary perfusion pressure is low, as in sudden hypotension, or when oxygen demands are greatly elevated, such as with aortic stenosis. Pathogenic mechanisms that may cause acute chest pain due to ischemia include the following: atherosclerosis; platelet aggregation in diseased vessels; transient coronary artery thrombosis; hemorrhage into atheromatous plaque; abnormal vasoconstriction (spasm) of a coronary artery; and extracardiac factors, such as anemia or thyrotoxicosis.

ASSESSMENT

General signs and symptoms: Pain that usually is precipitated by exertion or emotional upset; subsides with rest; lasts for 1-4 minutes, but not longer than 30 minutes; subsides gradually when precipitating factor is removed; and is relieved by nitroglycerin, usually within 45-90 seconds.

Chest pain with myocardial ischemia: Abrupt or gradual onset of substernal discomfort described as deep, visceral, and squeezing. Many patients will deny the presence of chest ''pain'' but will admit to severe chest ''discomfort.''

Chest pain with transmural myocardial infarction: More severe, of longer duration (i.e., >30 min), unrelieved by nitroglycerin.

Forms of angina

- *Stable:* Has not increased in frequency or severity over a period of several months.
- *Unstable:* Quality of pain has changed or increased in frequency, duration, or severity; can occur with lessened exertion or at rest.
- *Preinfarction or crescendo:* Unstable angina with the potential for progression to infarction.
- *Prinzmetal's (variant):* May occur at rest, long after exercise, and during sleep; usually caused by coronary vasospasm.
- *Intractable:* Frequent or continued; unresponsive to therapy.

Physical assessment: BP may be elevated owing to chest pain, or decreased if pain is caused by ischemia, which can result in decreased cardiac output. HR may increase in response to hypoxia and enhanced sympathetic tone. S_4 heart sound may be audible during ischemic episodes.

History and risk factors: Familial history of coronary artery disease

(CAD), age over 65, male sex (risk for females increases after menopause), cigarette smoking, hypercholesterolemia, hypertension, diabetes, obesity, increased stress, sedentary lifestyle.

DIAGNOSTIC TESTS

1. *EKG:* May establish diagnosis of ischemic heart disease if characteristic changes are present, although the absence of abnormality does not rule out this disease. In the absence of pain and with the patient at rest, the 12-lead EKG may be normal; therefore this test must be obtained during an episode of chest pain. ST and T-wave changes, which occur during spontaneous chest pain and disappear with relief of the pain, are significant. The most characteristic change is depression of the ST segment with or without T-wave inversion. These EKG changes are similar to those induced during a positive stress test. In variant or Prinzmetal angina, the ST segments may be elevated during the chest pain episode.

2. *Stress test:* Patient is exercised while being monitored with an EKG. Its purpose is to elicit chest pain and document any EKG changes associated with this symptom. A positive stress test elicits at least 1.0 mm horizontal depression or downsloping ST segment in one or more leads lasting 0.08 seconds. In addition, frequent PVCs or runs of ventricular tachycardia are suggestive of ischemia.

3. *Thallium treadmill:* Normal myocardial tissue will take up thallium, while infarcted or ischemic areas will have decreased uptake, appearing as "cold spots" on the scan. To identify areas of decreased uptake, the patient is exercised after an injection of thallium. A scan is done both immediately after exercise and 4 hours later to determine if areas with decreased uptake fill in after 4 hours. Ischemic areas that fill in are considered to have viable tissue and reversible damage, while areas that remain as "cold spots" are diagnosed as infarcted.

4. *Serum enzymes:* To rule out the occurrence of myocardial infarction.

5. *Chest x-ray:* May reveal cardiac enlargement. In patients with ischemic heart disease, cardiomegaly signals the presence of myocardial ischemia and decreased myocardial contractility.

6. *Cardiac catheterization:* To determine presence and extent of coronary artery disease as the etiology of the chest pain.

MEDICAL MANAGEMENT AND SURGICAL INTERVENTIONS

1. **Relief of acute pain:** Drugs are administered and titrated to reduce or eliminate chest pain.
   - *IV nitroglycerin (NTG):* For unstable angina, it is titrated until relief is obtained.
   - *IV morphine sulfate:* Given in small increments (i.e., 2 mg) until relief is obtained.
   - *Oral, sublingual, and topical forms of nitroglycerin:* Can be used for short-term use or longer-lasting effects.
   - *Calcium-channel blocking agents* (e.g., nifedipine): Block the movement of calcium into the cells, causing vasodilatation of the coronary and peripheral arteries to relieve chest pain caused by coronary artery spasm. In addition, they decrease contraction and oxygen demand.

2. **Reduction of cardiac workload**
   - *Beta-adrenergic blocking agents:* To decrease HR, BP, myocardial contractility, and myocardial oxygen demand.

- *Limit activities:* Bed rest or specific restrictions based on patient's activity intolerance.
- *Oxygen:* Usually 2-4 L/min by nasal cannula, or mode and rate as directed by ABG values.

3. **Percutaneous transluminal coronary angioplasty:** To improve blood flow through stenotic coronary arteries for surgical candidates whose angina is refractory to medical treatment and whose lesions are amenable to the procedure. For discussion, see p. 136.

4. **Percutaneous balloon valvuloplasty:** To dilate stenotic aortic valves for patients who are not candidates for surgery because of advanced age (>80) or who refuse surgery. These patients may have chest pain due to critical stenosis of the aortic valve with decreased blood flow through coronary arteries. For discussion, see p. 140.

NURSING DIAGNOSES AND INTERVENTIONS

Alteration in comfort: Chest pain related to decreased oxygen supply to the myocardium

---

Desired outcome: Patient verbalizes a relief from or decrease in severity and frequency of chest pain and does not exhibit signs of uncontrolled discomfort.

---

1. Assess and document the character of patient's chest pain, including location, duration, quality, intensity, precipitating and alleviating factors, presence or absence of radiation, and associating symptoms.
2. Measure BP and HR with each episode of chest pain. BP and HR may increase due to sympathetic stimulation secondary to pain. If the chest pain is caused by ischemia, the heart muscle may not be functioning normally and cardiac output may decrease, resulting in a low BP. In addition, dysrhythmias such as bradycardia and ventricular ectopy may be noted with ischemia.
3. Take 12-lead EKG during patient's episode of chest pain. In an angina attack, ischemia usually is demonstrated on the EKG by ST-segment depression and T-wave inversion.
4. Administer nitrates as prescribed, titrating IV nitroglycerin so that chest pain is relieved, yet systolic BP remains >90 mm Hg.
5. As prescribed, administer beta blockers and calcium channel blockers, which relieve chest pain by diminishing coronary artery spasm and decreasing myocardial contractility and oxygen demand.
6. Administer oxygen per nasal cannula at 2-4 L/min, as prescribed.
7. Position patient according to his or her comfort level.
8. Provide care in a calm and efficient manner; reassure and support patient during chest pain episodes.
9. Maintain a quiet environment and group patient care activities to allow for periods of uninterrupted rest.
10. Ensure that activity restrictions and bed rest are maintained; teach patient the importance of activity limitation and its rationale: to minimize oxygen requirements, and hence, decrease chest pain.
11. Instruct patient to report any further episodes of chest pain.

Activity intolerance related to episodes of chest pain

Desired outcome: Patient exhibits cardiac tolerance to increasing levels of activity as evidenced by RR <24 breaths/min, normal sinus rhythm on EKG, BP within 20 mm Hg of patient's normal range, HR ≤120 bpm (or within 20 bpm of resting HR for patients on beta-blocker therapy), and absence of chest pain.

---

1. Assist patient with identifying activities that precipitate chest pain and teach patient to utilize NTG prophylactically prior to the activity.
2. Assist patient as needed in progressive activity program, beginning with Level I and progressing to Level IV, as tolerated (see Table 2-1).
3. Assess patient's response to activity progression. Be alert to presence of chest pain, SOB, excessive fatigue, and dysrhythmias. Monitor for a decrease in BP >20 mm Hg and an increase in HR to >120 bpm (or >20 bpm above resting HR in patients on beta-blocker therapy).
4. Teach patient about measures that prevent complications of decreased mobility, such as active ROM exercises. For more detail, see section "Caring for the Critically Ill on Prolonged Bed Rest," p. 506.

Knowledge deficit: Disease process and its lifestyle implications

---

Desired outcome: Patient verbalizes understanding of his or her disease as well as the necessary lifestyle changes that must be made.

---

1. Teach patient about ischemia and its resultant chest pain, referred to as "angina pectoris."
2. Discuss the pathophysiology underlying patient's angina, using drawings or heart models as indicated.
3. Assist patient with identifying his or her own risk factors, for example, cigarette smoking, high-stress lifestyle.
4. Teach patient about risk factor modification:
   • *Diet low in cholesterol:* Provide sample diet plan for meals that are low in

---

TABLE 2-1
Activity level progression in hospitalized patients

Level I: Bedrest	Flexion and extension of extremities qid, 15 times each extremity; deep breathing qid, 15 breaths; position change from side to side q2h.
Level II: OOB to Chair	As tolerated, tid for 20-30 minutes.
Level III: Ambulate in room	As tolerated, tid for 20-30 minutes.
Level IV: Ambulate in hall	Initially, 50-200 feet bid; progressing to 50-200 feet qid.
Signs of activity intolerance:	Decrease in BP >20 mm Hg; increase in HR to >120 bpm (or >20 bpm above resting HR in patients on beta-blocker therapy).

cholesterol. Teach patient about foods that are high and low in cholesterol (see Table 2-3, p. 84).
- *Smoking cessation:* Teach patient that smoking causes the coronary arteries to constrict, thus decreasing blood flow to the heart.
- *Activity program:* See Table 2-1.
- *Stress management:* Discuss the role that stress plays in angina. Explain that stress increases sympathetic tone, which can cause the BP and HR to increase, resulting in increased oxygen demand. By employing relaxation techniques such as imagery, meditation, or biofeedback, one can decrease the effects of stress on the heart. For a sample relaxation technique, see **Knowledge deficit:** Relaxation technique effective for stress reduction and facilitation of decreased sympathetic tone, p. 98.

5. Teach patient about the prescribed medications, including name, purpose, dosage, action, schedule, precautions, and potential side effects.
6. Teach patient the actions that should be taken if chest pain is unrelieved or increases in intensity. If chest pain occurs:
- Stop and rest.
- Take one NTG; wait 5 minutes. If pain is not relieved, take a second NTG; wait 5 minutes. If pain is not relieved, take a third NTG.
- If the pain is not relieved after three NTGs taken over a 15-minute period, call physician or dial 911.
- Explain to patient that it is no more beneficial to be in the emergency room than it is to be at home during episodes of chest pain due to angina, and that therefore, taking emergency action at the first sign of chest pain usually is unnecessary.

REHABILITATION AND PATIENT-FAMILY TEACHING CONCEPTS

Give patient and significant others verbal and written information for the following:
1. Activity limitations and prescribed progressions. Provide the following information:

When you are discharged from the hospital, it is important that you continue your walking program. The guidelines in Table 2-2 are to help you plan a program that is right for you. Don't overestimate your ability; rather, start off slowly and build up. Depending on how you feel, you may only be able

---

T A B L E 2 - 2

Guidelines for a progressive at-home walking program

Week	Distance	Time
1	100-200 feet	2 times a day
2	200-400 feet	2 times a day
3	¼ mile	8-10 minutes
4	½ mile	15 minutes
5	1 mile	30 minutes
6	1¾ mile	30 minutes
7	2 miles	40 minutes

to stay at one level or you may progress to 2 miles quickly. Remember to warm up and cool down with stretches for 5-7 minutes and to walk 3-5 times each week. In addition:
- Avoid sudden energetic activities.
- Plan for regular rest periods in the afternoon.
- Let your body guide you regarding whether to increase or decrease activity.
- Inform your physician of any changes in activity tolerance, such as the development of new symptoms with the same activity.

2. Sexual activity guidelines: Because sexual activity is a physical activity, certain guidelines can help the patient and his or her partner enjoy a satisfying sexual relationship while minimizing the workload of the heart.
- Rest is beneficial before engaging in intercourse.
- Find a position that is comfortable for you and your partner. Assuming a different position that is uncomfortable to both may increase the workload of the heart.
- Medications such as nitroglycerin may be taken prophylactically by the patient before intercourse to prevent chest pain.
- Postpone intercourse for 1-1½ hours after eating a heavy meal.
- Report the following symptoms to your physician if they are experienced after sexual relations: SOB, increased HR that persists for more than 15 minutes, unrelieved chest pain.

3. Medications, including drug name, purpose, dosage, schedule, precautions, and potential side effects.

4. Low-cholesterol diet modifications, including sample recipes and menus. See Table 2-3, p. 84, for a list of foods that are allowed and avoided in a low-cholesterol diet.

5. Techniques for stress reduction and relaxation (see **Knowledge deficit:** Relaxation technique effective for stress reduction and facilitation of decreased sympathetic tone, p. 98).

6. Organizations that aid with smoking cessation, for example, Smoke Enders, Shick, YMCA smoking cessation program.

7. Importance of community CPR training for significant others.

8. Activation of the community emergency medical system (EMS): 911 is the number to call in most communities.

9. Signs and symptoms that necessitate medical attention: unrelieved chest pain after 3 NTG tablets taken over a 15-minute period.

10. Also see **Knowledge deficit:** Disease process and its lifestyle implications, p. 76.

Acute myocardial infarction

Myocardial infarction (MI) is necrosis of myocardial tissue due to relative or absolute lack of blood supply to the myocardium. Most MIs are caused by atherosclerosis (e.g., fat deposits, fibrosis, calcification, and platelet aggregation), which results in a progressive narrowing of the coronary artery, thrombus formation, and ultimately, occlusion of blood flow. Occlusion also can be caused by coronary artery spasm. The site of infarction is determined by the location of the occluded artery.

ASSESSMENT

Signs and symptoms: Substernal, pressure-like chest pain that can radiate anywhere within the 6-dermatome pathway, from the jaw to the epigastrum. Classically, the pain radiates to the left arm, down the inner aspect along the ulnar nerve. The chest pain differs from angina, in that it is constant and unrelieved by rest, position, or nitrates; duration is ≥30 minutes. Other associated signs and symptoms include nausea, vomiting, dyspnea, orthopnea, anxiety, apprehension, denial, cyanosis, and unexplained weakness and fatigue.

Physical assessment: HR may be increased because of enhanced sympathetic tone; or the patient may have dysrhythmias, such as bradycardia, AV block, or ventricular ectopy. BP may be decreased due to a decrease in cardiac output; an increase in temperature may occur because of the inflammatory process. Auscultation may reveal any of the following: presystolic gallop (S_4); pericardial friction rub; murmurs; crackles (rales); and split S_1, S_2, and S_3 heart sounds if failure has occurred.

History and risk factors: Familial history of coronary artery disease, age over 65 years, male sex (risk for females increases after menopause), cigarette smoking, hypercholesterolemia, hypertension, diabetes, obesity, increased stress, sedentary lifestyle.

DIAGNOSTIC TESTS

1. *Serum enzymes:* Elevation of CPK will peak within 24 hours following MI. However, CPK elevation alone is not indicative of MI because it can be elevated for a variety of reasons, such as trauma or surgery. Isoenzymes are more diagnostic of cardiac muscle damage. CPK-MB should be 10% greater than total CPK for definitive diagnosis of MI. However, this criterion may vary from one institution to another. If the patient's history is strongly suggestive of MI and CPK total and MB are within normal limits, then LDH isoenzyme may be helpful. LDH_1 is more specific for MI than LDH_{2-5}. If the total LDH is elevated and LDH_1 is the predominant isoenzyme, this is diagnostic of MI.

2. *Lipid tests*
   - *Cholesterol:* A total cholesterol test measures the circulating levels of free cholesterol and cholesterol esters, reflecting the level of the forms of cholesterol that appear in the body. Total cholesterol is the only cholesterol routinely measured. Concentrations vary with age. Most cardiologists prefer cardiac patients to have a cholesterol level of <200 mg/dl.
   - *Lipoprotein-cholesterol fractionation:* Measures the major lipids in the serum. These include very low-density lipoproteins (VLDL), low-density lipoproteins (LDL), and high-density lipoproteins (HDL). Cholesterol in HDL is inversely related to the incidence of coronary artery disease (CAD): the higher the HDL, the lower the incidence of CAD. Normal HDL levels range from 29 to 77 mg/100 ml; normal LDL levels range from 62 to 185 mg/100 ml. High LDL levels increase the risk of CAD.
   - *Triglycerides:* This test analyzes the storage form of lipids, which constitute 95% of fatty tissue. Although not in itself diagnostic of CAD, serum triglyceride analysis enables early identification of those individuals who may have increased risk of CAD. Triglyceride values are age-related, but a generally accepted range is 10-190 mg/dl in the 50-59 year-old population.

3. *Leukocyte count and erythrocyte sedimentation rate (ESR):* Although they are not diagnostic of MI, patients with MI will have increased values of these laboratory tests due to the inflammatory process.

4. *EKGs:* Lead changes identify the area of infarct. Changes include the following
   - *Q waves:* Are indicative of MI and meet one of two criteria. Either they are too wide (>.04 seconds) or too deep (>25% of the total voltage of the QRS).
   - *ST-segment changes:* Will be elevated in the lead over or facing the infarcted area. Reciprocal changes (ST segment depressions) will be found in leads 180 degrees from the area of infarction.
   - *T-wave changes:* May occur hours to weeks after infarction. Within the early hours of infarction, "giant" upright T waves may be seen in leads over the infarct. Within several hours to days, the T wave becomes inverted. Gradually over time, the ST segment becomes isoelectric and the T wave may remain inverted. T-wave changes may last for weeks and return to normal or remain inverted for the rest of the patient's life.

5. *Chest x-ray:* Usually reveals cardiomegaly and signs of left ventricular failure (interstitial pulmonary edema), but also may be normal.

6. *Technetium pyrophosphate:* May help to localize area of infarction and demonstrate necrotic tissue. IV pyrophosphate will bind with calcium, which is found in high concentrations within the cells of necrotic tissue, and appears as a darkened area or "hot spot" on the scan up to 10 days post-MI.

7. *Multiple-gated acquisition (MUGA) scanning:* IV injection of the isotope technetium pertechnetate to evaluate left ventricular function and detect aneurysms, wall-motion abnormalities, and intracardiac shunting. In the stress MUGA test, the same test is performed at rest and after exercise.

8. *Echocardiogram:* To detect abnormalities of left ventricular wall motion and measure ejection fraction and valve function.

9. *Positron emission tomography:* Use of isotopes to assess metabolic activity of areas of infarction to determine if viable, but jeopardized, tissue is present. Viable tissue has metabolic activity as seen by increased uptake of the glucose tracer and decreased uptake of the blood flow tracer, which is ammonia.

10. *Hemodynamic monitoring:* Used in patient with a complicated MI that results in failure with possible progression to cardiogenic shock. Pulmonary artery and capillary pressures are measured, along with cardiac output determinations and SVR calculations. With MI, the following are likely to be found: increased PAP, increased PAWP, decreased CO, and increased SVR.

11. *Coronary angiography:* To locate areas of myocardium that may be in danger of infarction. It is used as a diagnostic tool in patients post MI with recurrent or refractory chest pain.

MEDICAL MANAGEMENT AND SURGICAL INTERVENTIONS

1. **Relief of acute pain:** IV nitroglycerin is titrated until relief of chest pain occurs, while ensuring that systolic pressure remains >90 mm Hg. IV morphine sulfate may be used in conjunction with nitrates to relieve chest pain and reduce anxiety and sympathetic tone. Usual dosage is 2-4 mg initially, in 2 mg increments.

2. **Reduction of cardiac workload:** Achieved with bed rest and use of beta-adrenergic blockade.

3. **Oxygen:** Usually 2-4 L/min *via* nasal cannula or mask.
4. **Prevention and treatment of dysrhythmias:** Patients may be given lidocaine prophylactically to prevent primary ventricular dysrhythmias (protocol varies from institution to institution).
5. **Management of fluid imbalance:** Oral and IV fluids are given for dehydration; diuretics and vasodilators are given for volume overload.
6. **Reperfusion to limit infarction**
   - *Medical:* Thrombolytic therapy with streptokinase or tissue plasminogen activator to lyse the clot in selected patients (see "Coronary Artery Thrombolysis," p. 160). Percutaneous transluminal coronary angioplasty may be performed for individuals with residual stenosis post thrombolytic therapy. See discussion, p. 136.
   - *Surgical:* Coronary artery bypass graft is performed for patients with multivessel disease or a large area of jeopardized myocardium. See discussion, p. 150.

NURSING DIAGNOSES AND INTERVENTIONS

The following nursing diagnoses address care for the individual with uncomplicated MI. For patients with complicated MI, see additional sections in "Congestive Heart Failure," p. 86; "Dysrhythmias and Conduction Disturbances," p. 96; "Acute Cardiac Tamponade," p. 107; "Acute Pericarditis," p. 118; and "Cardiogenic Shock," p. 134.

Alteration in comfort: Chest pain related to decreased oxygen supply to the myocardium

---

Desired outcome: Patient verbalizes that relief or reduction in chest pain has occurred and does not exhibit nonverbal indicators of discomfort.

---

1. Assess characteristics of chest pain, including location, duration, quality, intensity, presence of radiation, precipitating and alleviating factors, and associated symptoms.
2. Assess BP and HR with each episode of chest pain. Although BP may increase initially owing to increased sympathetic tone, myocardial damage can decrease heart function, resulting in decreased cardiac output and low BP. HR also may increase owing to sympathetic tone or patient may have dysrhythmias such as bradycardia, heart block, or tachycardia.
3. Run a 12-lead EKG daily for 3 days to document the evolutionary changes seen with MI. In addition, if chest pain recurs, take a 12-lead EKG during the chest pain to aid in evaluating whether the pain is caused by further ischemia or infarction.
4. Titrate nitroglycerin drip while also maintaining systolic BP at >90 mm Hg until complete relief of chest pain occurs. Nitroglycerin drip is 100 mg nitroglycerin in 250 mL D_5W. Begin with 3 ml/min, which is 19.8 µg/min. Titrate by increments of 3 ml q5min (or 19.8 µg q5min).
5. After each titration of IV nitroglycerin, evaluate patient's BP and the effects of therapy in relieving patient's chest pain. If slight hypotension occurs (80-90 mm Hg systolic), reduce the flow rate to 1/2 or less of the infusing dose.

If severe hypotension (<80 mm Hg systolic) occurs, stop the infusion, elevate the patient's lower extremities, and contact the physician for further directions. In both situations, the physician may prescribe a low-dose positive inotropic agent (e.g., dopamine or dobutamine), to enhance cardiac contractility.

6. Administer morphine sulfate as prescribed to reduce chest pain, preload, sympathetic tone, and patient's anxiety.
7. To determine and document the CPK rise seen in MI patients, send CPK total and MB to the lab q8h x3, or per hospital protocol. The CPK rises within 8 hours, peaks within 24 hours, and returns to normal in 2 days.
8. Administer oxygen by nasal cannula at 2-4 L/min as prescribed, or based on ABG results.
9. Give thrombolytic agent as prescribed. See section "Coronary Artery Thrombolysis," p. 160, for more information.
10. Instruct patient to report decreases or increases in chest pain.
11. Provide care in a calm, efficient manner that will reassure patient and minimize anxiety, and hence, chest pain.
12. Regulate visitations in accordance with patient's comfort level.
13. Enforce activity restrictions; maintain patient on bed rest to decrease oxygen demand.

Alteration in cardiac output: Decreased, related to life-threatening dysrhythmias secondary to injury to and enhanced automaticity of the myocardium

Desired outcome: Patient remains in sinus rhythm.

1. Orient patient to the monitor, its purpose, the alarms, and the need for continuous monitoring.
2. Monitor patient continuously in MCL-1 lead to detect ventricular ectopy versus aberrancy. Run lead II if supraventricular dysrhythmias are present or if it is imperative to identify axis deviations. Keep alarms on at all times (e.g., set at 50, 100).
3. Document rhythm strip every shift and prn if dysrhythmias occur. Measure PR, QRS, and QT intervals with each strip. Note and report any deviations from normal (i.e., PR >.10-.20 sec; QRS of .04-.10 sec; QT <.40 sec).
4. Administer antiarrhythmic agents as prescribed. Prophylactic lidocaine is used for the first 24 hours after MI. A usual protocol is a bolus of 1 mg/kg initially, followed by a drip of 1-4 mg/min, and another bolus 10 minutes after the initial bolus, using half the initial dose.
5. Monitor serum potassium for levels >5.5 mEq/L or <3.5 mEq/L. Hypokalemia or hyperkalemia can cause dysrhythmias. Replace potassium as prescribed.
6. Deliver oxygen *via* nasal cannula at 2-4 L/min or as prescribed. Oxygen may be beneficial for treating dysrhythmias caused by ischemia.

Alteration in cardiac output: Decreased, related to impaired contractility secondary to myocardial injury

Desired outcomes: Patient has adequate cardiac output, as evidenced by systolic BP >90 mm Hg; CO ≥4L/min; HR ≤100 bpm; RR 12-20 breaths/min with normal pattern and depth (eupnea); orientation to person, place, and time; warm and dry skin; and urinary output ≥30 ml/hr. PAWP remains ≤18 mm Hg.

1. Assess for and document the following as evidence of myocardial dysfunction with decreasing cardiac output: presence of jugular venous distention, dependent edema (i.e., sacral), hepatomegaly, fatigue, weakness, decreased activity level, and SOB with activity. In addition, assess and document the following:
   - *Mental status:* Be alert to restlessness and decreased responsiveness.
   - *Lung sounds:* Monitor for crackles (rales), rhonchi.
   - *Heart sounds:* Note presence of gallop, murmur, and increased HR.
   - *Urinary output:* Be alert to output <30 ml/hour.
   - *Skin:* Monitor for pallor, mottling, cyanosis, coolness, diaphoresis.
   - *Vital signs:* Note BP ≤90 mm Hg systolic, HR ≥100 bpm, RR >20 breaths/min, and temperature >38.5° C (101.4° F). Patients with MI may spike a temperature due to the body's reaction to necrotic tissue.
2. If a pulmonary artery catheter is present, record hemodynamic readings q1-2h and prn. Be alert to PAWP >18 mm Hg and CO <4 L/min.
3. Keep accurate I&O records and weigh patient daily. Be alert to a positive hydration state. A 1 kg acute weight gain can signal retention of 1 L of fluid.
4. Help minimize cardiac workload by administering prescribed beta blockers, positioning patient in Fowler's or semi-Fowler's position, and enforcing bed rest.
5. Have patient perform active ROM exercises, along with Level I activities (see Table 2-1, p. 76) to help prevent deleterious effects of bed rest on oxygen supplies.
6. Administer and titrate prescribed medications: nitrates and afterload reducing agents, such as nitroprusside and nitroglycerin, to maintain SVR within 900-1200 dynes/sec/cm^{-5} and PAWP ≤18 mm Hg; diuretics, such as furosemide and metolazone, to keep PAWP ≤18 mm Hg and urine output ≥30 ml/hour; and inotropic agents, such as dopamine and dobutamine, to keep systolic BP >90 mm Hg.

Knowledge deficit: Myocardial infarction and its implications for lifestyle changes

Desired outcome: Patient and significant others verbalize an understanding of heart attack and the necessary lifestyle changes that must be made.

1. Discuss the following with patient and significant others, providing both oral instructions and written materials:
   - Anatomy and functions of the heart muscle.
   - Coronary arteries and the atherosclerotic process.
   - Definition of "heart attack."
   - Healing process of the heart and the role of collateral circulation.
2. Assist patient with identifying his or her own risk factors.
3. Assist patient with devising a plan for risk factor modification, for example, diet, smoking cessation, stress-reduction techniques.
4. Provide guidelines for low-cholesterol diet (see Table 2-3); refer patient to dietician if necessary.

TABLE 2-3

Low-cholesterol dietary guidelines

Foods to avoid	Foods allowed
Egg yolks (no more than three per week)	Egg whites; cholesterol-free egg substitutes
Foods made with many egg yolks (e.g., sponge cakes)	Lean, well-trimmed meats; minimize servings of beef, lamb, and pork
Fatty cuts of meat; fat on meats	Fish (except shellfish), chicken and turkey (without the skin)
Skin on chicken and turkey	Dried peas and beans as meat substitutes
Luncheon meats or cold cuts	Nonfat (skim) or lowfat (2%) milk
Sausage, frankfurters	Partially skim-milk cheeses
Shellfish (e.g., lobster, shrimp, crab)	Ice milk and sherbet
Whole milk, cream, whole milk cheese	Polyunsaturated oils for cooking and food preparation: corn, safflower, cottonseed, sesame, and sunflower
Ice cream	Margarines that list one of the above oils as their first ingredient
Commercially prepared foods with *hydrogenated* shortening. This is saturated fat.	Foods prepared "from scratch" with the above suggested oils
Coconut and palm oils and products made with them (e.g., cream substitutes)	Meats (in acceptable quantity) and vegetables prepared by broiling, steaming, or baking (never frying)
Butter, lard, hydrogenated shortening	Spices, herbs, lemon juice, wine, flavored wine vinegars
Meats and vegetables prepared by frying	
Seasonings containing large amounts of sugar and saturated fats	
Sauces and gravies	
Salad dressings containing cream, cheeses, or mayonnaise	

5. Discuss activity progression post-MI, for example, a progressive walking program. See Rehabilitation and Patient-Family Teaching Concepts, p. 77, with "Chest Pain."

6. Discuss guidelines for resuming sexual activity post-MI. Explain that sexual activity requires the same amount of oxygen as that needed to walk briskly up two flights of stairs; consequently, patients usually are instructed to wait for two weeks after hospital discharge before resuming sexual activity.

7. Teach patient about medications that will be taken after hospital discharge, including name, purpose, dosage, schedule, precautions, and potential side effects.

In addition, see nursing diagnoses and interventions in the following: "Caring for the Critically Ill on Prolonged Bed Rest," pp. 506-511; "Caring for the Critically Ill with Life-Threatening Disorders," pp. 511-522; and "Caring for the Family of the Critically Ill," pp. 522-526.

REHABILITATION AND PATIENT-FAMILY TEACHING CONCEPTS

Give patient and significant others verbal and written instructions for the following:
1. See interventions with **Knowledge deficit:** Myocardial infarction and its implications for lifestyle changes, above.

2. Signs and symptoms that necessitate immediate medical attention: chest pain, SOB, severe fatigue/weakness, syncope, weight gain.
3. Community referrals, for example, American Heart Association.

Congestive heart failure/pulmonary edema

In this state the left ventricle is unable to maintain a cardiac output sufficient to meet the needs of the body. It begins when the diseased left ventricular myocardium cannot pump the blood returning from the lungs into systemic circulation. In addition, pressure increases in the lungs because of the accumulation of blood. If the pressure exceeds pulmonary capillary oncotic pressure (>30 mm Hg), fluid will leak into the pulmonary interstitial spaces. This results in pulmonary edema, which causes impairment of oxygen and carbon dioxide exchange. As pressure continues to increase in the lungs, pressure in the right side of the heart increases because of backflow of pressure in the pulmonary vasculature. Consequently, the right ventricle cannot pump blood into the pulmonary system and venous return to the right side of the heart is inhibited. As pressure continues to back up in the systemic circulation, body organs become congested with venous blood. This results in congestive heart failure.

ASSESSMENT

Left heart failure (pulmonary edema)
- *Signs and symptoms:* Anxiety, air hunger, nocturnal dyspnea, dyspnea on exertion, orthopnea, moist cough with frothy sputum, tachycardia, diaphoresis, cyanosis or pallor, insomnia, palpitations, weakness, fatigue, anorexia, and changes in mentation.
- *Physical assessment:* Decreased BP, tachycardia, dysrhythmias, crackles (rales), bronchial wheezes, S_3 or summation gallop, pulsus alternans.

Right heart failure (congestive heart failure)
- *Signs and symptoms:* Fluid retention, peripheral edema, decreased urinary output, abdominal tenderness, nausea, vomiting, and anorexia.
- *Physical assessment:* Hepatosplenomegaly, dependent pitting edema, jugular venous distention, positive hepatojugular reflex, bounding pulses, ascites.

Monitoring parameters: Elevated PAP, PAWP, and SVR with left heart failure; elevated RAP and CVP with right heart failure.

History and risk factors: Familial history of coronary artery disease, age over 65 years, male sex (risk for females increases after menopause), cigarette smoking, hypercholesterolemia, hypertension, diabetes, obesity, increased stress, and sedentary lifestyle. Other important data include noncompliance with low-sodium diet or medications, orthopnea, nocturia, decreased exercise tolerance, and increasing SOB.

DIAGNOSTIC TESTS

1. *Chest x-ray:* Will reveal pulmonary clouding, increased interstitial density, engorged pulmonary vasculature, and cardiomegaly.
2. *Serum electrolytes:* May reveal hyponatremia (dilutional); hyperkalemia if glomerular filtration is decreased; or hypokalemia, which can result from use of diuretics.
3. *Serum enzymes:* Liver function tests may be abnormal because of hepatic venous congestion.

4. *Serum bilirubin:* May reveal hyperbilirubinemia in the presence of liver dysfunction.
5. *Circulation time:* Although this test is not usually performed, in the presence of heart failure, circulation time often is increased at rest. In mild cases of heart failure, circulation time may be normal at rest but increased with exercise. Sodium dehydrocholate is given IV and the time is measured until the patient begins to experience a bitter taste in his or her mouth.
6. *CBC:* May reveal decreased hemoglobin and hematocrit in the presence of anemia or dilution.
7. *Arterial blood gas values:* May reveal hypoxemia due to the decreased oxygen available from fluid-filled alveoli and respiratory alkalosis because of the increase in respiratory rate, causing patient to blow off more CO_2.
8. *Digitalis levels:* The CHF patient may have been treated with digitalis in the past. With CHF, the patient is predisposed to digitalis toxicity due to the low cardiac output state, which also causes decreased renal excretion of the drug.

MEDICAL MANAGEMENT AND SURGICAL INTERVENTIONS

1. **Treatment of underlying cause and precipitating factors**
   - *Left heart failure:* Atherosclerotic heart disease, acute MI, dysrhythmias, cardiomyopathy, increased circulating volume, aortic stenosis, aortic regurgitation, mitral regurgitation, coarctation of the aorta, atrial septal defect, ventricular septal defect, cardiac tamponade, and constrictive pericarditis.
   - *Right heart failure:* Left heart failure, atherosclerotic heart disease, acute MI, dysrhythmias, pulmonary embolism, fluid overload or excess sodium intake, COPD, pulmonary hypertension, mitral stenosis, and pulmonary stenosis.
2. **Bed rest and stress reduction**
3. **Low-calorie diet** (if weight control is necessary) **and low-sodium diet:** Extra salt and water are held in the circulatory system, causing increased strain on the heart. Limiting sodium (see Table 2-4) will reduce the amount of fluid retained by the body. In addition, fluids may be limited to 1500 ml/day.
4. **Pharmacotherapy**
   - *Morphine:* To induce vasodilatation and decrease venous return, sympathetic tone, anxiety, myocardial oxygen consumption, and pain.
   - *Diuretics:* To reduce blood volume and decrease preload.
   - *Inotropic agents:* Digitalis to strengthen contractions; dopamine, dobutamine, or amrinone to support BP and enhance contractility.
   - *Vasodilators:* Nitrates (oral, topical, or IV) to dilate venous or capacitant vessels, thereby reducing preload and cardiac and pulmonary congestion. Nitroprusside, hydralazine, captopril, or prazosin hydrochloride will dilate the arterial or resistant vessels and reduce afterload, thus increasing forward flow.

NURSING DIAGNOSES AND INTERVENTIONS

Fluid volume excess: Pulmonary and peripheral edema related to retention secondary to decreased cardiac output

---

Desired outcome: Patient becomes normovolemic as evidenced by absence of adventitious lung sounds, presence of normal breath sounds over the airways, decreased peripheral edema, increased urine output, weight loss, PAWP ≤18 mm Hg

TABLE 2-4
Low-sodium dietary guidelines

Foods high in sodium	Foods low in sodium
Canned or packaged soups	Fresh fruits and vegetables
Vegetables in brine or cans	Fresh fish, chicken, turkey, veal,
Monosodium glutamate (e.g.,	beef, and lamb (if limiting fats,
Accent)	avoid the latter two)
Canned, smoked, or salted meats;	Dry or hot cereal
salted fish	Carbonated beverages
Celery salt, onion salt, garlic	Oil, margarine
salt, seasoned salt	Fresh or dried herbs
Sauerkraut	Tabasco sauce
Dill pickles	Bread
Olives	Jello
Bouillon cubes	Peanut butter
Soy sauce	Tuna packed in water
Packaged snack foods	
Processed cheese	
Pancake or waffle mix	
Beans and frankfurters	
Fried chicken dinners	

Other points: Don't add table salt to foods.
Season with fresh or dried herbs.
Avoid salts or powders.
Don't buy convenience foods. Remember that fresh is best.
Read all labels for salt, sodium, or NaCl content.

(reasonable outcome for these patients), SVR ≤ 1200 dynes/sec/cm^{-5}, and CO ≥ 4 L/min.

1. Auscultate lung fields for presence of crackles (rales) and rhonchi or other adventitious sounds.
2. Monitor I&O closely. Report positive fluid state or decrease in urine output to <30 ml/hr.
3. Weigh patient daily; report increases in weight. A 1 kg acute gain in weight can signal a 1 L gain in fluid.
4. Note changes in patient from baseline assessment to detect worsening of heart failure, such as increased pedal edema, increased jugular venous distention, development of S_3 heart sound or new murmur, and dysrhythmias.
5. Monitor hemodynamic status q1-2h and prn. Note response to drug therapy as well as indicators of the need for more aggressive therapy, including increasing PAWP and SVR and decreasing CO.
6. Limit oral fluids as prescribed, and offer patient ice chips or Popsicles to decrease thirst and discomfort of dry mouth.
7. Maintain bed rest restrictions to facilitate fluid movement from interstitial spaces in dependent extremities to the intravascular spaces.

Impaired gas exchange related to decreased diffusion of oxygen secondary to fluid collection in the lungs

---

Desired outcomes: Patient has improved gas exchange as evidenced by $Pao_2 \geq 80$ mm Hg. RR is 12-20 breaths/min with normal pattern and depth (eupnea) and adventitious breaths sounds are not present over the lung fields.

---

1. Monitor respiratory rate, rhythm, and character q1-2h. Be alert to RR >20 breaths/min, irregular rhythm, use of accessory muscles of respiration, or cough.
2. Auscultate breath sounds, noting presence of crackles (rales), wheezes, and other adventitious sounds.
3. Provide supplemental oxygen as prescribed.
4. Assess ABG findings; note changes in response to oxygen supplement or treatment of altered hemodynamics.
5. Suction patient as needed.
6. Establish a protocol for deep breathing, coughing, and turning q2h.
7. Place patient in semi- or high-Fowler's position to ensure maximal chest excursion.

Activity intolerance related to weakness and fatigue secondary to decreased functioning of the myocardium

---

Desired outcome: Patient exhibits cardiac tolerance to increasing levels of activity as evidenced by RR <24 breaths/min, normal sinus rhythm on EKG, HR ≤120 bpm (or within 20 bpm of resting HR), BP within 20 mm Hg of patient's normal range, and absence of chest pain.

---

1. Maintain prescribed activity level and teach patient the rationale for activity limitation.
2. Organize nursing care so that periods of activity are interspersed with extended periods of uninterrupted rest.
3. To help prevent complications of immobility, assist patient with active/passive ROM exercises, as appropriate. Encourage patient to do as much as possible within prescribed activity allowances. For interventions related to a progressive in-bed exercise program, see Table 2-1, p. 76, and the section "Caring for the Critically Ill on Prolonged Bed Rest," p. 506.
4. Note patient's physiologic response to activity, including BP, HR, RR, and heart rhythm. Signs of activity intolerance include chest pain, increasing SOB, excessive fatigue, increased dysrhythmias, palpitations, HR response >120 bpm, systolic BP >20 mm Hg from baseline or >160 mm Hg, and ST-segment changes.
5. If activity intolerance is noted, instruct patient to stop the activity and rest.
6. Administer medications as prescribed and note their effects on patient's activity tolerance. Examples of medications include isosorbide dinitrate (Isordil), prophylactic NTG, and nitroglycerin paste; all reduce preload.

7. As needed to help prevent muscle loss and wasting, refer patient to physical therapy department.

Knowledge deficit: Disease process with CHF and the prescribed diet and medications

---

Desired outcome: Patient and significant others verbalize understanding of patient's disease as well as the prescribed diet and medication regimens.

---

1. Teach patient the physiologic process of CHF, discussing in terms appropriate to the patient how fluid volume increases because of poor heart functioning.
2. Teach patient about the importance of a low-sodium diet and medications to help reduce volume overload. Provide patient with a list of foods that are high and low in sodium (see Table 2-4, p. 87)
3. Teach patient the signs and symptoms of fluid volume excess that necessitate medical attention: irregular or slow pulse, increased SOB, orthopnea, decreased exercise tolerance, and steady weight gain (≥ 1 kg/day for two successive days).
4. Advise patient about the need to keep a journal of daily weights. Explain that an increase of ≥ 1 kg/day on 2 successive days of normal eating necessitates notification of physician.
5. If patient is taking digitalis, teach the technique for measuring pulse rate. Provide parameters for holding digitalis (usually for pulse rate <60/min) and notifying the physician.

Also see nursing diagnoses and interventions in the following: "Caring for the Critically Ill on Prolonged Bed Rest," pp. 506-511; "Caring for the Critically Ill with Life-Threatening Disorders," pp. 511-522; and "Caring for the Family of the Critically Ill," pp. 522-526.

REHABILITATION AND PATIENT-FAMILY TEACHING CONCEPTS

Give patient and significant others verbal and written instructions for the following:
1. Medications, including drug name, action, dosage, schedule, precautions, and potential side effects. Stress the importance of taking diuretics and vasodilators. Explain that diuretics reduce the congestion in the heart and vasodilators relax the vessels and reduce the amount of blood returning to the heart, making it easier for the heart to pump.
2. Diet: List foods that are allowed and those to be avoided on a low-sodium diet (see Table 2-4, p. 87). Refer patient to dietician, if necessary, and provide materials from American Heart Association for low-sodium diet.
3. Signs and symptoms that necessitate medical attention.
4. Risk factor modification (see "Acute Chest Pain," p. 76).
5. Prescribed activity progression after hospital discharge, signs of activity intolerance that signal the need for rest, and use of prophylactic NTG to reduce congestion of the heart and lungs. General activity guidelines are as follows:
   • Get up and get dressed every morning.
   • Space your meals and activities to allow time for rest and relaxation.

TABLE 2-5
Activity progression after hospital discharge

Week	Distance	Time
1-2	¼ mile	Leisurely; 2 times/day
2-3	½ mile	15 minutes
3-4	1 mile	30 minutes
4-5	1½ miles	30 minutes
5-6	2 miles	40 minutes

- Perform activities at a comfortable, moderate pace. If you get tired during any activity, stop to rest for 15 minutes before resuming.
- Avoid activities that require straining (e.g., lifting >30 pounds, push-ups, pull-ups, straining during bowel movement). Use laxatives as needed.
- Plan at least 2 periods a day of walking outside when the weather is nice, following the guidelines in Table 2-5.
- Start out slowly, (e.g., 200-400 feet) and work up to ¼ mile in the first week. Progress according to your own ability. Let the way you feel be your guide. Walk a minimum of 3 times a week on nonsuccessive days. Exercise should be fun. Enjoy!
- Warning signals to stop your activity and rest: chest pain, shortness of breath, dizziness or faintness, unusual weakness.
6. Emergency telephone numbers (i.e., health-care provider's and 911) in the event of the need for immediate medical attention.
7. Importance of follow-up care; confirm date and time of next appointment, if known.
8. For more information, see **Knowledge deficit:** Disease process with CHF and the prescribed diet and medications, p. 89.

Cardiomyopathy

Cardiomyopathy is a subacute or chronic disorder of unknown or obscure etiology involving the heart muscle. It results in heart failure.

Functional classification

1. *Dilated (previously referred to as "congestive"):* The significant feature of this disease process is dilatation rather than congestion; therefore, the term "congestive" has been replaced with "dilated" cardiomyopathy. The majority of cases are termed idiopathic because of the unknown origin of the disease process. Heart failure occurs secondary to decreased systolic ejection fraction. There is little or no hypertrophy of the ventricles.
2. *Hypertrophic or obstructive:* Characterized by an abnormally stiff left ventricle during diastole, which restricts ventricular filling. There may be hypertrophy of the ventricular septum, which leads to obstruction of the ventricular outflow tract. This is called idiopathic hypertrophic subaortic stenosis (IHSS). Although cardiac function can remain normal for varying periods of time, deterioration and poor ventricular compliance usually occur.

3. *Restrictive or constrictive:* The ventricular walls are rigid from fibrosis and there is inadequate diastolic filling, resulting in abnormal diastolic function.
4. *Ischemic:* Results from coronary artery disease. There is greater than 70% luminal narrowing of at least one coronary artery, as well as multiple ventricular wall motion abnormalities. Cardiomegaly is present and left ventricular ejection fraction (LVEF) is decreased.

ASSESSMENT

Signs and symptoms: Forward failure and low cardiac output lead to fatigue, weakness, hypotension, ischemic chest pain, low urine output, altered mental status, palpitations, and syncope. Backward failure and pulmonary congestion can lead to SOB, dyspnea on exertion, orthopnea, peripheral edema, anorexia, and nausea.

Physical assessment: Presence of S_3 or S_4 heart sounds or a summation gallop, valvular murmurs of mitral and tricuspid regurgitation, murmur of IHSS, increased venous pressure pulsations, crackles (rales), decreased BP, increased HR, and presence of dysrhythmias. Peripheral hypoperfusion may be present and will manifest as diminished pulses, cool skin, and mottling or cyanosis. In addition, hepatomegaly and mild to severe cardiomegaly may be present, causing a displaced and diffuse PMI.

Monitoring parameters: See Table 2-6.

DIAGNOSTIC TESTS

1. *Chest x-ray:* May detect cardiomegaly with enlarged left ventricle, pulmonary venous congestion, and Kerley B lines of interstitial edema.
2. *EKG:* May reveal dysrhythmias, such as sinus tachycardia, atrial fibrillation, and ventricular ectopy. Other changes may include left ventricular hypertrophy, left bundle-branch block, left anterior hemiblock, left axis deviation, nonspecific ST-segment changes, and Q waves that resemble those that occur with myocardial infarction.
3. *Echocardiogram:* To assess degree of left ventricular impairment and dilatation of the cardiac chambers. Ventricular wall and septal contractility can be evaluated, as well as valvular motion. Two-dimensional echo can detect thrombus formation and estimate ejection fraction.
4. *Cardiac catheterization:* Does not confirm cardiomyopathy but can be used to

---

TABLE 2-6

Hemodynamic presentation with cardiomyopathy

Pressure	Cardiomyopathy	Normal
Right atrial pressure	Increased	4-6 mm Hg
Pulmonary artery pressure	Increased	20-30/8-15 mm Hg
Pulmonary wedge pressure	Increased	6-12 mm Hg
Cardiac output	Decreased	4-7 L/min
Cardiac index	Decreased	2.5-4 L/min/m^2
Pulmonary vascular resistance	Unchanged or increased	60-100 dynes/sec/cm^{-5}
Systemic vascular resistance	Increased	900-1200 dynes/sec/cm^{-5}

rule out other disorders, such as ischemic heart disease. Findings may include decreased cardiac output, ventricular wall motion, and ejection fraction; increased filling pressure; and valvular regurgitation.

5. *Endocardial biopsy:* May be necessary to identify the type of pathologic agent causing the cardiomyopathy. It can be done during cardiac catheterization.

6. *Radionuclide studies:* May show diffuse left ventricular hypokinesis, left ventricular ejection fraction <40%, and elevated end diastolic and systolic volumes.

MEDICAL MANAGEMENT AND SURGICAL INTERVENTIONS

1. **Pharmacotherapy:** To maintain or reestablish hemodynamic stability.
   - *Vasodilators:* To decrease preload and afterload, thus improving cardiac output.
   - *Diuretics:* To reduce preload and pulmonary congestion.
   - *Inotropic therapy:* To enhance contractility.
   - *Antiarrhythmic agents:* To control dysrhythmias.
   - *Calcium antagonists:* To produce vasodilatation and decrease cardiac workload.
   - *Beta blockers:* For hypertrophic cardiomyopathy to decrease outflow obstruction during exercise and reduce inappropriate sympathetic cardiac stimulation.
   - *Anticoagulants:* To prevent thrombus formation, as these patients often are at risk owing to their predisposition for atrial fibrillation.
   - *Potassium supplements:* To replace potassium lost in the urine due to diuresis.

2. **Activity level:** Initially it is reduced to decrease oxygen demand, but then is increased gradually to prevent complications of immobility.

3. **Intra-aortic balloon pump:** In the presence of a failing myocardium, may be used to decrease afterload and increase coronary artery perfusion. See discussion, p. 142.

4. **Heart transplant:** For patients refractory to medical therapy such as vasodilators and inotropic agents. Each institution has criteria that must be met before a transplant is considered as an alternative treatment.

NURSING DIAGNOSES AND INTERVENTIONS

Alteration in cardiac output: Decreased, related to impaired contractility secondary to myocardial dilatation

---

Desired outcomes: Patient has adequate cardiac output as evidenced by systolic BP >90 mm Hg; CO 4-7 L/min; CI 2.5-4 L/min/m^2; RR 12-20 breaths/min; HR <100 bpm; urinary output ≥30 ml/hr; intake equal to output plus insensible losses; warm and dry skin; and orientation to person, place, and time. PAWP is ≤18 mm Hg and RAP is 4-6 mm Hg.

---

1. Assess for and document the following as evidence of decreasing cardiac output: presence of jugular venous distention, dependent edema, hepatomegaly, fatigue, weakness, decreased activity level, and SOB with activity. In addition, assess and document the following:
   - *Mental status:* Be alert to restlessness and decreased responsiveness.

- *Lung sounds:* Monitor for crackles (rales), rhonchi, wheezes.
- *Heart sounds:* Note presence of gallop, murmur, and increased HR.
- *Urinary output:* Be alert to output <30 ml/hour.
- *Skin:* Monitor for pallor, mottling, cyanosis, coolness, diaphoresis.
- *Vital signs:* Note BP ≤90 mm Hg systolic, HR ≥100 bpm, RR >20 min, and elevated temperature.

2. If a pulmonary artery catheter is present, record hemodynamic readings q1-2h and prn. Be alert to PAWP >18 mm Hg and RAP >6 mm Hg. Although normal PAWP is 6-12 mm Hg, these patients may need increased filling pressures, with wedge pressure at 15-18 mm Hg.
3. Measure CO/CI q2-4h and prn. Optimally, CO should be within 4-7 L/min and CI should be 2.5-4 L/min/m^2.
4. Keep accurate I&O records and weigh patient daily, noting trends.
5. Help minimize patient's cardiac workload by assisting patient with ADLs when necessary.
6. Monitor for compensatory mechanisms, including increased HR and BP due to sodium and water retention.
7. Administer medications as prescribed, including nitrates and other vasodilators, diuretics, inotropic agents, and anticoagulants.
8. Position patient according to his or her comfort level.

Activity intolerance related to weakness and fatigue secondary to decreased myocardial contractions

---

Desired outcome: Patient exhibits cardiac tolerance to increasing levels of activity as evidenced by RR <24 breaths/min, normal sinus rhythm on EKG, BP within 20 mm Hg of patient's normal range, HR within 20 bpm of patient's resting HR, peripheral pulses >2+ on a 0-4+ scale, and absence of chest pain.

---

1. Monitor BP and VS; report changes such as dysrhythmias or decreasing BP.
2. Observe for and report any signs of decreased cardiac output, such as oliguria, changes in mentation, or decreased BP.
3. Assess peripheral pulses and rate on a scale of 0-4+.
4. Plan nursing care so that patient is assured of extended (at least 90 minutes) periods of rest.
5. Monitor patient's physiologic response to activity, reporting any symptoms of chest pain, new or increasing SOB, increases in HR >20 beats above resting HR, and increase or decrease in systolic BP >20 mm Hg.
6. To prevent complications of immobility, perform or teach patient and significant others active, passive, and assistive ROM exercises. For a discussion of in-bed exercise program, see Table 2-1, p. 76, and interventions in the section ''Caring for the Critically Ill on Prolonged Bed Rest,'' p. 506. Consult with MD to ensure that exercises are within patient's prescribed limitations.

Also see nursing diagnoses and interventions in the following: ''Caring for the Critically Ill on Prolonged Bed Rest,'' pp. 506-511; ''Caring for the Critically Ill with Life-Threatening Disorders,'' pp. 511-522; and ''Caring for the Family of the Critically Ill,'' pp. 522-526.

REHABILITATION AND PATIENT-FAMILY TEACHING CONCEPTS

Give patient and significant others verbal and written instructions for the following:
1. Medications, including drug name, dosage, action, schedule, precautions, and potential side effects.
2. Signs and symptoms that necessitate immediate medical attention: dyspnea, decreased exercise tolerance, alterations in pulse rate/rhythm, changes in mentation, and weight gain >2 lbs/day for 2 successive days.
3. Importance of abstaining from alcohol because of its cardiodepressant effects.
4. Reinforcement that cardiomyopathy is a chronic disease that requires ongoing treatment and management.
5. Names and addresses of community resources such as the American Heart Association, the YMCA or YWCA, and other resources such as VNA and home health-care nurses as the disease progresses.

Dysrhythmias and conduction disturbances

Dysrhythmias are abnormal rhythms of the heart's electrical system. They can originate in any part of the conduction system, such as the sinus node, atrium, AV node, His-Purkinje system, bundle branches, and ventricular tissue. Although a variety of diseases may cause dysrhythmias, the most common are coronary artery disease (CAD) and myocardial infarction (MI). Other causes include electrolyte imbalance, changes in oxygenation, and drug toxicity. Cardiac dysrhythmias may result from the following mechanisms:

Disturbances in automaticity: May involve an increase or decrease in automaticity in the sinus node (i.e., sinus tachycardia or sinus bradycardia). Premature beats may arise *via* this mechanism from the atria, junction, or ventricles. Abnormal rhythms, such as atrial or ventricular tachycardia, also may occur.

Disturbances in conductivity: Conduction may be too rapid, as in conditions caused by an accessory pathway (e.g., Wolff-Parkinson-White syndrome), or too slow (e.g., AV block). Reentry is a situation in which a stimulus reexcites a conduction pathway through which it already has passed. Once started, this impulse may circulate repeatedly. In order for reentry to occur, there must be two different pathways for conduction: one with slowed conduction and one with unidirectional block.

Combinations of altered automaticity and conductivity: Observed when several dysrhythmias are noted, for example, first-degree AV block (disturbance in conductivity) and premature atrial contractions, a disturbance in automaticity.

ASSESSMENT

Signs and symptoms: Can vary on a continuum from absence of symptoms to complete cardiopulmonary collapse. General indicators include alterations in LOC, vertigo, syncope, weakness, fatigue, activity intolerance, SOB, dyspnea on exertion, chest pain, palpitations, sensation of ''skipped beats,'' anxiety, and restlessness.

Physical assessment: Increases or decreases in HR, BP, and RR; dusky color or pallor; crackles (rales); cool skin; decreased urine output; and paradoxical pulse and abnormal heart sounds (e.g., paradoxical splitting of S_1 and S_2).

EKG and hemodynamic measurements: Decreased cardiac output, elevated PAP. Some EKG findings seen with various dysrhythmias include abnormalities in rate such as sinus bradycardia or sinus tachycardia, irregular rhythm such as atrial fibrillation, extra beats such as PACs and PJCs, wide and bizarre-looking beats such as PVCs and VT, a fibrillating baseline such as VT, and a straight line as with asystole.

History and risk factors: CAD, recent MI, electrolyte disturbances, drug toxicity.

DIAGNOSTIC TESTS

1. *12-lead EKG:* To detect dysrhythmias and identify possible etiology.
2. *Serum electrolytes:* To identify electrolyte abnormality, which can precipitate dysrhythmias. The most common are hyperkalemia and hypokalemia.
3. *Drug levels:* To identify toxicities (e.g., of digoxin, quinidine, procainamide) that can precipitate dysrhythmias.
4. *24-hour holter monitoring:* Records patient's EKG for 24 hours, during which time the patient keeps a diary of activities and symptoms. This allows documentation of subtle dysrhythmias and can associate abnormal rhythm with patient's symptomatology.
5. *Electrophysiologic study (EPS):* Invasive test in which 2-3 catheters are placed into the heart, giving the heart a pacing stimulus at varying sites and of varying voltages. The test determines origin of dysrhythmia, inducibility, and effectiveness of drug therapy in dysrhythmia suppression.
6. *Exercise stress testing:* Used in conjunction with 24-hour holter monitoring to detect advanced grades of PVCs (those caused by ischemia) and to guide therapy. During the test, EKG and BP reading are taken while the patient walks on a treadmill or pedals a stationary bicycle; response to a constant or increasing workload is observed. The test continues until the patient reaches target heart rate or symptoms such as chest pain, severe fatigue, dysrhythmias, or abnormal BP occur.

MEDICAL MANAGEMENT AND SURGICAL INTERVENTIONS

1. **Antiarrhythmic drugs**
   - *Group I drugs (lidocaine, quinidine, procainamide):* Decrease automaticity of ventricular conduction, delay ventricular repolarization, decrease conduction velocity, increase conduction *via* AV node, and suppress ventricular automaticity.
   - *Group II drugs (beta-adrenergic blockade, such as propranolol):* Slow sinus automaticity, slow conduction *via* AV node, control ventricular response to supraventricular tachycardias, and shorten the action potential of Purkinje fibers.
   - *Group III drugs (e.g., bretylium and amiodarone):* Experimental drugs, which increase the action potential and refractory period of Purkinje fibers, increase ventricular fibrillation threshold, restore injured myocardial cell electrophysiology toward normal, and suppress reentrant dysrhythmias.
   - *Group IV drugs (e.g., verapamil and other calcium-channel blockers):* Depress automaticity in the SA and AV nodes, block the slow calcium current

in the AV junctional tissue, reduce conduction *via* the AV node, and are useful in treating tachyarrhythmias due to AV junction reentry.

2. Experimental procedures

- *Ablation:* A procedure in which a catheter is placed in the heart *via* cardiac catheterization and an electrical heat stimulus is applied to the area in which the dysrhythmia originates. The heat stimulus causes controlled, localized necrosis of the area. This procedure is currently under investigation in several institutions and is used when the patient has not responded to antiarrhythmic drug therapy.
- *Automatic implantable defibrillator (AID):* Programmed to identify ventricular tachycardia and ventricular fibrillation and to deliver a defibrillatory charge of 25-30 joules. It is used in patients with sustained, recurrent ventricular tachycardia and history of sudden death with resistance to drug therapy. See discussion p. 157.

3. Dietary guidelines: Usually, patients with recurrent dysrhythmias are put on a diet that restricts or reduces caffeine and is low in cholesterol.

4. Surgical procedures

- *Left ventricular aneurysmectomy and infarctectomy:* Excision of possible focal spots of ventricular dysrhythmias.
- *Myocardial revascularization:* Done alone or in conjunction with electrophysiologic mapping, with excision or cryoablation of the dysrhythmia focus.
- *Encircling ventriculotomy:* Excises the diseased portion of the ventricle without compromising myocardial blood supply.
- *Stellate ganglionectomy and block:* Alters the electrical stability of the myocardium and predisposition to ventricular dysrhythmias.

NURSING DIAGNOSES AND INTERVENTIONS

Alteration in cardiac output: Decreased, related to dysrhythmias or impaired contractility secondary to cardiac disease

---

Desired outcomes: Patient has a normal cardiac output as evidenced by BP >90/60 mm Hg, HR 60-100 bpm, and normal sinus rhythm on EKG. PAP is 20-30/8-15 mm Hg; PAWP is ≤18 mm Hg (a reasonable outcome for these patients); RAP is ≤7 mm Hg; and CO is 4-7 L/min.

---

1. Monitor patient's heart rhythm continuously; note BP and symptoms if dysrhythmias occur or increase in occurrence.
2. If a pulmonary artery catheter is present, note PAP, PAWP, and RAP; and monitor for a reduced cardiac output in response to dysrhythmias.
3. Document dysrhythmias with rhythm strip. Use a 12-lead EKG as necessary to identify the dysrhythmia.
4. Monitor patient's lab data, particularly electrolytes and digoxin levels. Serum potassium levels <3.5 mEq/L or >5.5 mEq/L can cause dysrhythmias.
5. Administer antiarrhythmic agents as prescribed; note patient's response to therapy.
6. Provide oxygen as prescribed. Oxygen may be beneficial if dysrhythmias are caused by ischemia.

7. Maintain a quiet environment and administer pain medications promptly. Both stress and pain can increase sympathetic tone and cause dysrhythmias.

8. If life-threatening dysrhythmias occur, initiate immediate unit protocols or standing orders for treatment, as well as CPR and ACLS procedures as necessary.

9. When dysrhythmias occur, stay with patient; provide support and reassurance while performing assessments and administering treatment.

10. Administer inotropic agents (e.g., dopamine, dobutamine, amrinone, isoproterenol) as prescribed to support patient's BP and cardiac output.

Knowledge deficit: Mechanism by which dysrhythmias occur and lifestyle implications

---

Desired outcome: Patient and significant others verbalize knowledge about causes of dysrhythmias and the implications for patient's lifestyle modifications.

---

1. Discuss causal mechanisms for dysrhythmias, including resulting symptoms. Use a heart model or diagrams, as necessary.

2. Teach the signs and symptoms of dysrhythmias that necessitate medical attention: unrelieved, prolonged palpitations; chest pain; SOB; rapid pulse (>150); dizziness; syncope.

3. Teach patient and significant others about medications that will be taken after hospital discharge, including drug name, purpose, dosage, schedule, precautions, and potential side effects. Stress that patient will be maintained on long-term antiarrhythmic therapy and that it could be life-threatening to stop or skip these medications without physician approval because doing so may decrease blood levels effective for dysrhythmia suppression.

4. Advise patient and significant others about the availability of support groups and counseling; provide appropriate community referrals. Patients who survive sudden cardiac arrest may experience nightmares or other sleep disturbances at home. Explain that anxiety and fear, along with periodic feelings of denial, depression, anger, and confusion, are normal following this experience.

5. Stress the importance of leading a normal and productive life, even though patient may fear breakthrough of life-threatening dysrhythmias. If patient is going on vacation, advise him or her to take along sufficient medication and to investigate health-care facilities in the vacation area.

6. Advise patient and significant others to take CPR classes; provide addresses of community programs.

7. Teach the importance of follow-up care; confirm date and time of next appointment, if known. Explain that outpatient holter monitoring is performed periodically.

8. Explain that individuals with recurrent dysrhythmias should follow a general low-cholesterol diet (see Table 2-3, p. 84) and reduce intake of products containing caffeine, including coffee, tea, chocolate, and colas.

9. As indicated, teach patient relaxation techniques, which will reduce stress and enable patient to decrease sympathetic tone (see next nursing diagnosis).

Knowledge deficit: Relaxation technique effective for stress reduction and facilitation of decreased sympathetic tone

---

Desired outcome: Patient verbalizes and demonstrates the following relaxation technique.

---

1. Explain that to decrease sympathetic tone, some patients with dysrhythmias may benefit from practicing a relaxation response. Many different techniques can be used, including use of breathing alone or in conjunction with muscle group contraction and relaxation. Other techniques incorporate use of imagery. The following is a relaxation response that can facilitate a hypometabolic state of decreased sympathetic nervous system outflow. Give patient the following instructions:
   - Sit quietly in a comfortable position. Close your eyes.
   - Relax all your muscles, starting at your feet and progressing to your facial muscles.
   - Breathe through your nose. As you breathe out, say the word "one" silently to yourself. Become aware of your breathing and continue this process for approximately 20 minutes.
   - Do not worry whether you are achieving a deep level of relaxation. Maintain a passive attitude and permit relaxation to occur at its own pace. Expect distractions to occur, but just ignore them. Continue breathing and repeating the word "one."
2. Encourage patient to practice this technique once or twice a day. Reassure patient that relaxation is a learned skill that takes practice and will become easier over time.

Also see nursing diagnoses and interventions in the following: "Caring for the Critically Ill with Life-Threatening Disorders," pp. 511-522; and "Caring for the Family of the Critically Ill," pp. 522-526.

REHABILITATION AND PATIENT-FAMILY TEACHING CONCEPTS

See both **Knowledge deficit** nursing diagnoses, above.

Cardiac arrest

Cardiac arrest occurs when the heart stops beating (asystole) or when the contraction is ineffective in maintaining cardiac output, as with ventricular tachycardia or ventricular fibrillation. Many conditions can precipitate cardiac arrest, including myocardial infarction, heart failure, shock, severe electrolyte disturbances, drowning, electrocution, drug overdose, and respiratory arrest. Any of these factors can set the stage for further deterioration of other vital organs. For example, a dysrhythmia can lead to a low cardiac output, which can cause decreased myocardial perfusion, chest pain due to ischemia, and myocardial hypoxia, which in turn can lead to a life-threatening dysrhythmia such as ventricular tachycardia or fibrillation.

Although cardiac arrest can occur without prior warning, effective and prompt treatment must be administered early to interrupt a potentially life-threatening cycle.

ASSESSMENT

Signs and symptoms: Loss of consciousness—inability to be aroused by shaking and shouting.

Physical assessment: Absence of carotid pulse, loss of audible or palpable BP, absence of respirations.

MEDICAL MANAGEMENT

Medical management of cardiac arrest should include basic cardiopulmonary resuscitation (CPR), advanced cardiac life support (ACLS) guidelines set by the American Heart Association, and procedures established by each institution.

1. **Management of prearrest phase:** Includes treatment of any of the precipitating factors listed above, airway support and oxygen therapy, antiarrhythmic drugs, inotropic support, and pain management.

2. **Basic life support:** Cardiopulmonary resuscitation (CPR) is performed to provide and maintain a patent airway, oxygenation *via* mouth-to-mouth technique, and cardiac compression, which if effective can provide 25-30% of normal cardiac output. Once ventilation has been established and equipment and personnel arrive, oxygen can be delivered by oral airway and bag-valve-mask unit at a 100% flow rate. In addition, endotracheal intubation and mechanical ventilation can be used.

3. **Advanced cardiac life support (ACLS):** Once airway, breathing, and circulation (ABCs) have been established by basic life support, ACLS can be instituted. ACLS generally includes the following:
   - *Recognition and management of dysrhythmias:* EKG monitoring should be established immediately. ACLS providers must be familiar with the following dysrhythmias: sinus tachycardia, sinus bradycardia, premature atrial complexes, paroxysmal supraventricular tachycardia, atrial flutter, atrial fibrillation, junctional rhythms, AV blocks, PVCs, ventricular tachycardia, ventricular fibrillation, and ventricular asystole (cardiac standstill).
   - *Establishment of IV access* (preferably an antecubital vein unless a central vein access already is established): For administration of appropriate medications and fluids. Usually, D_5W is used to keep the line open. In the presence of acute blood loss, volume expansion is achieved with packed cells, crystalloid solutions (e.g., Ringer's solution), or colloid solutions (e.g., albumin).
   - *Pharmacotherapy:* The following are general guidelines.
     —Oxygen therapy: Administered according to ABG results.
     —Morphine sulfate: Given for acute pain and to reduce myocardial oxygen demands.
     —Lidocaine: For treatment of ventricular tachycardia (VT) and ventricular fibrillation (VF). A bolus of 1 mg/kg is given initially, followed by a drip of 1-4 mg/min. After initial bolus, 1/2 the initial bolus is given.
     —Procainamide: Used as second line therapy for VT or VF if dysrhythmias are not controlled with lidocaine. 50 mg is given q5min at a rate of 20 mg/min, not to exceed 1 gram/hr. This is followed by an infusion drip of 1-4 mg/min.

—Bretylium: To treat VT and VF that are refractory to lidocaine and procainamide. 500 mg is mixed with 50 ml D_5W with delivery of 5-10 mg/kg over 8-10 minutes. This is followed by a drip of 2 mg/min.

—Atropine: To treat severe symptomatic sinus bradycardia and complete heart block. Dosage is 0.5 mg IV, repeated at 5 minute intervals. Generally, the total does not exceed 2.0 mg.

—Isoproterenol: Used after atropine for severe bradycardia or complete heart block, isoproterenol is a temporary therapy until a pacemaker can be inserted. Two mg is mixed in 500 ml D_5W and infused at 1-2 μg/min. Infusion can be increased until the desired heart rate response occurs.

—Sodium bicarbonate: Given, based on pH results from ABGs.

• *Precordial thump:* To restore sinus rhythm in the early onset of VT and VF. It is administered by using the fleshy part of the closed fist (hypothenar eminence) to deliver a quick blow to the precordium from a height of 8-12 inches (20-30 cm) above the sternum.

• *Defibrillation and synchronized cardioversion techniques:* With defibrillation, a current is passed through the heart to depolarize the myocardium, terminating the dysrhythmia. Cardioversion is restoration of the heart's normal sinus rhythm *via* delivery of a synchronized current. Cardioversion is used to treat VT and supraventricular rhythms.

• *Management of metabolic acidosis:* During cardiac arrest or when low cardiac output states are present (e.g., after external cardiac compression), anaerobic metabolism occurs, causing a buildup of lactic acid. Metabolism of lactic acid requires oxygen. In the absence of adequate tissue oxygenation, lactic acid cannot be metabolized and will increase in quantity in the blood and body tissues, resulting in metabolic acidosis. For treatment, see ''Metabolic Acidosis,'' p. 53.

< N O T E :   For a detailed description of actions for treatment of specific dysrhythmias, see ''ACLS Algorithms,'' p. 527, in the Appendix.

4. Postarrest management

• *EKG:* To monitor cardiac rhythm.

• *Supplemental oxygen: Via* nasal cannula, face mask, or mechanical ventilation as indicated.

• *Provision of patent IV access:* For delivery of antiarrhythmic agents if arrest was due to VT or VF, morphine if patient is in pain, and atropine if HR is <50.

• *Determine precipitating cause of arrest, if possible*

• *Ongoing assessment of hemodynamic status: Via* pulmonary artery catheter, if necessary.

• *12-lead EKG:* To determine if any new changes occurred postarrest, including ST-segment changes (may signal myocardial damage) and dysrhythmias.

• *Laboratory values:* CPK totals and MB; ABG to check acid-base balance and oxygenation.

• *Chest x-ray:* For evaluation of endotracheal tube and pulmonary artery catheter positions.

NURSING DIAGNOSES AND INTERVENTIONS

Alteration in cardiac output: Absent/decreased, related to cardiac arrest

Desired outcome: Patient has an adequate cardiac output as evidenced by responsiveness to commands, palpable pulses, and systolic BP >90 mm Hg.

< N O T E : The following interventions should be performed after an assessment of breathlessness and pulselessness has been made.

1. Ensure that patient's airway is patent by maintaining the head-tilt/chin-lift maneuver and then oxygenate patient adequately *via* mouth-to-mouth respiration. Give two initial breaths of 1-1 1/2 seconds each. Ensure that each breath is of sufficient volume to cause the patient's chest to rise and that air is heard and felt during patient's exhalation.

2. Deliver serial and rhythmic compressions to the lower half of the sternum, while keeping patient in a supine position. To ensure adequate compression, depress the sternum 3.8-5.0 cm (1.5-2 in) for an adult of normal size, releasing the pressure completely between compressions to allow blood to flow into the heart. Provide 80-100 compressions per minute, allowing as much time between compressions as it takes to deliver each compression. If alone, deliver 15 compressions followed by two ventilations. If assisted, deliver 5 compressions to 1 ventilation. Evaluate effectiveness of the compressions by palpating for carotid pulses during compression.

3. Ensure that cardiac monitoring is in place for dysrhythmia recognition and prompt treatment with antiarrhythmic agents/electric shock when appropriate.

4. Establish and maintain IV line. Unless a central line is already in place, use antecubital vein. Usually, D_5W is used to keep the vein open.

5. When pulses are palpated, check BP q1-5min; support BP with inotropic drugs as prescribed.

6. Evaluate acid-base status *via* ABG results. ABG results during cardiac arrest can vary. The following are examples of findings and their implications.
   • *Respiratory acidosis* (e.g., pH 7.28, Pao_2 70, $Paco_2$ 65). Need to increase oxygenation and ventilation.
   • *Respiratory alkalosis* (e.g., pH 7.58, Pao_2 100, $Paco_2$ 22). Need to decrease ventilation.
   • *Metabolic acidosis* (e.g., pH 7.3, Pao_2 100, $Paco_2$ 40, HCO_3^- 15). Needs bicarbonate.
   • *Metabolic alkalosis* (e.g., pH 7.6, Pao_2 100, $Paco_2$ 40, HCO_3^- 32). Too much bicarbonate.

7. After pulse and BP have been established, assess LOC and monitor respirations. The patient may be responsive and have some spontaneous respirations.

8. For a detailed discussion of interventions made in relation to specific dysrhythmias, see "ACLS Algorithms," pp. 527-534, in the Appendix.

9. Ensure that family members and significant others are notified of critical changes in the patient's condition. Prepare them before they visit the patient by providing simple and brief explanations of changes in patient's color and responsiveness and presence of tubes.

For other nursing diagnoses and interventions, see the following: "Caring for the Critically Ill with Life-Threatening Disorders," pp. 511-522; and "Caring for the Family of the Critically Ill," pp. 522-526.

REHABILITATION AND PATIENT-FAMILY TEACHING CONCEPTS

Refer to discussion under patient's primary diagnosis.

Cardiac Trauma

Cardiac trauma is caused by blunt or penetrating injuries to the heart. *Blunt cardiac trauma* commonly is caused by acceleration-deceleration injury in a motor vehicle accident, during which the driver slams forward against the steering wheel. When this occurs, the heart muscle is injured by one or more of four mechanisms: compression of the heart between the sternum and vertebrae, bruising of heart tissue by bony structures, rupture or compression of coronary arteries by the blow, or cardiac rupture due to intrathoracic or intra-abdominal pressure. Blunt cardiac trauma can be classified as cardiac concussion or cardiac contusion. With cardiac concussion, the less severe injury, the patient will demonstrate many of the clinical signs and symptoms of cardiac trauma, without any evidence of cellular injury. In comparison, cardiac contusion involves the demonstrable cellular necrosis of myocardial infarction. Blunt injuries also may damage the ventricular septum, valves, and papillary muscle attachment.

Penetrating cardiac trauma is caused by gunshot wounds, stab wounds, or foreign bodies in the heart. The right ventricle, which rests below the junction of the sternum and xiphoid process, is thin-walled and forms the largest percentage of the anterior portion of the heart. Because of its anterior location, the right ventricle is the chamber most commonly involved in this type of injury. Penetrating injuries are the most common cause of intrapericardial hemorrhage (see "Acute Cardiac Tamponade," p. 105).

ASSESSMENT

Signs and symptoms
- *Blunt injury:* Precordial chest pain (difficult to distinguish from angina), bradycardia or tachycardia, SOB, guarded breathing.
- *Penetrating injury:* Tachycardia, SOB, weakness, diaphoresis, acute anxiety, cool and clammy skin.

Physical assessment
- *Blunt injury:* Contusion marks on chest (may outline shape of steering wheel), flail chest (loss of continuity of bony thorax because of rib fracture) with resulting paradoxical respiratory movement of the chest wall, murmurs indicating valvular injury, atrial or ventricular gallops (if cardiac injury has decreased ventricular contractility).
- *Penetrating injury:* Protrusion of penetrating instrument (e.g., knife, ice pick), external puncture wound, signs of cardiac tamponade (see "Acute Cardiac Tamponade," p. 105).

History and risk factors: Motor vehicle accident, assault, sporting accident, auto-pedestrian accident.

EKG and hemodynamic monitoring measurements
- *Cardiac monitor:* Sinus tachycardia, sinus bradycardia, ventricular tachycardia, ventricular fibrillation, asystole, and ST and T-wave changes.
- *Arterial blood pressure:* Decreased.

DIAGNOSTIC TESTS

There is no clear agreement on the diagnostic criteria for the medical diagnosis of cardiac contusion. Elevations of the creatinine phosphokinase MB fraction, echocardiography, electrocardiography, and myocardial scanning are considered reliable aids in making the diagnosis, but no single test is widely accepted as the definitive diagnostic tool. The following diagnostic tests may demonstrate abnormal results with cardiac contusion.

1. *Chest x-ray:* Although heart muscle damage will not appear on routine chest x-ray, x-ray may reveal damage to bony structures of the chest.
2. *Cardiac enzymes:* Myocardial band isoenzymes phosphokinase (CPK) will be increased >7-8% of the total CPK in the presence of cardiac cellular injury.
3. *EKG:* Cardiac injury causes alterations in depolarization, repolarization, and in muscle perfusion. The following abnormalities occur: ST-segment changes, T-wave changes, prolongation of QT interval, sinus tachycardia, heart block, and ventricular dysrhythmias.
4. *Multiple gated acquisition (MUGA) scan:* In the presence of a contusion, detects decreased ability of the heart to pump efficiently.
5. *Echocardiogram:* Detects abnormalities in wall motion and valvular function and presence of intracavity thrombi or pericardial effusion.
6. *Technetium pyrophosphate myocardial scan:* Identifies localized area(s) of radioisotope uptake by damaged myocardial cells, revealed as ''hot spot(s)'' on the scan.

MEDICAL MANAGEMENT AND SURGICAL INTERVENTIONS

For blunt injuries

1. **Treatment of dysrhythmias:** Antiarrhythmic agents (e.g., lidocaine for ventricular dysrhythmias and digitalis for pump failure or tachycardia) or temporary pacemakers for heart block. If rhythm disturbances do not appear in the first five days following trauma, they rarely occur later.
2. **Relief of acute pain:** Usually with IV morphine sulfate in small increments unless hypotension occurs.
3. **Restriction of activity and institution of continuous observation**
4. **Immediate corrective surgical repair:** For ruptured valve, torn papillary muscle, or torn intraventricular septum accompanied by hemodynamic instability.
5. **Treatment of shock:** With fluid resuscitation, pressor agents.
6. **Treatment of myocardial failure:** Oxygen, diuretics, positive inotropic agents, and monitoring with a pulmonary artery catheter for right- and left-sided heart pressures.

For penetrating injuries

1. **Surgical intervention:** Foreign bodies of reasonable size are localized by fluoroscopic examination and removed surgically.

< C A U T I O N :   Because of the potential for hemorrhage or pneumothorax, never remove a penetrating object until a surgeon is present.

< E X C E P T I O N :   If life-threatening signs of tension pneumothorax are present, the pressure must be relieved.

2. **Antimicrobial agents:** To control infections that occur secondary to contamination by the penetrating instrument.
3. For more information, see interventions in ''Acute Cardiac Tamponade,'' p. 106.

NURSING DIAGNOSES AND INTERVENTIONS

Alteration in tissue perfusion: Peripheral, cardiopulmonary, renal, and cerebral related to impaired circulation (ischemia) secondary to decreased cardiac contractility

---

Desired outcome: Patient has adequate perfusion as evidenced by systolic BP ≥100 mm Hg; HR ≤100 bpm; urine output ≥30 ml/hr; brisk capillary refill (<3 seconds); peripheral pulses >2+ on a 0-4+ scale; normal sinus rhythm; and orientation to person, place, and time.

---

1. Perform a complete cardiac assessment q4h, noting peripheral pulses, heart sounds, and capillary refill; assess heart rate and rhythm and BP hourly. For more assessment information, see **Alterations in cardiac output,** p. 107, in "Acute Cardiac Tamponade" and **Impaired gas exchange,** p. 30, in "Pneumothorax."
2. Notify MD of changes in mental status, systolic BP <100 mm Hg or a drop of >20 mm Hg from trend, delayed capillary refill, or absent or thready peripheral pulses.
3. Administer fluids as prescribed to maintain systolic BP at ≥100 mm Hg and urine output at ≥30 ml/hour.
4. Maintain continuous cardiac monitoring for the first 3-4 days following cardiac trauma.
5. If dysrhythmias occur, prepare to administer antiarrhythmic agents or assist with insertion of a temporary pacemaker.
6. If hemodynamic instability occurs, place patient in supine position, if injuries allow, and prepare for initiation of pulmonary artery pressure monitoring.

Alteration in comfort: Precordial chest pain related to myocardial damage and chest wall injuries

---

Desired outcome: Patient states that a reduction in discomfort has occurred and does not exhibit signs of uncontrolled pain.

---

1. Assess and document location, type, severity, and duration of patient's discomfort. Administer analgesia as prescribed and record its effectiveness. Pain may begin immediately after injury or after approximately eight hours. Usually, it is not affected by coronary vasodilators.
2. Place patient in a position of comfort. Often, patients prefer the HOB elevated at 30°-45°.
3. If bony structures are damaged and pain limits coughing and deep breathing, assist patient with chest splinting during chest physiotherapy. For some patients, intercostal nerve blocks may be necessary.
4. Teach patient to recognize signs of posttraumatic pericarditis (see "Rehabilitation and Patient-Family Teaching Concepts," on p. 105).

For other nursing diagnoses and interventions, see "Caring for the Critically Ill on Prolonged Bed Rest," pp. 506-511; "Caring for the Critically Ill with Life-Threatening Disorders,'' pp. 511-522; and ''Caring for the Family of the Critically Ill,'' pp. 522-526.

REHABILITATION AND PATIENT-FAMILY TEACHING CONCEPTS

Give patient and significant others verbal and written instructions for the following:

1. Indicators of posttraumatic pericarditis, which can occur shortly after the injury or as long as months later. Signs and symptoms include fever, diaphoresis, and precordial chest pain; if they occur, patient should notify MD promptly.
2. Medications, including name, purpose, dosage, route, schedule, precautions, and potential side effects.
3. Type and dates of follow-up treatment.
4. Activity after hospital discharge. Generally, activity is limited for 2-4 weeks.

Acute cardiac tamponade

Acute cardiac tamponade is the sudden accumulation of blood or fluid in the pericardial space, resulting in compression of the heart muscle and interference with cardiac filling during diastole and cardiac ejection during systole. Tamponade may occur as a result of blunt or penetrating cardiac trauma or as a complication following cardiac catheterization, anticoagulant therapy, myocardial infarction, or acute pericarditis.

The primary effect of sudden cardiac tamponade is hemodynamic compromise, with inadequate cardiac ouput and decreased tissue perfusion. Normally, the pericardial sac contains 10-20 ml of fluid that protects the myocardium. Because the pericardial sac has minimal stretching ability, the sudden addition of as little as 50-100 ml of fluid can increase intrapericardial pressure markedly. As intrapericardial pressure increases and exceeds central venous pressure, the atria, ventricles, and coronary arteries become compressed. The compressed heart chambers, which no longer can hold their usual volume, cause a reduction in end diastolic volume and end diastolic fiber stretch and a decrease in stroke volume. Ultimately, decreased cardiac output and poor tissue perfusion occur.

ASSESSMENT

Signs and symptoms: Tachycardia, decreased BP, shock, pallor, confusion, restlessness, cold and clammy skin, dyspnea, oliguria, thready pulse.

Physical assessment: See Table 2-7.

< C A U T I O N : In severe hypovolemic states, physical signs may be masked.

EKG and hemodynamic measurements

- *Cardiac monitor:* May show evidence of sinus tachycardia.
- *Pulmonary artery catheter:* Elevation of right atrial pressure (early sign if severe hypotension does not occur); elevation of left ventricular end diastolic pressure (late sign).

DIAGNOSTIC TESTS

1. *EKG:* May reveal ST-segment elevation, nonspecific ST and T-wave changes (representing myocardial ischemia), and electrical alternans (alternation of the QRS axis from beat to beat) caused by the heart's movement like a pendulum

TABLE 2-7
Physical signs of acute cardiac tamponade

Physical sign	Explanation for findings in cardiac tamponade
Muffled heart sounds	Accumulation of fluid surrounding the heart diminishes the sounds of valve closure.
CVP elevated to >12 mm Hg	The mean right atrial pressure is elevated because diastolic filling is impeded by atrial compression.
Decreased blood pressure	Compression by the tamponade reduces ventricular filling, decreasing cardiac output and blood pressure.
Jugular venous distention	As the atria and ventricles become compressed, there is less space for diastolic filling, causing impairment of venous return.
Pulsus paradoxus: A fall of ≥10 mm Hg in systolic BP during inspiration	Two possible explanations: 1) During each inspiration, blood pools in the pulmonary veins, reducing left ventricular filling and output. 2) With inspiration, the intraventricular septum shifts toward the left ventricle, causing more volume to be drawn to the right heart rather than to the left heart.
Absence of Kussmaul's sign (a rise, rather than a fall, in venous pressure during inspiration)	On inspiration, blood is accelerated toward the right atrium because of the septal shift toward the left ventricle.

within the pericardial effusion. The underlying mechanism for this movement is not understood.

2. *Chest x-ray:* May reveal normal cardiac silhouette, clear lung fields, dilatation of the superior vena cava, and an enlarged mediastinum.

3. *Echocardiogram:* May show echo-free space anterior to the right ventricular wall and posterior to the left ventricular wall, with a decrease in right ventricular chamber size. There will be right-to-left intraventricular septal shift during inspiration.

MEDICAL MANAGEMENT AND SURGICAL INTERVENTIONS

1. **Pericardiocentesis:** Needle aspiration of the pericardium by the subxiphoid or left parasternal approach to drain the pericardial space of the excess fluid. Often, the blood removed from the pericardium will not clot due to breaking down of clotting factors (defibrination) within the pericardial sac by heart action. Evidence exists that pericardiocentesis alone does not manage acute pericardial tamponade; surgical exploration is recommended following this procedure because of the high incidence of recurrent bleeding if surgery is not performed.

2. **Surgical procedures:** Subxiphoid pericardiostomy involves a resection of the xiphoid process to drain the pericardial sac; it can be done under local anesthesia. In addition, other, more extensive surgical procedures such as a pericardiectomy can be used to decompress a pericardial tamponade.

3. **Fluid resuscitation:** To increase filling pressures during diastole, resulting in increased cardiac output and blood pressure. Blood products, colloids, or crystalloids may be used.

4. Inotropic agents: To increase myocardial contractility and support cardiac output. Examples include dopamine, norepinephrine, phenylephrine, isoproterenol, and amrinone.

5. Oxygen, intubation, mechanical ventilation, as necessary: To correct hypoxia.

NURSING DIAGNOSES AND INTERVENTIONS

Alterations in cardiac output: Decreased, related to diminished ventricular filling secondary to compression of ventricles by fluid in the pericardial sac

---

Desired outcome: Patient has adequate cardiac output as evidenced by mean RAP 4-6 mm Hg, mean PAWP 6-12 mm Hg, PAP 20-30/8-15 mm Hg, CO 4-7 L/min, systolic BP ≥100 mm Hg, HR 60-100 bpm, normal sinus rhythm on EKG, and absence of new murmurs or gallops, distended neck veins, and pulsus paradoxus.

---

1. Assess cardiovascular function by evaluating heart sounds and neck veins hourly. Notify MD of muffled heart sounds, new murmurs, new gallops, irregularities in rate and rhythm, and distended neck veins.
2. Evaluate patient for pulsus paradoxus (an abnormal decrease in arterial systolic BP during inspiration compared to that with expiration).
   - After placing BP cuff on patient, inflate it above the known systolic BP. Instruct patient to breathe normally.
   - While slowly deflating the cuff, auscultate BP.
   - Listen for the first Korotkoff sound, which will occur during expiration with cardiac tamponade.
   - Note the manometer reading when the first sound occurs and continue to deflate the cuff slowly until Korotkoff sounds are audible throughout inspiration and expiration.
   - Record the difference in mm Hg between the first and second sounds. This is the pulsus paradoxus.
3. Measure and record hemodynamic parameters. Notify MD of abnormalities or changes in trend.
4. Evaluate EKG for ST-segment changes, T-wave changes, rate, and rhythm. The optimal is sinus rhythm or sinus tachycardia. Maintain patient on continuous cardiac monitoring.
5. Administer blood products, colloids, or crystalloids through large-bore intravenous lines in the periphery, if possible. Compared to the longer and narrower central catheters, peripheral IV catheters provide less resistance to rapid infusion during fluid resuscitation. Be prepared to administer pressor agents if fluid resuscitation does not support patient's BP.
6. Have emergency equipment available for immediate pulmonary artery catheterization, central line insertion, pericardiocentesis, or surgical drainage of blood accumulation in the pericardial sac.

Alteration in tissue perfusion: Cardiovascular, peripheral, cerebral, and renal, related to impaired circulation secondary to acute cardiac tamponade

Desired outcome: Patient has adequate perfusion as evidenced by orientation to person, place, and time; systolic BP ≥100 mm Hg; peripheral pulses >2+ on a 0-4+ scale; equal and normoreactive pupils; warm and dry skin; brisk capillary refill (<3 seconds); and urine output ≥30 ml/hr.

1. Assess tissue perfusion by evaluating the following at least qh: LOC, BP, pulses, pupillary response, skin temperature, and capillary refill.
2. Evaluate urine output hourly to ensure that it is at least 30 ml/hour. Assess urine specific gravity q4h; elevations (>1.030) may signal inadequate kidney perfusion.
3. Maintain tissue perfusion by delivering prescribed blood products, colloids, or crystalloids.
4. If hypotension occurs, be prepared to administer pharmacotherapy to maintain BP. Be familar with dosage, side effects, and calculations necessary for administration. At frequent intervals, assess peripheral intravenous lines for evidence of infiltration. Pressor agents, which infiltrate subcutaneous tissues, jeopardize future tissue perfusion.

< N O T E :   When feasible, all pressor agents (e.g., dopamine) should be infused through a central line.

For other nursing diagnoses and interventions, see "Caring for the Critically Ill on Prolonged Bed Rest," pp. 506-511; "Caring for the Critically Ill with Life-Threatening Disorders," pp. 511-522; and "Caring for the Family of the Critically Ill," pp. 522-526.

REHABILITATION AND PATIENT-FAMILY TEACHING CONCEPTS

Give patient and significant others verbal and written instructions for the following:
1. Medications, including name, purpose, dosage, route, schedule, precautions, and potential side effects.
2. Type and dates of follow-up treatment and procedures, particularly EKGs.
3. Activity limitations after hospital discharge: Activity is usually kept at a minimum for 2-4 weeks.

Acute infective endocarditis

Infective endocarditis (IE) is infection of the endocardium (the innermost layer of the heart), which often involves the natural or prosthetic valve. It is caused by bacteria, viruses, fungi, or rickettsiae. Four mechanisms are known to contribute to the development of IE. One is a congenital or acquired defect of the heart valve or the septum. Frequently, it is accompanied by a jet-venturi stream of blood flowing from a high- to low-pressure area through a narrow opening. This occurs when there is a septal defect or a stenotic or insufficient valve. The low-pressure sink beyond the narrowed jet flow site provides an area that is ideal for colonization by any infecting organism. The second mechanism is the formation of a sterile platelet fibrin thrombus at the low-pressure site, which gives rise to vegetation. Third, a bacteremia occurs secondary to colonization in the vegetation. Finally, a high level of agglutinating antibodies promotes the growth of the vegetation.

Portals of entry for the infecting organism include the mouth and gastrointestinal (GI) tract, upper airway, skin, and external genitourinary (GU) tract. Any heart valve can become infected, but the aortic and mitral valves are more common sites than the right-sided pulmonic and tricuspid valves. Once the infection process begins, valvular dysfunction, manifested by insufficiency with regurgitant blood flow, can occur, ultimately resulting in a decrease in cardiac output. The vegetation may become so large that it obstructs the valve orifice, mimicking valvular stenosis, and reducing cardiac output further. At times, pieces of the vegetation may break off and embolize to vital organs. In severe cases, the affected valve may necrose, develop an aneurysm, and rupture; or the infection may extend through the myocardium and epicardium to cause a pericarditis (see ''Acute Pericarditis,'' p. 116). Mortality rates between 20% and 50% have been reported with IE. Recurrence of the infection occurs at a rate of 10-20%.

ASSESSMENT

Acute infective stage: Fever, diaphoresis, fatigue, anorexia, joint pain, weight loss, and abdominal pain. The severity of symptoms will vary, depending on the infective organism. For example, *Staphylococcus albus* will produce more severe symptoms than will *Streptococcus viridans*.

Physical assessment: A new or changed murmur may be heard, owing to the valvular dysfunction. See Table 2-8 for a description of the types of murmurs that can be heard, depending on the valve affected and the type of dysfunction present. If heart failure has resulted from the valvular disorder, fine crackles may be auscultated at the bases of the lungs and an S_3 or S_4 heart sound may be heard. The skin is often pale, but if right-sided heart failure is present, owing to valvular insufficiency, jaundice of the skin and sclera may be present, as well as edema, neck vein distention, a positive hepatojugular reflex, and ascites. Later, anemia, petechiae, and clubbing of the fingers may occur.

Classic findings

- *Splinter hemorrhages:* Small red streaks on the distal third of the fingernails or toenails.
- *Janeway lesions:* Painless, small, hemorrhagic lesions found on the fingers, toes, nose, or earlobes, probably occurring as the result of immune complex deposition with inflammation.
- *Osler's nodes:* Painful, red, subcutaneous nodules found on the pads of the fingers or on the feet, probably occurring as a result of emboli producing small areas of gangrene or vasculitis.
- *Roth's spots:* Retinal hemorrhages with pale centers seen on fundoscopic exam.

< N O T E : If emboli of the vegetations occur in other areas, signs and symptoms of CVA; peripheral obstruction; or myocardial, renal, or mesenteric infarct will be seen.

Hemodynamic measurements: Invasive monitoring devices are used cautiously with these patients to prevent further valvular dysfunction, embolization, and infection. However, when warranted, a pulmonary artery (PA) catheter may be used to assess hemodynamic function. Elevations of PAP or RAP can be expected in most patients with IE. In addition, reduced CO usually is present.

TABLE 2-8

Assessment findings with infective endocarditis

Valve dysfunction	Murmur	Pathology	Hemodynamic changes
Aortic stenosis	Systolic, blowing murmur at 2nd ICS, right sternal border (RSB); may radiate to the neck.	Reduced flow across aortic valve with increased left ventricular volume and pressure with diminished CO. Left ventricular hypertrophy eventually occurs.	Increased left ventricular (LV) pressure; increased PA end diastolic pressure (PAEDP). Decreased CO and aortic pressure with a narrow pulse pressure reflecting the decreased stroke volume.
Aortic insufficiency	Diastolic blowing murmur at 2nd ICS, RSB, beginning immediately with S_2.	Regurgitant blood flow from aorta to left ventricle during diastole.	Increased LV pressure; increased PAEDP. Decreased CO, increased systolic BP, and widened pulse pressure.
Mitral stenosis	Loud, long, diastolic rumbling murmur at 5th ICS, midclavicular line (MCL); may radiate to axilla. S_1 is loud; there is opening snap with S_2.	Reduced flow across mitral valve with left atrial and pulmonary congestion.	Increased mean PAP; decreased CO.
Mitral insufficiency	Systolic murmur at 5th ICS, MCL.	Regurgitant blood flow from left ventricle to left atrium, resulting in pulmonary congestion.	Giant V waves in PA occlusive tracing; increased systolic PAP; decreased CO. Mean PAP may be normal.
Pulmonic stenosis	Systolic blowing murmur at 2nd ICS, left sternal border (LSB); may radiate to neck.	Reduced flow across pulmonic valve with increased right ventricular (RV) volume and pressure with diminished LV return, resulting in reduced CO.	Increased RV systolic pressure, mean RAP, PAEDP, and mean PAP.
Pulmonic insufficiency	Diastolic murmur at 2nd ICS, LSB that starts later and is lower pitched than an aortic murmur.	Regurgitant blood flow from pulmonary artery to right ventricle during diastole, resulting in right ventricular overload.	Increased systolic RV pressure with wide pulse pressure. LVEDP and CO often normal but may decrease if disorder is severe.

Continued.

T A B L E 2 - 8 cont'd.

Assessment findings with infective endocarditis

Valve dysfunction	Murmur	Pathology	Hemodynamic changes
Tricuspid stenosis	Diastolic murmur at 4th ICS.	Reduced flow across tricuspid valve with increased right atrial and venous congestion.	CVP elevated with accentuated A wave on the RA waveform.
Tricuspid insufficiency	Pansystolic murmur at 4th ICS, LSB that increases in intensity with inspiration.	Regurgitant blood flow from right ventricle to right atrium. Right atrial and venous congestion occurs.	Increased CVP with prominent V wave on the RA tracing. Normal or low PAP, LVEDP, and CO.

History and risk factors: Invasive procedures, such as temporary pacemaker insertion, PA catheter insertion, transurethral resection, endoscopy, surgery, or dental work, put the patient with a preexisting valvular disorder at greater risk of developing the bacteremia that can lead to IE. The increase in IV drug abuse over the past few years has led to an increase in IE, especially IE involving the tricuspid valve. An immunosuppressed patient (i.e., one with a transplant, carcinoma, burns, or diabetes mellitus) also is at risk for developing IE.

DIAGNOSTIC TESTS

1. *Blood cultures:* Provide the definitive diagnosis of the infecting organism. If the results are negative, the patient may be past the acute infective phase, and cultures may be repeated later.

2. *Echocardiogram:* Reveals valvular involvement and vegetation size and defines the severity of the valvular dysfunction. M-mode, two-dimensional, or Doppler echocardiograms may be used.

3. *EKG:* While not useful in diagnosing IE, it is frequently performed to determine if conduction system defects are present. AV node or bundle of His may be affected as the area of infection spreads. Right or left atrial or ventricular enlargement may be seen, owing to prolonged hemodynamic effects on chamber size or muscle wall thickness (see Table 2-9). Atrial dysrhythmias frequently are seen as that chamber enlarges from volume overload. Premature atrial contractions (PACs), paroxysmal atrial tachycardia (PAT), supraventricular tachycardia (SVT), atrial flutter, or atrial fibrillation may be seen on the EKG or monitor strip.

4. *Hematology studies:* Will show an increase in the WBC count and eosinophil rate. Frequently, anemia is present.

5. *Cardiac enzymes:* Will be elevated if a myocardial infarction occurs due to emboli of vegetations that migrate to the coronary arteries.

6. *ABG values:* Evaluated to determine the degree of pulmonary dysfunction secondary to the cardiac disorder.

7. *Additional studies:* May be performed to assess for embolization to other or-

TABLE 2-9
EKG changes seen with ventricular and atrial hypertrophy

Chamber	EKG change
Left ventricular enlargement (LVE)	"R" voltage increases in V_{4-6}; "S" voltage increases (deeper inflection in V_{1-2}). The sum of "S" in V_1 or V_2 and "R" in V_5 or V_6 will be >35 mm; or "R" in any V lead will be >25 mm.
Left atrial enlargement (LAE)	"P mitrale" in leads II, III, aVF, and V_1. The P wave is m-shaped with a duration >0.1 second.
Right ventricular enlargement (RVE)	"R" voltage increased in V_{1-2}. "S" voltage increased in V_{5-6}. The sum of "R" in V_1 or V_2 and "S" in V_5 or V_6 will be ≥35 mm.
Right atrial enlargement (RAE)	"P pulmonale" in leads II, III, aVF, and V_1. The P wave is >2.5 mm voltage and <0.1 second duration.

gans. Studies such as renal, mesenteric, or peripheral arteriograms or CT scan may be done.

MEDICAL MANAGEMENT AND SURGICAL INTERVENTIONS

1. **Antibiotic treatment:** Patients usually require 6-8 weeks of IV antibiotics. The antibiotic selected is based on the results of the blood culture and sensitivity studies.
2. **Fluid and sodium limitations:** Often required to promote optimal hemodynamics. Specific restrictions must be individualized, based on severity of symptoms and impairment of hemodynamic function.
3. **Bed rest:** Recommended initially, with activity limitations throughout the remainder of the treatment.
4. **Diet:** High in protein and calories to prevent cardiac cachexia.
5. **Pharmacotherapy**
   - *Diuretics and vasodilators:* May be required to decrease the symptoms of congestive heart failure by decreasing preload.
   - *Positive inotropic agents* (e.g., digoxin, dobutamine, amrinone): May be needed to increase contractility and cardiac output.
   - *Nitroprusside:* To reduce afterload.
   - *Sedation:* May be necessary to allay patient's anxiety during this long period of hospitalization.
6. **Oxygen therapy:** Administered as needed at an FIO_2 that maintains PaO_2 >60 mm Hg and oxygen saturation at >95%.
7. **Treatment of other signs and symptoms:** If heart failure has resulted from the valvular disorder, see "Congestive Heart Failure," p. 86, for treatment of those signs and symptoms. See "Cardiogenic Shock," p. 132, for the medical treatment that may be necessary if the valvular dysfunction deteriorates to the point that it is life-threatening.
8. **Surgical valve replacement:** Required when hemodynamic function deteriorates or if the infection does not respond to antibiotic therapy. See "Valvular Heart Disease and Valve Surgery," p. 153.

NURSING DIAGNOSES AND INTERVENTIONS

Alterations in cardiac output: Decreased, related to altered preload, afterload, or contractility secondary to valvular dysfunction

---

Desired outcomes: Patient has adequate hemodynamic function with controlled atrial fibrillation as evidenced by normal sinus rhythm, HR ≤100 bpm, BP >90/60 mm Hg, stable weights, intake equal to output plus insensible losses, RR ≤20 breaths/min with normal depth and pattern (eupnea), and absence of S_3 or S_4 heart sounds, crackles, distended neck veins, and other clinical signs of heart failure. Optimally, the following normal parameters will be achieved: CO 4-7 L/min, CVP 2-6 mm Hg, PAP 20-30/8-15 mm Hg, RAP 4-6 mm Hg, and MAP 60-105 mm Hg.

---

1. Assess heart sounds q2-4h. A change in the characteristics of a heart murmur may signal progression of valvular dysfunction, which can occur with insufficiency, stenosis, or dislodgement of vegetation.
2. Assess for the presence of an extra heart sound. A new S_3 or S_4 sound may signal heart failure.
3. Monitor heart rhythm continuously. Report dysrhythmias or conduction defects, which may be indicative of the spread of infection to the conduction system or atrial volume overload.
4. Monitor for signs of left-sided heart failure secondary to valvular dysfunction: crackles (rales), S_3 or S_4 sounds, dyspnea, tachypnea, digital clubbing, decreased BP, increased pulse pressure, increased left ventricular end diastolic pressure (LVEDP), and decreased CO.
5. Monitor for signs of right-sided heart failure secondary to valvular dysfunction: increased CVP, distended neck veins, positive hepatojugular reflex, edema, jaundice, ascites.
6. Monitor I&O hourly and measure weight daily. To help prevent miscalculations of patient's weight, use the same scale and amount of clothing and weigh patient at the same time of day. Notify MD if patient's weight increases by more than 1 kilogram (2 pounds) per day.
7. If patient's PAP or RAP is high, decrease preload by limiting fluid and sodium intake and administering diuretics and venous dilators as prescribed.
8. If patient's MAP is high, decrease afterload with prescribed arterial dilators.
9. If afterload is low, increase afterload with vasopressors, as prescribed.

< N O T E :   See "Cardiogenic Shock," p. 134, for a discussion of preload and afterload medications.

10. If afterload is low, prevent further reductions caused by vasodilation, for example, by avoiding administration of morphine sulfate or rapid warming of the hypothermic patient.
11. Increase contractility with positive inotropes, as prescribed.
12. Limit patient's activities to reduce myocardial oxygen needs; schedule patient care activities according to patient's tolerance.
13. Help patient reduce stress by teaching stress-reduction techniques, such as imagery, meditation, or progressive muscle relaxation. For description of a relax-

ation technique, see **Knowledge deficit:** Relaxation technique effective for stress reduction and facilitation of decreased sympathetic tone, p. 98.

14. Provide sedation as needed.
15. Prevent orthostatic hypotension by changing patient's position slowly.

Impaired gas exchange related to decreased diffusion of oxygen secondary to pulmonary congestion

---

Desired outcome: Patient has adequate gas exchange as evidenced by RR ≤ 20 breaths/min with normal pattern and depth (eupnea), SVO_2 60-80%, $PaO_2 \geq 80$ mm Hg, oxygen saturation $\geq 95\%$, and natural skin color.

---

1. Assess rate, effort, and depth of patient's respirations. Tachypnea may be indicative of pulmonary congestion, as the respiratory rate increases to compensate for the decreased depth caused by pulmonary congestion or airway obstruction.
2. Assess color of skin and mucous membranes, being alert to pallor as a signal of impaired oxygenation.
3. Auscultate lungs q2h. Report presence of crackles (which are most often found at the lung bases), rhonchi, and wheezing.
4. If hemodynamic monitoring with oximetry is used, assess mixed venous oxygen saturation (SVO_2). SVO_2 will fall below normal when oxygen uptake is increased owing to increased metabolic demands or if extraction is increased owing to reduced oxygen delivery. This change occurs before there is a change in symptoms and it correlates with cardiac output.
5. Monitor ABG values for evidence of hypoxemia (PaO_2 <80 mm Hg), respiratory acidosis ($PaCO_2$ >45 mm Hg, pH <7.35), or respiratory alkalosis ($PaCO_2$ <35 mm Hg, pH >7.45), which may be present with pulmonary congestion.
6. Deliver humidified oxygen, as prescribed.
7. Assess arterial oxygen saturation with a transcutaneous pulse oximeter. Normal oxygen saturation is 95-100%. Levels of 90-95% necessitate frequent assessment. Levels <90% require aggressive interventions to increase oxygen saturation. This is accomplished by increasing FIO_2, decreasing preload, and increasing the number of coughing and deep-breathing exercises.
8. Unless contraindicated, place patient in high-Fowler's position to facilitate gas exchange.
9. Schedule coughing, deep breathing, and incentive spirometry q2-4h to prevent atelectasis.

Potential for infection (secondary) related to vulnerability secondary to prolonged antibiotic use and presence of invasive catheters and lines

---

Desired outcomes: Patient is free of secondary infection as evidenced by urine that is clear with characteristic odor, wound healing within acceptable timeframe, and absence of erythema, warmth, and purulent drainage at insertion sites for IV lines. Upon resolution of acute stage of IE, patient remains normothermic with WBC count $\leq$11,000 μl, negative cultures, and HR $\leq$100 bpm. SVR is $\geq$900 dynes/sec/cm^{-5}, CO is $\leq$7 L/min, and SVO$_2$ is 60-80%.

1. Ensure strict aseptic technique for insertion site care for all invasive monitoring devices and IV lines.
2. Change tubing, collection containers, and peripheral needles and catheters q48-72hrs, per agency protocol.
3. Provide mouth care q4h to minimize the potential for fungal infections.
4. For patients with in-dwelling urinary catheters, cleanse urinary meatus with soap and water with the daily bath. Inspect urine for evidence of infection, such as casts, cloudiness, or foul odor. Be alert to patient complaints of burning with urination.
5. Monitor temperature, WBC count, and HR. Increases may be signs of infection.
6. Calculate SVR whenever CO measurements are obtained. Septic shock is demonstrated by an increase in CO and a drop in SVR during the early stages. In addition, SVO$_2$ may increase.
7. Teach patient and significant others the signs and symptoms of infection and the importance of notifying staff promptly if they occur.

Potential alteration in tissue perfusion: Renal, GI, peripheral, cerebral, and cardiopulmonary related to impaired circulation secondary to emboli caused by vegetations

Desired outcome: Patient has adequate perfusion as evidenced by urine output $\geq$30 ml/hr; 5-34 bowel sounds/min; peripheral pulses >2+ on a 0-4+ scale; warm and dry skin; BP >90/60; RR 12-20 breaths/min with normal pattern and depth (eupnea); normal sinus rhythm on EKG; and orientation to person, place, and time.

< N O T E : Unlike peripheral venous emboli, these emboli are caused by the vegetations; therefore, there is nothing that can be done by physicians or nurses to prevent their occurrence.

1. Monitor I&O at frequent intervals. Be alert to urinary output <30 ml/hr for two consecutive hours. Report oliguria, as it may be a sign of renal infarct.
2. Monitor bowel sounds q2h. Report hypoactive or absent bowel sounds, as they may be the result of mesenteric infarct.
3. Assess peripheral pulses, color, and temperature of extremities. Be alert to pulses $\leq$2+ (on a 4+ scale) and extremities that are pale and cool, as these findings may denote embolization to the extremities.
4. Monitor patient for confusion, changes in sensorimotor capabilities, or changes in cognition. Alterations can occur with cerebral emboli.
5. Assess for chest pain, decreased BP, SOB, ischemic or injury pattern on 12-lead EKG, or elevated cardiac enzymes. These may be signs of myocardial infarction due to emboli of vegetations that have migrated to the coronary arteries. See "Acute Myocardial Infarction," p. 79.
6. Assess for and report appearance of splinter hemorrhages, Osler's nodes, Janeway's lesions, and Roth's spots.

As appropriate, see nursing diagnoses and interventions in the following: "Congestive Heart Failure," pp. 86-89; "Cardiogenic Shock," pp. 134-136; "Management of the Adult with Hemodynamic Monitoring," pp. 168-170; "Providing Nutritional Support," pp. 490-505; "Caring for the Critically Ill on Prolonged Bed Rest," pp. 506-511; "Caring for the Critically Ill with Life-Threatening Disorders," pp. 511-522; and "Caring for the Family of the Critically Ill," pp. 522-526.

REHABILITATION AND PATIENT-FAMILY TEACHING CONCEPTS

Give patient and significant others verbal and written instructions for the following:

1. Importance of reporting signs and symptoms of recurring infections (e.g., fever, malaise, flushing, anorexia) or heart failure (e.g., dyspnea, tachypnea, tachycardia, digital clubbing, edema, ascites, weight gain, jaundice).

2. Medications, including drug name, purpose, dosage, schedule, precautions, and potential side effects.

3. Importance of prophylactic antibiotics prior to invasive procedures such as dental exams or surgery. The American Heart Association publishes general guidelines for prophylactic antibiotic treatment for preventing IE. This information may be obtained from the local chapter of this organization and should be provided to all consulting physicians.

Acute pericarditis

Pericarditis is the general term for an inflammatory process involving the epicardial surface of the heart and the protective covering, the pericardium. The inflammatory process can occur as the result of a myocardial infarction; infection; or an immunologic, chemical, or mechanical event. Often, early pericarditis manifests as a dry irritation, while late pericarditis (after 6 weeks) involves pericardial effusions that can lead to cardiac tamponade if severe. Most often, pericarditis is seen in ICU as a secondary finding in the critically ill patient. Because it can be masked by the primary condition, astute assessment and recognition are essential for appropriate treatment. Occasionally, patients are admitted to ICU with cardiac decompensation caused by the effusions.

Initial pathophysiology of pericarditis includes infiltration of polymorphonuclear leukocytes, increased vascularity, and fibrin deposit. The inflammation may spread from the pericardium to the epicardium or pleura. Eventually, the visceral layer develops exudates, and in some cases, adhesions may develop. See Table 2-10 for conditions that are associated with the development of pericarditis.

ASSESSMENT

Signs and symptoms: The chief complaint is chest pain, but location and quality can vary. Usually the pain is aggravated by a supine position, coughing, deep inspiration, and swallowing. Dyspnea develops because of shallow breathing to prevent pain.

- *Early indicators:* Fatigue, pallor, fever, and anorexia.
- *Late indicators* (evident after development of effusions): Increased dyspnea, crackles (rales), and neck vein distention. Heart sounds will be distant and the pulmonic component of the second heart sound will be accentuated. Joint pain may be present when inflammation is generalized.

TABLE 2-10

Conditions associated with the development of pericarditis

Idiopathic	Rheumatologic disease
Infection	• Rheumatic fever
Myocardial infarction (MI)	• Rheumatoid arthritis
Autoimmune cardiac injury	• Systemic lupus erythematosus
• Dressler's syndrome (post MI)	Neoplasms
• Post pericardiotomy syndrome	Radiation injury
Trauma	Drug-induced
Uremia	• Procainamide, hydralazine

Physical assessment: Auscultation of heart sounds often will reveal an intermittent friction rub composed of one, two, or three components: atrial systole, ventricular systole, and rapid ventricular filling. The rub is heard best with the patient sitting and leaning forward and the diaphragm of the stethoscope positioned at the left lower sternal border.

< N O T E :   Pericarditis may persist, yet a friction rub may never be heard.

• *Pulsus paradoxus:* The BP should be checked for a paradox >10 mm Hg pressure. Normally, the systolic pressure is slightly higher during the inspiratory portion of the respiratory cycle. When effusions are present, arterial systolic BP will be decreased during inspiration and the difference will be >10 mm Hg. For procedure, see "Acute Cardiac Tamponade," p. 107.

EKG findings: During acute episodes, atrial dysrhythmias such as PAT, PACs, atrial flutter, or atrial fibrillation may occur. Late dysrhythmias include ventricular ectopy or bundle-branch blocks if the inflammatory process involves the ventricles. Diffuse ST-segment elevation can be documented as described in Table 2-11.

Hemodynamic measurements: If a pulmonary artery catheter is in place, it will reveal that the CVP, PAP, and PAWP are elevated. As effusions increase, cardiac output will decrease. If adhesions are present, the filling of the chambers may be restricted, resulting in lower volumes and pressure.

DIAGNOSTIC TESTS

1. *EKG:* Will show ST- or T-wave changes, which often are confused with ischemic changes. In pericarditis they are more diffuse and follow a four-stage pattern (see Table 2-11).

2. *Echocardiogram:* Will show absence of echoes in the areas of effusion. This test is essential for quantifying and evaluating trend of effusions, but will appear normal if the pericarditis is present without effusions.

3. *CT scan:* Will differentiate restrictive pericarditis from constrictive myopathy *via* appearance of thickened pericardium on the cross-sectional views of the thorax occurring with pericarditis.

4. *Cardiac enzymes:* May reveal elevation of the CPK and MB bands if the epicardium is inflamed.

5. *Cardiac technetium pyrophosphate scan:* May show a diffuse regional uptake in an area of epicardial inflammation.

6. *Hematologic studies:* ASO titer is elevated when the cause of the pericarditis is

TABLE 2-11

EKG changes with pericarditis

Stage	Time of change	Pattern
Stage One	Onset of pain	ST segments have a concave elevation in all leads except aVL and V_1. T waves are upright
Stage Two	1 to 7 days	Return of ST segments to baseline with T-wave flattening
Stage Three	1 to 2 weeks	Inversion of T waves without R or Q changes
Stage Four	Weeks to months	Normalization of T waves

an immunologic disorder. If the pericarditis is the result of an infection, blood cultures will identify the infecting organism.

MEDICAL MANAGEMENT

1. **Bed rest:** Enforced until pain and fever have disappeared. Activity limitations continue if effusions are present.
2. **Pharmacotherapy**
   - *Nonsteroidal anti-inflammatory medications:* Preferred for reducing inflammation, particularly if the patient has had MI or cardiac surgery, as these medications do not delay healing. In addition, these medications have fewer side effects than steroids. Examples include ASA 650 mg q3-4h, indomethacin 25-75 mg q6h, or ibuprofen.
   - *Prednisone:* Given if there is no response to the above medications. It is begun at 60-80 mg qd for 5-7 days and then tapered gradually.

< N O T E :   In the presence of effusions, anticoagulants are contraindicated because of the high risk of cardiac tamponade, which can result from bleeding into the pericardium.

3. **Subxiphoid pericardiocentesis:** If effusions persist and cardiac status begins to decompensate, this procedure is performed to remove fluid that is compressing the heart. The pericardial catheter may be removed after the fluid has been withdrawn or may be left in place for several days to allow for gradual removal of fluid. Usually, 100 ml is withdrawn q4-6h. Strict aseptic technique is essential for preventing infection.
4. **Pericardiectomy:** To prevent cardiac compression or relieve the restriction. It may be necessary in chronic pericarditis for patients with recurrent effusions or adhesions.

NURSING DIAGNOSES AND INTERVENTIONS

Ineffective breathing pattern related to guarding secondary to chest pain

Desired outcome: Patient demonstrates RR 12-20 breaths/min with normal depth and pattern (eupnea) and verbalizes that chest pain is controlled.

1. Assess the character and intensity of the chest pain. Provide prescribed pain medication as needed.
2. Teach patient to avoid aggravating factors such as a supine position. Encourage patient to alter his or her position to minimize the chest pain. The following positions may be helpful: side-lying, high Fowler's, or sitting and leaning forward.
3. Assess lung sounds q4h. If breath sounds are decreased, encourage patient to perform incentive spirometry exercises q2-4h along with coughing and deep-breathing exercises.
4. To facilitate coughing and deep-breathing, support patient's chest by splinting with pillows or teach patient to press his or her arms against the chest for added support.

Activity intolerance related to weakness and fatigue secondary to impaired cardiac function, ineffective breathing pattern, or deconditioning

---

Desired outcome: Patient exhibits cardiac tolerance to increasing levels of exercise as evidenced by peak HR $\leq$20 bpm over patient's resting HR, peak systolic BP $\leq$20 mm Hg over patient's resting systolic BP, systolic BP during peak exercise $\leq$20 mm Hg under patient's resting systolic BP, SVO_2 $\geq$60%, RR <24 breaths/min, normal sinus rhythm, warm and dry skin, and absence of crackles, murmurs, and chest pain.

< N O T E : Steroid myopathy may develop in patients on high doses of or long-term treatment with steroids. Muscle weakness occurs predominately in the large proximal muscles. Patients experience difficulty in lifting objects and moving from a sitting position to a standing position.

1. Assess the patient for evidence of muscle weakness; assist with activities as needed.
2. Modify the activity plan for the patient with post-MI pericarditis who is on steroids. A lower activity level may help prevent thinning of the ventricular wall and reduce the risk of an aneurysm or rupture of the ventricle.
3. For other interventions, see the same nursing diagnosis in ''Caring for the Critically Ill on Prolonged Bed Rest,'' p. 506.

See ''Acute Cardiac Tamponade'' for the following: **Alteration in cardiac output:** Decreased, related to diminished ventricular filling secondary to compression of ventricles by fluid in the pericardial sac, p. 107. See ''Renal Transplant'' for the following: **Knowledge deficit:** Immunosuppressive medications and their side effects, pp. 195-197; **Impairment of skin integrity** related to herpetic lesions, skin fungal rashes, pruritus, and capillary fragility secondary to immunosuppression with corticosteroids, p. 198; and **Potential for infection** related to increased susceptibilty secondary to immunosuppression, pp. 197-198. For other nursing diagnoses and interventions, see ''Caring for the Critically Ill on Prolonged Bed Rest,'' pp. 506-511.

REHABILITATION AND PATIENT-FAMILY TEACHING CONCEPTS

Give patient and significant others verbal and written instructions for the following:
1. Importance of reporting episodes of pain or fever promptly to MD. Have patient return demonstration for temperature measurement.
2. Medications, including drug name, purpose, dosage, schedule, precautions, and potential side effects. Teach patient the potential side effects of steroids, including delayed healing, masking of signs of infection, GI upset, GI bleeding, mood swings, elevation of blood sugar, and fluid retention.
3. Activity level: Teach patient to resume activities gradually, as prescribed, allowing for adequate periods of rest between activities.

Hypertensive crisis

Hypertension is sustained elevation of the resting arterial pressure. In 1986 the American Heart Association defined hypertension as elevation of blood pressure (BP) above 140/90 mm Hg. Over 37,000,000 Americans have hypertension and 190,000 will have a fatal stroke or other cardiac event annually; thus, the impact of this disease on mortality is greater than that of any other health problem.

Most often, hypertension occurs as a primary disorder; however, its etiology is unknown. Secondary hypertension is the result of other disorders that alter the mechanisms that control BP. Many factors contribute to the development of secondary hypertension: (1) increase in secretion of catecholamines; (2) increase in secretion of renin by the kidneys; (3) increase in serum sodium and blood volume; (4) increase in plasma and extracellular fluid volume; (5) reduction in kidney perfusion pressure; (6) impairment of control mechanisms in the kidney; and (7) alteration in adrenal cortical hormone secretion. Table 2-12 lists the causes of secondary hypertension.

Hypertensive crisis is seen in about 1% of the hypertensive population. When it occurs, there is a threat of immediate vascular necrosis, which can occur if the diastolic pressure exceeds 140 mm Hg, although necrosis also has been seen with

---

T A B L E 2 - 1 2
Causes of secondary hypertension

Renal disease	Endocrine disorders	Congenital disorders
Acute glomerulonephritis	Primary aldosteronism	Coarctation of the aorta
Renal tumors	Cushing's syndrome	Adrenal hyperplasia
Hydronephrosis	Pheochromocytoma	
Chronic pyelonephritis	Hyperparathyroidism	
Renovascular hypertension		

Pregnancy-induced disorders	Drug-induced disorders
Preeclampsia	Birth control pills
Eclampsia	Steroids
	Cyclosporine

mean arterial pressures (MAP) ≥150 mm Hg. MAP is calculated using the following formula:

$$MAP = \frac{Systolic\ Pressure\ +\ 2\ (Diastolic\ Pressure)}{3}$$

The rapidity of the rise in pressure may be more destructive than the actual BP level recorded. If left untreated, hypertensive crisis is fatal to 75% of affected individuals within one year. With current treatment techniques, there is a 30% one-year mortality rate and 50% five-year mortality rate. Hypertensive crisis can lead to hypertensive encephalopathy as cerebral blood vessels dilate owing to their inability to autoregulate. Blood flow is increased and the excessive pressure drives fluid into the perivascular tissue, resulting in cerebral edema. The extreme pressure can cause arteriolar damage, as demonstrated by fibrinoid necrosis of the intima and media of the vessel wall. Although any organ is vulnerable, the eyes and kidneys are most likely to suffer damage, leading to blindness and renal failure.

Hypertensive patients admitted to the ICU may experience a rebound elevation of the BP if their usual antihypertensive regimen is interrupted. These patients also may experience a loss of BP control owing to the nature of their primary disorder, trauma, or stress of the ICU. Complications of hypertension include nephrosclerosis, aortic dissection (see p. 128), coronary artery disease, congestive heart failure (see p. 85), strokes, and peripheral vascular disease.

ASSESSMENT

Early indicators: Although most patients are asymptomatic, vague discomfort, fatigue, dizziness, and headache can occur.

Late indicators (nearly always present during a hypertensive crisis): Throbbing suboccipital headache, confusion, somnolence, stupor, visual loss, focal deficits, and coma. The patient also may present with signs of heart failure, including dyspnea on exertion, orthopnea, and paroxysmal nocturnal dyspnea. If coronary artery disease is present, the patient may experience angina owing to increased myocardial oxygen consumption caused by the high BP. Renal symptoms include hematuria, nocturia, and azotemia. Nausea and vomiting also may be present.

Physical assessment: An accurate cuff pressure must be obtained, with three resting measurements taken at least 3-5 minutes apart. A well-calibrated manometer and a properly fitting cuff should be selected for use. The bladder of the cuff must encircle the arm and cover two-thirds of the length of the upper arm. Note when the patient last smoked or used any nicotine product, how much caffeine was consumed during the past 4 hours, and whether adrenergic stimulants (e.g., over-the-counter decongestants or bronchodilators) have been used within the past 24 hours, as these factors elevate BP.

- *Cardiac assessment:* Evaluates left ventricular hypertrophy, which results from the need of the heart to pump against the high systemic vascular resistance (SVR) or afterload. A left ventricular heave may be palpated with the palm of the hand at the mitral area (5th ICS at the MCL). A fourth heart sound or S_4 gallop may be auscultated in the same site with the stethoscope bell. If cardiac failure is present, the apical impulse will be felt at the anterior axillary line (AAL) instead of the MCL, demonstrating heart enlargement. In addition, crackles (rales) may be auscultated in the presence of cardiac failure.

Pulsus alternans, an alteration in pulse pressure with a regular rhythm, may be palpated at any of the major pulse points. All peripheral pulses should be palpated bilaterally. With coarctation of the aorta, the femoral pulses will be bilaterally weak with a slow up-stroke; while the radial and brachial pulses will be normal or bounding.

- *Eye assessment:* A fundoscope is used to determine whether hemorrhage, fluffy cotton exudates, or arterial-venous nicking of the vessels has occurred. When these changes occur, visual perception is decreased. Nurses should assess the patient's ability to read and recognize objects and people.
- *Neurologic assessment:* May reveal evidence of a residual neurologic deficit from a cerebral infarct or ischemic event, as manifested by a positive Babinski (up-going toe), hemiparesis, hemiplegia, ataxia, confusion, or cognitive alterations.

History and risk factors: Psychologic stress, diet high in sodium, and cigarette smoking increase the risk of developing high BP. Hypertension is a familial disease; genetic and environmental factors contribute to its etiology. Hypertension is a risk factor for angina and MI. See "Acute Chest Pain," p. 73 and "Myocardial Infarction," p. 78.

DIAGNOSTIC TESTS

The definitive test for hypertension is blood pressure measurement. Once hypertension has been documented, many tests may be performed to determine the amount of end organ damage or diagnose the condition responsible for the development of secondary hypertension.

1. *EKG:* Left ventricular hypertrophy (LVH) is demonstrated by an increase in voltage in the LV precordial lead (V_{5-6}). In addition, a strain pattern of ST-segment depression and T-wave inversion reflects repolarization abnormalities due to the endocardial fibrosis that accompanies hypertrophy. General voltage criteria for LVH are: (1) "R" in V_5 or V_6 plus "S" in V_1 >35 mm; or (2) voltage of "R" in any precordial lead >25 mm.

2. *Echocardiogram:* LVH with or without dilatation will be demonstrated on echo by increase in the wall thickness with or without increased chamber size.

3. *Chest x-ray:* If dilatation of the left ventricle is present, the cardiac silhouette will be enlarged. If failure is present, there will be evidence of pulmonary congestion and pleural effusions. Notching of the aorta and a distended aortic root are indicative of coarctation of the aorta. If widening of the aorta is seen, dissection is suspected (see p. 128).

4. *Urinalysis/Urine culture:* Urinalysis will be normal until hypertension causes renal impairment. Specific gravity may be low (<1.010) and proteinuria may be present. Glomerulonephritis is suspected if the urine contains granular or red cell casts or the patient has hematuria. Pyelonephritis is suspected if there is bacterial growth in the urine. An elevation of the 24-hour urine vanillylmandelic acid (VMA) is indicative of pheochromocytoma, a rare catecholamine-producing tumor found in or near the adrenal glands. If the patient has Cushing's disease, the urine cortisol or ACTH level will be elevated.

5. *Blood chemistry:* If renal parenchymal disease is present, the patient may have serum creatinine >1.3 mg/dl and BUN >20 mg/dl. The RBC count may fall owing to hematuria.

MEDICAL MANAGEMENT AND SURGICAL INTERVENTIONS

1. **Lifestyle alterations:** Dietary changes, exercise, smoking cessation, and stress reduction are the cornerstones of medical treatment for early and established hypertension. Daily intake of sodium for the average adult is 4 grams but should be modified to 2 or 3 grams for the hypertensive individual (see Table 2-4, ''Low-Sodium Dietary Guidelines,'' p. 87). Smoking cessation is imperative to halt the injury to the intima of the coronary and peripheral vessels, which leads to the development of atherosclerosis, and to reduce the workload of the heart. A regular aerobic program has been proven beneficial in maintaining better control of blood pressure.

2. **Treatment of hypertensive crisis:** Necessitates immediate and rapid reduction in pressure.

   • *Nitroprusside:* Drug of choice because of its almost immediate vasodilation effects. It is supplied in 50 mg vials, which must be reconstituted with 2-3 ml of sterile water, mixed in a 250 ml bag of D_5W, and infused *via* mechanical controller device. Usual initial dose is 10-25 μg/min, with increases of 5-10 μg q5min. Until oral treatment is effective, the maintenance dose for nitroprusside ranges from 0.5-8.0 μg/kg/min. This drug has a short action time and BP will rise almost immediately if the drip is stopped. Direct arterial pressure monitoring is essential for the titration of this drug, with constant vigilance to prevent hypotension. When oral antihypertensives begin to affect the BP, nitroprusside will require careful weaning to prevent hypotensive episodes. Because nitroprusside is unstable in light, the bag should be wrapped with the aluminum foil provided by the manufacturer. Nitroprusside is metabolized to thiocyanate, which can cause fatigue, nausea, tinnitus, blurred vision, and delirium. Serum thiocyanate levels should be drawn after 48 hours of use and regularly thereafter. Levels <10 mg/dl are considered safe.

   • *Diazoxide:* A vasodilator that acts on the smooth muscle of the arterioles, is another agent that can be administered during a hypertensive crisis. It is administered in a bolus of 75-300 mg. Within minutes the SVR drops by about 25%, but the HR can increase by 30 bpm. The effects can last for hours.

   • *Labetalol hydrochloride:* A fast-acting alpha and beta blocker, which also can be used to treat the patient in hypertensive crisis. It is less likely to cause hypotension than diazoxide. It is administered IV push slowly, beginning with a 20 mg dose. This can be repeated q10min. The usual cumulative dose is 50-200 mg. Keep the patient supine during the injection and for up to 1 hour afterward. Maintain BP checks q5min × 6 and then q30min × 4.

3. **Pharmacotherapy:** Maintenance pharmacotherapy for hypertension is approached in a stepwise fashion. This approach has been accepted and promoted by the American Heart Association. After an adequate trial on Step 1, the patient is advanced to Step 2 if the BP remains refractory to treatment. An adequate trial of various medications for each step is attempted. Table 2-13 identifies the steps, medications, usual dosage, schedule, and potential side effects of the antihypertensive agents commonly used.

4. **Surgical treatment:** Although there is no surgical intervention for primary hypertension, several forms of secondary hypertension respond well to the surgical correction of the primary problem. A coarctation of the aorta can be repaired *via* removal of the narrowed area of the vessel with insertion of a Teflon aortic

TABLE 2-13
Stepwise approach to the treatment of hypertension

Step	Medication	Dosage	Schedule	Side effects
Step 1 Diuretics	*Thiazides*			Hypokalemia and hyperuricemia (found with all of the first 3 categories of diuretics); hypercholesterolemia, hypoglycemia, impotence, and indigestion (found with all diuretic categories)
	• Chlorothiazide	250-500 mg	q6-12 hrs	
	• Hydrochlorothiazide	25-100 mg	q12-18 hrs	
	Related compounds			
	• Chlorthalidone	25-50 mg	q24-72 hrs	
	• Quinethazone	50-200 mg	q18-24 hrs	
	• Metolazone	1.0-10 mg	q24 hrs	
	Loop diuretics			
	• Furosemide	40-120 mg	q4-6 hrs	
	• Ethacrynic acid	50-400 mg	q12 hrs	
	Potassium-sparing agents			Gynecomastia; menstrual abnormalities
	• Spironalactone	25-100 mg	q8-12 hrs	
	• Triamterene	100-300 mg	q12 hrs	
	• Amiloride	5-10 mg	q24 hrs	
Step 2 Adrenergic inhibiting agents	*Beta blockers*			Drowsiness, depression, fluid retention, heart failure, impotence, hypoglycemia, flushing (for all beta blockers)
	• Propranolol	40-100 mg	qid	
	• Atenolol	50-100 mg	qd	
	• Nadolol	40-320 mg	qd	
	• Metaprolol	50-100 mg	bid-tid	
	• Timolol	10-30 mg	bid	
	Central alpha receptor blockers			
	• Clonidine hydrochloride	0.1-0.4 mg	bid	Hypotention

Step 2 cont'd.			
• Methyldopa	250 mg-1 Gm	bid-qid	Hemolytic anemia, depression, dry mouth, nasal stuffiness, impotence
Alpha receptor blockers			
• Prazosin hydrochloride	1-7 mg	tid	First-dose syncope, blurred vision
• Phentolamine	50 mg	qid	Hypoglycemia, diarrhea, hypotension, flushing
Peripheral neuronal inhibitors			
• Reserpine	0.1-0.5 mg	qd	Hypotension, hyperacidity
• Guanethidine	10-50 mg	qd	Hypotension, impotence, weight gain
Step 3 Vasodilators			
Hydralazine	20-40 mg IV push 10-50 mg PO	qid	Lupus syndrome, angina, sodium retention
Minoxidil	5-40 mg PO	qd	Edema, pericardial effusions, increased hair growth
Diazoxide	50-300 mg IV push		Hypotension, fluid retention
Nitroprusside	0.5 μg/kg/min IV (immediate effect with 1-5 minute duration)		Hypotension; thiocyanate toxicity (if >20 mg/%) as evidenced by fatigue, anorexia, weakness, delirium
Step 4 Converting enzyme inhibitors			
Captopril	25-100 mg PO	tid	Dizziness, tachycardia, loss of ability to taste, urinary frequency, renal failure

graft. Renal artery stenosis may be corrected by grafting or by renal artery angioplasty. Pheochromocytoma is a rare epinephrine- and norepinephrine-producing tumor found near the adrenal medulla, resulting in hypertensive crisis precipitated by stress, postural change, or abdominal pressure. Surgical removal of the tumor(s) returns the patient to a normotensive state.

NURSING DIAGNOSES AND INTERVENTIONS

Alteration in tissue perfusion: Cardiopulmonary, cerebral, ophthalmic, and renal, related to impaired circulation secondary to vasoconstriction that occurs with interruption of the normal BP control mechanism; or vasodilatation with tissue edema that occurs with loss of autoregulation

---

Desired outcomes: Tissue perfusion is normal as evidenced by systemic arterial BP 110-140/70-90 mm Hg (or within patient's normal range); MAP 70-105 mm Hg; equal and normoreactive pupils; strength and tone of the extremities bilaterally equal and normal for patient; orientation to person, place, and time; urinary output ≥30 ml/hr; stable weight; and absence of hemorrhages and fluffy cotton exudates on fundoscopic exam. BUN is ≤20 mg/dl, creatinine clearance is ≥9.5 ml/min, and serum creatinine is ≤1.5 mg/dl.

---

1. Monitor BP and MAP q1-5min during titration of the medications. As patient's condition stabilizes, perform these assessments q15min-1h. Be alert to sudden drops or elevations in the BP. As the oral medications begin to affect the BP, wean nitroprusside gradually to prevent hypotensive episodes. Continuous monitoring by arterial cannulation or automatic BP apparatus is recommended.
   - Correlate cuff pressure with pressure from arterial cannulation.
   - Determine ideal range for BP control and maximal nitroprusside dose with MD. Usually, the following guidelines are used: systolic BP <140-160 mm Hg, MAP <110 mm Hg, or diastolic BP <90 mm Hg.
2. Assess patient for neurologic deficit by performing hourly neurochecks. Be alert to sensorimotor deficit if MAP is >140 mm Hg. As patient's condition stabilizes and BP becomes controlled, perform neurochecks at least q4h.
3. Assess patient for evidence of decreasing renal perfusion by monitoring I&O and weighing patient daily. Notify MD of urinary output<30 ml/hr for two consecutive hours or weight gain of ≥1 kg (2 pounds). Also be alert to azotemia (increasing BUN), decreasing creatinine clearance, and increasing serum creatinine.
4. Monitor patient for changes in fundoscopic examination. Notify MD if hemorrhages or fluffy cotton exudates are present.

Alteration in comfort: Headache related to cerebral edema occurring with high perfusion pressures

---

Desired outcome: Patient relates that headache is absent or reduced in intensity and does not exhibit nonverbal indicators of discomfort.

---

1. Monitor patient for pain at frequent intervals.
2. Provide pain medications as prescribed. A variety of analgesics may be used, ranging from acetaminophen with codeine to morphine, depending on severity of the symptoms. Assess effectiveness of the pain medication.
3. Teach patient relaxation techniques to use in conjunction with the medications. Guided imagery, meditation, and progressive muscle relaxation often are effective. See **Knowledge deficit:** Relaxation technique effective for stress reduction and facilitation of decreased sympathetic tone, p. 98.
4. Maintain a quiet, low-lit environment that is free of extensive distraction and stimulation. Limit visitations, as indicated.

Sensory-perceptual alterations related to decreased visual acuity secondary to retinal damage occurring with high perfusion pressures

---

Desired outcome: Patient reads print, recognizes objects or people, and demonstrates coordination of movement.

---

1. Assess patient for signs of decreased visual acuity by monitoring patient's ability to read and recognize objects or people. Evaluate patient's coordination of movement to determine depth perception. If considered a part of the nursing physical assessment practice by agency, perform a fundoscopic exam q8h for evidence of findings discussed on p. 122. Report significant findings.
2. If patient has decreased visual acuity, assist with feeding and other ADLs and keep patient's personal effects within his or her visual field.
3. Reassure patient and signficant others that visual problems usually resolve when the BP is lowered sufficiently.

For other nursing diagnoses and interventions, see the following as appropriate: "Management of the Adult with Hemodynamic Monitoring," pp. 168-170; "Caring for the Critically Ill with Life-Threatening Disorders," pp. 511-522; and "Caring for the Family of the Critically Ill," pp. 522-526.

REHABILITATION AND PATIENT-FAMILY TEACHING CONCEPTS

Give patient and significant others verbal and written instructions for the following:
1. Pathophysiology of hypertension and risk factor management as they relate to patient's condition.
2. Rationale for low-sodium dietary intake, low-sodium dietary guidelines (see Table 2-4, p. 87), and "heart-smart" shopping and cooking techniques. Provide pamphlets from American Heart Association or the National Heart, Lung, and Blood Institute.
3. If patient smokes, the reason that smoking cessation is essential. Provide counselling regarding cessation techniques and refer patient to community programs.
4. Methods for stress reduction, such as imagery, meditation, progressive muscle relaxation.
5. Initiation of low-level aerobic exercise program after patient's BP has been controlled: 5-10 minutes of brisk walking 3-5 times a week, with gradual increase

in duration to 30 minutes, with the intensity increased to 70-80% of the maximal heart rate achieved on an exercise test.

6. Technique for BP measurement and importance of maintaining a diary of daily readings.

7. Importance of continuing treatment, even if feeling well.

8. Medications, including drug name, purpose, dosage, schedule, precautions, and potential side effects.

Aortic dissection

An aortic dissection is a longitudinal tear in the medial layer of the aortic wall caused by the driving pressure of a column of blood. The column of blood drives the dissection distally with the force of systole and the diastolic recoil within the aorta forces the dissection in the proximal direction. Precipitating factors include medial necrosis from other disorders, trauma (e.g., blunt injury due to motor vehicle accident), or hypertension (see p. 120). The three types of aortic dissections first described by Debakey are differentiated by the site of the intimal tear and the direction of dissection. In Type I, which accounts for 60-80% of all cases, the tear begins in the ascending aorta and the dissection extends beyond the aortic arch. Type II is the rarest form, with the intimal tear and entire dissection confined to the ascending aorta. Type III occurs in 20-30% of all cases and involves a tear in the descending aorta, with distal dissection only.

Aortic dissection is a sudden and very serious threat to life because the disruption of the vessel may continue along any arterial branch of the aorta, compromising organs such as the heart, brain, and kidneys if the coronary, subclavian, innominate, and renal arteries are involved. Approximately 2000 episodes occur annually, with mortality rate approaching 100% if the dissection is left untreated.

ASSESSMENT

Signs and symptoms: The major symptom is a sudden onset of severe, tearing chest pain that is unrelieved by position or respiratory change. The pain may radiate to the back if the dissection is moving distally, or to the neck if the dissection is moving proximally. Vasovagal responses such as diaphoresis, apprehension, nausea, vomiting, and faintness may occur. Signs of congestive heart failure may be seen if the dissection involves the coronary arteries or the aortic valve. Neurologic deficits such as confusion, sensorimotor changes, and lethargy may be the result of a dissection along the branches of the ascending aorta. Urine output will fall if the renal arteries dissect.

Physical assessment: Pulse deficits or BP differences between extremities are classic findings. A drop in BP or pulse at a site helps identify the location of the dissection, as both will be decreased beyond the area of dissection. Usually the skin is pale and cool and there is sluggish capillary refill due to poor tissue perfusion. If bleeding extends to the pericardium, cardiac tamponade can occur (see p. 105).

History and risk factors: Hypertension, connective tissue disorders such as Marfan's syndrome or Ehlers-Danlos syndrome, coarctation of the aorta, blunt chest trauma, medial necrosis of the aorta, or pregnancy.

DIAGNOSTIC TESTS

1. *Chest x-ray:* Will demonstrate widening of the aortic arch or descending aorta. An upright film is necessary to demonstrate widening of the mediastinum.

2. *Echocardiograms of the aortic arch or descending aorta:* Will locate the site of dissection, as the hemorrhage within the vessel will be an area of absent echoes and the total diameter of the vessel will be enlarged.

3. *Aortogram:* Will locate actual site of the tear and dissection *via* use of contrast material.

4. *CT scan:* Often as useful as aortogram in locating the dissection. Its advantage over aortogram is that it is noninvasive.

MEDICAL MANAGEMENT AND SURGICAL INTERVENTIONS

1. Antihypertensive therapy: Initiated as soon as possible to prevent further aortic dissection. Usually nitroprusside is started, as described with "Hypertensive Crisis," p. 123. A MAP of 70-80 mm Hg is desired. After control of the pressure is achieved, oral antihypertensive therapy is begun, along with gradual weaning from the IV infusion.

2. Propranolol therapy: To reduce velocity of the left ventricular ejection, HR, and BP. Usually it is administered IV in increments of 1 mg at 5-minute intervals until the HR is reduced to 60-80 bpm. The maximal initial dose should not exceed 0.15 mg/kg/body weight. Additional doses of 2-6 mg q4-6h are then administered until the patient can be managed with oral medications.

3. Absolute bed rest: To prevent further dissection. This may continue for weeks until the dissection has stabilized.

4. Pain relief: Usually achieved with IV morphine sulfate, 2-10 mg.

5. Sedation: To prevent sympathetic stimulation, which can increase BP. Diazepam 2-10 mg may be given q4-6h.

6. Long-term medical management: Aimed at maintaining systolic BP under 130 mm Hg to prevent redissection.

7. Surgical treatment: Recommended for proximal dissection, distal dissection when vital organ compromise occurs, impending rupture, or when pain and BP are refractory to medications. The surgery involves removal of the dissected vessel sections and replacement of the vessel sections with Teflon grafts.

NURSING DIAGNOSES AND INTERVENTIONS

Alteration in tissue perfusion: Peripheral, cardiopulmonary, renal, and cerebral, related to mechanical impairment to blood flow secondary to narrowed aortic lumen

---

Desired outcome: Patient has adequate tissue perfusion as evidenced by distal pulses equal and >2+ on a 0-4+ scale; brisk capillary refill (<3 seconds); warm skin; bilaterally equal systolic BP; BP within patient's normal range; HR ≤100 bpm; normal sinus rhythm on EKG; urine output ≥30 ml/hr; bilaterally equal sensations in the extremities; equal and normoreactive pupils; and orientation to person, place, and time.

---

1. Perform bilateral assessment of BP and distal pulses (particularly, radial, femoral, and dorsalis pedis) qh during the initial phase of dissection, and then q4h as the patient's condition stabilizes. Note changes in strength or symmetry of the distal pulses. Correlate cuff pressures with arterial monitor recordings. Be alert to any change in color, capillary refill, and temperature of each extremity. Report significant findings.

2. If the difference in systolic BP between the extremities exceeds 10 mm Hg, notify MD immediately.
3. Assess for signs of pericardial tamponade: distended neck veins, muffled heart sounds, decreased systolic BP (BP <90 mm Hg or a greater than 20 mm Hg drop in systolic trend), and paradoxical pulse.
4. Monitor for paresthesias of the extremities, a sign of decreased peripheral perfusion.
5. Monitor urine output hourly. Notify MD if urine output is <30 ml/hr for 2 consecutive hours.
6. Assess neurologic status hourly. Report restlessness and changes in LOC, pupil size, or reaction to light.
7. Assess cardiovascular status by monitoring heart rate and rhythm, EKG, and cardiac enzymes. A dissection along the coronary arteries will result in a myocardial infarction.

Alteration in comfort: Pain related to necrosis at the aortic media and distal tissue hypoperfusion

---

Desired outcome: Patient relates a reduction in or absence of pain and does not exhibit signs of uncontrolled discomfort.

---

1. Monitor patient at frequent intervals for the presence of discomfort; medicate with analgesics as prescribed.
2. Teach patient relaxation techniques to use in conjunction with analgesics. Examples include guided imagery, meditation, and progressive muscle relaxation. For guidelines, see **Knowledge deficit:** Relaxation technique effective for stress reduction and facilitation of decreased sympathetic tone, p. 98.
3. During episodes of pain, assess for a change in peripheral pulses or altered hemodynamics (i.e., BP, PAP, PAWP, CO, SVR), as this often is associated with an increase in aortic dissection.
4. Control BP during episodes of pain by titrating nitroprusside to maintain specified parameters.
5. Immediately report any increase in the severity of pain, as this may be indicative of the need for emergency surgery.

For other nursing diagnoses and interventions, see the following as appropriate: "Management of the Adult with Hemodynamic Monitoring," pp. 168-170; "Caring for the Critically Ill on Prolonged Bed Rest," pp. 506-511; "Caring for the Critically Ill with Life-Threatening Disorders," pp. 511-522; and "Caring for the Family of the Critically Ill," pp. 522-526.

REHABILITATION AND PATIENT-FAMILY TEACHING CONCEPTS

Because hypertension is a precipitating factor with aortic dissection, see rehabilitation and patient-family teaching discussion, p. 127. All the information applies, except for the discussion about aerobic exercise.

Cardiogenic shock

Shock is a state in which blood flow to peripheral tissue is inadequate to sustain life. It can be caused by hemorrhage, hypovolemia, sepsis (see p. 433), neurologic impairment with decreased sympathetic stimulation, anaphylaxis (see p. 443), or cardiogenic impairment. Usually, cardiogenic shock is caused by a massive myocardial infarction (MI) that renders 40% or more of the myocardium dysfunctional due to necrosis or ischemia. As a result, cardiac output is reduced and all tissues suffer from inadequate perfusion. With decreased perfusion to the heart, coronary flow is reduced, which further impairs cardiac function, decreasing cardiac output even further. Cardiogenic shock occurs with 15-20% of all MIs and carries a mortality rate of 80% or more. Other causes of cardiogenic shock include depressed cardiac function, postcardiac surgery, massive pulmonary embolus, severe valvular dysfunction, end-stage cardiomyopathy, congestive heart failure, and cardiac tamponade.

The first stage of shock is characterized by increased sympathetic discharge as the baroreceptors at the carotid sinus and aortic arch become stimulated by the drop in blood pressure. The release of epinephrine and norephinephrine is a compensatory mechanism that increases cardiac output by increasing the heart rate and contractility of the uninjured myocardium. Vasoconstriction, a mechanism that increases blood pressure, occurs. The second or middle stage of shock is characterized by decreased perfusion to the brain, kidney, and heart. Lactate and pyruvic acid accumulate in the tissues and metabolic acidosis occurs due to anaerobic metabolism. Blood is diverted to the skin, gut, and skeletal muscles. In the late stage of shock, which usually is irreversible, compensatory mechanisms become ineffective and multiple organ failure occurs.

At the cellular level, injury begins with hypoxia and loss of adenosine triphosphate (ATP), the energy source for all cellular functions. This leads to condensations in the mitochondria and swelling of the endoplasmic reticulum. The final phase of cellular damage is marked by swelling, rupture of the membrane, and complete cellular degradation. Cellular changes are similar in all body organs and types of tissue.

ASSESSMENT

Signs and symptoms: The assessment of MI (see p. 79) describes the early stage of cardiogenic shock. As cardiogenic shock progresses, mentation is decreased due to poor cerebral perfusion. This is evidenced by agitation, restlessness, lethargy, confusion, or unresponsiveness. Urine output drops to <30 ml/hr as renal perfusion pressure drops and the kidneys attempt to compensate by triggering the renin-angiotensin system to retain more fluid.

Physical assessment: HR is elevated and the pulses are equal bilaterally, but weak and often irregular. Systolic BP is <90 mm Hg or at least 30 mm Hg below the patient's normal resting level. The skin is cold, clammy, and mottled due to compromised peripheral perfusion. Cardiac auscultation usually reveals S_3 or S_4 sounds due to the overdistended and noncompliant ventricle. Crackles (rales) are auscultated over the lung fields due to pulmonary congestion; hyperventilation is common.

Hemodynamic measurements: Cuff pressures are very inaccurate during shock, mandating the use of arterial pressure monitoring. PAP monitoring is essential for guiding therapy during the early stage of shock. Arterial systolic and mean arterial pressures are decreased, with a decreased or narrow pulse pressure.

Because contractility is greatly reduced, the stroke volume, ejection fraction, and cardiac output are decreased. RAP, PAP, PAEDP, and PAWP all are elevated as evidence of increased preload secondary to pulmonary congestion. SVR is increased owing to vasoconstriction, which occurs as a compensatory mechanism when flow to an organ is reduced.

An oximetric catheter may be used to provide continuous measurement of the oxygen saturation of the mixed venous blood (SVO_2) in the pulmonary artery. The SVO_2 reflects the adequacy of oxygen supply in meeting tissue demands. When demand is increased (as in anemia) or supply is decreased (as in cardiogenic shock), the SVO_2 will fall below normal range of 60-80%. The SVO_2 has a positive correlation with the cardiac output, thus continuous monitoring of SVO_2 provides an indirect but continuous assessment of CO. For detailed parameters for assessment, see Table 2-14.

DIAGNOSTIC TESTS

The diagnosis of cardiogenic shock is made by physical assessment and analysis of the hemodynamic profile. The primary problem, myocardial infarction, is diagnosed by EKG and enzyme changes (see discussion, p. 79). Other diagnostic tests are useful in assessing the effect of hypoperfusion on other organs.

1. *ABG values:* Hypoxemia (Pao_2 <80 mm Hg) and metabolic acidosis (pH <7.35, $Paco_2$ usually <35 mm Hg) are seen due to impaired oxygen diffusion in the alveoli and tissue lactic acidosis from anaerobic metabolism.
2. *Serum chemistries:* Moderate hyperglycemia may be found, owing to epinephrine-induced glycogenolysis. Because the pancreas is hypoperfused, inadequate insulin is released to meet this need. Serum lactate levels may be elevated due to anaerobic metabolism. Electrolyte studies may reveal hypernatremia, which is reflective of a water deficit; hypokalemia, which may be associated with the cause of shock; or hyperkalemia, which may be seen with renal failure secondary to the shock state.
3. *Urinalysis:* Urine sodium, osmolality, and creatinine levels are reflective of the patient's renal status.
4. *Coagulation profile:* Although coagulation studies often are abnormal, there is no established pattern with cardiogenic shock.

MEDICAL MANAGEMENT AND SURGICAL INTERVENTIONS

1. **Oxygen therapy:** For oxygenation of the tissues. If dyspnea, hypoxemia, acidosis, or pulmonary congestion worsens, intubation and mechanical ventilation will be necessary. Morphine sulfate 2 mg IV push may assist in reducing pulmonary congestion, thereby relieving dyspnea and increasing Pao_2.
2. **Correction of acidosis:** Sodium bicarbonate delivered by IV push, guided by serial ABG checks to assess effectiveness of treatment.
3. **Correction of electrolyte imbalance:** For example, replacement of potassium, sodium, chloride, or calcium as indicated by serum chemistry findings.
4. **Institution of hemodynamic monitoring:** Arterial and pulmonary artery catheters are inserted to guide pharmacologic therapy.
5. **Diuretics:** To decrease preload and improve stroke volume and cardiac output. Diuretics such as furosemide 40-200 mg IV push or ethocrinic acid 25-100 ml IV push may be given. Morphine sulfate also reduces preload. Nitrates such as oral, topical, or IV nitroglycerin and IV nitroprusside (Nipride) may be used to decrease filling pressures *via* venous dilatation.

TABLE 2-14
Hemodynamic profile of shock

	RAP mm Hg	RVP mm Hg	PAP mm Hg	PAWP mm Hg	SVR dynes/sec/cm^{-5}	SVO$_2$ %	CO L/min	CI L/min/m^2
Normal value	4-6	25/0-5	20-30/8-15	6-12	900-1200	60-80	4-7	2.5-4
Cardiogenic shock	6-10	40-50/6-15	50/25-30	25-40	>1200	≤50	<4	≤1.5
Hypovolemic shock	0-2	15-20/0-2	15-20/2-8	2-6	>1200	65	<4	2.5
Neurogenic shock	0-2	20-25/0-2	20-25/0-8	0-6	≤1000	60-80	≥4-7	≥2.5
Septic shock *Early*	0-2	20-25/0-2	20-25/0-8	0-6	≤900	≥60	>7	≥4.0
Late	0-4	25/0-4	25/4-10	>12	>1200	≤60	<4	<2.5

< N O T E : It may be necessary to increase preload if the patient is hypovolemic. In this situation, fluids are increased cautiously, the patient is monitored carefully, and diuretics are discontinued or avoided.

6. **Positive inotropic agents:** To improve contractility of the uninjured myocardium and increase cardiac output. Dopamine infusions at 2.0-20 μg/kg/min are titrated to accomplish the desired effect. Higher doses increase HR and SVR, which increase the myocardial workload. Dobutamine infusions of 2.0-20 μg/kg/min increase contractility and decrease preload with less of an increase in HR, but may decrease renal perfusion. Amrinone infusions of 1-10 μg/kg/min provide the same inotropic effect. Isoproterenol will increase HR and contractility but it is used with caution because it increases myocardial workload.

7. **Vasopressors:** To increase BP to an adequate mean level (usually ≥70 mm Hg) that will perfuse the tissues. This is accomplished by stimulating the alpha adrenergic receptors in the blood vessels, which causes vasoconstriction. Vasopressors frequently used include norepinephrine, epinephrine, phenylephrine hydrochloride, and methoxamine hydrochloride.

8. **Intra-aortic balloon pump:** To increase coronary perfusion and decrease afterload (see discussion, p. 142).

9. **Heart-assist device:** To increase perfusion pressure (see discussion, p. 147).

10. **Emergency cardiac catheterization:** To determine patient's suitability for emergency percutaneous transluminal coronary angioplasty or coronary artery bypass graft.

11. **Emergency coronary artery bypass graft:** To reperfuse areas with reversible injury patterns. This procedure will not be beneficial if the tissue already is necrotic, as evidenced by Q waves on the EKG. See discussion, p. 150. At the time of surgery, a left ventricular aneurysmectomy may be done to remove the thin-walled, dysfunctional sac.

12. **Emergency percutaneous transluminal coronary angioplasty:** To reperfuse areas of the myocardium with reversible injury pattern. See discussion, p. 136.

13. **Thrombolytic therapy:** For reperfusion of the injured and uninfarcted myocardium. See discussion, p. 160.

14. **Heart transplant:** To replace the failing heart with a suitably matched donor organ. The recipient is screened carefully to ensure that all other organs are still functional.

NURSING DIAGNOSES AND INTERVENTIONS

Alteration in cardiac output: Decreased, related to decreased or increased afterload, increased preload, or decreased contractility secondary to loss of ≥40% of myocardial functional mass

---

Desired outcome: Hemodynamic function is as near the acceptable limits as possible as evidenced by CO ≥4 L/min, BP >90/60 mm Hg, and PAWP <12 mm Hg.

---

1. On a continuous basis, monitor arterial BP, PAP, SVO₂, and heart rate and rhythm. Titrate vasoactive drugs to achieve a CO between 4-7 L/min, arterial BP >90/60, and PAWP <12 mm Hg.

2. Assess cardiac output q1-4h and after every change in pharmacologic therapy.
3. Auscultate lung sounds q1-2h. Report changes, including an increase in crackles (rales), as additional diuretics may be necessary.
4. To prevent further decreases in BP, do not increase the angle of the HOB more than 30 degrees.
5. Treat ventricular dysrhythmias with prescribed lidocaine, procainamide hydrochloride, or bretylium infusions.
6. Be prepared to pace the patient if bradycardia or a second- or third-degree heart block is found. Either temporary transcutaneous or transvenous pacing may be used.
7. If preload is low, administer prescribed crystalloid IV fluids according to fluid challenge protocol. See Table 2-15 for sample protocol.
8. If medical management is ineffective, prepare patient for insertion of intra-aortic balloon pump (see p. 142) or left ventricular assist device (see "Heart-Assist Device," p. 147).

Alteration in tissue perfusion: Cerebral, renal, peripheral, and cardiopulmonary related to impaired circulation to vital organs secondary to inadequate arterial pressure

---

Desired outcome: Patient has adequate tissue perfusion as evidenced by orientation to person, place, and time; equal and normoreactive pupils; normal reflexes; urine output ≥30 ml/hr; warm and dry skin; peripheral pulses >2+ on a 0-4+ scale; brisk capillary refill (<3 seconds); and BP >90/60 or within patient's normal range.

---

1. Perform neurochecks q1-2h to assess cerebral perfusion. Be alert to changes in LOC, orientation, perception, motor activity, reflexes, and pupillary response to light. Notify MD of any changes.
2. Monitor I&O hourly to assess renal perfusion; report urine output <30 ml/hr for two consecutive hours.
3. Assess extremities q1-2h, noting changes in skin color, temperature, capillary refill, BP, and distal pulses.

TABLE 2-15

Fluid challenge guidelines in cardiogenic shock

Assessment	PAWP	Fluids
CO low and PAWP as follows	<6	200 ml infused over 10 minutes
	6-12	100 ml infused over 10 minutes
	≥12	50 ml infused over 10 minutes
PAWP status during infusion	>6	Return to keep vein open (KVO) rate
	≤3	Continue infusion
Assess PAWP after 10 minutes	if >3 or <6	Repeat challenge

4. Notify MD if SVR increases (>1200 dynes/sec/cm^{-5}), as nitroprusside or similar medication may be needed to decrease excessive afterload.

5. Titrate vasoactive drugs to maintain systolic BP >90 mm Hg.

Impaired gas exchange related to decreased diffusion of oxygen secondary to pulmonary congestion and acidosis occurring with anaerobic metabolism

---

Desired outcome: Patient has adequate gas exchange as evidenced by Pao$_2$ ≥80 mm Hg, RR 12-20 breaths/min with normal depth and pattern (eupnea), oxygen saturation ≥95%, and SVO$_2$ 60-80%.

---

1. At least hourly, assess rate, depth, and effort of patient's respirations for tachypnea or labored breaths. Also inspect skin and mucous membranes for pallor or cyanosis (a late sign of hypoxia). Notify MD promptly of significant findings.

2. Auscultate lung fields q1-2h. Be alert to rales (crackles), rhonchi, or wheezes.

3. Monitor ABG values for hypoxemia (Pao$_2$ <80 mm Hg) or metabolic acidosis (pH <7.35 and HCO$_3^-$ <22 mEq/L).

4. Deliver humidifed oxygen as prescribed.

5. Monitor transcutaneous oxygen saturation with a pulse oximeter. Alert MD if oxygen saturation falls below 90%.

6. Monitor SVO$_2$. When cardiac output drops, SVO$_2$ will decrease, indicating increased oxygen extraction, which occurs when perfusion is decreased. Alert MD to SVO$_2$ <60%.

7. If patient's condition continues to deteriorate, prepare patient for entubation and mechanical ventilation.

For other nursing diagnoses and interventions, see the following as appropriate: "Adult Respiratory Distress Syndrome," pp. 20-21; "Acute Respiratory Failure/Management of the Adult on Mechanical Ventilation," pp. 66-70; "Acute Myocardial Infarction," pp. 81-84; "Acute Cardiac Tamponade," pp. 107-108; "Management of the Adult with Hemodynamic Monitoring," pp. 168-170; "Caring for the Critically Ill with Life-Threatening Disorders," pp. 511-522; and "Caring for the Family of the Critically Ill," pp. 522-526.

Percutaneous transluminal coronary angioplasty

Percutaneous transluminal coronary angioplasty (PTCA) is an invasive procedure for improving blood flow through stenotic coronary arteries. A balloon-tipped catheter is inserted into the coronary arterial lesion and the balloon is inflated to compress the plaque material against the vessel wall, thereby opening the narrowed lumen. PTCA is indicated for the surgical candidate whose angina is refractory to medical treatment. It is also being performed for individuals with postinfarction angina, postbypass angina, and chronic stable angina. The ideal candidate has single vessel disease with a discrete, proximal, noncalcified lesion.

During the procedure, the patient is sedated lightly; given a local anesthetic at the insertion site, usually the femoral artery; and EKG electrodes are placed on the chest. A pulmonary artery catheter is passed through the right side of the heart to measure heart pressure, and a pacing wire may be inserted as well. A sheath is inserted into the artery, a guide wire is passed into the aorta and coronary artery, and the balloon catheter is passed over the guide wire to the stenotic site. The patient may be asked to take deep breaths and cough to facilitate passage of the catheter. Heparin is given to prevent clot formation, and intracoronary nitroglycerin and sublingual nifedipine are administered to dilate coronary vessels and prevent spasm. The balloon is inflated repeatedly for 60-90 seconds at 4-11 atmospheres pressure. At this time the patient may experience mild, transient chest discomfort. Radiopaque dye is injected to determine whether the stenosis has been reduced to less than 50% of the vessel diameter, which is the goal of the procedure. The introducer sheath is left in the femoral artery for up to 12 hours post-PTCA for heparin infusion or in the event of the need for repeat angiography. To minimize the risk of hemorrhage, the patient must lie flat in bed for at least 6 hours and should not bend the knee and hip or sit up.

Complications following PTCA include acute coronary artery occlusion, myocardial infarction, coronary artery spasm, bleeding, circulatory insufficiency, renal hypersensitivity to contrast material, hypokalemia, vasovagal reaction, dysrhythmias, and hypotension. Restenosis can occur 6 weeks to 6 months post-PTCA, although the patient may not experience angina.

NURSING DIAGNOSES AND INTERVENTIONS

Knowledge deficit: Angioplasty procedure and postprocedure care

---

Desired outcome: Patient describes the rationale for the procedure, how it is performed, postprocedure care, and discharge instructions.

---

1. Assess patient's understanding of coronary artery disease and the purpose of angioplasty. Evaluate patient's style of coping and degree of information desired.

2. As appropriate for coping style, discuss the following with patient and significant others:
   - Location of patient's coronary artery disease, using heart drawing.
   - Use of local anesthesia and sedation during procedure.
   - Insertion site of catheter: groin or arm.
   - Sensations that may occur: mild chest discomfort.
   - Use of fluoroscopy during procedure. Determine patient's history of sensitivity to contrast material.
   - Ongoing observations made by nurse postprocedure: BP, HR, EKG, leg or arm pulses, blood tests.
   - Importance of lying flat in bed 6-12 hours postprocedure.
   - Necessity for nurse assistance with eating, drinking, and toileting needs postprocedure.
   - Need for increased fluid intake postprocedure to wash dye out of system.
   - Discharge instructions: Importance of taking antiplatelet drugs to prevent restenosis, avoidance of strenuous activity during first few weeks at home, follow-up visit with cardiologist one week after hospital discharge, signs and symptoms to report to physician (i.e., GI upset, new angina, fainting).

3. If patient and significant others express or exhibit evidence of anxiety regarding the upcoming procedure, try to arrange for them to meet with another patient who has had a successful angioplasty.

Alteration in comfort: Chest pain related to decreased myocardial oxygen supply due to coronary artery disease

---

Desired outcome: Patient verbalizes relief or improvement in chest pain and does not exhibit signs of uncontrolled discomfort.

---

1. Assess location, quality, duration, intensity, and precipitating and relieving factors of chest pain.
2. Administer sublingual or IV nitroglycerin (NTG) as prescribed.
3. Monitor for side effects of NTG: headache, hypotension, syncope, facial flushing, nausea. If side effects occur, reduce dose and place patient in a supine position. Confer with MD regarding need for alteration of dose.
4. Administer oxygen *via* nasal cannula or mask as needed.
5. Administer beta-blocker drugs as prescribed. Monitor for side effects, including bradycardia and hypotension. Also be alert to indicators of heart failure (i.e., fatigue, SOB, weight gain, ankle edema) and heart block (i.e., syncope and dizziness).
6. Provide an environment conducive to relaxation. Teach patient about relaxation techniques, including progressive relaxation, biofeedback, music therapy. See **Knowledge deficit:** Relaxation technique effective for stress reduction and facilitation of decreased sympathetic tone, p. 98.
7. For other interventions, see the same nursing diagnosis in "Acute Myocardial Infarction," p. 81.

Potential alteration in cardiac output: Decreased, related to risk of vessel occlusion, myocardial infarction, coronary artery spasm, dysrhythmias, bleeding, or cardiac tamponade secondary to complications of angioplasty

---

Desired outcomes: Patient exhibits a normal cardiac output, as evidenced by BP within normal limits for patient; HR 60-100 bpm; normal sinus rhythm on EKG; peripheral pulses >2+ on a 0-4+ scale; warm and dry skin; hourly urine output ≥30 ml; measured cardiac output 4-7 L/min; RAP 4-6 mm Hg, PAP 20-30/8-15 mm Hg, PAWP 6-12 mm Hg; creatinine phosphokinase-myocardial band (CPK-MB) 0-5% of total CPK; and patient awake, alert, oriented, and free from anginal pain.

---

1. Monitor BP, RAP, and PAP continuously; monitor PAWP and cardiac output hourly. Be alert to the following indicators of decreased cardiac output: decreased BP, increased HR, increased PAP, increased PAWP, decreased measured cardiac output, and decreased RAP.
2. Monitor EKG continuously for evidence of dysrhythmias and ST- and T-wave changes. Observe for bradyarrhythmias during sheath removal. Run 12-lead EKG daily.

3. Monitor urinary output hourly for the first 4 hours, and thereafter according to agency protocol. Alert MD to output <30 ml/h for two consecutive hours.

4. Measure CPK-MB immediately after PTCA procedure and then q8h x3; report elevations.

5. Monitor patient responses to antianginal and coronary vasodilator medications given for hypotension; report BP below desired range. Hypotension also can occur secondary to vessel occlusion. Treat hypotension immediately, as prescribed. Usually, fluids are given and the patient is placed in Trendelenberg's position.

6. When patient first sits up, ensure that it is done in stages to minimize the likelihood of postural hypotension.

7. Monitor patient continuously for bleeding at sheath insertion site. Monitor hematocrit for decrease from baseline values.

8. Monitor patient for evidence of cardiac tamponade: hypotension, tachycardia, pulsus paradoxus, jugular venous distention, elevation and plateau pressuring of PAWP and RAP, and, possibly, an enlarged heart silhouette on chest x-ray.

9. Do not discontinue heparin or antiplatelet drugs without physician directive. When these drugs are discontinued, monitor patient closely for indicators of coronary occlusion: ST-segment elevation on EKG, angina, hypotension, tachycardia, dysrhythmias, and diaphoresis.

10. Monitor peripheral pulses (radial and pedal) and color and temperature of extremities q4h for first 4 hours.

11. Monitor patient's mental alertness on an ongoing basis.

12. If patient develops angina, check BP and heart rate and rhythm; obtain 12-lead EKG reading; deliver oxygen; and administer NTG as prescribed, noting patient's response to the drug. Notify MD of significant findings.

Potential alteration in tissue perfusion: Peripheral (involved limb), related to impaired circulation secondary to presence of angioplasty sheath or risk of clot formation in vessel following sheath removal

---

Desired outcome: Patient has adequate tissue perfusion in the involved limb as evidenced by warm skin, peripheral pulses >2+ on a 0-4+ scale, natural skin color, ability to move the toes, and complete sensation.

---

1. Monitor circulation to affected limb q30 min x4 and then q2h thereafter. Assess pulses, temperature, color, sensation, and mobility of toes. Be alert to weak or thready pulses, coolness and pallor of the extremity, and patient complaints of numbness and tingling. Notify MD immediately if any of these signs or symptoms is present.

2. Inspect sheath site for signs of external or subcutaneous bleeding.

3. Keep sandbag at insertion site until discontinued by MD.

4. Maintain immobilization of limb at least 6 hours or until discontinued by MD.

5. Keep HOB no higher than 15 degrees to prevent kinking of sheath.

6. Monitor sheath patency by evaluating for continuous IV infusion into the involved vessel.

7. Instruct patient to notify staff immediately if numbness, tingling, or pain occurs at the affected extremity.

Potential fluid volume deficit related to decreased circulating volume secondary to diuresis occurring in response to contrast material

---

Desired outcomes: Patient is normovolemic as evidenced by intake equal to output plus insensible losses, urine specific gravity 1.010-1.030, HR ≤100 bpm, BP within patient's normal range, MAP ≥70 mm Hg, CVP ≥2 mm Hg, CO ≥4 L/min, moist mucous membranes, good skin turgor, and absence of thirst. BUN is ≤20 mg/dl, serum creatinine is ≤1.5 mg/dl, and serum potassium is ≥3.5 mEq/L.

---

1. Measure I&O hourly for the first 4 hours, and thereafter as indicated. Assess for urine output >80-125 ml/hr (depending on intake) or output out of proportion to intake.
2. Monitor hemodynamic values for decreases in MAP, CVP, and CO. Also be alert to tachycardia, hypotension, poor skin turgor, dry and sticky mucous membranes, decreases in urine specific gravity, and patient complaints of thirst.
3. Monitor BUN and creatinine values qd; be alert to elevations.
4. Provide parenteral fluids as prescribed until patient is taking fluids orally. Encourage oral fluids when patient is able, explaining that fluids will help flush contrast material out of the system.
5. Monitor potassium levels. Be alert to hypokalemia, which can occur with diuresis (see "Hypokalemia," p. 226).

See "Intra-Aortic Balloon Pump" for the following: **Potential for injury** related to risk of bleeding/hemorrhage secondary to mechanical coagulopathy and IV anticoagulants, p. 146. As appropriate, see nursing diagnoses and interventions in the following: "Management of the Adult with Hemodynamic Monitoring," pp. 168-170; "Caring for the Critically Ill with Life-Threatening Disorders," pp. 511-522; and "Caring for the Family of the Critically Ill," pp. 522-526.

REHABILITATION AND PATIENT-FAMILY TEACHING CONCEPTS

Because the hospital stay rarely exceeds 3 days, the nurse has limited time in which to prepare the patient for hospital discharge; therefore, discharge teaching should begin at admission. Give patient and significant others verbal and written instructions for the following:
1. See content in **Knowledge deficit,** p. 137.
2. Risk factor modification: smoking cessation, diet low in fat and cholesterol (see Table 2-3, p. 84), alteration in type A behavior, control of hypertension, and increase in exercise. Provide materials by American Heart Association, which has many excellent booklets on these topics.

Percutaneous balloon valvuloplasty

Percutaneous balloon valvuloplasty (PBV) is a recently developed procedure for the dilatation of stenotic heart valves. Candidates for this procedure are individuals with aortic or mitral stenosis who: (1) are high-risk surgical candidates; (2) refuse surgery; (3) are elderly (often >80 years of age); or (4) are informed of treatment choices and choose this procedure over others. The procedure parallels the technique for percutaneous transluminal coronary angioplasty. The femoral artery and vein are cannulated and the patient is anticoagulated with 5,000 units of heparin. For aortic valve dilatation, a catheter is passed into the femoral artery to measure supravalvular and left ventricular pressures prior to valvuloplasty. A 12 mm balloon valvuloplasty catheter is then passed over a guidewire into the left ventricle. It is inflated three times for 12-30 seconds at 12 atmospheres pressure. Additional heparin is administered and the valve gradient is measured again. To reach the mitral valve, the balloon valvuloplasty catheter is passed *via* the femoral vein and through the atrial septum to the mitral valve opening. The inflation procedure is the same.

Currently there are three theories to explain how this procedure improves cusp motion: (1) the dilatation results in separation of fused commissures; (2) there is fracturing and redistribution of nodular calcium deposits within the valve leaflets; and (3) there is stretching of the rigid leaflet and annulus structure. With both aortic and mitral dilatation, significant improvement has been demonstrated in the valve gradient and blood flow across the valve. Complications that have been observed include embolization to the brain, disruption of the valve ring, acute valve regurgitation, valvular restenosis, hemorrhage at the catheter insertion site, guidewire perforation of the left ventricular, and dysrhythmias.

NURSING DIAGNOSES AND INTERVENTIONS

Knowledge deficit: Procedure for percutaneous balloon valvuloplasty and postprocedure assessment

---

Desired outcome: Patient verbalizes rationale for the procedure, the technique, and postprocedure care.

---

1. Assess patient's understanding of aortic stenosis and the purpose of valvuloplasty. Evaluate patient's style of coping and degree of information desired.
2. As appropriate for patient's coping style, discuss with patient and significant others the valvuloplasty procedure, including:
   - Location of diseased valve, using heart drawing.
   - Use of local anesthesia and sedation during procedure.
   - Insertion site of catheter: femoral artery and vein.
   - Use of fluoroscopy during procedure. Evaluate patient for a history of sensitivity to contrast material.
   - Observations made by nurse postprocedure: BP, HR, EKG, pulses, and catheter insertion site.
   - Importance of lying flat 6-12 hours postprocedure to minimize the risk of bleeding.

Potential alteration in cardiac output: Decreased, related to risk of dysrhythmias, valve regurgitation, tamponade, or hemorrhage secondary to PBV procedure

---

Desired outcomes: Patient has normal cardiac output as evidenced by normal sinus rhythm; CO 4-7 L/min; HR 60-100 bpm; RAP 4-6 mm Hg; PAWP 6-12 mm Hg; PAP 20-30/8-15 mm Hg; BP within patient's normal range; urinary output ≥30 ml/hr; peripheral pulses >2+ on a 0-4+ scale; orientation to person, place, and time; and absence of new murmurs, pulsus paradoxus, or jugular venous distention. Hematocrit is >37% (female) or >40% (male), partial thromboplastin time is 30-40 seconds (activated), and serum potassium is 3.5-5.5 mEq/L.

1. Monitor EKG continuously during and after procedure. Document any changes. Report dysrhythmias to MD and treat according to type of dysrhythmia and hospital protocol.
2. Monitor CO, HR, RAP, PAWP, and PAP hourly or as prescribed. Report a fall in CO, change in HR, and increase or decrease in RAP, PAWP, or PAP.
3. Monitor hematocrit, clotting studies, and electrolyte values. Observe for a decrease in hematocrit, prolonged clotting results, or any change in electrolytes (particularly potassium) that could precipitate dysrhythmias.
4. Assess heart sounds immediately after procedure and q4h. Report the development of a new murmur.
5. Monitor patient for evidence of cardiac tamponade: hypotension, tachycardia, pulsus paradoxus, jugular venous distention, elevation and plateau pressuring of PAWP and RAP, and possibly, an enlarged heart silhouette on chest x-ray. For more information, see "Acute Cardiac Tamponade," p. 105.

Also see "Percutaneous Transluminal Coronary Angioplasty" for the following: **Potential alteration in tissue perfusion:** Peripheral (involved limb), related to impaired circulation secondary to presence of angioplasty sheath or risk of clot formation in vessel following sheath removal, p. 139.

Intra-aortic balloon pump

The intra-aortic balloon pump (IABP) is a counterpulsation device that assists the failing heart by decreasing afterload and increasing coronary artery perfusion. It is indicated in any clincial condition in which the myocardium is failing or has the potential for failure, or there is an imbalance between myocardial oxygen supply and demand. These clinical conditions include heart failure, cardiogenic shock, unstable angina, pre- and post-cardiac surgery, refractory ventricular dysrhythmias, cardiomyopathy, and post-PTCA complications, as well as patients awaiting heart transplantation. IABP is a temporary measure, which supports the heart and circulation for up to 30 days. It is used as an adjunct to medical therapy.

Balloon insertion can be performed emergently at the bedside or under controlled conditions during fluoroscopy. A local anesthetic agent is injected over the right or left femoral artery, the introducer sheath is inserted, and the balloon is passed through the sheath into the thoracic aorta. The balloon is then unwrapped and connected to the pump console. Pumping is timed according to the EKG or arterial pressure waveform. Balloon inflation occurs with diastole and deflation occurs with systole. The balloon's location is confirmed by x-ray to ensure that there is no obstruction of the left subclavian, mesenteric, or renal arteries.

The patient derives benefits from both phases of balloon pumping. Balloon inflation, the first phase, is termed *diastolic augmentation*. During this phase there is an increase in blood flow antegrade and retrograde within the aorta. Coronary artery blood flow is increased, resulting in increased oxygen supply to the myocardium. There also is increased blood flow to the kidneys, improving urinary output. *Systolic unloading* or balloon deflation is the second phase. Aortic pressure decreases rapidly, reducing afterload and resistance to blood flow out of the left ventricle and decreasing ventricular wall tension. With reduced afterload, the ventricle empties more completely, stroke volume rises, and myocardial oxygen usage diminishes. Clinical signs of the balloon's benefits include increased BP, increased measured cardiac output, increased urinary flow, improved mental alertness, warm extremities, palpable peripheral pulses, decreased chest pain, and improvement of the EKG changes that denote ischemia.

Complications of IABP therapy include aortic dissection, thrombus formation, impaired circulation to the balloon leg, sepsis, obstruction to the left subclavian artery blood flow, obstruction to the renal and mesenteric arteries, and paraplegia (due to spinal artery thrombosis). In addition, problems such as pneumonia and dermal ulcers can occur as a result of prolonged immobility.

NURSING DIAGNOSES AND INTERVENTIONS

Knowledge deficit: Procedure for and purpose of IABP

Desired outcome: Patient and/or significant others verbalize the purpose for IABP and describe the procedure for insertion of IABP.

< N O T E : These patients often are severely ill and may require simple and repeated instructions.

1. Teach patient and significant others about IABP, explaining the following: the balloon assists the pumping action of the heart, but it does not replace the heart's function. Use drawings to illustrate the process.
2. Explain that IABP is a temporary assistive device and that it will be removed within a few days.
3. Explain that the patient will be restricted to bed rest while the balloon is in place and that he or she may not bend the leg in which the balloon is inserted.
4. Describe the insertion procedure:
   • Patient will be given a local anesthetic.
   • An introducer sheath will be passed into the artery.
   • The balloon will be passed through the sheath and connected to a pump console.
   • The patient will be awake during the procedure but should not feel pain or discomfort.

Potential alteration in cardiac output: Decreased, related to impaired contractility and rhythm disturbances secondary to myocardial ischemia or cardiac injury

---

Desired outcomes: Patient has a normal cardiac output as evidenced by BP within patient's normal range; normal sinus rhythm on EKG; HR 60-100 bpm; peripheral pulses >2+ on a 0-4+ scale; warm and dry skin; hourly urinary output ≥30 ml; measured CO 4-7 L/min; CI ≥3.5 L/min/m^2; PAWP ≤12 mm Hg; SVR ≤1200 dynes/sec/cm^{-5}; SVO$_2$ 60-80%; and patient awake, alert, oriented, and free from anginal pain. CPK-MB is within normal limits (0-5% CPK).

---

1. Monitor BP, PAP, RAP, SVO_2, and heart rate and rhythm on a continuous basis. Monitor PAWP, SVR, and CO hourly. Be alert to and report to MD the following: elevation in PAWP, decreased CO, ST-segment changes, ectopic heartbeats, decreased SVO_2, or elevated SVR.

2. Monitor hourly urinary output, noting output that is <30 ml/h for 2 consecutive hours. Monitor BUN and creatinine values daily. Be alert to increased BUN (>20 mg/dl) and serum creatinine (>1.5 mg/dl), which can occur with low urinary output and acute tubular necrosis.

3. Monitor bilateral peripheral pulses and color and temperature of extremities q2h.

4. Provide oxygen therapy as prescribed.

5. Regulate IV inotropic agents, such as dobutamine, dopamine, amrinone, and isoproterenol to maintain cardiac index >3.5-4 $L/min/m^2$. Monitor for side effects, including tachyarrhythmias, ventricular ectopy, headache, and angina.

6. Regulate afterload reducing agents such as nitroprusside and nitroglycerin to maintain SVR <1200 $dynes/sec/cm^{-5}$. Monitor for drug side effects, including hypotension, headache, dizziness, nausea, vomiting, and cutaneous flushing.

7. Administer diuretic agents as prescribed for elevated PAWP (>12 mm Hg). Monitor for signs and symptoms of hypokalemia (e.g., weakness, dysrhythmias), a potential side effect of diuretics.

8. Provide a quiet environment conducive to stress reduction.

9. Administer prescribed pain medications as needed to reduce sympathetic response, which increases afterload.

10. Monitor hemoglobin and hematocrit values daily for decrease, which may signal bleeding and reduced blood volume, along with reduced oxygen-carrying capacity of the blood.

Potential alteration in tissue perfusion: Peripheral (balloon leg), related to risk of obstruction or hemorrhage of femoral artery secondary to arterial wall dissection by sheath or thrombus formation

---

Desired outcomes: Patient has adequate perfusion in the balloon leg as evidenced by peripheral pulses >2+ on a 0-4+ scale; normal color and sensation; warmth; full motor function; and absence of bleeding, abdominal pain, and tingling in the involved leg. Hematocrit is ≥37% (female) or ≥40% (male), partial thromboplastin time (PTT) is 30-40 seconds (activated), and prothrombin time (PT) is 11-15 seconds.

---

1. Monitor circulation in affected leg q30 minutes ×4 and q2h thereafter if assessment is within normal limits. Assess pulses, temperature, color, sensation, and mobility of the toes in the involved leg. Promptly report significant changes to MD.

2. Instruct patient to notify staff if pain, numbness, or tingling occurs in the involved leg.

3. Provide protection to heel of involved foot, using sheepskin, occlusive opaque (e.g., Duoderm) dressing, or heel protector. Place lambswool between the toes to minimize the pressure of the toes against each other.

4. To enhance perfusion in the involved leg, have patient perform passive foot

exercises without bending leg at the hip. The following should be performed qid: foot flexion/extension, foot circles, quadriceps setting. Antiembolism hose also may be beneficial.

5. Administer IV dextran or heparin as prescribed to prevent clots from forming on the balloon. Monitor patient for signs of bleeding, including abnormal PT or PTT, decreased hematocrit, abdominal pain, hematuria, oral bleeding, or blood-tinged mucus. Maintain adequate hydration (2-3 L/day) to minimize the risk of clot formation.

6. Keep HOB at 30 degrees or less to prevent upward migration of catheter, which would occlude subclavian artery.

7. Assess for the following signs of balloon migration: decreased left radial pulse, sudden decrease in urine output (<30 ml/hr), flank pain, and dizziness.

8. When the balloon is no longer needed, maintain regular balloon inflation to prevent clot formation until balloon can be removed.

Potential for impaired skin or tissue integrity related to vulnerability secondary to prolonged bed rest, diminished circulation, and decreased protein intake due to NPO status

---

Desired outcome: Patient's skin and tissue remain intact.

---

1. Position patient on protective bed, for example, Flexicare, Medicus, or Kin-Air. These beds reduce the capillary pressure to less than closing pressure, thereby enhancing blood flow to dependent areas. In addition, they also circulate air around the patient to promote evaporation of moisture.

2. Reposition patient q2h, particularly at night when spontaneous movement is diminished. When turning patient, keep balloon leg extended and logroll patient onto side.

3. Ensure meticulous skin care to keep skin clean and dry. Massage vulnerable areas (e.g., coccyx, ischial tuberosity, calcaneus, and malleoli) at least tid.

4. If skin over the bony prominences becomes reddened, apply an occlusive opaque dressing (e.g., Duoderm), according to manufacturer's instructions, to prevent further breakdown.

5. Ensure that patient's diet is high in protein and calories to promote nitrogen balance. If patient's oral intake is inadequate or patient is intubated, confer with MD regarding need for nutritional support such as enteral feedings or parenteral nutrition.

6. As patient's condition improves, teach patient to move self in bed while minimizing flexion of balloon hip.

Potential for impaired gas exchange related to hypoventilation secondary to prolonged bed rest and restricted chest excursion (HOB no higher than 30 degrees)

Desired outcomes: Patient has adequate gas exchange as evidenced by $Pao_2 \geq 80$ mm Hg, presence of normal breath sounds, and absence of adventitious sounds. RR is 12-20 breaths/min with normal pattern and depth (eupnea).

---

1. Monitor breath sounds q2h. Assess anterior and posterior lung fields for adventitious (e.g., crackles, rhonchi) or absent sounds.
2. Monitor respiratory rate, rhythm, and breathing pattern hourly.
3. Be alert to indicators of atelectasis (e.g., dyspnea, elevated temperature, weakness, absent or decreased breath sounds) and respiratory infection (elevated temperature, SOB, increased sputum production or coughing, altered color of sputum).
4. Monitor temperature q4h and WBC count daily for signs of infection. Be alert to low-grade fever of ≤37.8° C (≤100° F) and increased WBC count.
5. Provide supplemental oxygen and chest physiotherapy as prescribed.
6. Encourage patient to perform deep-breathing exercises or incentive spirometry q1-2h to promote gas exchange, followed by coughing to raise secretions.
7. If coughing is ineffective in raising secretions, suction patient as indicated, using aseptic technique.
8. Reposition patient at least q2h to minimize stasis of lung secretions.
9. Monitor patient's fluid volume status to ensure that hydration is adequate to keep secretions thin and mobile. Unless contraindicated, maintain patient's fluid intake at 2-3 L/day.
10. As often as it is allowed, elevate HOB 30 degrees to promote optimal gas exchange.

Potential for injury related to risk of bleeding/hemorrhage secondary to mechanical coagulopathy and IV anticoagulants

---

Desired outcomes: Patient is asymptomatic of bleeding as evidenced by secretions and excretions negative for blood and absence of abdominal pain or ecchymoses. Hematocrit (Hct) is ≥37% (female) or ≥40% (male), prothrombin time (PT) is 11-15 seconds, partial thromboplastin time (PTT) is 30-40 seconds (activated), activated clotting time (ACT) is ≤120 seconds, and platelet count is 150,000-400,000 μl.

---

1. Monitor PT, PTT, ACT, platelets, and Hct daily. Be alert to increased PT and PTT; ACT >120 sec; decreased platelets; and decreased Hct.
2. Test secretions and excretions daily for blood.
3. Protect patient from injury. Pad side rails, if necessary, and turn patient carefully. Use toothettes or swabs for oral care.
4. Test gastric pH q4h. Administer gastric-acid neutralizing drugs as prescribed to maintain gastric pH >5.0.

Also see the following, as appropriate: "Management of the Adult on Mechanical Ventilation," pp. 61-70; "Management of the Adult with Hemodynamic Monitoring," pp. 163-170; "Providing Nutritional Support," pp. 490-505; "Caring for the Critically Ill on Prolonged Bed Rest," pp. 506-511; "Caring for the Critically Ill with Life-Threatening Disorders," pp. 511-522; and "Caring for the Family of the Critically Ill," pp. 522-526.

Heart-assist device

A mechanical heart-assist device is indicated for the patient who has refractory heart failure that is unresponsive to drug therapy or the intra-aortic balloon pump. This includes the patient with cardiogenic shock, low cardiac output syndrome following heart surgery, or cardiomyopathy awaiting heart transplant.

There are a number of heart-assist devices available, ranging from simple to complex. Most are external to the body but a few are implanted into the abdomen. Most heart-assist devices consist of two cannulas: an outflow cannula to divert blood away from the heart and an inflow cannula that returns blood to the pulmonary artery (for right ventricular assist) or aorta (for left ventricular assist). At this time, these cannulas must be placed *via* a surgical approach. Future devices may be inserted *via* a percutaneous approach. The cannulas attach to a pump that uses a roller head, centrifugal force, pneumatic drive, or electrically powered pusher plate to propel the blood back into the body. The pump has the ability to produce a cardiac output of up to 10 L/min. The operator of the device increases or decreases the amount of blood flow according to the patient's changing needs. The assist device empties the ventricle almost totally, allowing it to recover and rest. With use of this device, the hemodynamic picture improves immediately: CO increases, BP increases, SVR decreases, PAWP or RAP decreases, and urinary output increases. As the patient's overall condition improves, the goal is gradual weaning of the patient from the device by decreasing the flow rate.

Complications of the assist device include coagulopathy, bleeding, embolization, infection, sepsis, right ventricular failure (with left heart assist only), and renal failure. Because of the critical nature of these patients and their need for constant monitoring using multiple assessment modalities, highly specialized nursing care is imperative.

NURSING DIAGNOSES AND INTERVENTIONS

Potential for injury related to risk of bleeding secondary to mechanical coagulopathy, therapeutic anticoagulation, and effects of cardiopulmonary bypass on blood components

---

Desired outcome: Patient is asymptomatic of internal or external bleeding as evidenced by hematocrit ≥37% (female) or ≥40% (male); secretions and excretions negative for blood; chest tube drainage within acceptable amounts (<100 ml/h); and absence of ecchymoses and abdominal or back pain.

---

1. Monitor hematocrit daily for a decrease in value.
2. Test gastric drainage and stool daily for blood; report positive results.
3. Monitor daily clotting studies (PT, PTT), platelets, and ACT. Report elevations of PT, PTT, or ACT above desired range, which will depend on whether or not patient is anticoagulated. Anticoagulation of patients on a heart-assist device is desirable but may not be feasible if the patient is bleeding actively from the surgical site. Monitor platelets and be alert to a decrease to <100,000 μl, which represents a significant drop.
4. Inspect all drainage for evidence of bleeding.
5. Administer coagulation factors as prescribed, for example platelets, fresh frozen plasma, cryoprecipitate, vitamin K, protamine sulfate, and aminocaproic acid.

6. Test gastric pH q4h and administer prescribed antacids for pH >5.0.
7. Administer prophylactic acid neutralizing drugs (i.e., antacids) as prescribed, as well as H_2 receptor antagonists, which block the release of histamine. Examples include cimetadine, ranitidine, and famotidine.

Impaired physical mobility related to precautions against movement secondary to presence of assist device or debilitated state

---

Desired outcome: Patient has complete range of motion without evidence of muscle atrophy, contracture formation, skin breakdown, or pulmonary infection.

---

1. Be aware that patient *can* be turned gently from side to side when the heart-assist device is in place. Do this q2h, observing assist device cannulas closely to ensure that tension is not placed on them during patient repositioning.
2. Provide passive ROM to extremities qid.
3. For interventions related to skin and tissue integrity, see **Potential for impairment of skin or tissue integrity,** p. 145, in "Intra-Aortic Balloon Pump."
4. Monitor temperature q4h and WBC count daily for signs of infection: low-grade fever ≤37.8° C (≤100° F) and WBC count >11,000 µl.
5. Monitor breath sounds q2h. Assess for the presence of crackles (rales) and rhonchi. If patient is extubated, establish hourly deep-breathing and coughing exercises.
6. If patient is incapable of raising secretions independently, suction patient as often as need is determined by auscultation. Inspect the mucus, noting color and consistency. Be alert to secretions that are yellow, green, or thickened.
7. Provide gentle chest physiotherapy as prescribed. Percussion and vibration can be performed over the posterior and lateral lung lobes during every positioning change, or at least qid.

Potential alteration in cardiac output: Decreased, related to risk of right ventricular failure secondary to reduced right ventricular contraction occurring with left-heart-assist device

< N O T E : This is a complication of the left-heart-assist device, particularly when the outflow cannula is located in the left ventricle. When the left ventricle is decompressed, septal wall motion is diminished, thereby reducing right ventricular contraction. Patients who have pulmonary hypertension or impaired right ventricular function due to MI or cardiopulmonary bypass are especially prone to this problem.

Desired outcome: Patient's cardiac output is adequate as evidenced by measured CO 4-7 L/min, RAP 4-6 mm Hg, and PVR 60-100 dynes/sec/cm^{-5}.

---

1. Monitor patient for a decrease in CO with associated increases in RAP and PVR, which are diagnostic of the complication described above.
2. Ensure that patient attains prescribed IV fluid intake to maintain a minimal LAP of 10 mm Hg. An adequate preload is necessary to prevent a vacuum effect from the device, which would aggravate this problem.

Potential for infection related to vulnerability secondary to presence of multiple invasive lines, cannulas, and debilitated state

---

Desired outcome: Patient is free of infection as evidenced by normothermia, WBC ≤11,000 μl, negative cultures, and absence of erythema, swelling, warmth, tenderness, and purulent drainage at incision or cannulation sites.

---

1. On a daily basis, monitor temperature, WBC count, and all incisions and cannulation sites for evidence of infection. Be alert to low-grade temperature of ≤37.8° C (≤100° F), WBC count >11,000 μl, and incision that is erythematous, warm, swollen, tender to the touch, and has purulent discharge.
2. Culture any suspicious drainage or secretions; report positive findings.
3. Change IV tubing q48-72h (or per agency protocol), using aseptic technique.
4. Change all dressings per agency protocol, using aseptic technique. Apply antimicrobial (e.g., povidone-iodine) ointment.
5. Administer prophylactic IV antibiotics as prescribed.
6. Provide nutritional support to ensure that nitrogen balance is attained.

Alteration in nutrition: Less than body requirements related to decreased intake secondary to oral intubation and increased need secondary to debilitated state and impaired tissue perfusion with concomitant nitrogen malabsorption

---

Desired outcome: Patient has adequate nutrition as evidenced by a balanced nitrogen state, stable weights, urine nitrogen 10-20 g/24 hr, thyroxine-binding prealbumin 200-300 μg/ml, and retinol-binding protein 40-50 μg/ml.

---

1. Provide nutrition *via* tube feedings or total parenteral nutrition to ensure minimum of 1-5 g protein/kg/day and a calorie intake of 100 kcal/kg/day, along with other essential elements. Have dietician monitor daily calorie and protein intake.
2. Weigh patient daily for trend. Report continuing decreases in weight.
3. Monitor 24-hour urinary nitrogen every 3 days for increase in excretion.
4. Monitor I&O qh. Report positive or negative fluid state of 300 ml/hr.
5. Assess patient for signs of cardiac cachexia: muscle atrophy, weakness, anorexia, and weight loss.
6. For more information, see section "Providing Nutritional Support," p. 490.

For other nursing diagnoses and interventions, see the following: "Management of the Adult on Mechanical Ventilation," pp. 66-70; "Management of the Adult with Hemodyamic Monitoring," pp. 168-170; "Caring for the Critically Ill on Prolonged Bed Rest," pp. 506-511; "Caring for the Critically Ill with Life-Threatening Disorders," pp. 511-522; and "Caring for the Family of the Critically Ill," pp. 522-526.

Coronary artery bypass graft

Coronary artery bypass graft (CABG) for coronary artery disease (CAD) may be indicated when medical treatment (e.g., nitrates, calcium-channel blockers, thrombolysis, and angioplasty) are unsuccessful or disease progression is evident. A patient with significant CAD is evaluated with angiography before surgery and the decision for surgery is based on the patient's symptoms and angiography results. Surgical indications include the following: (1) stable angina with 50% stenosis of the left main coronary artery; (2) stable angina with three-vessel coronary artery disease; (3) unstable angina with three-vessel disease or severe two-vessel disease; (4) recent myocardial infarction; (5) ischemic heart failure with cardiogenic shock; and (6) signs of ischemia or impending MI postangiography.

The surgical technique for CABG involves the use of a conduit such as a saphenous vein graft (SVG), internal mammary artery (IMA), brachial vein, or gortex graft to bypass the obstructed portion of the coronary artery. When the IMA conduit is used, the mammary artery is released from its intercostal branches and anastomosed distally past the coronary stenosis. The major advantage of the IMA is its long-term patency rate, which exceeds all other grafts. With the other conduits, the proximal anastomosis is to the aorta and the distal anastomosis to the coronary artery. The saphenous vein is by far the most common of these, with a patency rate far superior to the brachial vein or gortex graft.

The operative procedure requires the use of general anesthesia, cardiopulmonary bypass, a medial sternotomy incision, one or more incisions (e.g., on the leg for saphenous vein) for the graft, and placement of pulmonary artery, systemic arterial, or left atrial catheters for postoperative monitoring. Postoperatively, the patient is monitored in an intensive care unit for the following complications: low cardiac output syndrome, hemorrhage, cardiac tamponade, dysrhythmias, atelectasis, hypertension/hypotension, neurologic dysfunction, paralytic ileus, GI bleeding, infection or sepsis, renal failure, or postpericardiotomy syndrome. Mortality rate for CABG is approximately 2%.

NURSING DIAGNOSES AND INTERVENTIONS

Potential alteration in cardiac output: Decreased, related to altered contractility secondary to intraoperative subendocardial ischemia and administration of myocardial depressant drugs

---

Desired outcomes: Patient exhibits a normal cardiac output as evidenced by normal sinus rhythm on EKG; measured CO 4-7 L/min; peripheral pulses >2+ on a 0-4+ scale; warm and dry skin; and hourly urine output ≥30 ml/hr. Patient is awake, alert, and oriented.

---

1. Monitor EKG continuously for presence of dysrhythmias, which can alter cardiac output. Symptomatic junctional rhythms or atrial fibrillation can decrease cardiac output by 20%. Junctional rhythms are treated by pacing the heart. Atrial fibrillation can be treated wih drug therapy, including digitalis and procainamide.
2. Assess I&O hourly for evidence of decreasing output.
3. For other interventions, see the same nursing diagnosis in "Intra-Aortic Balloon Pump," p. 143.

Potential fluid volume deficit related to decreased circulating volume secondary to postoperative diuresis and excessive bleeding

< N O T E :   Diuresis is common in the early postoperative period because of the hormonal changes that accompany surgery.

Desired outcomes: Patient is normovolemic as evidenced by intake equal to output plus insensible losses, RAP ≥4 mm Hg, and PAWP ≥6.0 mm Hg. Prothrombin time (PT) is 11-15 seconds, partial thromboplastin time (PTT) is 30-40 seconds (activated), activated clotting time (ACT) is ≤120 seconds, platelet count is 150,000-400,000 μl, and fibrinogen is 200-400 mg/dl.

---

1. Measure I&O qh. Report urinary output ≥120 ml/hr and excessive chest tube drainage (>100 ml/hr). Replace excessive chest tube drainage with packed red blood cells as prescribed.
2. Monitor RAP and PAWP qh. Report PAWP <6 mm Hg and RAP <4 mm Hg.
3. As prescribed, administer IV fluids in the early postoperative period to equal the amount of diuresis.
4. Monitor clotting studies (i.e., PT, PTT, ACT, and platelet count) immediately postoperative and then q12 h × 2. Be alert to prolongation of PT, PTT, ACT; decreased platelet count; and low fibrinogen value.
5. Replace clotting factors as prescribed with platelets, fresh frozen plasma, cryoprecipitate, protamine, or aminocaproic acid.
6. Assess chest x-ray immediately after surgery and daily for signs of bleeding into the pericardial sac and mediastinum, as evidenced by an increase in the cardiac silhouette.

Hypothermia related to prolonged cooling of body during surgery

---

Desired outcome: Patient's body temperature is returned to normal gradually, as evidenced by warm extremities and absence of shivering.

< C A U T I O N :   The danger of postoperative hypothermia in heart surgery is that the patient will warm too quickly and shiver, causing hyper- or hypotension, increased or decreased SVR, metabolic acidosis, and hypoxia. All of these problems can increase cardiac workload and may potentiate ischemia, dysrhythmias, or hemorrhage in the early postoperative period.

1. On a continuous basis, measure core temperature rectally or *via* thermodilution catheter. If temperature is <36° C (96.8° F), initiate warming measures such as warm blankets, thermal garment, heating lamps, heating blankets, or warm inspired gases.
2. Continue to monitor patient during rewarming phase, maintaining rewarming rate at 1 degree Centigrade per hour.
3. Monitor skin temperature, particularly that of the extremities, q30min-1 hr during rewarming. Once extremities are warm, patient should be close to normothermia and warming measures should be discontinued.

4. Monitor BP, pulse, CO, and SVR continuously during rewarming for sudden changes related to rewarming. SVR may fall along with BP as the peripheral vascular bed dilates. This can precipitate sudden hypotension, which may require changes in patient's treatment plan. For example, if patient is on nitroprusside, the drug *may* need to be discontinued temporarily. Optimally, BP will be within patient's normal range, HR will be 60-100 bpm, CO will be 4-7 L/min, and SVR will be $\geq$900 dynes/sec/cm^{-5}.

5. If shivering due to hypothermia develops, treat immediately with warming measures and drug therapy as prescribed. Drugs used to treat shivering may include morphine sulfate, meperidine, diazepam, or pancuronium bromide. During shivering episodes, monitor VS for changes and assess oxygen saturation continuously with oximeter.

Potential for impaired gas exchange related to decreased diffusion of oxygen secondary to postoperative atelectasis, guarding of respirations, diminished activity, retained secretions, or use of anesthesia

---

Desired outcomes: Patient has adequate gas exchange as evidenced by Pa_{O_2} $\geq$80 mm Hg, Pa_{CO_2} 35-45 mm Hg, ph 7.35-7.45, presence of normal breath sounds, and absence of adventitious breath sounds. RR is 12-20 breaths/min with normal pattern and depth (eupnea).

---

1. While patient is intubated, provide supportive measures to ensure optimal aeration: suction patient when its need is determined by auscultatory findings, provide chest physiotherapy to posterior and lateral lobes as prescribed, turn patient q2h, and maintain HOB at an elevation of 45 degrees, if tolerated.

2. Assess breath sounds, RR, and amount and character of mucus production qh during the first 12 hours after surgery. Be alert to crackles (rales) and rhonchi, labored breathing, and subjective complaints of breathing difficulties. Copious, tenacious secretions put the patient at risk for airway obstruction due to mucus plugging.

3. Assess ABG values upon admission and prn during periods of respiratory distress. Report significant findings to MD, including a decreasing Pa_{O_2}, increased Pa_{CO_2}, and the presence of acidosis or alkalosis.

4. Consult with MD regarding need for ventilation changes if the above assessments are suggestive of their need.

5. As prescribed, wean and extubate patient as early as possible. It may be necessary to withhold sedation or narcotics while weaning patient.
   - Explain weaning procedure to patient. Stay with patient during first 15 minutes after each ventilatory change and reassure patient about his or her ability to breathe independently. Instruct patient to take slow, deep breaths.
   - Monitor patient's RR, tidal volume, expiratory pressure, BP, HR, and EKG during weaning. Report changes to MD, as they may be indicative of weaning intolerance.

6. Following extubation, turn patient q2h. Have patient deep breathe and cough q2h and use incentive spirometry qh. As prescribed, perform chest physiotherapy qid.

7. As soon as tolerated, have patient dangle lower extremities over the side of bed and sit in chair.

8. Instruct patient to sit upright as much as possible and to perform deep-breathing exercises. In addition, teach patient the following procedure for basal expansion exercises, which are indicated for patients recovering from chest surgery for whom pain on the surgical side inhibits bilateral chest expansion.
   • With patient sitting upright, position your palms on the midaxillary lines in the area of the 8th ribs.
   • Instruct patient to inhale as you apply moderate pressure.
   • Instruct patient to attempt to move your hands outward while expanding the lower ribs.
   • Instruct patient to maintain maximum inspiration for 1-2 seconds to achieve optimal aeration of the alveoli.
   • Have patient exhale in a relaxed, passive manner.
   • Teach patients to perform this exercise independently by positioning their own palms against the 8th ribs. Explain that performing this technique correctly and at frequent intervals will promote lower chest wall mobility.

As appropriate, see nursing diagnoses and interventions in the following: ''Management of the Adult on Mechanical Ventilation,'' pp. 66-70; ''Management of the Adult with Hemodynamic Monitoring,'' pp. 168-170; ''Providing Nutritional Support,'' pp. 490-505; ''Caring for the Critically Ill on Prolonged Bed Rest,'' pp. 506-511; ''Caring for the Critically Ill with Life-Threatening Disorders,'' pp. 511-522; and ''Caring for the Family of the Critically Ill,'' pp. 522-526.

Valvular heart disease and valve surgery

Valvular heart disease involves obstruction to forward flow (stenosis) or insufficiency of the valve, allowing backward flow (regurgitation). One or more valves may be affected by one or both processes. When the effectiveness of a valve is compromised, the patient may develop symptoms of valvular incompetency or the heart may begin to show signs of failure.

Usually, stenosis of a valve is caused by sclerosing, thickening, and calcification of the valve leaflets. A stenotic valve obstructs blood flow from the affected atria or ventricle, which leads to heart chamber hypertrophy. With a stenotic aortic or pulmonic valve, intramyocardial wall tension increases; this increase enables the heart to pump more blood through the highly resistant valve opening. If the stenosis is unrelieved, the ventricle eventually fails. When the left ventricle fails, blood backs up into the left atrium and pulmonary capillary bed, leading to pulmonary congestion and edema. In addition, with ventricular hypertrophy and high intramyocardial wall tension, blood flow to the endocardium may be diminished. These patients therefore, may have angina and ventricular dysrhythmias. When the mitral or tricuspid valve is stenotic, the atria hypertrophy and atrial pressure increases. Acute mitral stenosis results in pulmonary congestion and edema. Long-term mitral stenosis results in elevated pulmonary artery resistance and stiffening of the lung tissues. Eventually, right ventricular failure occurs. With tricuspid stenosis, systemic venous return cannot flow to the right ventricle. This results in systemic venous congestion with liver enlargement, ascites, and peripheral edema. Both mitral and tricuspid stenosis can be severely debilitating, causing easy fatigability and limited activity.

Regurgitation of a valve may be caused by rheumatic heart disease, dilatation of the valve ring, or damage to the nearby valve structures. Regurgitation results in increased volume into the affected chamber. With aortic regurgitation there is a backwash of blood into the left ventricle during diastole. The ventricle becomes volume overloaded, dilates, and eventually fails. With mitral regurgitation, there is retrograde leakage of blood into the left atrium during diastole. If the regurgitation is severe, the patient may develop pulmonary edema and low cardiac output.

Valve surgery: Methods of surgical treatment include valve repair (valvuloplasty), commissurotomy, and replacement. For patients with regurgitation, *valve repair* is the treatment of choice. In this procedure, parts of the leaflets are removed, supportive structures are shortened, or excess tissue of the dilated valve ring is gathered up. *Commissurotomy,* one of the oldest heart surgery techniques, is a procedure in which the stenotic valve is opened by a dilating instrument. When performed early in the course of the disease, chances of success are good, although it may result in valve regurgitation and recurrent stenosis. *Valve replacement* is performed in patients with moderate to severe calcification, mixed stenosis and insufficiency, and pure insufficiency and has a mortality rate of about 6%. Three types of valve replacement are used for replacement: homografts, heterografts, and artificial grafts. Homografts are human cadaver valves that have been specially treated for surgical use. Because they are not readily available, they are seldom used. A heterograft is a valve from an animal, usually a pig or cow, that has been prepared for surgical use. These valves are readily available and in common use. Artificial valves are made from stainless steel, carbon, and other durable materials. Tissue grafts are advantageous because they are natural and hence blood elements do not tend to form on them. Their disadvantage is their short duration of use, which is about 5-8 years. There is a tendency for clots to form on the artificial graft, and therefore the patient must be on lifetime anticoagulant therapy; however, the graft can be used for 10-15 years. Postoperative care of the valve surgery patient is similar to that of the patient who has undergone coronary artery bypass grafting (see p. 150). Postoperative considerations specific to these patients are discussed under the nursing diagnoses and interventions.

NURSING DIAGNOSES AND INTERVENTIONS

Potential fluid volume deficit related to decreased circulating volume secondary to hemorrhage

< C A U T I O N :   Patients undergoing aortic valve replacement are at a higher risk for postoperative hemorrhage than those undergoing CABG.

Desired outcomes: Patient is asymptomatic of bleeding or hemorrhage as evidenced by RAP ≥4 mm Hg, PAWP ≥6 mm Hg, BP within patient's normal range, CO ≥4 L/min, urine output ≥30 ml/hr, urine specific gravity 1.010-1.030, and chest tube drainage ≤100 ml/hr. Hematocrit is ≥37% (female) or ≥40% (male), prothrombin time (PT) is 11-15 seconds, partial thromboplastin time (PTT) is 30-40 seconds (activated), platelet count is 150,000-400,000 μl, and activated clotting time (ACT) is ≤120 seconds.

---

1. Measure chest tube drainage hourly. Report chest tube drainage >100 ml/hr. Maintain patency of chest tubes at all times.
2. Monitor clotting studies. Be alert to and report prolonged PT, PTT, and ACT and decreased platelet count. For patient with prolonged PT, PTT, or ACT, administer IV protamine sulfate as prescribed.
3. Assess VS qh and monitor patient for physical indicators of hemorrhage or hypovolemia: RAP <4 mm Hg, PAWP <6 mm Hg, decreased BP, decreased measured CO, urine output <30 ml/hr, increased urine specific gravity, and excessive chest tube drainage (>100 ml/hr). Be alert to a decreased hematocrit.
4. Assess postoperative chest x-ray for a widened mediastinum, which may be indicative of hemorrhage and possible cardiac tamponade.
5. As prescribed, administer platelets, fresh frozen plasma, or cryoprecipitate to replace clotting factors and blood volume.
6. Administer packed red blood cells as prescribed to replace blood volume.
7. To correct hyperfibrinolytic state (increased fibrin degradation products), administer aminocaproic acid slowly per IV bolus as prescribed.

Potential alteration in cardiac output: Decreased, related to altered contractility secondary to intraoperative subendocardial ischemia and administration of myocardial depressant drugs

< N O T E : After cardiac surgery there is always some myocardial depression present, usually lasting 48-72 hours. Patients with long-standing aortic stenosis or ventricular failure due to mitral valve disease are at an even greater risk for postoperative low cardiac output.

Desired outcomes: Patient has adequate cardiac output as evidenced by normal sinus rhythm on EKG, a measured CO of 4-7 L/min, CI >3.5 $L/min/m^2$, BP within patient's normal range, PAP 20-30/8-15 mm Hg, PAWP 6-12 mm Hg (or range specified by MD), SVO_2 60-80%, SVR 900-1200 dynes/sec/cm^{-5}, peripheral pulses >2+ on a 0-4+ scale, warm and dry skin, and hourly urine output ≥30 ml/hr. Patient is awake, alert, and oriented.

---

1. Monitor BP, PAP, RAP, SVO_2, HR, and heart rhythm continuously. Monitor PAWP, SVR, and CO hourly. Be alert to and report the following: elevation in PAWP, decreased CO, decreased SVO_2, or elevated SVR.
2. Monitor urinary output, noting output that is <30 ml/hr for two consecutive hours.
3. Monitor peripheral pulses and color and temperature of extremities q2h.
4. Provide oxygen therapy as prescribed.
5. Maintain an adequate preload (i.e., PAWP >6 mm Hg, RAP >4-6 mm Hg) *via* administration of IV fluids.

< N O T E : With aortic stenosis and severe left ventricular hypertrophy, a high filling pressure (i.e., PAWP >18 mm Hg) may be necessary to ensure an adequate cardiac output.

6. Maintain a normal or reduced afterload (SVR <1200 dynes/sec/cm^{-5}) by admin-

istering prescribed IV vasodilating drugs, such as nitroprusside and nitroglycerin.

7. Maintain normal sinus rhythm by administering antiarrhythmic agents as prescribed. Atrial fibrillation is common in aortic and mitral valve disease and may result in a 20% decrease in CO. If a junctional rhythm or bradycardia occurs, a pacemaker usually becomes necessary.

8. Administer inotropic agents as prescribed to maintain CI >3.5 L/min/m^2 and systolic BP >90 mm Hg. Commonly used agents include dobutamine, dopamine, amrinone, and isoproterenol. Monitor for side effects, including tachyarrhythmias, ventricular ectopy, headache, and angina.

Potential alteration in tissue perfusion: Cerebral, related to impaired circulation to the brain secondary to embolization resulting from cardiac surgery

< C A U T I O N :   Air embolism, particulate embolism from calcified valves, and thrombotic emboli from prosthetic valves may lodge in the brain, leading to varying degrees of stroke.

Desired outcome: Patient has adequate brain perfusion as evidenced by orientation to person, place, and time; equal and normoreactive pupils; and ability to move all extremities, communicate, and respond to requests.

---

1. Monitor patient immediately after surgery and qh for signs of neurologic impairment: diminished LOC, pupillary response, ability to move all extremities, and response to verbal stimuli.

2. Assess patient's orientation and ability to communicate, answer yes-no questions, point to objects, write a response on a piece of paper, write sentences and appropriate requests, identify family members, and identify where he or she is. Inform other health-care personnel about patient's LOC and communication deficits.

3. If CNS impairment is suspected, administer urea solutions, mannitol, and corticosteroids as prescribed.

4. In the presence of CNS impairment, implement the following measures:
   • Assist patient with turning and moving as needed. Teach patient to use unaffected extremities to assist with moving.
   • Perform ROM to all extremites qid. Have patient assist as much as possible.
   • Progress patient's activity level, as tolerated, with the assistance of a physical therapist.

5. When patient is able to take oral foods and fluids, assess patient's ability to swallow. If patient's voice is hoarse or patient coughs when swallowing, alert MD. Patient may require NPO status and an enteric tube until the swallowing reflex has improved.

Knowledge deficit: Risk of infective endocarditis following valve surgery and precautions that must be taken to prevent it

< N O T E :   All patients with valve surgery are at risk for infective endocarditis as a result of bacteria entering the bloodstream and traveling to the heart, leading to destruction of a new tissue valve or obtruction of a new artificial valve.

Desired outcome: Patient verbalizes knowledge about the risk of infective endocarditis following valve surgery and the precautions that must be taken to prevent it.

1. Teach patient about infective endocarditis (see ''Acute Infective Endocarditis,'' p. 108), describing what it is, how it develops, and how it may affect the repaired valve.
2. Teach patient that antibiotics are prescribed as a prophylaxis against endocarditis following valve surgery. Explain that they must be taken prior to any dental work or scopic exam, including teeth cleaning, fillings, extractions, cystoscopy, endoscopy, or sigmoidoscopy. Caution patient to notify dentists and other physicians about the valve surgery so that antibiotics can be prescribed prior to any invasive procedure.
3. Instruct patient to cleanse all wounds and apply antibiotic ointments to help prevent infection.

See ''Perfusion Disorders'' for the following: **Knowledge deficit:** Oral anticoagulant therapy, potential side effects, and foods and medications to avoid during therapy, p. 27. See ''Coronary Artery Bypass Graft'' for the following: **Potential impairment of gas exchange** secondary to postoperative atelectasis, guarding of respirations, diminished activity, retained secretions, and anesthesia, p. 152. Also see nursing diagnoses and interventions in the following: ''Management of the Adult with Hemodynamic Monitoring,'' pp. 168-170; ''Caring for the Critically Ill on Prolonged Bed Rest,'' pp. 506-511; ''Caring for the Critically Ill with Life-Threatening Disorders,'' pp. 511-522; and ''Caring for the Family of the Critically Ill,'' pp. 522-526.

Automatic implantable cardioverter-defibrillator

The automatic implantable cardioverter-defibrillator (AIC-D) is a pulse generator used to correct lethal cardiac dysrhythmias. It is recommended for patients who have had at least two episodes of cardiac arrest or for patients with coronary artery disease who have had a cardiac arrest and are not CABG candidates. The pulse generator, made of titanium and powered by lithium batteries, is surgically inserted into a ''pocket'' formed in the umbilical region. The leads of the AIC-D consist of two sets of electrodes. The first set includes an apical ''mesh'' patch, which is sutured to the epicardium, and a superior vena cava (SVC) lead, which is utilized to sense morphology and deliver defibrillatory ''shocks.'' The second set serves as the rate sensing lead and consists either of a bipolar right ventricular endocardial catheter or two epicardial screws placed on the exterior of the left ventricle. The AIC-D is programmed to ''shock'' either at a pre-determined cut-off rate or after assessing the morphology of the EKG.

The surgical procedure for AIC-D insertion can be accomplished *via* one of three approaches. Usually, a median sternotomy incision is used, allowing other forms of cardiac surgery (i.e., valvular surgery, aneurysmectomy, CABG) to be performed concurrently. The lateral thoracotomy incision is reserved for those patients who have undergone CABG, and subsequently, are prone to adhesions. The

subxiphoid approach has the fewest complications, but because perioperative visualization is poor, it is used rarely. Postoperative complications include atelectasis,
pneumonia, seroma at the generator "pocket," pneumothorax, or thrombosis. Lead
migration and lead fracture are the two most common structural problems. Interference from unipolar pacemakers and "myopotentials" (electrical interference) are
common mechanical complications.

NURSING DIAGNOSES AND INTERVENTIONS

Knowledge deficit: AIC-D procedure and follow-up care

Desired outcome. Patient describes rationale for the procedure, method of insertion, postinsertion care, and need for continued physician and nurse follow-up.

---

1. Assess patient's understanding of his or her medical condition (dysrhythmias)
   and the amount of detailed information desired.
2. Discuss the following with the patient and significant others:
   - Type of dysrhythmia patient has, using rhythm strip and heart model to pro-
     mote understanding.
   - Need for temporary transvenous pacemaker insertion prior to AIC-D proce-
     dure, which is utilized to induce ventricular tachycardia or ventricular fibril-
     lation or for emergency use should the patient require pacing prior to insertion
     of AIC-D.
   - Use of general anesthesia throughout procedure.
   - Testing of the ability of the AIC-D to terminate lethal dysrhythmias, which
     will occur in the operating room after implantation, before the incision is
     closed. Explain that the patient will be given extra systoles *via* the temporary
     pacemaker to induce clinical rhythm.
   - Reassurance that should the mechanism fail to terminate the dysrhythmia, the
     patient can be paced in an overdrive mode to abort the dysrhythmia.
   - Continuous observation of patient in a cardiac care unit for 48-72 hours, with
     ongoing monitoring of BP, HR, and RR.
   - Importance of deep-breathing, coughing, and incentive spirometry exercises,
     which will be implemented immediately after surgery. Explain that patient is
     at increased risk for respiratory tract infection because of the thoracic surgery,
     which tends to cause patient to avoid deep breathing and coughing to guard
     against pain. Have patient return demonstrations of breathing exercises that
     will be implemented immediately following surgery. Reassure patient that an-
     algesics can be administered prior to pulmonary toilet exercises.
   - Discharge instructions: Follow-up visit within 10-14 days, need for obtaining
     "home defibrillator," and importance of CPR/defibrillator classes for signifi-
     cant others.

Potential for infection related to vulnerability secondary to invasive procedure into
thorax

Desired outcome: Patient is free of infection as evidenced by normothermia, WBC count ≤11,000 μl, negative cultures, and absence of the clinical indicators of infection at the incision site and of the respiratory tract.

1. Because of the thoracic incision site, the patient is at risk for atelectasis and pneumonia following the AIC-D insertion procedure. Enforce deep-breathing, coughing, and incentive spirometry exercises q2h and encourage early ambulation to the chair. As indicated, assist patient with splinting the incision site with hands or pillow to promote optimal excursion. Provide prescribed analgesics 20 minutes before scheduled breathing exercises to facilitate compliance. For more information, see this nursing diagnosis in "Pneumonia," p. 13.
2. Assess incision site q2h for warmth, erythema, swelling, and drainage. The presence of a seroma, which has the same symptomatology as incision site infection, is confirmed by decubitus chest films or CT scan.
3. Monitor patient's temperature q2-4h, being alert to elevation >38.6° C (101.5° F).
4. Monitor CBC for elevation of WBCs.
5. Notify MD of significant findings.
6. Teach patient and significant others the signs and symptoms of infection, both of the incision site (see #2, above) and respiratory tract: cough, sputum production, fever, dyspnea, chills, headache, myalgias. Explain that elderly individuals may be confused, disoriented, and run low-grade fevers, but present with few other indicators.

Potential for altered sexuality patterns related to fear of inducing dysrhythmias during sexual activity

Desired outcome: Patient and significant other verbalize understanding of interventions during and alternatives for sexual intercourse.

1. Assess patient for symptomatology (dysrhythmias) during presurgical sexual experiences.
2. Explain the following interventions or alternatives that can be made if patient continues to experience dysrhythmias during sexual intercourse:
   • Patient may need to take on a less dominant role.
   • Patient may find that taking a prescribed vasodilator prior to engaging in sexual intercouse will prevent dysrhythmias.
   • Suggest that during periods of time when dysrhythmias are problematic, less stressful forms of sexual activity, such as caressing and hugging, are positive alternatives.
3. As appropriate, advise patient that stressful situations, such as extramarital relations or unfamiliar environment, may contribute to symptomatology during sexual activity.
4. Explain that the device may "shock" at any time. If the patient's significant other is in contact with the patient's body at that time, the shock may be experienced as a tingling sensation by the significant other.

The patient is at risk for pneumothorax. As indicated, see "Pneumothorax," p. 28, for information related to this disorder.

REHABILITATION AND PATIENT-FAMILY TEACHING CONCEPTS

Patient education should begin upon admission and continue throughout hospitalization. Provide patient and significant others with verbal and written instructions for the following:

1. Importance of CPR training for all family members and significant others.
2. Importance of physician and nurse follow-up visits after hospital discharge.
3. Procedure should AIC-D device fire a "shock": patient should be taken to the emergency department *via* ambulance and physician notified at once. Teach patient to record the number of "shocks" experienced.
4. The home defibrillator, which is available commercially from several companies. It is designed to allow the nonmedical person to defibrillate the AIC-D patient and its purpose is to convert lethal dysrhythmias should the AIC-D fail. Explain that a yes-no format is utilized to answer questions asked by the defibrillator and that the family is trained in its use by the company representative prior to hospital discharge.
5. Explain that interference can occur in unipolar systems. If it occurs in a bipolar system, it is a sign of lead fracture. Any patient receiving "shocks" while in sinus rhythm may have lead fracture in his or her AIC-D system. Usually, this is detected while patient is being monitored (e.g., with EKG in physician's office, hospital monitor, or holter monitor).

Coronary artery thrombolysis

The formation of a thrombus in the atherosclerotic coronary vessel may be the last of a series of events that result in myocardial infarction (MI). Research has shown that early reperfusion of an ischemic myocardium can prevent or reduce myocardial injury. Therefore, the ability to dissolve (lyse) fresh coronary thromboses early in the course of infarction is a logical course for the treatment of MI. The goal of thrombolysis is to reduce infarct size, improve left ventricular function, and minimize morbidity and mortality. Currently, three thrombolytic agents are in use: streptokinase, urokinase, and tissue type plasminogen activator.

Streptokinase, an enzyme derived from group C beta-hemolytic streptococcus, acts as a catalyst for the conversion of plasminogen to plasmin, which lyses the clot. Streptokinase can be administered IV or *via* the intracoronary route. Because it is an antigen, patients who have had previous exposure to streptococcal organisms may have built up antibodies against streptokinase. Therefore, steroids or antihistamines are administered before streptokinase therapy to prevent a hypersensitivity reaction. Usual dose is 20,000 IU as a bolus and 4,000 IU/min as a continuous drip. The infusion is continued until a predetermined dose has been given, usually 150,000-500,000 IU. *Urokinase* is an enzyme derived from human renal cells. It activates plasminogen directly to form plasmin. Urokinase is administered in a manner similar to streptokinase, although desired dosages have not yet been well established. Both urokinase and streptokinase have some systemic lytic effects and may result in bleeding complications in other areas of the body. ***Tissue type*** *plasminogen activator* is produced by the body and converts plasminogen to plasmin after binding to the fibrin clot. This mechanism of action is advantageous because there are no systemic lytic effects. In addition, it is nonantigenic. It has a shorter half-life than the other two enzymes and has been shown in initial studies to be more effective than streptokinase and urokinase in lysing coronary thromboses. The suggested dose is 0.5-1.0 mg/kg IV infused over 60-90 minutes.

Specific protocols have been established for use of all three agents. Eligibility criteria include (1) chest pain of ≤3 hours duration; (2) ST-segment elevation and reciprocal ST depression, reflecting transmural ischemia; (3) chest pain and ST elevation unrelieved by nitroglycerin; (4) no evidence of impending cardiogenic shock; (5) under 75 years of age; and (6) no contraindications to thrombolytic or anticoagulant therapy, such as bleeding disorders or surgery within the last 6 months. (Source: UCLA streptokinase protocol.)

Thrombolytic therapy can be performed in an emergency room, where the thombolytic agents are administered peripherally, or in the catheterization lab under fluoroscopy, where it is administered *via* the intracoronary route. During the procedure, blood is drawn, lidocaine is administered prophylactically, the EKG is monitored continuously, and emergency drugs and equipment are made available. Indications that lysis has taken place include the following: decreased chest pain, rapid resolution of ST depression, and a new onset of dysrhythmias. Up to 80% of patients are reported to have had reperfusion dysrhythmias, primarily idioventricular rhythm and PVCs (Lewicki). Bradycardia and heart block also are seen.

NURSING DIAGNOSES AND INTERVENTIONS

Knowledge deficit: The atherosclerotic process and the rationale, procedure, and expected outcomes of thrombolytic therapy

---

Desired outcome: Patient verbalizes knowledge about the atherosclerotic process and thrombolytic therapy.

---

1. Assess patient's knowledge about the atherosclerotic process and the rationale, procedure, and expected outcome of thrombolytic therapy. Explain the goal of therapy: to reduce injury to the heart muscle.
2. Explain the need for monitoring and close observation post-procedure.
3. Provide emotional support during the procedure, keeping the patient informed about the events that are taking place.
4. After the procedure, discuss potential long-term outcomes and the possibility of re-stenosis, including interventions patient can take to prevent this: take prescribed antiplatelet medications, exercise, enforce dietary modifications, and manage or eliminate risk factors such as smoking, hyperlipidemia, hypertension, stress, and obesity.
5. Before discharge, instruct patient to report any signs and symptoms of MI that occur after patient leaves the hospital: unrelenting chest heaviness or pressure; pain that radiates to the arm, neck, or jaw; accompanying nausea and diaphoresis; and lightheadedness or dizziness.

Potential fluid volume deficit related to loss (hemorrhage) secondary to systemic lytic effects of streptokinase or urokinase

Desired outcome: Patient is asymptomatic of bleeding as evidenced by BP within patient's normal range, HR $\leq$100 bpm, secretions and excretions negative for blood, natural skin color, and absence of hematoma and back and abdominal pain.

1. When patient is admitted, obtain a thorough history, assessing for the following:
   - Risk factors for intracranial hemorrhage: hypertension >5 years duration, cerebrovascular pathology, CNS surgery within last 6 months.
   - Bleeding risks: peptic ulcer, recent trauma, recent surgery, bleeding diathesis, advanced liver or kidney disease.
   - Risk of systemic embolization: suspected left-heart thrombus.
   - High titers of anti-SK antibodies.
2. Monitor clotting studies per agency protocol. Regulate heparin drip to maintain PTT of at least 80-100 seconds, or according to protocol. *Never* discontinue heparin without physician directive.

< N O T E : During the first 24 hours, PTT tends to be higher than normal.

3. Apply pressure dressing over puncture site if cardiac catheterization was performed. Inspect site at frequent intervals for evidence of hematoma formation.
4. Monitor patient for other indicators of bleeding: back pain, abdominal pain, decreased BP, pallor, and bloody stool or urine. Report significant findings to MD.
5. Avoid giving injections, venipuncture, or arterial puncture.
6. Use care with oral hygiene and when shaving patient. For more information about safety precautions, see **Potential for injury** related to risk of bleeding or hemorrhage secondary to anticoagulation or thrombolytic therapy in "Perfusion Disorders," p. 26, in "Respiratory Dysfunctions."

Potential for injury related to risk of allergic response to streptokinase secondary to presence of antibodies in the body

Desired outcome: Patient is asymptomatic of allergic response as evidenced by normothermia, RR 12-20 breaths/min with normal pattern and depth (eupnea), HR $\leq$100 bpm, natural skin color, and absence of itching, hives, headache, muscular and abdominal pain, and nausea.

1. Before treatment, question patient about history of previous streptokinase therapy or streptococcal infection. Report findings to MD.
2. Administer prophylactic hydrocortisone as prescribed.
3. Monitor patient postinfusion for indicators of allergy: hives, fever, itching, flushing, nausea, headache, muscular pain, bronchospasm, abdominal pain, dyspnea, or tachycardia. These indicators can appear immediately after or as long as several days following streptokinase therapy.
4. Treat allergic response with diphenhydramine or other antihistamine, as prescribed.

Potential alteration in cardiac output: Decreased, related to risk of dysrhythmias secondary to thrombolytic therapy

---

Desired outcomes: Patient has normal cardiac output as evidenced by normal sinus rhythm on EKG, peripheral pulses >2+ on a 0-4+ scale, warm and dry skin, and hourly urine output ≥30 ml/hr. Patient is awake, alert, and oriented without palpitations, chest pain, or dizziness.

---

1. Monitor EKG continuously during thrombolytic therapy for evidence of dysrhythmias. Report findings to MD.
2. Monitor patient for signs of reocclusion: chest pain, ST-segment elevation.
3. With any dysrhythmia, check VS and note accompanying signs and symptoms such as dizziness, lightheadedness, syncope, and palpitations.
4. Ensure availability of emergency drugs and equipment: lidocaine, atropine, isoproterenol, epinephrine, defibrillator-cardioverter, pacemaker.
5. Evaluate patient response to medications and emergency treatment.

Management of the adult with hemodynamic monitoring

Many critically ill adults have a history of cardiovascular disease or are at risk for cardiovascular complications; therefore, it is important to be able to assess the heart's function as well as factors that regulate cardiac muscle mechanics. There are four major cardiac mechanisms that determine cardiac output (CO), which is the amount of blood ejected by each ventricle per minute. These mechanisms are preload, afterload, contractility, and heart rate.

Preload can be defined as the degree of myocardial fiber stretch at the end of diastole just prior to contraction. Preload is an important concept because of Starling's law of the heart, which states that within physiologic limits, the greater the stretch of the myocardial muscle, the greater the force of contraction. As the end-diastolic volume increases, the pressure generated in the ventricle increases, resulting in an increased amount of blood ejected by the ventricle. This mechanism enables the heart to pump varying volumes of blood and to keep the output of the two ventricles matched. Since myocardial stretch cannot be measured directly, it is measured indirectly by changes in pressure. The clinical measure for right ventricular preload is the central venous pressure (CVP) or right atrial pressure (RAP) and for the left ventricle, the pulmonary artery wedge pressure (PAWP) or left atrial pressure (LAP). Preload is influenced by the circulating blood volume, distribution of the volume, atrial contraction, and ventricular contraction. Therefore, any problem that influences one of these factors will result in a change in preload with a concomitant change in CO.

Afterload refers to the tension that develops within the ventricular myocardium during systole. In order for the heart to eject its contents, it must overcome any resistant forces. The aortic and pulmonary artery pressures are the main impediments to flow for the left and right ventricles. Other resistant forces include blood viscosity, vascular resistance, distensibility of the vascular system, and the valves themselves. Because vascular resistance plays a major role in determining pressure, afterload is evaluated by calculating the pulmonary vascular resistance (PVR) for right ventricular afterload and systemic vascular resistance (SVR) for left ventricular afterload. The significance of these measures is that the higher the afterload, the greater the myocardial wall tension. This work is achieved at the expense of oxygen utilization. In the abnormal heart where there is diminished blood flow, an increased afterload may result in ischemic myocardial injury and possible infarction.

Contractility is an inherent property of the myocardium and is a factor of the number of contractile units working together. This mechanism functions independently of variations in preload and afterload. Although contractility cannot be measured directly, a change can be inferred when there is a decreased CO and a normal PAWP, SVR, and heart rate. Several factors influence contractility: adrenaline, calcium, digitalis, and beta-adrenergic drugs increase it; while hypoxia, beta-blocker drugs, and antiarrhythmic drugs decrease it.

Heart rate (HR) is the final determinant of cardiac output. A rapid HR may result in decreased diastolic filling time and a drop in CO. In addition, atrial fibrillation with loss of atrial kick can decrease CO by 20%. Bradycardia may increase CO.

Hemodynamic monitoring refers to the specialized methods of evaluating cardiovascular performance. It provides information about tissue perfusion, blood volume, cardiac performance, tissue oxygenation, and vascular tone. Indirect methods of hemodynamic monitoring include measurement of arterial pressure *via* blood pressure (BP) cuff or Doppler and measurement of cardiac output (CO) with an echo Doppler. Direct methods of measuring hemodynamics include arterial catheter, central venous catheter, and pulmonary artery catheter. This section focuses on direct methods of hemodynamic monitoring.

TYPES OF DIRECT HEMODYNAMIC MEASUREMENT CANNULATION

1. **Arterial catheters:** Generally inserted *via* the radial artery because this artery is readily accessible and collateral blood flow usually is adequate. The arterial pressure waveform is displayed on a bedside monitor for continuous observation of systolic, diastolic, and mean arterial pressures. Changes in arterial pressure waveform may be due to mechanical factors such as thombosis of the catheter, catheter whip or fling (movement within the vessel), faulty instrumentation, infiltration, or cardiac disorders such as aortic stenosis, cardiac tamponade, low cardiac output, and dysrhythmias. Complications of arterial catheters include hand ischemia, exsanguination, infection, and infiltration. Continuous observation of the arterial line insertion site is an important nursing responsibility.

   • *Systolic blood pressure:* Determined by (1) the amount of blood ejected by the ventricle per beat (stroke volume), (2) wall compliance of the arterial system, and (3) peripheral resistance. Elevations in systolic pressure often reflect changes in vascular compliance, such as the hypertension seen in individuals with vascular atherosclerosis. A decrease in systolic pressure will be seen with heart disorders that result in decreased stroke volume or with the use of arterial vasodilators such as nitroprusside, hydralazine, and prazosin.

   • *Diastolic blood pressure:* Determined by (1) volume of blood within the arterial system, (2) compliance of the arterial wall, and (3) peripheral resistance. Because coronary artery blood flow occurs during diastole and a drop in diastolic pressure may result in ischemia of the subendocardium, diastolic blood pressure is an important measure, particularly when administering vasodilating drugs.

   • *Mean arterial pressure (MAP):* The average pressure within the arterial tree throughout the cardiac cycle. It can be calculated by the following formula:

$$MAP = \frac{systolic \ + \ 2 \ diastolic}{3}$$

Normal value is 70-105 mm Hg. MAP reflects the average force that pushes blood through the systemic circulation throughout the cardiac cycle, therefore, it is an important indicator of tissue blood flow. Since MAP is the product of CO × SVR, an increase in CO or SVR will increase MAP and a decrease in either value will decrease MAP.

2. **Central venous catheters:** Central venous pressure (CVP) is the measurement of systemic venous pressure at the level of the right atrium (RA). CVP can be measured by a catheter that is threaded into the jugular or subclavian vein or by a separate port of a pulmonary artery (PA) catheter. Normal value is 2-6 mm Hg. Because 60% of the blood volume is contained in the venous bed, the CVP is valuable in assessing fluid volume excess or deficit. In addition, it provides information regarding right ventricular (RV) function and venous tone. Disease processes that may increase CVP include right ventricular failure, cardiac tamponade, fluid volume overload, pulmonary hypertension, tricuspid valve disease, and chronic left ventricular failure. Usually, decreased CVP is caused by hypovolemia; however, venodilatation due to sepsis, drugs, or neurogenic causes also may decrease CVP.

3. **Pulmonary artery (PA) catheters:** These have become a vital link in the management of critically ill patients. They are inserted *via* the jugular, subclavian, antecubital, or femoral vein and passed through the right heart into the pulmonary artery, where the tip of the catheter is positioned in the pulmonary capillary bed. This catheter provides a wide variety of information that can be used in the assessment or treatment of heart disease, pulmonary disease, trauma, shock, complex surgeries, obstetrical emergencies, and other situations during which management of blood volume and heart function are important. Assessment data derived from this catheter include right atrial pressure (RAP); right ventricular pressure (RVP); pulmonary artery pressure (PAP), including systolic, diastolic, and mean pressures; pulmonary artery wedge pressure (PAWP); cardiac output (CO); core temperature; and mixed venous oxygen saturation (SVO_2). Although the risk of major complications with this catheter is low (3%), it is important for the nurse to be familiar with the possibilities: ventricular or atrial dysrhythmias, pulmonary ischemia or infarction, pulmonic valve injury, endocarditis, tricuspid valve damage, pulmonary artery rupture, and infection.

- *Right atrial pressure (RAP):* This is essentially the same as central venous pressure (CVP). With the PA catheter, RAP can be monitored continuously and displayed on a bedside screen. In addition, the catheter lumen can be used for fluid or drug administration. Normal mean RAP is 4-6 mm Hg.
- *Right ventricular pressure (RVP):* Measured during catheter insertion only and can provide information about the function of the right ventricle and the tricuspid and pulmonic valves. Normal RVP is 25/0-5 mm Hg. Elevation of RV systolic pressure may be seen in pulmonic stenosis, pulmonary hypertension, or ventricular septal defect (VSD) with left-to-right shunt. Elevation of RV diastolic pressure may occur with right ventricular failure, cardiac tamponade, or constrictive pericarditis. It is important for the nurse to identify the normal RV waveform because a complication of the PA catheter is redi-

rection of the catheter tip into the right ventricle, causing ventricular ectopy to occur.

- **Pulmonary artery pressure (PAP):** Used to evaluate left heart function and pulmonary vascular disease. Normal PAP is 20-30/8-15 mm Hg. PA diastolic pressure (PAD) corresponds closely to the pulmonary artery wedge pressure (PAWP) because the mitral valve is open during diastole and the catheter has a clear view to the left ventricle, thereby providing an indirect measurement of left ventricular end-diastolic pressure. A significant difference (i.e., >5 mm Hg) between the PAD and PAWP is seen with pulmonary disease or a pulmonary embolus. When this occurs, PA systolic and diastolic pressures are elevated, while the PAWP remains normal. Specific disease states that elevate PAP include pulmonary hypertension, pulmonary embolism, hypoxia, left ventricular failure due to valve disease, MI, cardiomyopathy, and left-to-right intracardiac shunt. A decreased PAP is seen with hypovolemia.

- **Pulmonary artery wedge pressure (PAWP):** Reflects left ventricular end-diastolic pressure (LVEDP) and is used to evaluate cardiac performance. Normal mean PAWP is 6-12 mm Hg. An elevated PAWP may be seen with left ventricular failure, acute mitral regurgitation, acute VSD, and acute cardiac tamponade. A decreased PAWP is seen with hypovolemia.

- **Left atrial pressure (LAP).** The most direct measure of left ventricular end-diastolic pressure (LVEDP). A left atrial catheter is inserted during heart surgery and brought through the chest wall or epigastric area. When connected to a transducer, a continuous display of left atrial pressure is possible. The normal value for LAP is 8-12 mm Hg.

- **Cardiac output (CO):** The volume of blood in liters ejected by the heart each minute and is the product of the stroke volume and heart rate (HR). Normal value is 4-7 L/min. *Stroke volume* (SV) is the volume of blood ejected by the heart per beat. Normal SV is 55-100 ml/beat. To compare individual differences in CO in relation to body size, the CO is divided by the body surface area (BSA) to obtain the value known as *cardiac index*. Normal cardiac index is 2.5-4 L/min/m^2.

- **Systemic vascular resistance (SVR):** The major factor that determines left ventricular afterload and therefore is the clinical measurement used to evaluate it. The formula for SVR is the following:

$$SVR = \frac{(MAP - RAP)}{CO} \times 80.$$

Normal value for SVR is 900–1200 dynes/sec/cm^{-5}. Any factor that increases SVR will increase the workload of the heart; therefore, measures are taken (e.g., vasodilator therapy) to keep SVR within normal limits.

- **Pulmonary vascular resistance (PVR):** The clinical measure of right ventricular overload. The formula for PVR is the following:

$$PVR = \frac{(MPAP - LAP)}{CO} \times 80$$

The normal value is 60–100 dynes/sec/cm^{-5}. PVR may be elevated as a result of mitral or aortic valve disease, congenital heart disease, long-standing left ventricular heart failure, hypoxia, COPD, or pulmonary embolus. Drugs also

TABLE 2-16
Normal hemodynamic values

Systemic arterial pressure	110-120/70-80 mm Hg
Central venous pressure (CVP)	2-6 mm Hg (5-12 cm H_2O)
Right atrial pressure (RAP)	4-6 mm Hg
Left atrial pressure (LAP)	8-12 mm Hg
Right ventricular pressure (RVP)	25/0-5 mm Hg
Pulmonary artery pressure (PAP)	20-30/8-15 mm Hg
Pulmonary artery wedge pressure (PAWP)	6-12 mm Hg
Mean arterial pressure (MAP)	70-105 mm Hg
Cardiac output (CO)	4-7 L/min
Cardiac index (CI)	2.5-4 L/min/m^2
Systemic vascular resistance (SVR)	900-1200 dynes/sec/cm^{-5}
Pulmonary vascular resistance (PVR)	60-100 dynes/sec/cm^{-5}
Stroke volume (SV)	55-100 ml/beat
Mixed venous oxygen concentration (SVO$_2$)	60-80%

may affect the PVR, for example, norepinephrine and the prostaglandins increase it, while isoproterenol and acetylcholine decrease it.

- *Mixed venous oxygen saturation (SVO$_2$):* Can be measured using mixed venous blood samples from the PA catheter or by continuous monitoring *via* a special fiberoptic PA catheter. While venous oxygen saturation is affected by arterial oxygen saturation, CO, oxygen consumption, and hemoglobin, SVO$_2$ is the average percentage of hemoglobin bound with oxygen in the venous blood and is reflective of the overall tissue utilization of oxygen. Normal range for SVO$_2$ is 60-80%. Measurement of SVO$_2$ is valuable in the critical care setting as it can aid in the diagnosis and treatment of life-threatening conditions that are common to critically ill patients. When it is monitored continuously, it can be used to evaluate the effects of medical and nursing interventions on tissue oxygen utilization. For example, the simple maneuver

TABLE 2-17
Formulas for obtaining common hemodynamic values

$$MAP = \frac{\text{systolic} + 2 \text{ diastolic}}{3}$$

$$CO = HR \times SV$$

$$CI = \frac{CO}{BSA}$$

$$SVR = \frac{(MAP - RAP)}{CO} \times 80$$

$$PVR = \frac{(MPAP - LAP)}{CO} \times 80$$

$$SV = \frac{CO}{HR}$$

of weighing a patient on a bed scale may cause a dramatic decline in SVO_2. Clinical conditions in which this can occur include heart failure, dysrhythmias, respiratory failure, hyperthermia, shivering, seizures, and fever. An increased SVO_2 may be the result of hypothermia, anesthesia, septic shock, increased FIo_2, polycythemia, and left-to-right shunt.

NURSING DIAGNOSES AND INTERVENTIONS

Knowledge deficit: Rationale for hemodynamic monitoring and procedure for catheter insertion

---

Desired outcome: Patient verbalizes knowledge of the rationale for hemodynamic monitoring, procedure for insertion of lines, and sensations that are experienced during and after the procedure.

---

1. Assess patient's knowledge about hemodynamic monitoring. As indicated, explain to patient that hemodynamic monitoring is useful in guiding medical therapy and that the PA catheter can measure pressures in the heart similar to the way in which pressures are measured in the arm *via* a BP cuff.
2. Teach patient about the insertion procedure, emphasizing that a local anesthetic will be used, he or she will not be able to move during the procedure, frequent x-rays will be taken, and a large dressing will be applied to the insertion site.
3. Explain the sensations that may be felt during the procedure: a stick from the local anesthetic, pressure as the catheter advances, coldness from the cleansing solution, burning from the injection of lidocaine, claustrophobia from drapes over the face, dull pushing and pulling sensations in the neck, and coldness from the injection of cardiac output iced solution.
4. Instruct patient to inform MD if anxiety or discomfort is felt during the procedure, as medications can be given as necessary.

Potential for infection related to vulnerability secondary to presence of hemodynamic lines

---

Desired outcome: Patient is free of infection as evidenced by normothermia, WBC count $\leq$11,000 μl, negative cultures, and absence of erythema, heat, swelling, or purulent drainage at the insertion site.

---

1. On a daily basis, monitor temperature for elevations $>37°$ C (99° F); WBC count for elevation; and catheter insertion site for erythema, tenderness to the touch, local warmth, and purulent drainage.
2. As prescribed, culture any suspicious drainage and report positive findings.
3. Use normal saline rather than D_5W for hemodynamic flush solution.
4. Change hemodynamic tubing, transducer, and solution q48h.
5. Change dressing at insertion site per agency protocol, using aseptic technique. Apply antimicrobial ointment such as povidone-iodine to insertion site.
6. Record date of catheter insertion and ensure that catheter is changed per agency protocol.

Potential for alteration in tissue perfusion: Pulmonary, related to risk of pulmonary infarction secondary to migration of PA catheter into a wedged position, overwedging of balloon, or continuous wedge position

---

Desired outcomes: Patient has adequate pulmonary perfusion as evidenced by normal PA waveform and RR 12-20 breaths/min with normal depth and pattern (eupnea). The following signs of pulmonary infarction are absent: acute onset of pleuritic chest pain, SOB, tachypnea, hemoptysis, or wedge-shaped infiltrate on chest x-ray.

---

1. Monitor PA waveform continuously. Report any change in configuration, particularly if the waveform becomes decreased in amplitude and flattened in appearance.
2. On a daily basis, evaluate position of catheter *via* chest x-ray.
3. Monitor PA waveform when wedging balloon. Inject only enough air to obtain a wedge configuration, but no more than the amount recommended by catheter manufacturer. Never pull back on syringe to remove air; disconnect syringe and allow passive deflation of balloon.
4. Deflate balloon after obtaining wedge pressure.
5. Pay special attention to PA waveform when patient moves about (e.g., when being taken to x-ray or getting up and into a chair).

Potential alteration in tissue perfusion: Peripheral (hand), related to risk of impaired circulation secondary to presence of arterial catheter or thrombosis caused by catheter

---

Desired outcome: Patient has adequate perfusion to the hand as evidenced by brisk capillary refill (<3 seconds), natural color, warm skin, sensation, and the ability to move the fingers.

---

1. On a continuous basis, monitor capillary refill, hand color, temperature, sensation, and movement. Be alert to indicators of hand ischemia and teach them to the patient, stressing the importance of notifying staff promptly should they occur.
2. Maintain arterial line on continuous flush at 3 ml/hr with heparinized normal saline (1 unit heparin/ml saline); ensure that pressure bag remains inflated at 300 mm Hg.
3. Support patient's wrist with armboard or other supportive device to prevent flexion and movement of the catheter.

Potential for injury related to risk of insertion complications secondary to patient movement during insertion procedure or difficult anatomy

< N O T E : With PA or CVP catheter insertion, the following complications may occur: carotid artery puncture, air embolism, RV perforation, hemorrhage, thoracic duct injury, pneumothorax, and cardiac tamponade.

Desired outcome: Patient is asymptomatic of PA or CVP catheter insertion complications as evidenced by normal sinus rhythm on EKG, BP within patient's normal range, HR ≤100 bpm, RR ≤20 breaths/min with normal pattern and depth (eupnea), normal breath sounds, and absence of adventitious breath sounds or muffled heart sounds.

1. During preprocedure teaching, caution patient about the importance of remaining still during insertion of catheter. Provide sedation as prescribed.
2. Perform a baseline assessment, monitoring BP, HR, RR, breath sounds, heart sounds, and EKG. Perform a postprocedure assessment, comparing it to baseline findings. Be alert to decreased BP, pulsus paradoxus (see p. 107), increased HR or RR, diminished or absent breath sounds, and muffled heart sounds, as well as dysrhythmias on EKG. Report significant findings.
3. After the procedure, obtain a chest x-ray as prescribed.

SELECTED REFERENCES

American Heart Association: Standards and Guidelines for Cardiopulmonary Resuscitation and Emergency Cardiac Care. *JAMA* June 1986; 225 (21): 2841-3044.

Alspach JG, Williams S: *Core Curriculum for Critical Care Nursing,* 3rd ed. Saunders, 1985.

Andreoli KG, et al. *Comprehensive Cardiac Care,* 5th ed. Mosby, 1983.

Brannon PH, Towner SB: Ventricular failure: New therapy using the mechanical assist device. *Crit Care Nurs* 1986; 6: 70-85.

Braunwald E (ed): *Heart Disease: A Textbook of Cardiovascular Disease,* Vols 1 and 2. Saunders, 1984.

Carolan J: *Shock: A Nursing Guide.* Medical Economics, 1984.

Constant J: *Bedside Cardiology,* 2nd ed. Little, Brown, 1986.

Echt DS: Clinical experience, complications, and survival in 70 patients with the automatic implantable cardioverter/defibrillator. *Circulation* 1985; 71: 289-296.

Erickson BA: Detecting abnormal heart sounds. *Nursing 86* 1986; 16(1): 58-63.

Estes ME: Management of the cardiac tamponade patient. A nursing framework. *Crit Care Nurs* 1985; 5(5): 17-26.

Flores B, Hildebrandt M: The automatic implantable defibrillator. *Heart Lung* 1984; 13: 608-613.

Frazee RC, et al: Objective evaluation of blunt cardiac trauma. *J Trauma* 1986; 26: 510-520.

Goldberger E: *Treatment of Cardiac Emergencies,* 4th ed. Mosby, 1986.

Goldman MJ: *Principles of Clinical Electrocardiology,* 11th ed. Lange, 1982.

Gore J, et al: *Handbook of Hemodynamic Monitoring.* Little, Brown, 1985.

Guzzetta C, Dossey B: *Cardiovascular Nursing: Body Mind Tapestry.* Mosby, 1984.

Holmes DR, Vlietstra RE: Percutaneous transluminal coronary angioplasty; Current status and future trends. *Mayo Clin Proc* 1986; 61: 865-876.

Hurst JM (ed): *The Heart,* 5th ed. McGraw-Hill, 1985.

Isner JM, et al: Treatment of aortic stenosis by balloon valvuloplasty. *Am J Cardiol* 1987; 59: 313-317.

Kenner B, Guzzetta C, Dossey B: *Critical Care Nursing: Body, Mind, Spirit.* Little, Brown, 1985.

Kern LS : Advances in the surgical treatment of coronary artery disease. *J Cariovasc Nurs* 1986; 1: 1-14.

Kern LS: Surgical treatment of underlying heart disease and mechanical support of the failing heart. In: Michaelson CR: *Congestive Heart Failure.* Mosby, 1983.

Kern LS, Gawlinski A: Stage-managing coronary artery disease. *Nurs 83* 13: 34-40.

Lanoue AS, et al: Percutaneous transluminal coronary angioplasty: Nonoperative treatment of coronary artery disease. *J Cardiovasc Nurs* 1986; 1: 30-44.

Lewicki L: Medical management of coronary artery disease. In: Kern L (ed): *Cardiac Critical Care Nursing*. Aspen, 1988.

McKay RG, et al: Balloon dilatation of calcific aortic stenosis in elderly patients: Postmortem, intraoperative, and percutaneous valvuloplasty studies. *Circulation* 1986; 74: 119-125.

Quaal S: Thrombolytic therapy: An overview. *J Cardiovasc Nurs* 1986; 1: 45-56.

Sokolow M, McElroy M: *Clinical Cardiology*. Lange, 1986.

Sommers MS: Cardiac tamponade after non-penetrating cardiac trauma. *Dim Crit Car Nurs* 1986; 5(4): 206-215.

Sommers MS: Nursing care of patients with blunt cardiac trauma. *Crit Care Nurs* 1985; 5(6): 58-66.

Tiongson JG, Woods A: Cardiac isoenzymes: Clinical implications and limitations. *Crit Car Qu* 1979; 2: 47-51.

Tueller BL: Cardiovascular Disorders. In: *Manual of Nursing Therapeutics: Applying Nursing Diagnoses to Medical Disorders*. Swearingen PL (ed). Addison-Wesley, 1986.

Underhill S, et al: *Cardiac Nursing*. Lippincott, 1982.

White KM: Completing the hemodynamic picture. SVO_2. *Heart Lung* 1985; 14: 272-280.

Winkle RA, et al: Practical aspects of automatic cardioverter-defibrillator implantation. *Am Heart J* 1984; 108: 1335-1346.

Yee B, Zorb S: *Cardiac Critical Care Nursing*. Little, Brown, 1986.

Zuidema GD, Rutherford RB, Ballinger WF: *The Management of Trauma*. Saunders, 1985.

3
RENAL-URINARY DYSFUNCTIONS

Acute renal failure

Lower urinary tract trauma

Renal trauma

Renal transplant

Dialytic therapy

Continuous arteriovenous hemofiltration

Fluid and electrolyte disturbances

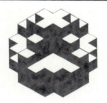

Acute renal failure

Acute renal failure (ARF) is a syndrome characterized by an abrupt deterioration of renal function, resulting in the accumulation of metabolic wastes and water, usually accompanied by a marked decline in urinary output. If it is undetected or treated inadequately, ARF can lead to parenchymal damage and progress to chronic renal failure. ARF is caused by decreased renal perfusion, nephrotoxic injury, ischemic injury, or obstruction. It is categorized as prerenal, intrarenal, and postrenal (see Table 3-1). The most common cause of ARF is acute tubular necrosis (ATN).

TABLE 3-1
Causes of acute renal failure

Prerenal (decreased renal perfusion)	Intrarenal (parenchymal damage; acute tubular necrosis)	Postrenal (obstruction)
Hypovolemia	Nephrotoxic agents	Calculi
• GI losses	• Antibiotics (aminoglycosides, sulfonamides, methicillin)	Tumor
• Hemorrhage		
• Third space (interstitial) losses (burns, peritonitis)	• Diuretics (e.g., furosemide)	Benign prostatic hypertrophy
• Dehydration from diuretic use	• Nonsteroidal anti-inflammatory drugs (e.g., ibuprofen)	Necrotizing papillitis
Hepatorenal syndrome	• Contrast media	Urethral strictures
Edema-forming conditions	• Heavy metals (lead, gold, mercury)	Blood clots
• Congestive heart failure	• Organic solvents (carbon tetrachloride, ethylene glycol)	Retroperitoneal fibrosis
• Cirrhosis		
• Nephrotic syndrome	Infection (gram-negative sepsis) pancreatitis, peritonitis	
Renal vascular disorders	Transfusion reaction (hemolysis)	
• Renal artery stenosis	Rhabdomyolysis with myoglobinuria (severe muscle injury)	
• Renal artery thrombosis	• Trauma	
• Renal vein thrombosis	• Exertion	
	• Seizures	
	• Drug-related: heroin, barbiturates, IV amphetamines, succinylcholine	
	Glomerular diseases	
	• Poststreptococcal glomerulonephritis	
	• IgA nephropathy (e.g., Berger's disease)	
	• Lupus glomerulonephritis	
	• Serum sickness	
	Ischemic injury	

ATN is the result of nephrotoxic injury or a prolonged compromise in renal perfusion (ischemic injury). In the acutely ill adult, both factors may be operative since renal ischemia tends to potentiate the injury produced by nephrotoxins.

Generally, there are three identifiable phases or stages of ARF. Phase one usually is characterized by oliguria, a drop in the 24-hour urinary output to 400 ml or less. This phase lasts approximately 7-21 days, depending on the underlying pathology. There are, however, approximately 30% of patients who present with a syndrome of nonoliguric renal failure. The diuretic phase is evidenced initially by a doubling of the urinary output from the previous 24-hour total. During this phase, the patient may produce as much as 3-5 liters of urine in 24 hours. The recovery phase is marked by a return to a normal 24-hour volume (1500-1800 ml). Usually, renal function continues to improve and may take 6 months to a year from the initial insult to return to baseline functional status.

ASSESSMENT

ARF can dramatically affect fluid, electrolyte, and acid-base balances.

Fluid volume alterations
- *Excess:* Peripheral edema, jugular vein distention, S_3 or S_4 gallop, crackles (rales), increased BP, oliguria.
- *Deficit:* Decreased BP, poor skin turgor, flushed skin, dry mucous membranes, oliguria.

Electrolyte imbalances: Dysrhythmias, altered mental status, gastrointestinal disturbances, neuromuscular dysfunction.

Metabolic acidosis: Weakness, disorientation, SOB, Kussmaul's respirations.

Uremic manifestations: Accumulation of urea, creatinine, uric acid; anemia and bleeding tendencies; fatigue and pallor; increased BP, congestive heart failure, pericarditis with tamponade, pulmonary edema; anorexia, nausea, vomiting, diarrhea; behavioral changes; decreased wound healing ability; increased susceptibility to infection.

Physical assessment
- *Cardiovascular:* S_3 or S_4 gallop, pericardial friction rub, jugular vein distention, tachycardia, dysrhythmias, increased BP, pulsus paradoxus in the presence of fluid volume excess, edema (peripheral, periorbital, sacral), capillary fragility, purpura.
- *Respiratory:* Crackles (rales), hyperventilation.
- *Neuromuscular:* Weakness, lethargy, muscle irritability, muscle tenderness, asterixis.
- *Cutaneous:* Pallor; presence of uremic frost in severely uremic individuals.

History and risk factors: Chronic illness (e.g., hypertension, diabetes), recent infections (e.g., streptococcal), recent episodes of hypotension (major bleeding, major surgery), exposure to nephrotoxic drugs or other agents (e.g., carbon tetrachloride, diuretics, aminoglycoside antibiotics, dyes), recent blood transfusion, urinary tract disorder, toxemia of pregnancy or abortion, recent severe muscle damage (rhabdomyolysis with myoglobinuria).

DIAGNOSTIC TESTS

1. *Serum BUN, creatinine, uric acid, and electrolytes:* Creatinine is the most reliable indicator of renal function. BUN is influenced by hydration, catabolism, presence of bleeding, infection, fever, and antianabolic agents (corticoste-

roids). BUN, creatinine, and uric acid will be elevated in the presence of ARF, as will potassium, phosphorus, and magnesium.

2. *Creatinine clearance test:* For clinical purposes, this is the most reliable estimation of glomerular filtration rate. Accuracy depends on complete collection. Creatinine clearance decreases with age. Normal creatinine clearance is 95-125 ml/min. In the presence of ARF, it usually is <50 ml/min.

3. *Urinalysis:* The presence of sediment-containing tubular epitheleal cells, cellular debris, and tubular casts supports a diagnosis of ARF. Large amounts of protein and many RBC casts are common in ARF when it is secondary to parenchymal (intrarenal) disease. Sediment is normal when the causes are categorized as prerenal.

4. *Urinary sodium:* A prerenal cause is signalled by a sodium count <10 mEq/L.

5. *CBC and coagulation studies (PT, PTT):* To evaluate for hematologic complications. Baseline hematocrit may be low owing to ARF, and hematocrit and hemoglobin will fall steadily if the ARF patient experiences bleeding.

6. *ABG values:* Because ARF patients have metabolic acidosis, $Paco_2$ and plasma pH will be low.

7. *Ultrasound:* Identifies hydronephrosis, fluid collection, and masses.

8. *Intravenous pyelograms (IVP, both retrograde and antegrade):* Diagnose partial or complete obstruction.

9. *Renal scan:* Provides information about renal perfusion.

10. *Renal angiography and venography:* Assess for the presence or absence of thrombotic or stenotic lesions in the main renal vessels.

MEDICAL MANAGEMENT AND SURGICAL INTERVENTIONS

Prerenal ARF

1. **Volume replacement:** Replacement solutions include free water plus electrolytes lost through the urine, wounds, drainage tubes, diarrhea, and vomiting. Usually, losses are replaced on a volume for volume basis. Maintenance fluids total approximately 1500 ml/24 hours. With a moderate fluid deficit (5% weight loss), at least 2400 ml are given over a 24-hour period. A severe deficit (>5% weight loss) requires a replacement of at least 3000 ml/24 hours.

2. **Diuretics** (furosemide and ethacrynic acid): Decrease filtrate reabsorption and enhance water excretion. They may be used, after adequate hydration, to increase urine output or in an attempt to prevent onset of oliguria. Mannitol or low-dosage dopamine may be used to increase renal blood flow and urine output in an attempt to prevent oliguria.

Intrarenal ARF

1. **Removal or discontinuation of causative agent** (e.g., aminoglycosides, dye load, chemicals)

2. **Dialytic therapy:** Maintains homeostasis (see discussion, p 199).

3. **Nutrition therapy:** Involves a diet high in carbohydrates to prevent endogenous protein catabolism and muscle breakdown, low in sodium for individuals retaining sodium and water, high in sodium for those who have lost large volumes of sodium and water owing to diuresis or other bodily drainage, low in potassium if the patient is retaining potassium, and low in protein to maintain daily requirements while minimizing increases in azotemia. Nutrition is delivered either *via* oral, enteral, or total parenteral nutrition (TPN). See Table 3-14, p. 219,

for a list of foods high in sodium and Table 3-15, p. 228, for a list of foods high in potassium.

4. **Blood transfusions:** If indicated, to maintain a stable hematocrit. There are two major hematologic complications of renal failure:
   - *Anemia:* Caused by decreased erythropoietin, low-grade GI bleeding from mucosal ulceration, blood drawing, and shortened life of the RBCs.
   - *Prolonged bleeding time:* Caused by decreased platelet adhesiveness.

   As renal failure progresses, anemia becomes more profound and platelet adhesiveness decreases further.

5. **Pharmacotherapy**
   - *Antihypertensives.*
   - *Phosphate binders (aluminum hydroxide antacids and calcium carbonate antacids):* Bind phosphorus and control hyperphosphatemia.
   - *Sodium bicarbonate:* Controls metabolic acidosis and promotes shift of potassium back into the cells.
   - *Sodium polystyrene sulfonate (Kayexalate):* Oral or rectal preparation that exchanges sodium for potassium in the GI tract to help control hyperkalemia.
   - *Water-soluble vitamin supplements:* For patients receiving dialytic therapy. Water-soluble vitamins are diffused across the membrane and are dialyzed out during treatments.

$<$ N O T E : See Table 3-2 for a list of drugs that require dosage modification for patients with ARF. Drugs that require dosage modification in renal failure are those that are excreted primarily by the kidneys. Dosage must be governed by clinical responses as well as serum levels, if available. Drugs that should be avoided are those that are nephrotoxic; those (or their metabolites) that are toxic to other organs if they accumulate; those that aggravate uremic symptoms; and those that accentuate metabolic derangements of renal failure.

Postrenal

1. **Relief of obstruction:** Achieved *via* catheterization with in-dwelling urinary catheter, ureteral stent to relieve obstruction prior to surgical intervention, lithotripsy to disintegrate stones, or prostatectomy if benign prostatic hypertrophy is the cause of the obstruction.
2. **Monitoring of fluid and electrolyte balance:** Postobstructive diuresis may result in hypovolemia (see p. 215), hyponatremia (see p. 222), hypokalemia (see p. 226), hypocalcemia (see p. 232), and hypomagnesemia.
3. **Culturing of urine and administration of antibiotics** if indicated

NURSING DIAGNOSES AND INTERVENTIONS

Fluid volume excess: Edema related to retention of sodium and water secondary to acute renal failure

---

Desired outcome: Patient is normovolemic as evidenced by balanced I&O, urinary output $\geq$30 ml/hr, stable weights, absence of edema and other physical indicators of volume overload, BP within patient's normal range, CVP $\leq$6 mm Hg, and HR $<$100 bpm.

TABLE 3-2
Drugs that require dosage modification in renal failure

Antimicrobials	Cardiovascular agents	Analgesics	Sedatives	Miscellaneous
amikacin	digoxin	meperidine	phenobarbital	insulin
gentamicin	digitoxin	methadone	meprobamate	cimetidine
kanamycin	procainamide			clofibrate
tobramycin	guanethidine			neostigmine
amphotericin B				
vencomycin				
lincomycin				
sulfonamides				
ethambutol				
penicillins				

Drugs to avoid

tetracycline
nitrofurantoin
spironolactone
amiloride
aspirin
lithium carbonate
cisplatin
phenylbutazone
nonsteroidal anti-inflammatory agents
magnesium-containing medications

< N O T E :   Although patient is retaining sodium, his or her serum sodium may be within normal limits or decreased from baseline due to the dilutional effect of the fluid overload.

1. Document I&O hourly. Notify MD if urinary output falls to <30 ml/h.
2. Weigh patient daily; notify MD of significant weight gain, (e.g., 0.5-1.5 kg/24 hrs).
3. Assess for and document the presence of basilar crackles (rales), jugular vein distention, tachycardia, pericardial friction rub, gallop, increased BP, increased CVP, or SOB, any of which are indicative of fluid volume overload.
4. Assess for and document the presence of peripheral, sacral, or periorbital edema.
5. Restrict patient's total fluid intake to 1200-1500 ml/24 hrs, or as prescribed.
6. Provide ice chips or chewing gum to help patient quench thirst and moisten mouth.
7. Monitor serum osmolality and serum sodium values. These values may be decreased due to the dilutional effect of fluid overload.
8. Recognize that if it is delivered, TPN should be the largest volume of fluid given. If total fluid intake is >2000 ml/day, ultrafiltration with dialysis (see p.

199) or continuous arterial-venous hemofiltration (CAVH) (see p. 207) may be necessary to maintain fluid balance.

9. If patient is retaining sodium, restrict sodium-containing foods (see Table 3-14, p. 219) and avoid diluting IV medications with high-sodium diluents. Also avoid sodium-containing medications, such as sodium penicillin.

Fluid volume deficit related to decreased circulating volume secondary to diuresis, vomiting, diarrhea, hemorrhage, or fluid shift to interstitial compartments

---

Desired outcomes: Patient is normovolemic as evidenced by urinary output ≥30 ml/hr with specific gravity of 1.010-1.030; stable weights; CVP ≥2 mm Hg; HR 60-100 bpm; BP within patient's normal range; and absence of thirst and other indicators of hypovolemia. BUN is ≤20 mg/dl and serum creatinine is ≤1.5 mg/ dl (or within acceptable range, given patient's underlying condition); hematocrit is within acceptable range.

< N O T E :　A patient with ARF has a hematocrit in the range of 20-30%, owing to the anemia that occurs with renal failure.

1. Weigh patient daily. Notify MD of weight loss of ≥1-1.5 kg/24 hrs.

2. Monitor and document I&O hourly. Notify MD if patient's output is <30 ml/ hr. With deficit, intake should exceed output by 0.5-1 L (depending on severity of dehydration) q24h.

3. Notify MD if there is an increase in losses from vomiting, diarrhea, or wound drainage or sudden onset of diuresis.

4. Observe for and document indicators of dehydration and hypovolemia, e.g., poor skin turgor, dry and sticky mucous membranes, thirst, increasing girth (from interstitial spacing), hypotension, tachycardia, decreasing CVP.

5. Encourage oral fluids, if they are allowed. Ensure that IV fluid rates are maintained as prescribed.

6. Be aware that approximately 30% of patients with ARF have GI bleeding. Monitor hemoglobin, hematocrit, and BUN. In the presence of bleeding with ARF, hemoglobin and hematocrit will fall steadily (rapidly if there is massive bleeding). BUN will increase in the presence of GI bleeding without a concomitant rise in serum creatinine.

7. Test all stools, urine, emesis, and peritoneal dialysate drainage for occult blood. Check urine and dialysate drainage at least q8h.

8. To minimize the risk of bleeding, keep siderails up and padded, use small-gauge needles for injections, minimize blood drawing, and promote the use of electric razors and soft-bristled toothbrushes. Limit invasive procedures as much as possible. If possible, avoid injections for 1 hour post hemodialysis. Apply gentle pressure to injection sites.

9. Inspect gums, mouth, nose, skin, and perianal and vaginal areas q8h for bleeding. Also inspect hemodialysis insertion and peritoneal access sites for evidence of bleeding q8h. Apply a soft, occlusive sterile dressing to peritoneal, subclavian, or femoral access sites daily to protect skin from irritation and bleeding due to catheter movement.

Alteration in nutrition: Less than body requirements related to increased catabolism or dietary restrictions secondary to acute renal failure

---

Desired outcomes: Patient has adequate nutrition as evidenced by stable weights and a state of nitrogen balance (estimated). Patient's caloric intake ranges from 35-45 calories/kg of normal body weight.

---

1. Infuse enteral feedings and hyperalimentation as prescribed.
2. Assess and document patient's intake of nutrients every shift.
3. Weigh patient daily. Notify MD of significant findings (i.e., loss of >1.5 kg/24 hrs).
4. As prescribed, utilize cooling blanket or antipyretics to control fever. Fever increases tissue catabolism, which in turn increases energy needs.
5. The end products of protein metabolism that accumulate in renal failure are reflected by an increase in BUN level. Low-protein diets are used to decrease the nitrogenous load and attempt to control uremia to some extent. Ensure intake of high-biologic value protein, which contains the more essential amino acids necessary for cell building (e.g., eggs, meat, fowl, milk, and fish).
6. Be sure that caloric intake ranges from 35-45 calories/kg of normal body weight. The exact amount will vary with age, sex, activity, and the degree of preexisting malnutrition. Foods that may be used to increase caloric intake include honey, hard candy, gum drops, and sherbet.
7. Restrict high-potassium foods, such as bananas, citrus fruits, fruit juices, nuts, tea, coffee, legumes, and salt substitute. In ARF, the kidneys are unable to excrete potassium effectively.
8. Sodium requirements will vary greatly. If oliguria is present, sodium may be restricted from the diet. If diuresis is present, sodium intake may be increased because of excess sodium loss in the urine. Intervene accordingly.
9. Hypocalcemia may be present early in ARF as a result of decreased absorption of calcium from the gut. As prescribed, replace calcium orally (e.g., with dairy products) or intravenously.

Potential for injury related to sensorimotor and mentation alterations secondary to electrolyte disturbances, metabolic acidosis, or uremia occurring with ARF

Desired outcomes: Patient does not exhibit evidence of injury due to sensorimotor or mentation alterations that can occur with electrolyte disturbances, metabolic acidosis, or uremia. Patient and significant others verbalize knowledge of the signs and symptoms of complications that can occur with ARF, as well as dietary restrictions and other interventions that can be made to prevent or allay their occurrence.

Hyperkalemia (serum potassium >5.5 mEq/L): Occurs because of the kidneys' decreasing ability to excrete potassium, and the release of potassium that occurs with protein catabolism and metabolic acidosis.

< N O T E :   Hyperkalemia can be a fatal complication, especially during the oliguric phase of ARF, because of its adverse effect on cardiac status.

1. Assess patient for signs and symptoms of hyperkalemia; monitor EKG and serum potassium levels. Notify MD of significant findings including serum potassium level >5.5 mEq/L, paresthesias, muscle weakness or flaccidity, bradycardia (HR <60 bpm), tall and peaked T waves, loss of P waves, ventricular fibrillation, and cardiac arrest (usually seen with potassium concentrations >6.5 mEq/L).
2. Teach patient and significant others the indicators of hyperkalemia and the importance of notifying staff promptly should they occur.
3. Provide a list of foods that are high in potassium (see Table 3-15, p. 228), and stress the importance of avoiding these foods.
4. Implement and teach interventions that will help minimize the cellular release of potassium:
   • Ensure that patient consumes only the amount of protein allotted by MD, enforce sound infection control techniques to minimize the risk of infection, and treat fevers promptly (catabolism of protein, which occurs in the above situations, causes potassium to be released from the tissues).
   • Ensure that patient consumes the allotted amounts of carbohydrates and enforce bedrest or limit patient activities as prescribed, both of which will spare protein.
5. Have emergency supplies (i.e., manual resuscitator bag, crash cart, and emergency drug tray) readily available.
6. Also see discussion of metabolic acidosis, below. For a more detailed discussion, see "Hyperkalemia," p. 229.

Hypokalemia (serum potassium <3.5 mEq/L): May result from prolonged, inadequate oral intake; use of potassium-losing diuretics without proper replacement; excessive loss from vomiting or diarrhea; excessive loss through NG or intestinal suction. With a severe deficit, paralysis and heart block can occur. EKG changes are more likely to occur at serum levels <3 mEq/L and neuromuscular symptoms are seen at levels of approximately 2.5 mEq/L.

< N O T E :   Hypokalemia can be fatal, causing apnea or heart block.

1. Assess patient for indicators of hypokalemia; monitor EKG and serum potassium levels. Notify MD of signficant findings including serum potassium level <3.5 mEq/L, muscle weakness, soft and flabby skeletal muscles, ileus, decreased bowel sounds, paresthesias, weak and irregular pulse, prolonged P-R interval, flattened or inverted T wave, depressed ST-segment, presence of U wave, and distant heart sounds.
2. Teach patient and significant others to recognize and report indicators of hypokalemia.
3. Provide a list of foods high in potassium (see Table 3-15, p. 228); assist patient and significant others with planning menus that incorporate high-potassium foods.
4. Avoid administration of diuretics that cause potassium loss, such as chlorothiazide (Diuril), chlorthalidone (Hygroton), ethacrynic acid (Edecrin), furosemide (Lasix), hydrochlorothiazide (Esidrix), and metolazone (Zaroxolyn).
5. Administer oral or IV potassium supplements as prescribed.

- For oral replacement, administer with at least 4 ounces of water or juice to decrease gastric irritation.
- Monitor flow rate of IV replacement to ensure precise delivery.
6. For more detail, see "Hypokalemia," p. 226.

Hypernatremia (serum sodium >147 mEq/L): Precipitating events include the kidneys' inability to excrete excess sodium, decreased water intake, increased water losses *via* osmotic diuresis, and excessive parenteral administration of sodium-containing solutions (e.g., sodium bicarbonate, 3% sodium chloride).
1. Monitor VS and I&O hourly. Assess patient for dry mucous membranes, flushed skin, firm and rubbery tissue turgor, elevated temperature, agitation, oliguria, or anuria.
2. Monitor serum sodium levels.
3. Assess sensorium for restlessness and agitation; institute seizure precautions as indicated.
4. Administer prescribed IV replacement fluids.
5. Administer diuretics if prescribed.
6. For more information, see "Hypernatremia," p. 225.

Hyponatremia (serum sodium <137 mEq/L): Loss occurs through vomiting, diarrhea, profuse diaphoresis; use of potent diuretics; salt-losing nephropathies; and administration of large amounts of sodium-free intravenous fluids. Hyponatremia may be associated with fluid volume excess or seen with postobstructive diuresis.
1. Monitor I&O hourly; measure weight daily for trend. Assess patient for abdominal cramps, diarrhea and nausea, dizziness with changing position, postural hypotension, cold and clammy skin, and apprehension.
2. Monitor serum sodium levels.
3. Provide parenteral replacement as prescribed.
4. Institute a safe environment for individuals with altered LOC.
5. For more information, see "Hyponatremia," p. 222.

Hypocalcemia (serum calcium <8.5 mg/dl): In the presence of renal failure, dietary calcium is poorly utilized. With an elevated phosphorus level, calcium may precipitate out into the tissues. Lack of conversion of vitamin D to its usable form causes inadequate absorption and utilization of calcium. A calcium deficit requires the administration of activated vitamin D (Rocaltrol) and calcium supplements.
1. Monitor serum calcium levels.
2. Monitor for numbness and tingling around the mouth as well as muscle twitching, facial twitching, and tonic muscle spasms. Assess for Trousseau's sign (carpopedal spasm) and Chvostek's sign (spasm of lip and cheek). Notify MD of signficant findings.
3. Administer calcium and vitamin D supplements as prescribed.
4. Teach patient and significant others the indicators of hypocalcemia.
5. Reinforce the necessity of taking vitamin D and calcium supplements as prescribed.
6. Teach the importance of continued follow-up to check serum calcium levels.
7. For more information, see "Hypocalcemia," p. 232.

Hyperphosphatemia (serum phosphorus >4.5 mg/dl): Occurs chiefly in acute and chronic renal disease. Although most foods contain generous amounts of

- For oral replacement, administer with at least 4 ounces of water or juice to decrease gastric irritation.
- Monitor flow rate of IV replacement to ensure precise delivery.
6. For more detail, see "Hypokalemia," p. 226.

Hypernatremia (serum sodium >147 mEq/L): Precipitating events include the kidneys' inability to excrete excess sodium, decreased water intake, increased water losses *via* osmotic diuresis, and excessive parenteral administration of sodium-containing solutions (e.g., sodium bicarbonate, 3% sodium chloride).
1. Monitor VS and I&O hourly. Assess patient for dry mucous membranes, flushed skin, firm and rubbery tissue turgor, elevated temperature, agitation, oliguria, or anuria.
2. Monitor serum sodium levels.
3. Assess sensorium for restlessness and agitation; institute seizure precautions as indicated.
4. Administer prescribed IV replacement fluids.
5. Administer diuretics if prescribed.
6. For more information, see "Hypernatremia," p. 225.

Hyponatremia (serum sodium <137 mEq/L): Loss occurs through vomiting, diarrhea, profuse diaphoresis; use of potent diuretics; salt-losing nephropathies; and administration of large amounts of sodium-free intravenous fluids. Hyponatremia may be associated with fluid volume excess or seen with postobstructive diuresis.
1. Monitor I&O hourly; measure weight daily for trend. Assess patient for abdominal cramps, diarrhea and nausea, dizziness with changing position, postural hypotension, cold and clammy skin, and apprehension.
2. Monitor serum sodium levels.
3. Provide parenteral replacement as prescribed.
4. Institute a safe environment for individuals with altered LOC.
5. For more information, see "Hyponatremia," p. 222.

Hypocalcemia (serum calcium <8.5 mg/dl): In the presence of renal failure, dietary calcium is poorly utilized. With an elevated phosphorus level, calcium may precipitate out into the tissues. Lack of conversion of vitamin D to its usable form causes inadequate absorption and utilization of calcium. A calcium deficit requires the administration of activated vitamin D (Rocaltrol) and calcium supplements.
1. Monitor serum calcium levels.
2. Monitor for numbness and tingling around the mouth as well as muscle twitching, facial twitching, and tonic muscle spasms. Assess for Trousseau's sign (carpopedal spasm) and Chvostek's sign (spasm of lip and cheek). Notify MD of signficant findings.
3. Administer calcium and vitamin D supplements as prescribed.
4. Teach patient and significant others the indicators of hypocalcemia.
5. Reinforce the necessity of taking vitamin D and calcium supplements as prescribed.
6. Teach the importance of continued follow-up to check serum calcium levels.
7. For more information, see "Hypocalcemia," p. 232.

Hyperphosphatemia (serum phosphorus >4.5 mg/dl): Occurs chiefly in acute and chronic renal disease. Although most foods contain generous amounts of

Uremia: Syndrome that occurs when the kidneys fail to excrete urea, creatinine, uric acid, and other metabolic waste products.

1. Monitor patient for signs and symptoms of uremia. Be alert to chronic fatigue
   bleeding tendency, muscular twitching, involuntary leg movements, decreasing
   attention span,

   daily and are very subtle. Explain that they should notify staff of sudden worsening of the symptoms that may be present.

3. Monitor and record dietary intake of protein, potassium, and sodium.

   unpleasant taste.

6. Encourage isometric exercises and short walks, if patient is able, to help maintain patient's muscle strength and tone, especially in the legs.

7. Teach family that because of patient's decreasing concentration level, they
   should communicate

8. Teach patient to maintain good nutrition by ingesting the allotted amounts of
   carbohydrates and high biologic value proteins

9. Explain that profuse bleeding can occur with uremia and that knives, scissors
   and other sharp instruments should be used with caution.

10. Stress that OTC medications, such as aspirin, may

11. Emphasize the importance of follow-up visits to evaluate the progression of
    uremia.

12. Stress that dialysis schedule should be maintained to temper the symptoms of
    uremia and correct many of the metabolic abnormalities that occur.

state associated with the high serum level of

renal failure

NOTE:

in ARF.

1. Monitor and record patient's temperature q8h. If it is elevated >37° C (99° F),
   monitor temperature q2-4h and q2h if it is >38° C (101° F).

   example, be alert to cloudy or blood-tinged peritoneal dialysate return, cloudy

and foul-smelling urine, foul-smelling wound exudate, purulent drainage from any catheter site, foul-smelling and watery stools, foul-smelling vaginal discharge, or purulent sputum. Send sample of any suspicious fluid or drainage for culture and sensitivity tests as prescribed.
3. Monitor WBC count for elevations.
4. Ensure aseptic technique when manipulating central lines, peripheral IV lines, and in-dwelling catheters.
5. Avoid use of in-dwelling urinary catheter in oliguric and anuric patients. The presence of a catheter in these patients further increases the risk of infection.
6. To help maintain the integrity of the oral mucous membranes, provide oral hygiene q2h.
7. Reposition patient q2-4h to help maintain the barrier of an intact integumentary system. Provide skin care at least q8h.

For patients undergoing dialytic therapy, see nursing diagnoses and interventions in "Dialytic Therapy," pp. 203-207. Also see the following as appropriate: "Providing Nutritional Support," pp. 490-505; "Caring for the Critically Ill on Prolonged Bed Rest," pp. 506-511; "Caring for the Critically Ill with Life-Threatening Disorders," pp. 511-522; and "Caring for the Family of the Critically Ill," pp. 522-526.

REHABILITATION AND PATIENT-FAMILY TEACHING CONCEPTS

Give patient and significant others verbal and written instructions for the following:
1. Prescribed dietary plan, including foods that are to be avoided.
2. Medications, including name, dosage, purpose, schedule, precautions, and potential side effects.
3. Indicators of infection, bleeding, electrolyte imbalance, and alterations in fluid volume.
4. Care of peritoneal or hemodialysis access site, if appropriate.
5. Importance of follow-up appointments with MD for checking renal function; confirm date and time of next appointment if known.

Lower urinary tract trauma

Injuries to the ureters, urinary bladder, and urethra are relatively uncommon, occurring in approximately 3% of patients hospitalized with trauma. If unrecognized and untreated, however, lower urinary tract (LUT) injuries may result in serious complications, and even death. Blunt injuries are responsible for most LUT trauma. They are caused by motor vehicle accidents, falls, sports-related injuries, and assaults. Penetrating injuries often are caused by violence, such as gunshot wounds and stabbings, or by iatrogenic injuries during surgery.

Ureteral injury occurs most frequently at the uretero-pelvic junction, where the upper ureter joins the renal pelvis. *Bladder injury,* particularly bladder rupture, occurs most often in motor vehicle accidents and is frequently accompanied by pelvic fractures. Bladder rupture may be intraperitoneal, with the bladder dome rupturing into the peritoneal cavity, or extraperitoneal, close to the bladder base without extravasation into the peritoneum. Motor vehicle accidents with deceleration may cause *urethral injury,* particularly in a male, whose urethra is longer and more rigidly fixed than that of a female.

ASSESSMENT

Signs and symptoms: Suprapubic tenderness, inability to void, microscopic or gross hematuria.

< N O T E : Urologic injury frequently exists without hematuria.

Physical assessment: Blood at the urethral meatus, bruised or discolored genitalia, palpable and overdistended bladder, tracking of urine into tissues of the thigh or abdominal wall.

History: Recent traumatic injury.

DIAGNOSTIC TESTS

< N O T E : Also see "Renal Trauma," p. 190, for a discussion of BUN, creatinine, clearance tests, and KUB x-ray.

1. *Retrograde urethrogram:* A small urinary catheter is inserted and the balloon inflated to 2 ml in the distal anterior urethra, 2 cm from the urinary meatus. Five to ten ml of contrast material is injected and a single x-ray is taken to outline the inner size and shape of the urethra. In urethral rupture, extravasation of the contrast material occurs, usually near the membranous urethra.

2. *Cystogram:* If no urethral tear is found on retrograde urethrogram, a catheter is inserted into the bladder. The bladder is filled with 300 ml of contrast material. Following x-rays to determine if intraperitoneal or extraperitoneal extravasation of contrast material occurs, the bladder is drained and repeat x-rays are taken to check for small posterior ruptures.

3. *Excretory urogram/intravenous pyelogram (IVP):* Contrast material is administered intravenously and is filtered by the kidneys before excretion through the urinary tract. X-rays provide visualization of the normal or injured structures of the kidneys, ureters, or bladder.

< C A U T I O N : Check patient for a history of allergy to iodine, iodine-containing foods, or contrast material. Adequate hydration is needed to rid the body of contrast material following this test.

4. *Renal ultrasound:* A transducer transmits high frequency sound waves through the urinary tract. The resultant echoes are amplified and converted into electrical impulses that are displayed on an oscilloscope. The sound waves demonstrate the presence or absence of fluid accumulation, blood clots, and LUT structural damage.

5. *Radionuclide imaging:* After IV injection of a radionuclide, a radioactivity detecting device scans and records the radioactive uptake to evaluate for injured LUT structures and alterations in renal blood flow.

< C A U T I O N : Wear gloves when handling urine after this procedure. It takes 6-24 hours for the substance to be excreted from the patient's body.

MEDICAL MANAGEMENT AND SURGICAL INTERVENTIONS

1. **Pharmacotherapy**
   - *Antibiotics:* For positive urine cultures, penetrating injuries, or peritonitis.
   - *Analgesics:* For pain.
2. **Catheterization** if patient is unable to void: Catheter should be passed only as far as it will progress without undue force. If any resistance is met during

catheterization, a urethrogram is indicated. If blood is present at the urethral meatus, the patient should not be catheterized under any circumstances prior to the urethrogram as the blood may signal ureteral injury. In the presence of ureteral injury, an improperly placed catheter can cause subsequent incontinence, impotence, and ureteral strictures.

3. **Suprapubic catheter for urinary diversion:** May be used to manage severe urethral lacerations and urethral disruption. Urethral splinting and surgical reconstruction are usually delayed for 3-6 months to allow for a reduction in bruising and swelling, which could delay healing of urinary structures.

4. **Ureteral stents:** Internal ureteral catheters, which are indicated for gunshot wounds to maintain ureteral alignment, ensure urinary drainage, and provide support during anastomosis.

5. **Surgical correction:** Indicated for transected ureter, partial ureteral tears of more than a third of the circumference of the ureter, bladder perforation with associated abdominal injuries or intraperitoneal rupture, and injuries accompanied by rapidly expanding, pulsating hematomas. The following are examples of procedures for the various types of LUT injuries:

- *Proximal ureteral injury:* Primary ureterostomy with end-to-end anastomosis.
- *Distal ureteral injury:* Ureteral stenting or percutaneous nephrostomy, depending on location and extent of injury.
- *Bladder injury:* Use of suprapubic drainage versus in-dwelling urethral catheter drainage is controversial. However, use of a suprapubic catheter avoids the complications of prolonged urethral catheterization, particularly in males who may develop urinary strictures.
- *Urethral injury:* Suprapubic cystotomy and drainage for temporary urinary evacuation, followed by surgical repair in 3-6 months.

NURSING DIAGNOSES AND INTERVENTIONS

Alteration in pattern of urinary elimination related to inadequate urinary outflow secondary to injury of LUT structures

---

Desired outcomes: Patient has a urinary output of ≥ 30 ml/hour. Serum BUN is ≤ 20 mg/dl and serum creatinine is ≤ 1.5 mg/dl.

---

1. Ensure adequate urinary outflow by encouraging patient to void. If patient is unable to void, assess for the need for urinary catheterization or suprapubic drainage by palpating gently for a full bladder. As indicated, discuss the need for a urinary catheter with MD.

2. Do not catheterize patient if there is blood at the urethral meatus unless a urethrogram has indicated that catheterization can be performed safely. Do not force a catheter if resistance is felt. Call for a physician consult if urethral injury is suspected.

3. Monitor serum BUN and creatinine. Elevations reflect ineffective removal of waste products.

4. Document I&O hourly. Assess patency of urinary collection system hourly to determine if clots are occluding the system. If indicated, obtain prescription for catheter irrigation or call MD to irrigate catheter, according to agency policy.

5. Sudden cessation of urine flow through the collection system (particularly if past output was >50 ml/hr) indicates possible catheter obstruction. If catheter irri-

gation does not resume urine drainage, consider changing the urinary catheter following discussion with MD.

Potential fluid volume deficit related to abnormal blood loss secondary to LUT injury

---

Desired outcome: Patient is normovolemic as evidenced by BP >90/60 (or within patient's normal range); HR ≤100 bpm; urine specific gravity 1.010-1.030; PAWP ≥6 mm Hg; RAP ≥4 mm Hg; warm and dry skin; absence of gross hematuria; hemoglobin 14-18 g/dl (male) or 12-16 g/dl (female); and hematocrit 40%-50% (male) or 37%-47% (female).

---

1. Observe for signs of hemorrhage. Gross hematuria may occur following LUT trauma. In rarer instances, pulsating hematomas in the flank or pelvic region cause hypotension and shock.
2. Monitor BP for drops of 10-20 mm Hg below trend. Assess for signs of sympathetic nervous stimulation indicative of shock and hemorrhage, e.g., cool and clammy skin, rapid pulse rate, confusion, pallor, and diaphoresis.
3. Assess for signs of fluid volume deficit, including decreased pulmonary artery wedge pressure (PAWP) or right atrial pressure (RAP), flattened jugular veins with patient in a supine position, and increased specific gravity of urine. If these signs appear, notify MD and be prepared to provide rapid fluid resuscitation and administration of pressor agents.
4. Monitor hematocrit and hemoglobin for drops, indicating excessive bleeding.

Potential for infection related to high risk secondary to bacterial contamination of the urinary tract system occurring with penetrating trauma, rupture of the bladder into the perineum, or instrumentation

---

Desired outcome: Patient is free of infection as evidenced by normothermia, WBC ≤11,000 μl, and urine and wound drainage testing free of infective organisms.

---

1. Use aseptic technique when caring for urinary drainage systems. Maintain catheters and collection container at a level lower than the bladder to prevent reflux; keep drainage tubing unkinked.
2. Record the color, odor, and specific gravity of urine each shift. Culture urine when infection is suspected.
3. Monitor patient's WBC count every day and temperature q4h for elevations.
4. Assess patient each shift for signs of peritonitis: abdominal pain, abdominal distention with rigidity, nausea, vomiting, fever, malaise, and weakness.
5. Assess catheter exit site each shift for the presence of erythema, swelling, or drainage.
6. Assess thigh, groin, and lower abdomen for indicators of urinary extravasation: swelling, pain, mass(es), erythema, and tracking of urine along fascial planes.
7. Assess surgical incision for approximation of suture line and evidence of wound healing, noting presence of erythema, swelling, and drainage. Note and record color, odor, and consistency of wound drainage. Culture drainage that is purulent and notify MD of results.

Alteration in comfort: Pain occurring with LUT structural injury, procedures for urinary diversion, or surgical incisions

---

Desired outcomes: Patient states that a reduction in discomfort has occurred and does not exhibit signs of uncontrolled pain.

---

1. Assess patient for pain at least q4h, medicating promptly, as prescribed. Be alert to shallow breathing in the presence of abdominal pain, which can cause inadequate pulmonary excursion. Document patient's perception of the severity of the pain, as well as response to analgesia. IV narcotics may be indicated if the injury is severe.
2. Explain the cause of the pain to the patient.
3. Assist patient into a position of comfort. Often, knee flexion will relax lower abdominal muscles and help reduce discomfort.

Potential impairment of skin integrity related to irritation secondary to suprapubic catheter placement and maintenance

---

Desired outcome: Patient's skin at the suprapubic catheter entrance site is free of swelling and erythema.

---

1. At least q8h assess skin at suprapubic catheter entrance site for indicators of irritation from contact with urine, including erythema and swelling.
2. Cleanse the insertion site q8h with antimicrobial solution. Apply sterile gauze pad(s) over the catheter exit site and tape securely with paper tape.
3. Change dressing q24h or as soon as it becomes wet.
4. If erythema and swelling occur as a result of maceration from contact with the urine, consider the use of a pectin wafer skin barrier for extra protection.

Potential for sexual dysfunction related to altered body image or physical limitations secondary to LUT injury

---

Desired outcome: Patient verbalizes accurate information regarding long-term effects of his or her LUT trauma.

---

1. Encourage patient to express feelings, concerns, and fears about sexual functioning in relationship to the individual's LUT trauma.
2. Provide correct information, based on the short- and long-term effects of the individual's LUT trauma.
3. Evaluate responses of significant others regarding the patient's potential for sexual dysfunction; provide accurate information as needed.
4. Initiate referrals to social workers, therapists, clinical nurse specialists, and MDs if significant or unusual problems are identified.
5. See "Rehabilitation and Patient-Family Teaching," for further information.

REHABILITATION AND PATIENT-FAMILY TEACHING CONCEPTS

Give patient and significant others verbal and written instructions for the following:

1. Severe urethral injury may result in urethral strictures, impotence, and incontinence. Often, impotence or incontinence is not caused by the original injury, but rather, attempts at early repair when structures are distorted by bruising and swelling. If indicated, prepare patient and significant others for the possibility of stricture, impotence, or incontinence.

2. In males, potency may be delayed for up to two years before sexual functioning returns to normal. As indicated, explain to patient that if functioning does not return, a penile prosthesis may be considered after that time period has elapsed.

3. Suprapubic cystotomy may be used for urinary drainage following severe urethral injury, with delayed urethral reconstruction 3-6 months following injury. As indicated, teach patient and significant others catheter care prior to discharge.

Renal trauma

Penetrating or blunt injuries to the kidney can result in hemorrhage, shock, infection, or loss of organ function. The kidneys are well protected from injury posteriorially by the muscles of the back, and anteriorly by the intestines, liver, spleen, and diaphragm. However, they are fixed in the retroperitoneal space by only the renal pedicle (vascular stem at the renal hilum) and ureters, making them prone to dislocation by sudden disruptive forces, such as motor vehicle accidents.

Blunt injuries, caused by motor vehicle accidents, sports-related trauma, or occupational injuries, are responsible for most renal trauma. Blunt trauma often is a

TABLE 3-3
Classification of blunt renal trauma

	Minor trauma	Major trauma	Critical trauma
Definition	Bruising of renal parenchyma; superficial lacerations of renal cortex without rupture of renal capsule.	Major lacerations through cortex and medulla. Continuation of laceration through renal capsule.	Renal vascular trauma in which kidney is shattered and renal pedicle is injured.
Type of injury	Renal contusion. Subscapular hematoma. Shallow lacerations.	Major lacerations.	Fragmentation. Renal pedicle injury.
Frequency of injury	85%	10–15%	Less than 5%
Symptoms	Hematuria, flank tenderness.	Hematuria, flank pain, hypotension.	Severe blood loss, shock, rapidly expanding flank mass.
Interventions	Rest and observation.	Observation or surgical intervention.	Immediate surgical exploration.
Outcome	Usually, a full recovery.	Nephrectomy may be necessary in 10% of cases.	Chance of saving kidney is 10-30%.

result of direct compression of the kidney by the twelfth rib, which rotates inward and squeezes the kidney into the lumbar spine. Blunt renal trauma can be categorized as minor, major, or critical (vascular) trauma (see Table 3-3). Renal damage often is accompanied by trauma to the spleen, liver, colon, and pancreas. *Penetrating injuries* disrupt renal circulation, lacerate functional tissue, and can cause renal fragmentation.

ASSESSMENT

Signs and symptoms: Abdominal or flank pain, colicky pain with the passage of blood clots, hemorrhage (pallor, diaphoresis, hypotension, tachycardia, restlessness, confusion), gross or microscopic hematuria.

< N O T E : Gross hematuria is present in slightly more than half of patients with renal trauma and is considered an unreliable diagnostic sign.

Physical assessment: Hematoma over the flank of the eleventh or twelfth ribs, Grey Turner's sign (bruising over the lower back and flank due to a retroperitoneal hemorrhage), pain at the costovertebral angle.

< N O T E : Physical signs may be masked because of the protection of the kidneys by abdominal organs, back muscles, and bony structures.

History: Previously abnormal kidneys (polycystic kidney disease), recent traumatic injury.

DIAGNOSTIC TESTS

See ''Lower Urinary Tract Trauma,'' p. 185, for a discussion of retrograde urethrogram, cystogram, excretory urogram, renal ultrasound, and radionuclide imaging.

1. *Blood urea nitrogen (BUN)*: Measurement of the nitrogen fraction of urea, the end product of protein metabolism. Renal dysfunction causes insufficient excretion of urea, elevating nitrogenous wastes in the blood. In renal trauma, BUN also may increase because of body catabolism or dehydration. Normal value = 10-20 mg/dl.

2. *Serum creatinine:* Measurement of a nonprotein end product of creatinine metabolism. Creatinine measures renal damage more accurately than the BUN because renal impairment is virtually the only cause of elevated serum creatinine. Creatinine production is fairly constant day to day because production is proportional to muscle mass. Creatinine is freely filtered at the glomerulus and minimally reabsorbed, causing creatinine excretion to be roughly proportional to glomerular filtration rate. Normal value = 0.7-1.5 mg/dl.

3. *Clearance tests:* Clearance is the volume of plasma that can be cleared of a specific substance during a specified period of time. Clearance tests evaluate the extent of injury by assessing renal filtration, reabsorption, secretion, and renal plasma flow. Creatinine, inulin (a plant starch), and urea are the substances usually tested.

4. *Kidney-ureter-bladder (KUB) radiography*: Evaluates position, size, structure, and defects of kidney and LUT structures. Abnormal findings include retroperitoneal hematoma, fracture of the lower ribs or pelvis, foreign bodies, organ displacement, or fluid accumulation.

5. *Computed tomography (CT):* Imaging of the kidneys *via* a series of cross-sectional slices that are then interpreted by computer. CT scanning following

renal trauma may reveal hematomas, renal lacerations, renal infarcts, or extravasation of urine.

6. *Renal angiography:* Arterial injection of a contrast medium, permitting identification on x-ray of renal vasculature and functional tissue. Following renal trauma, angiography permits identification of renal pedicle injury, renal infarct, intrarenal hematoma, lacerations, and shattered kidney.

< N O T E : Assess patient for allergy to contrast medium.

MEDICAL MANAGEMENT AND SURGICAL INTERVENTIONS

1. **Management of complications**
   - *Hemorrhagic shock:* Rapid volume replacement; pressor agents if unresponsive to volume replacement.
   - *Infections:* Blood and urine cultures, antibiotics.
   - *Renal dysfunction:* Evaluation of need for fluid restriction; dietary restriction of protein, sodium, or potassium; peritoneal dialysis; hemodialysis.
   - *Hypertension:* Antihypertensives, nephrectomy.

< N O T E : Hypertension is a potential complication following renal injury.

2. **Surgical indications:** Dependent on extent of injury.
   - *Minor trauma:* Rest and observation with careful followup to prevent progressive deformity and to evaluate BP.
   - *Major trauma:* Surgical intervention if hypotension and hemodynamic instability occur.
   - *Critical trauma:* Immediate surgical exploration (low renal salvage rate.)
3. **Catheterization:** See guideline with ''Lower Urinary Tract Trauma,'' p. 185.
   - *Nephrostomy tube:* Diversion of urine may be required, depending on location of injury, or in cases of coexisting pancreatic and duodenal injury.
4. **Pharmacotherapy:** See ''Lower Urinary Tract Trauma,'' p. 185.

NURSING DIAGNOSES AND INTERVENTIONS

Alteration in pattern of urinary elimination related to inadequate urinary outflow secondary to damaged functional renal tissue or side effects from diagnostic testing

---

Desired outcome: Patient has a urinary output of at least 30 ml/hour, serum BUN of ≤20 mg/dl, and serum creatinine ≤1.5 mg/dl.

---

1. Encourage patient to void to promote adequate urinary outflow. If patient is unable to void, consult with MD regarding the need for urinary catheterization or nephrostomy tube drainage.
2. Document I&O hourly to evaluate renal function.
3. Monitor serum BUN and creatinine. Elevations reflect ineffective removal of waste products. Notify MD of significant findings.
4. Ensure that the nephrostomy tube is not occluded by patient's weight or external pressure. Irrigate the nephrostomy tube *only* if prescribed, and with ≤5 ml of fluid, as the renal pelvis can hold no more than 10 ml fluid.
5. Assess entrance site of the nephrostomy tube for bleeding or leakage of urine. Catheter blockage with clots or catheter dislodging can cause a sudden decrease in urine output. Notify MD if urine output is <30 ml/hour.

6. Assess urine for color and presence or absence or clots. Expect hematuria for the first 24-48 hours following nephrostomy tube insertion. Notify MD if gross bleeding (with or without clots) occurs.

7. Ensure adequate hydration to allow for clearing of contrast material from patient's system following diagnostic testing. Wear gloves when handling urine until radioactive substances have been cleared from patient's urine (usually 6-24 hours).

See "Lower Urinary Tract Trauma" for the following: **Potential fluid volume deficit** related to abnormal blood loss, p. 187, **Potential for infection** secondary to bacterial contamination, p. 187, **Potential impairment of skin integrity** secondary to suprapubic (nephrostomy) catheter placement and maintenance, p. 188.

REHABILITATION AND PATIENT-FAMILY TEACHING CONCEPTS

Give patient and significant others verbal and written instructions for the following:

1. Medications, including drug name, purpose, dosage, frequency, precautions, and potential side effects, particularly of the antihypertensives.
2. Care of postoperative or postprocedure incisions, urinary drainage systems.
3. Indications of progressive renal dysfunction leading to acute renal failure: edema, hypertension, weakness, pruritis, oliguria, lethargy.

Renal transplant

Renal transplant has become an accepted mode of treatment for end-stage renal disease, owing, to a large extent, to advances in the development of immunosuppressive medications in the late 1960s and the 1970s. Approximately 30-40% of individuals needing transplant have chronic renal failure caused by glomerulonephritis; 20-30% have pyelonephritis or other interstitial disease; 15-20% have multi-system disease; and approximately 10% have cystic kidney disease. There are two types of transplant donors, living and cadaveric. The success rate with live donor transplant is 90-95%. The success rate with cadaveric transplant since the advent of cyclosporine has improved to 75-85%. The majority of patients do not have a viable (medically or psychologically) live donor and are therefore placed on a cadaveric waiting list. The demand exceeds the supply, with approximately 6000-7000 patients awaiting transplant in the United States alone.

Rejection and infection remain the major complications following transplant. Rejection is the phenomenon that represents the recipient's immunologic response to the transplanted kidney. There are two types of lymphocytes involved in the rejection response and either or both may participate: B lymphocytes, which form antibodies (humoral immunity), and T lymphocytes, which produce cell-mediated immunity. The rejection response can be categorized into four distinct types: hyperacute, accelerated acute, acute, and chronic. See Table 3-4 for characteristics.

ASSESSMENT FOR REJECTION

1. **Sudden drop in urine output:** Oliguria or anuria may develop.

< N O T E : A sudden drop in output in the first 24 hours postoperative, when a Foley catheter is in place, may signal the presence of clot obstruction and should be ruled out as the first cause of oliguria.

TABLE 3-4
Types of renal rejection

Type	Mechanism	Clinical presentation	Treatment
Hyperacute	Preformed antibodies against donor antigens.	Occurs in the operating room. Kidney turns blue and becomes soft and flabby.	Removal of kidney.
Accelerated acute	May be mediated by humoral antibody or primed lymphocytes (possible presensitization in the recipient).	Occurs 48-72 hours after transplant. Abrupt fall in urine output; leukocytosis or leukopenia; tenderness over kidney; decreased flow on renal scan; profound thrombocytopenia.	Bolus IV steroids for 3-4 days; antilymphocyte preparations. Prognosis for reversal is poor.
Acute	Cell-mediated T lymphocytes infiltrate renal tissue. Humoral mediated antigen-antibody complexes, platelets, and fibrin aggregates are present in glomerular and peritubular capillaries. May be a combination of cell mediated and humoral mediated.	Occurs from 1-2 weeks to several months after transplant. Fever, leukocytosis, an enlarged and tender kidney, drop in urine output, weight gain (1-1.5 kg/24 hrs), hypertension, elevated BUN and creatinine.	Bolus steroids, antilymphocyte preparations, and monoclonal antibody treatments are most effective in reversing this type of rejection. Prognosis is good.
Chronic	Probably a combined effect of antibody and cell-mediated components.	Occurs months to years after transplant. Slow, progressive decrease in renal function; hypertension; proteinuria.	None known. Prognosis for graft survival is poor.

2. **Elevated temperature:** Low-grade, persistent temperatures of 37.2°-37.8° C (99°-100° F) can occur with rejection. In the presence of accelerated or acute rejection, the patient may have temperatures ranging from 37.8°-40° C (100°-104° F).

3. **Edema:** May increase in grade from 1+ (slight indentation over bony areas, such as the shin) to 3+ and 4+, with the degree of indentation increasing significantly.

4. **Hypertension:** BP that increases ≥10 mm Hg over baseline.

5. **Weight gain:** Increase of 2-3 pounds over a 24-hour period.

6. **BUN and creatinine:** Will increase from previous 24-hour levels (e.g., BUN, 25-52 mg/100 ml; creatinine, 1.3-1.8 mg/100 ml).

7. **24-hour urine collection:** Will exhibit a change in components, for example,

decreases in creatinine clearance, total amount of creatinine excreted, and urinary sodium excretion, and an increase in protein excretion.

< N O T E :   In the early postoperative period, the urine will remain bloody for several days, causing urinary protein concentration to be falsely elevated due to hemoglobin breakdown in the urine.

8. Renal scan: Will exhibit decreased blood flow.

9. Kidney assessment: Will reveal a firm, large kidney that is tender on palpation.

DIAGNOSTIC TESTS

1. *Renal scan:* Evaluates blood flow to the kidney and rate of excretion of substances into the bladder.

2. *Renal biopsy:* Determines presence, type, and severity of rejection.

3. *Renal ultrasound:* To rule out possibility of obstruction.

TREATMENT OPTIONS FOR REJECTION

1. **Megadoses of IV methylprednisolone (Solumedrol):** Block the production of interleukin-2, thereby barring essential factors for activated T-cells, and prevent transcription of interleukin-1. The release of interleukin-1 and -2 is part of the process of helper T-cell and cytotoxic T-cell differentiation, which occurs during the immune response that is triggered when foreign antigens are present in the body. For more information, see Table 8-9, Immune Response with Organ Transplantation, p. 473. Methylprednisolone also is used for its anti-inflammatory properties. See Table 3-5 on the next page.

2. **Antithymocyte or antilymphocyte preparations:** See Table 3-5 on the next page.

3. **Monoclonal antibody (Orthoclone OKT-3):** Reacts with and blocks the function of the T-3 complex on the surface of the T-lymphocytes, causing their entrapment by cells in the spleen and liver and leading to their destruction. The T-3 complex is responsible for the T-lymphocytes' identification of a transplanted organ as foreign. See Table 3-5 on the next page.

4. **Graft irradiation:** Destroys lymphyocytes within the graft. Irradiation is done with 150 rads for approximately 3 days in succession.

NURSING DIAGNOSES AND INTERVENTIONS

Fear and anxiety related to threat of loss of the kidney from rejection

---

Desired outcome: Patient verbalizes accurate information about the signs and symptoms of rejection. Patient's fear and anxiety are controlled as evidenced by HR ≤100 bpm, BP within patient's normal range, and RR ≤20 breaths/min.

---

1. Provide opportunities for patient to express fears, concerns, and anxieties about kidney rejection.

2. Assess patient's knowledge of the signs and symptoms of rejection. Ensure that patient and significant others can verbalize knowledge of the following indicators of rejection
   • Persistent, low-grade temperature of 37.2°-37.8° C (99°-100° F).
   • Increased swelling of feet, ankles, hands, or face.

TABLE 3-5

Immunosuppressives (standard agents and prophylaxis)

Drug name	Action	Dosage
Azathioprine (e.g., Imuran)	Blocks proliferation of immuno-competent lymphoid cells; affects the rapidly-dividing B and T cells.	Ranges from 1.5-2 mg/kg day; given IV or PO.
Corticosteroids (prednisone)	Suppress the body's inflammatory and allergic processes.	Varies; total dose tapered to 20-30 mg/day by first postoperative month.
Cyclophosphamide (e.g., Cytoxan)	See azathioprine.	1 mg/kg day; given IV or PO.
Cyclosporine (e.g., Sandimmune)	Interferes with helper T-lymphocyte function; used in combination with corticosteroids and azathioprine.	8-14 mg/kg day; usually given PO.
Antilymphocyte sera (e.g., ATGAM)	Immunoglobulin preparations that coat the T-cells, making them susceptible to phagocytosis.	*Prophylaxis:* 10-15 mg/kg IV for 5-10 days. *Rejection:* 10-15 mg/kg IV for 10-14 days.
Monoclonal antibody (Orthoclone OKT-3)	Reacts with T-3 complex on the surface of the T-cells, causing their removal from the circulation.	5 mg IV push for 10-14 days to treat rejection.

< N O T E :   All of these agents, when used individually or in combinations, lead to an increased incidence of infection and malignancy secondary to their immunosuppressive properties.

- Weight gain of >1 kg/24 hours.
- Painful and swollen kidney.

3. Reassure patient that several medication regimens (e.g., corticosteroids, antilymphocyte preparations, and monoclonal antibody) are available to treat rejection episodes.
4. Reassure patient that rejection does not necessarily mean kidney loss. Under most circumstances, rejection can be reversed.
5. Reassure patient that retransplant is a viable option if kidney loss occurs.

Knowledge deficit: Immunosuppressive medications and their side effects

---

Desired outcome: Patient and significant others verbalize accurate information regarding the prescribed immunosuppressive medications, the side effects that can occur, and precautions that should be taken.

---

1. Provide patient with verbal and written information for the type of immunosuppressive agent that has been prescribed. Discuss the generic name, trade name, purpose, usual dosage, route, side effects, and precautions (see Table 3-5, above, for purpose, usual dosage, and route).

Azathioprine (Imuran)
- Major side effects include leukopenia and thrombocytopenia, nausea and vomiting, and diarrhea. In addition, it increases the risk of cancer and can contribute to an increased susceptibility toward infection and hepatotoxicity.
- Instruct patient to report fever, chills, cough, muscle or joint pain, rapid heartbeat, stomach pain with nausea and vomiting, sores on lips.
- Teach patient that blood should be tested at frequent intervals for evaluation of WBCs and platelets, and that jaundice should be reported promptly to MD.
- Explain that hair loss can occur early in the treatment course but that it usually lessens in occurrence over time.

Corticosteroids
- Major side effects include Cushingoid features, hypertension, bone disease, muscle wasting, cataracts, steroid-induced diabetes, acne, and capillary fragility.
- Teach patient to notify MD for the following: swelling of ankles, hands, or face; BP >20 mm Hg over baseline; swollen or bleeding gums; night sweats; change in eyesight; muscle weakness.

Cyclophosphamide (e.g., Cytoxan)
- Major side effects include hemorrhagic cystitis (manifested by hematuria and dysuria); alopecia; and bone marrow depression, often appearing during 9-14th day of treatment.
- Teach patient the importance of increasing fluid intake and voiding frequently to minimize the potential for hemorrhagic cystitis and getting WBCs checked as prescribed to detect bone marrow suppression.
- Instruct patient to report presence of rashes or lesions (warts) on skin or genital area.

Cyclosporine (Sandimmune)
- Major side effects include nephrotoxicity, hepatotoxicity, leukopenia, thrombocytopenia, hirsutism, muscle pain, fluid retention, edema, tremors, hypertension, nausea, vomiting, diarrhea, gum hyperplasia, anorexia, and anaphylaxis (rare, but can occur with IV route). Teach these to patient and instruct him or her to report the symptoms to the MD if they occur.
- Teach patient that blood levels of cyclosporine must be monitored at frequent intervals to ensure that absorption of oral solution is maximal. This is particularly important for patients experiencing malabsorption from the GI tract.
- Explain that to make oral solutions more palatable, they should be mixed with orange juice or milk and drunk immediately. Teach patient to stir the mixture well and to use a glass container, as plastic, foam, or paper will absorb the medication.
- Instruct patient to rinse syringe and container with milk or orange juice and drink the remaining solution to ensure that all medication has been taken.
- Instruct patient to take medication 1 hour before or 2 hours after meals, and if taking twice a day, to space the doses 12 hours apart.
- Explain that tolerance to the medication, with a decrease in side effects, occurs over time.
- Because of gum hyperplasia, teach patient to brush teeth with soft-bristled toothbrush and nonabrasive tooth paste after meals and snacks.

- Teach patient to report nausea and vomiting that occur after dose of cyclosporine and *not* to repeat dose unless told to do so by MD.
- Instruct patient to report headache, breast enlargement, flushing, and presence of any skin lesions.
- Teach patient to protect skin from freezing temperatures, for example, by wearing a mitten when taking foods out of the freezer.
- Caution patient about taking OTC medications without first consulting MD.

Antilymphocyte sera
- Major side effects include serum sickness (manifested as fever, chills, and joint pain), local phlebitis, thrombocytopenia, and pruritis.
- Teach patient to report rashes on the skin or genital area, joint pain and swelling, fever and chills, and night sweats.

Monoclonal antibody
- Major side effects include chills and fever, headache, photophobia, nausea, vomiting, diarrhea, dyspnea, and bronchospasm.

< C A U T I O N :   Intensive monitoring is required during the first two doses, owing to the high frequency of side effects (first-dose reaction). In addition, there is an increased risk of pulmonary edema in the presence of fluid volume excess.

- Reassure patient that premedication, usually with acetaminophen and diphenhydramine, is given to minimize potential side effects.

Potential for infection related to increased susceptibility secondary to immunosuppression

---

Desired outcome: Patient is free of infection as evidenced by normothermia; absence of erythema, swelling, and drainage of catheter and wound sites; absence of adventitious breath sounds and cloudy and foul-smelling urine; negative cultures of urine, wound drainage, and blood; and WBC count 4500-11,000 μl.

---

1. Assess and record patient's temperature q4h; notify MD of elevations ≥37.8° C (100° F).
2. Assess and document condition of in-dwelling IV sites and other catheter sites q8h. Be alert to swelling, erythema, tenderness, and drainage. Notify MD of any of these findings.
3. As prescribed, obtain blood, urine, and wound cultures when infection is suspected.
4. Be alert to WBC count >11,000 L or <4500 L. A below normal WBC count with increased band neutrophils on differential (shift to the left) may signal acute infection.
5. Inspect transplant wound for erythema, swelling, and drainage. Notify MD of significant findings.
6. Record volume, appearance, color, and odor of urine. Be alert to foul-smelling or cloudy urine, frequency and urgency of urination, and patient complaints of flank or labial pain, all of which are signs of renal-urinary infection.
7. Auscultate lung fields q shift, noting presence of rhonchi, crackles (rales), and decreased breath sounds.

8. Use meticulous aseptic technique when dressing and caring for wounds and catheter sites.
9. Obtain urine cultures once a week during patient's hospitalization and once a month after hospital discharge.

Potential alteration in oral mucous membranes related to stomatitis secondary to immunosuppression

Desired outcome: Patient's oral mucous membranes are intact and free of exudate and lesions.

1. Inspect the mouth daily for signs of exudate and lesions; notify MD if they are present. Teach patient to perform self-inspection of mouth.
2. Teach patient to brush with a soft-bristled toothbrush and nonabrasive toothpaste after meals and snacks.
3. To help prevent monilia, provide patient with mycostatin prophylactic mouthwash for "swish and swallow" after meals and at bedtime.

Impairment of skin integrity related to herpetic lesions, skin fungal rashes, pruritus, and capillary fragility secondary to immunosuppression with corticosteroids

Desired outcome: Patient's skin is intact and free of open lesions or abrasions.

1. Assess for and document daily the presence of erythema, excoriation, rashes, or bruises on patient's skin.
2. Assess for and document the presence of rashes or lesions in the perineal area, as herpetic lesions are common in the immunosuppressed patient.
3. Inspect the trunk area daily for the presence of flat, itchy rashes. Skin fungal rashes are common in the immunosuppressed.
4. Teach patient the importance of daily skin care with water, nondrying soap, and lubricating lotion.
5. Use nonallergic tape when anchoring IV tubing, catheters, and dressings.
6. Assist patient with changing position at least q2h; massage areas that are susceptible to breakdown, particularly areas over bony prominences.

Also see "Organ Rejection" for the following: **Powerlessness** related to actual and perceived inability to control organ rejection episodes, p. 475. For other nursing diagnoses and interventions, see the following sections, as appropriate: "Providing Nutritional Support," pp. 490-505; "Caring for the Critically Ill on Prolonged Bed Rest," pp. 506-511; "Caring for the Critically Ill with Life-Threatening Disorders," pp. 511-522; and "Caring for the Family of the Critically Ill," pp. 522-526.

REHABILITATION AND PATIENT-FAMILY TEACHING CONCEPTS

Give patient and significant others verbal and written instructions for the following:

1. Medications, including generic and brand names, purpose, usual dosage, frequency, side effects, and precautions.
2. Foods that are high in sodium, which should be avoided to minimize the effect of salt and water retention resulting from corticosteroid therapy. See Table 3-14, p. 219.
3. Care of incision, with special attention to the presence of pain, swelling, redness, or drainage, which can occur with infection and should be reported promptly to MD.
4. Signs and symptoms of upper respiratory infection (e.g., cough, sore throat, fever, chest pain during deep breathing, dyspnea, wheezing) and urinary tract infection (urinary burning, pain, hesistancy), which should be reported promptly to MD.
5. Importance of a graded exercise program for controlling weight gain and improving muscle strength.
6. Importance of checking with MD before taking any vaccines or immunizations while being immunosuppressed.
7. Necessity of recording weight and temperature daily to monitor graft function.

Dialytic therapy

The patient with renal dysfunction has an increasingly malfunctioning physiologic system. The goal of dialytic therapy is to restore dynamic equilibrium to that system. The four functions of dialysis are the removal of excess water, correction of electrolyte disturbances, removal of waste products, and correction of acid-base imbalances. In dialysis, water and electrolytes move across a semipermeable membrane from one fluid compartment to another. Dialysis is based on three principles: diffusion, osmosis, and ultrafiltration

- *Diffusion:* Movement of solutes from an area of greater concentration to an area of lesser concentration. Diffusion requires a concentration gradient. During dialysis, high concentrations of waste products and excess electrolytes diffuse into the dialysate, which contains much lower concentrations of these solutes.
- *Osmosis:* Passive movement of water from an area of low solute concentration to an area of high solute concentration. Thus, the use of high concentrations of glucose in the peritoneal dialysate causes movement of water from the patient's plasma into the dialysate.
- *Ultrafiltration:* Movement of water from an area of higher pressure to an area of lower pressure. In hemodialysis, negative pressure in the dialysate facilitates the rapid removal of excess water from the blood compartment, where positive pressure exists.

Indications for dialysis

1. Volume excess.
2. Hyperkalemia and other electrolyte disturbances.
3. Metabolic acidosis.
4. Uremic intoxication.
   - Central nervous system (encephalopathy).
   - Hematologic (bleeding due to platelet dysfunction).

- Gastrointestinal (anorexia, nausea, vomiting).
- Cardiovascular (pericarditis).

5. Need for removal of dialyzable substances (metabolites, drugs, toxins).

Determination for type of dialysis used

1. Availability of hemodialysis or peritoneal dialysis in the institution.
2. Type best suited for patient's clinical status. For example, the catabolic patient has rapid rises in BUN, creatinine, and potassium. These patients need rapid removal of metabolic wastes (i.e., hemodialysis). See Table 3-6.
3. Blood or peritoneal access route availability.
4. Ability to anticoagulate the patient safely.

PERITONEAL DIALYSIS

The semipermeable membrane utilized during peritoneal dialysis is the patient's peritoneum. A special catheter is placed in the peritoneal cavity and dialysate solution is instilled. Water, electrolytes, and waste products cross between the capillary bed of the peritoneum and the dialysate *via* osmosis and diffusion.

System components

1. **Catheter:** Two types are commonly used.
   - *Trocar:* A stiff Silastic catheter inserted at the bedside.
   - *Soft Silastic in-dwelling catheter* (e.g., Tenckkoff): Inserted in the operating room.

TABLE 3-6

Comparison of peritoneal dialysis and hemodialysis

	Peritoneal dialysis	**Hemodialysis**
Access route	Catheter, which may be used immediately.	Subclavian or femoral catheter or shunt, which may be used immediately.
Semipermeable membrane	Peritoneum; approximately 2.2 m² (the total area available for diffusion of solutes).	Cuprophan or cellulose acetate; 1.0-2 m².
Molecular movement	Diffusion by a concentration gradient.	Diffusion by a concentration gradient.
Water removal	Osmotic pressure, using high glucose concentration.	Hydrostatic pressure (pressure gradient across the membrane).
Duration	10-24 hrs, 3-4 × week, or continuous cycling.	4-5 hrs, 3 × week; a maximum of 3-4 hours daily.
Efficiency	Slow diffusion; less efficient than hemodialysis.	High efficiency.
Risk of infection	High.	Lower than peritoneal method.
Major problem	Development of peritonitis.	May not be tolerated by the hemodynamically unstable patient.

2. **Dialysate:** A premixed sterile electrolyte solution with a composition similar to normal plasma. The concentration of ionized calcium is high to maintain a positive calcium balance. Patients in renal failure tend to be hypocalcemic and the goal is to maintain serum calcium levels at 8.5-10 mg/dl. Glucose concentrations are variable, as hypertonic solutions are used to increase osmotic load for more filtration. Potassium is added according to patient need.

Methods of peritoneal dialysis
1. **Intermittent peritoneal dialysis (IPD):** Usually involves 3-4 treatments per week, lasting 8-10 hours each session. Inpatient acute renal failure patients may be dialyzed 24 hours every other day.
2. **Continuous ambulatory peritoneal dialysis (CAPD):** Involves extension of the time the fluid remains in the abdomen (dwell time) to 4 hours during the day and 8 hours during the night, with 4-5 exchanges during a day. Dialysis occurs 7 days a week, 24 hours a day, and is the most physiologic form of dialysis.

HEMODIALYSIS

With hemodialysis, an artificial semipermeable membrane is used to diffuse water, electrolytes, and waste products from the blood. The patient's blood is heparanized, passed through the dialyzer, and then returned to the circulation. For acutely ill patients, dialysis may be needed from 3 times a week to daily.

System components
1. **Dialyzer (artificial kidney):** Consists of the blood compartment, dialysate compartment, and the semipermeable membrane. Small molecules, such as electolytes, water, and waste products, pass through this membrane; but RBCs, protein, and bacteria are too large to cross.
2. **Dialysate:** Electrolyte solution similar to normal plasma. The potassium concentration varies according to patient need. Glucose may be necessary to prevent changes in the patient's serum glucose and osmolality. Although glucose is a large molecule, it can cross the semipermeable membrane, resulting in hypoglycemia. Use of a glucose bath reduces the risk of hypoglycemia.
3. **Vascular access:** Device used to deliver blood to the dialyzer at a rate of at least 200-300 ml/min.
   - *Arteriovenous (A-V) shunt:* Insertion of a Silastic tube into an artery and a vein, allowing blood to flow from the artery to the vein externally.
   - *Subclavian or femoral catheter:* Temporary access catheter (usually double lumen) that is placed in a large vein to enhance blood flow.
   - *Arteriovenous (A-V) fistula:* Anastomosis of an artery and vein to increase blood flow.
   - *Graft:* Bovine, Gortex, or saphenous vein. The graft connects the artery and vein internally in the arm or thigh.
   - *Hemasite:* A ''T''-shaped device inserted into an arterialized vein with a Gortex graft. The ''T'' projects out of the skin, resulting in an external entry point.

MEDICAL THERAPY FOR PATIENTS RECEIVING DIALYSIS
1. **Dietary restrictions**
   - *Hemodialysis:* Between dialysis treatments the main products of protein metabolism and potassium and sodium will accumulate, owing to the kidneys'

TABLE 3-7
Advantages and disadvantages of dialysis methods

Advantages	Disadvantages
Peritoneal Dialysis Simple equipment; rapid initiation of treatment. No anticoagulation needed. Slow dialysis; less risk of hypotension.	**Hemodialysis** Special equipment and trained staff. Heparinization usually required. Disequilibrium may occur from too rapid fluid and biochemical shifts. Maintaining vascular access may be difficult. Blood loss may necessitate transfusion.
Hemodialysis Very efficient; requires short, frequent treatments. As needed, fluid and chemical balance may be altered rapidly.	**Peritoneal Dialysis** Time consuming. Desired effects slower to occur. Protein loss. Some patient discomfort. Risk of peritonitis and pneumonia.

inability to excrete excesses of these products. Therefore, it is necessary to restrict the intake of protein to decrease the amount of urea generated, restrict potassium to prevent hyperkalemia, and restrict sodium to prevent hypernatremia and curb thirst. Recommended guidelines include: protein 1.0-1.2 g/kg/day; sodium 80-100 mEq/day (individualized); and potassium 40-80 mEq/day (individualized).

TABLE 3-8
Complications of dialysis

Hemodialysis	Peritoneal dialysis
Hypotension Angina and dysrhythmias Disequilibrium syndrome Hemorrhage Septicemia Blood loss (dialyzer rupture) Air embolus Hemolysis	Peritonitis Bowel or bladder perforation Hyperglycemic hyperosmolar coma Hypernatremia Metabolic alkalosis Hypovolemia
Access complications	
Bleeding Clotting Infection Phlebitis Venous spasm High output congestive heart failure	Abdominal distention: failure to drain due to • Catheter obstruction from clots or fibrin • Catheter becoming wrapped in omentum Cuff erosion Catheter malposition Tunnel infection

- *Peritoneal dialysis:* Patients on peritoneal dialysis tend to lose more protein through the peritoneal membrane. Therefore, protein restriction is liberalized to 1.2-1.5 g/kg/day to compensate for the extra loss. If peritonitis develops, protein loss can increase from around 10 g/day to 50 g/day. CAPD patients may need calorie restrictions due to the added calories they absorb from the glucose contained in the dialysate. If hypertonic solutions are used several times a day, these patients can absorb as much as 600 calories or more from the dialysate. Potassium may be less restricted in CAPD patients because the dialysate is potassium free and allows better diffusion of potassium with less accumulation that would lead to hyperkalemia. Sodium restriction in peritoneal dialysis is approximately 80-100 mEq/day to prevent hypernatremia and control thirst to prevent fluid overload.

2. **Fluid restriction:** To prevent fluid overload secondary to the kidneys' inability to excrete excess water. Weight gain between dialysis treatments usually is the result of fluid retention. An attempt is made to limit interdialytic weight gain to 1.5-2.0 kg by limiting fluid intake to 1500-1800 ml in 24 hours. This restriction also is individualized.

3. **Phosphate binders:** To prevent or control hyperphosphatemia, which can occur because of the kidneys' inability to excrete excess dietary phosphates.

4. **Vitamin D analogs** (dihydrotachysterol—the active form of vitamin D) **and calcium replacement:** To prevent hypocalcemia and renal osteodystrophy, which may occur due to the body's inability to absorb calcium and maintain serum levels. If hypocalcemia occurs, the parathyroid glands are activated to release parathomone, which releases calcium from the bone to replenish serum levels. Over time this can lead to bone demineralization and osteodystrophy.

5. **Water-soluble vitamins and folic acid:** Are dialyzable and necessitate replacement after dialysis.

NURSING DIAGNOSES AND INTERVENTIONS

Potential for infection related to vulnerability to septicemia or peritonitis secondary to peritoneal or vascular access

---

Desired outcome: Patient is free of infection as evidenced by normothermia, WBC count ≤11,000 μl, blood and dialysate free of infective organisms, and absence of erythema, purulent drainage, abdominal or access site pain, or cloudy dialysate.

---

1. Assess and document condition of the access site daily. Be alert to the presence of erythema, purulent drainage, or tenderness.

2. Peritonitis accounts for a high incidence of failure with peritoneal dialysis. Use strict, aseptic technique when cleansing catheter site and connecting and disconnecting dialysate bags. Use an antiseptic solution such as hydrogen peroxide or povidone-iodine to cleanse the access site. Maintain aseptic technique when cleansing and drying the site. Cover the site with a dry, sterile dressing. Because moist surfaces breed bacteria, change the dressing immediately if it becomes wet.

3. Keep all external access devices (shunts, subclavian catheters, femoral catheters, peritoneal catheters) covered with a dry, sterile dressing between treatments.

4. Document the appearance of peritoneal dialysis effluent. If peritoneal drainage becomes cloudy or contains flecks of material, as prescribed send for a culture and obtain a cell count to check for increased white cells in the peritoneal effluent. Notify MD of changes in outflow.
5. Document and report to MD the presence of an elevated temperature, malaise, access site drainage, cloudy dialysate, and abdominal pain. Teach patient to notify staff if symptoms of infection occur.

Alteration in nutrition: Less than body requirements related to dietary restrictions and protein loss occurring with peritoneal dialysis

---

Desired outcomes: Patient has adequate nutrition as evidenced by stable weekly body weights and a state of nitrogen balance. Patient's caloric intake ranges from 35-45 calories/kg body weight/day (may not be appropriate for CAPD patient, who absorbs calories through the dialysate).

---

1. Document food intake; count calories consumed with each meal. Total caloric intake should be 35-45 calories/kg body weight/24 hrs.
2. Consult with MD and dietician regarding use of nutritional supplements for maintaining caloric intake.
3. For peritoneal dialysis patient, encourage intake of protein (e.g., milk shakes using nondairy cream substitutes, custards).
4. Weigh patient daily. Be alert to losses $\geq$10% of patient's normal body weight over a one-week period. Daily fluctuations reflect body fluid changes.
5. For the hemodialysis patient, encourage the intake of foods that are high in calories (e.g., butter, honey, hard candy, tapioca, sherbet, Karo syrup, ginger ale, jellies, jams, marshmallows). Peritoneal dialysis patients absorb extra calories from the glucose in the peritoneal dialysate.
6. Concentrate protein intake on high-biologic value protein foods (e.g., meats, milk, fish, fowl, and eggs).
7. Minimize the intake of protein from low-biologic value protein foods (e.g., breads, cereals, pastas, grains, fruits, and vegetables).
8. For hemodialysis patients in particular, suggest the intake of caloric substances that do not contain protein or electrolytes. Examples of commercial products available include Cal-Powder, Controlyte, Hycal, and Polycose.
9. As appropriate, provide a referral to the dietician, who can teach the patient and significant others meal planning techniques that will include restrictions while maintaining a high calorie intake.
10. If patient is anorexic or nauseated, provide small, frequent meals. Ensure that food looks appetizing and that meals are served in a pleasant atmosphere. As indicated, medicate patient with prescribed antiemetic ½ hour before meals.

Potential fluid volume excess: Edema related to oliguria, abnormal retention of peritoneal dialysate solution, and dietary indiscretions of sodium and water

---

Desired outcome: Patient is normovolemic as evidenced by balanced I&O; stable weights; HR ≤100 bpm; BP within patient's normal range; RR 12-20 breaths/min; and absence of edema, crackles, and other physical indicators of hypervolemia.

1. Monitor and record I&O q2h and weight daily; report significant findings to MD. Be alert to weight gain of >0.5-1 kg/24 hours.
2. Assess and record status of VS, lung sounds, and cardiac rate and rhythm. Be alert to crackles (rales), tachycardia, pericardial friction rub, and pulsus paradoxus.
3. Assess for presence of peripheral, periorbital, and sacral edema.
4. Maintain fluid restrictions, as prescribed.
5. Elevate HOB during peritoneal dialysis to relieve pressure of fluid against diaphragm.
6. If outflow is poor, change patient's position or irrigate catheter to determine patency.

Potential fluid volume deficit related to decreased circulating volume secondary to excessive fluid removal during peritoneal dialysis or hemodialysis or bleeding associated with heparinization

Desired outcomes: Patient is normovolemic as evidenced by balanced I&O, daily weight within 1-2 pounds of calculated dry weight (true body weight without any excess fluid), BP within patient's normal range, CVP ≥2 mm Hg, and HR ≤100 bpm. Hematocrit is 20-30% (a range expected for the dialysis patient, owing to anemia associated with renal failure), and there is no evidence of blood loss due to line separation or dialyzer rupture.

1. When using hypertonic dialysate for peritoneal dialysis, assess skin turgor, mucous membranes, CVP, BP, and HR for signs of dehydration, which can occur from excessive fluid loss. Be alert to sudden decrease in BP, tachycardia, poor skin turgor, dry mucous membranes, and change in mental status (e.g., restlessness or unresponsiveness).
2. When using hypertonic peritoneal dialysate, check fingerstick glucose q8h. Notify MD of blood glucose levels >200 mg/dl.
3. Weigh patient daily for trend. Monitor I&O q8h and notify MD of output >1500 ml over intake.
4. Monitor hematocrit results prior to each hemodialysis. Notify MD if a >2 point drop occurs.
5. If hypotension occurs during peritoneal dialysis, stop the dialysis, notify MD, and encourage oral fluids up to 1000 ml (or per protocol).
6. If hypotension occurs during hemodialysis, give normal saline or volume expanders as prescribed, and notify MD.
7. During hemodialysis, notify MD immediately if blood loss occurs due to line separation or dialyzer rupture. As prescribed, send type and screen to the laboratory.

Potential alteration in tissue perfusion: Access site, related to impaired circulation secondary to clots, pressure, or disconnection of shunt

Desired outcome: Patient's access site for dialysis has adequate perfusion as evidenced by palpation of thrill, auscultation of bruit, visualization of blood flow, and warmth of shunt tubing or A-V fistula.

1. Confirm patency of access site by palpating for a thrill (vibratory sensation) and auscultating for presence of bruit (buzzing sound) over shunt or A-V fistula.
2. Keep a small section of the shunt tubing exposed for visualization of blood flow. Ensure that the blood appears uniformly red and that the external tubing is warm to the touch. Dark strands or white serum in the tubing can signal clotting.
3. Notify MD promptly if patency cannot be confirmed. Streptokinase or embolectomy may be indicated to save the fistula.
4. Avoid taking BP, drawing blood, or using restrictive clothing, name bands, or restraints on fistula arm. Teach patient the importance of these restrictions.
5. If using a pressure dressing over the access site, make sure it is snug enough to prevent bleeding, but not so tight that it could stop blood flow and promote clot formation. Remove the pressure dressing after it has been on the site for 1-2 hours.
6. Maintain constant infusion of heparin (i.e., 10 units per ml, or as prescribed *via* piggyback) through subclavian or femoral line or flush with heparinized saline and cap as prescribed.
7. Keep shunt clamps or rubbershod hemostats at bedside to clamp line in the event of accidental disconnection.
8. Flush peritoneal catheter before and after dialysis with 30-50 ml normal saline to ensure patency.
9. Always check fistula, graft, or shunt for patency after any hypotensive episode.
10. If for any reason it is suspected that air has entered the vascular access, clamp the line and place the patient in a left side-lying Trendelenburg position, which will trap air at the apex of the right ventricle of the heart, away from the outflow tract. Call the MD *stat,* administer oxygen, and monitor VS carefully.

Potential sensory-perceptual alterations related to dialysis disequilibrium syndrome secondary to rapid removal of metabolic waste with changes in serum osmolality

Desired outcome: Patient verbalizes orientation to person, place, and time; and does not exhibit signs and symptoms of disequilibrium syndrome: headache, nausea, vomiting, restlessness, asterixis, stupor, coma, or seizures.

1. Monitor patient for indicators of disequilibrium syndrome.
2. Notify MD of changing LOC and other marked signs of disequilibrium.
3. Recognize predisposing factors: BUN >150 mg/dl; hypernatremia (serum sodium >147 mEq/L); severe metabolic acidosis (pH <7.35, $Paco_2$ <35 mm Hg, HCO_3^- <22 mEq/L); and history of neurologic problems (e.g., seizures). The

syndrome often is prevented by short, frequent dialysis exchanges and by increasing the osmolality of dialysate by adding glucose, glycerol, urea, or mannitol, or giving IV mannitol during treatment.

4. Monitor BUN pre- and postdialysis to evaluate for changes occurring along with signs and symptoms of disequilibrium.

5. Raise and pad side rails and keep an airway at the bedside as indicated.

REHABILITATION AND PATIENT-FAMILY TEACHING CONCEPTS

Give patient and significant others verbal and written instructions for the following:

1. Dietary restrictions. In addition, provide lists of supplements for maintaining optimal intake of calories.

2. Technique for listening for bruit and feeling the vibration in the A-V fistula or graft.

3. Importance of checking daily and reporting the presence of redness, swelling, tenderness, or drainage from the access site.

4. If patient has a shunt, the importance of attaching clamps to dressing and clamping both limbs of the shunt should separation occur.

5. Importance of applying pressure and going to emergency room immediately if excessive bleeding occurs at any access site.

6. Care of subclavian catheter or A-V shunt:
   • Keep dressing clean and dry.
   • Keep dressing secure to prevent tubing from catching on clothing and dislodging the access.

7. Signs and symptoms of uremia (see p. 183) and hyperkalemia (see p. 180).

8. Complications of dialysis: bleeding after dialysis related to heparinization, signs and symptoms of disequilibrium syndrome (see p. 206), and signs and symptoms of hypokalemia (see p. 180).

9. Importance of keeping scheduled dialysis appointments to help prevent worsening uremia, pulmonary edema, and hyperkalemia.

Continuous arteriovenous hemofiltration

Continuous arteriovenous hemofiltration (CAVH) is a type of renal therapy performed to manage fluid overload in critically ill patients. Its advantage over conventional dialytic therapies is that ultrafiltration occurs gradually, thus avoiding drastic volume changes and rapid fluid shifts. Treatment duration may be 24 hours or several days, depending on the total amount of fluid to be removed.

Principles

• Use of a highly permeable, hollow fiber filter (e.g., Amicon Diafilter 20).
• Removal of plasma water and unbound substances, such as urea, calcium, sodium, potassium, chloride, vitamins, and unbound drugs, with a molecular weight between 500 and 10,000 daltons.
• Filtration: Movement of fluid across a semipermeable membrane from an area of greater pressure to one of lesser pressure (pressure gradient).
• Convection: Some elements in plasma water (e.g., urea) conveyed across the membrane as a result of the differences in hydrostatic pressure. The removal of large amounts of plasma water results in the removal of large amounts of filterable solutes.

For ultrafiltration to occur, there must be a pressure gradient across the membrane that favors filtration. In CAVH, this is called transmembrane pressure

(TMP), and its major determinants are hydrostatic pressure and oncotic pressure. The higher pressure in the blood compartment is a function of the individual's blood pressure. There is adequate pressure in the blood compartment when the systolic pressure is 50-70 mm Hg. Higher pressures enhance ultrafiltration. Negative pressure for ultrafiltration can be achieved by lowering the collection container 20-40 cm below the hemofilter. The differences in hydrostatic pressure also cause the crossing of some elements, such as glucose and some vitamins. The longer it takes for blood to clear the filter, the more likely that intermediate molecules (vitamins and glucose) will be filtered out of the patient's system. Opposing the hydrostatic pressure is oncotic pressure, which is maintained by plasma proteins that do not pass through the membrane. When hydrostatic pressure exceeds oncotic pressure, filtration of water and solutes occurs.

Indications for CAVH

- Massive fluid overload: Congestive heart failure, acute renal failure, multiple trauma.
- Fluid overload in the presence of hemodynamic instability.
- Cardiogenic shock with pulmonary edema.
- Diuretic patient unresponsive oliguria.
- Anuric patient requiring large volumes of parenteral fluid: acts as a supplement to hemodialysis to maintain fluid balance.

Method

The hemofilter and lines are primed with normal saline before initiating the treatment. Blood flows from the arterial (usually femoral or radial) limb of the vascular access through the filter and returns through the venous (usually femoral or cephalic) limb of the access. A continuous infusion of heparin prevents clotting in the lines and filter. Because blood is driven through the system by the patient's blood pressure, no pump is used. As the blood flows through the filter, water, electrolytes, and most drugs not bound to plasma protein diffuse across the membrane and thus become part of the filtrate. If the objective is the removal of large amounts of fluid and solute (urea, potassium, and creatinine), it is necessary to infuse large volumes of filtration replacement fluid (FRF) to maintain electrolyte balance. Nursing responsibilities include initiation of treatment, monitoring of the patient and system, and discontinuing treatment.

TABLE 3-9

Advantages, disadvantages, and complications of hemofiltration

Advantages	Disadvantages	Complications
Physiologic process	Low-efficiency solute removal	Bleeding
Ideal for the patient who is hemodynamically unstable	Large volume fluid replacement	Infection
		Volume depletion
Allows administration of large volumes (e.g., hyperalimentation)	Potential for electrolyte imbalance	Blood leakage
		Decreased ultrafiltration
Technically simple	Increased responsibilities for ICU nurses	Filter clotting
		Electrolyte disturbances

ASSESSMENT DURING CAVH

1. **Access site:** Check for patency and signs of infection at least q8h.
2. **System connections:** Prepare with povidone-iodine and secure with tape every day.
3. **Patency of system:** Arterial and venous tubing should be warm, with no signs of blood separation in the line. Monitor for a darkened or streaked filter.
4. **Laboratory values:** Monitor daily, especially for hyperkalemia.
5. **Hourly I&O:** Notify MD if amount of ultrafiltrate drops to <60 ml/hour.
6. **VS q2h:** Notify MD if BP drops <100 mm Hg systolic.
7. **Daily weight measurements:** Notify MD of loss ≥2.5 kg/day.

Signs and symptoms of uremia: Elevated BUN and creatinine; elevated potassium; decreased serum calcium; increased serum phosphorus; metabolic acidosis; peripheral neuropathy; lethargy; pruritus; pale, yellowish, skin tone; anemia; nausea; and vomiting.

DIAGNOSTIC TESTS

1. *Serum electrolytes*: Determine amount and type of replacement fluid needed.
2. *BUN and creatinine*: To assess level of uremia as a baseline for changes that can occur as a result of hemofiltration.
3. *Prothrombin time (PT) and partial thromboplastin time (PTT):* Baseline values are taken to evaluate clotting status before heparinization.
4. *Activated clotting time (ACT) of whole blood*: During CAVH, ACT is maintained at 100-300 seconds.

MEDICAL MANAGEMENT

The goal is the removal of excess fluid *via* CAVH, while maintaining electrolyte balance and adequate fluid intake for homeostasis. In the critically ill adult, catabolic rate is 2-3 times normal, and this is balanced with total parenteral nutrition (TPN).

1. **TPN:** To maintain nutritional requirements.
2. **CAVH:** To correct hypervolemic state. Either a shunt or large-bore catheter is used for access.
3. **Predilution fluid replacement:** If increased solute removal is required. See Table 3-10 for differences between predilution and postdilution replacement.
4. **Filtration replacement fluid (FRF):** To maintain fluid and electrolyte balance during CAVH. See Table 3-11 for calculation of infusion rate of these fluids.

Standard fluids infused simultaneously include:
- 1 L 0.9 NS with 7.5 ml 10% CaCl.
- 1 L 0.9 NS with 1.6 ml 50% $MgSO_4$.
- 1 L 0.9 NS.
- 1 L D_5W with 150 mEq $NaHCO_3$.

Final composition of fluid for typical patient:
- Sodium—150 mEq/L
- Chloride—114 mEq/L
- Bicarbonate—37 mEq/L
- Magnesium—1.6 mEq/L
- Calcium—2.5 mEq/L

T A B L E 3 - 10
Approaches to fluid replacement

Predilution: replacement fluid infused proximal to the filter	Postdilution: replacement fluid infused distal to the filter
Patient population: Those with poor blood flow, elevated BUN, elevated hematocrit.	*Patient population*: All types.
Replacement fluid infused into arterial line.	Replacement fluid infused into venous line.
Used to enhance urea clearance to ≥18%; decreases oncotic pressure, increasing net TMP; moves urea from erythrocytes into plasma.	Used to maintain fluid and electrolyte balance.
Increases net fluid removal	Less replacement fluid required.
Potentially increases filter life.	Simplified clearance determination.
*Urea clearance 12.5 ml/min.	Urea clearance 10.6 ml/min.

*< N O T E : If increased urea clearance is desired, predilution mode of fluid replacement is utilized.

< N O T E : Concentration may vary, depending on the replacement needs of the patient.

5. **Heparin infusion solution:** To prevent clotting in the CAVH circuit.
6. **Vasopressors:** To maintain arterial pressure, which is necessary for driving the blood through the hemofilter.

NURSING DIAGNOSES AND INTERVENTIONS

Potential alteration in cardiac output: Decreased, related to risk of dysrhythmias secondary to fluid and electrolyte disturbances occurring with hemofiltration

Desired outcomes: Patient's cardiac output is adequate as evidenced by systolic BP ≥100 mm Hg (or within patient's normal range), HR <100 bpm, RR ≤20 breaths/min, peripheral pulses >2+ on a 0-4+ scale, brisk capillary refill (<3 seconds), and normal sinus rhythm on EKG. Serum electrolytes are within normal range:

T A B L E 3 - 11
Calculation of filtration replacement fluid (FRF) rate

Infusion rate	Equals ultrafiltrate plus other losses per hour minus all fluid infused minus net removal rate.
Example	Ultrafiltrate = 600 ml/hr + losses (urine, G1) = 100 ml/hr − hyperalimentation 100 ml/hr; vasopressors 50 ml/hr − net fluid removal rate 150 ml/hr
FRF rate	= (600 + 100) − (100 + 50 + 150) 700 − 300
FRF rate	= 400 ml/hour.

potassium 3.5-5.5 mEq/L, calcium 8.5-10.5 mg/dl, phosphorus 2.5-4.5 mg/dl, and bicarbonate 22-26 mEq/L.

1. Assess and document BP, HR, and respirations qh for the first four hours of hemofiltration, and then q2h. Be alert to indicators of fluid volume deficit, manifested by a drop in systolic BP to <100 mm Hg, tachycardia, and tachypnea.

2. Assess and document peripheral pulses and color, temperature, and capillary refill in the extremities q2h. Be alert to decreased amplitude of peripheral pulses and to coolness, pallor, and delayed capillary refill in the extremities as indicators of decreased perfusion.

3. Measure and record I&O hourly. Notify MD of a loss of ≥200 ml/hour over desired loss.

4. Monitor cardiac rhythm continuously; notify MD of decrease in BP of 20 mm Hg from baseline, tachycardia, depressed T waves and ST segments, and dysrhythmias, which can occur with hypovolemia, potassium changes, or calcium changes.

5. Ensure prescribed rates of ultrafiltration and replacement fluid infusion (see Table 3-11) and adjust if ultrafiltration rate changes. Use an infusion pump for replacement fluids to ensure precise rate of infusion. Also maintain TPN and IV rates, as well as oral intake, within 50 ml of the values used to calculate the filtration fluid replacement rate. If any parameters change more than 50 ml, recalculate filtration fluid replacement rate and adjust accordingly.

6. Monitor serum electrolyte values, being alert to changes in potassium, calcium, phosphorus, and bicarbonate. See "Acid-Base Imbalances," p. 41, and "Fluid and Electrolyte Disturbances," p. 214, for specific findings.

Potential fluid volume deficit related to loss secondary to excessive ultrafiltration during CAVH

Desired outcome: Ultrafiltration rate remains within 50 ml of the desired hourly rate.

1. Measure and record I&O q30min for the first two hours and then hourly. Ensure that it is within desired limits.

2. Weigh patient daily. Be alert to loss ≥2.5 kg.

3. Record cumulative ultrafiltrate loss hourly. Measure amount in the ultrafiltrate container. The difference between this value and total hourly intake is the cumulative loss per hour.

4. Check replacement fluid rate hourly to ensure it is within prescribed limits, usually 25 ml of the calculated rate.

5. Notify MD of unanticipated fluid loss from vomiting, diarrhea, fever, and wound drainage.

6. Notify MD of increased filtration rate, which may occur because of increased BP or increased negative pressure, which may be caused by lowering of the ultrafiltration collection device.

7. Monitor VS hourly; notify MD of increased arterial pressure (≥10 mm Hg

above baseline), which would increase flow through the hemofilter, thereby increasing the rate of ultrafiltration.

8. Adjust the filtration replacement fluid rate as prescribed when ultrafiltration rate increases.

9. Maintain intake (oral, IV, TPN) within 25-50 ml of the value used to calculate fluid replacement rate.

Potential fluid volume excess: Edema related to decreased ultrafiltration secondary to hypotension, clogged or clotted filter, or kinked lines

---

Desired outcomes: As prescribed, patient experiences a gradual loss of fluid per hour *via* hemofiltration. Patient's BP remains with acceptable range; activated clotting time (ACT) is at 2-3 times the baseline value; CVP is ≤6 mm Hg, HR is 60-100 bpm, RR is ≤20 breaths/min; and there is absence of edema, crackles, and other physical indicators of hypervolemia.

---

1. Monitor BP q30min for the first two hours and then hourly. Notify MD of a 10-mm Hg drop in BP, which would decrease the rate of ultrafiltration significantly.

2. If ultrafiltration rate is decreased to 50% of the baseline, notify MD and decrease filtration replacement fluid (FRF) rate as prescribed.

3. Check tubes qh to ensure that they are not kinked.

4. Maintain constant heparin infusion per infusion pump to maintain ACT at 2-3 times the baseline value.

5. Monitor clotting time q2h. Use of an activated clotting time device is advisable.

6. Inspect vascular access filter and lines for patency qh. If clotting or clogging with protein is suspected, flush the system with 50 ml normal saline to check patency.

7. If clots are present, notify MD. As prescribed change the filter and recheck ACT to ensure necessary adjustment in heparin infusion rate.

8. On an hourly basis, assess for and document the presence of elevated CVP, elevated BP, tachycardia, jugular venous distention, basilar crackles (rales), increasing edema (peripheral, sacral, periorbital), and tachypnea, which may signal fluid volume excess due to a dramatic decrease in ultrafiltration rate.

Knowledge deficit: Hemofiltration procedure

Desired outcome: Patient verbalizes accurate information about the hemofiltration procedure.

---

1. Assess patient's knowledge of the procedure and intervene accordingly.

2. Explain the necessity of vascular access and the sensations that can be anticipated during cannula insertion.

3. Explain the importance of and rationale for limited movement of the involved extremity after cannula placement.

4. Describe the equipment that will be used for the procedure (e.g., filter, lines, infusion pump).

5. Explain that VS and blood tests will be performed at frequent intervals to monitor patient's status during the procedure.
6. Explain to patient that his or her blood will be visible in the filter and lines.
7. Reinforce that a staff member will be close to patient at all times during the procedure and will explain each step as it occurs.
8. Explain that the procedure may take 24 hours or longer until fluid balance is attained.
9. Teach patient that the typical access sites are the femoral artery and femoral vein or the radial artery and cephalic vein.

Impairment of physical mobility related to movement restrictions secondary to access and equipment for hemofiltration

---

Desired outcomes: Patient exhibits ability to move about in bed with assistance without evidence of disruption of hemofiltration equipment. Patient's skin remains intact and there is no evidence of muscle atrophy or contracture formation due to imposed immobility.

---

1. Secure access catheters with gauze wraps (elastic wrap may compress access site and cause clotting) and tape to ensure safe movement of the involved limb without disruption of access cannula.
2. Explain to patient the need for care and assistance when moving the involved limb.
3. Use soft restraints if movement must be restrained markedly.
4. Turn and reposition patient at least q2h, maintaining good body alignment.
5. Massage bony prominences during every position change to promote comfort and circulation.
6. Support involved extremites with pillows.
7. Teach patient assisted ROM exercises on uninvolved extremities. Encourage isometric, isotonic, and quadriceps-setting exercises on uninvolved extremities, especially for patients whose CAVH lasts >24 hours.

Potential fluid volume deficit related to risk of blood loss secondary to line disconnection or membrane rupture

---

Desired outcome: Patient's membrane and line connections remain intact and ultrafiltrate tests negative for blood.

---

1. Tape and secure all connections within the system.
2. Check connections qh to ensure they are secure.
3. Avoid concealing lines, filter, or connections with linen.
4. Position filter and lines close to the access extremity; secure them with gauze wraps and tape to prevent traction on the connections.
5. Inspect ultrafiltrate hourly for any signs of blood. If unsure whether ultrafiltrate contains blood, check the solution with a hemastix.
6. If the hemastix is positive for blood, clamp the ultrafiltrate port and notify MD for further interventions.

See "Perfusion Disorders" for the following: **Potential for injury** related to risk of bleeding or hemorrhage secondary to anticoagulation or thrombolytic therapy, p. 26. See "Dialytic Therapy" for the following: **Potential for infection,** p. 203. For more information about fluid and electrolytes, see "Fluid and Electrolyte Disturbances," p. 214. Also see "Caring for the Critically Ill on Prolonged Bed Rest," pp. 506-511.

REHABILITATION AND PATIENT-FAMILY TEACHING CONCEPTS

For information, see patient's primary diagnosis.

Fluid and electrolyte disturbances

The major constituent of the human body is water. The average adult male is approximately 60% water by weight and the average female is 55% water by weight. Typically, body water decreases both with age and increasing body fat. Body water is distributed between two fluid compartments: approximately two-thirds is located within the cells (intracellular fluid—ICF) and the remaining one-third is located outside the cells (extracellular fluid—ECF). The ECF is further divided into interstitial fluid, which surrounds the cells, and intravascular fluid, which is contained within blood vessels. The body gains water through oral intake, fluid therapy, and oxidative metabolism. Water is lost from the body *via* the kidneys, GI tract, skin, and lungs.

In addition to water, body fluids contain two types of dissolved substances: electrolytes and nonelectrolytes. *Electrolytes* are substances that dissociate in solution and will conduct an electrical current. They dissociate into positive and negative ions and are measured by their capacity to combine (millequivalents/liter—mEq/L). *Nonelectrolytes* are substances, such as glucose and urea, that do not dissociate in solution and are measured by weight (milligrams per 100 milliliters—mg/dl). Each of the body fluid compartments is separated by a semipermeable membrane, which allows movement of these disolved substances to occur. However, the unique composition of each compartment is maintained (see Table 3-12 below).

Composition and concentration of ECF are regulated by a combination of renal, metabolic, and neurologic functions, providing an optimal bath for the body's cells.

TABLE 3-12
*Primary constituents of body water compartments

Intravascular	Interstitial	Intracellular (skeletal muscle cell)
Na^+ 142 mEq/L	Na^+ 145 mEq/L	K^+ 150 mEq/L; HPO_4^{2-} 40 mEq/L
Cl^- 104 mEq/L	Cl^- 117 mEq/L	Na^+ 12 mEq/L
HCO_3^- 24 mEq/L	HCO_3^- 27 mEq/L	HCO_3^- 12 mEq/L
K^+ 4.5 mEq/L	K^+ 4.5 mEq/L	Cl^- 4.0 mEq/L
HPO_4^{2-} 2.0 mEq/L	HPO_4^{2-} 2.0 mEq/L	

*This is a partial list. Other constituents include Ca^{++}, Mg^{++}, and proteins.

While ECF is altered and then modified as the body reacts with its surrounding environment, ICF remains relatively stable, which is important for maintaining normal cellular function. Composition of ECF is determined by measuring the individual electrolytes and nonelectrolytes. Osmolality, i.e., the number of particles in solution, determines the concentration. Two important mechanisms for maintaining volume and concentration of ECF are thirst and the release of antidiuretic hormone (ADH). ADH is released in response to a reduction in intravascular volume or an increase in extracellular osmolality. It acts on the kidney to increase urine concentration, thereby conserving water. Thirst is stimulated by similar changes in volume and osmolality. Aldosterone is another important regulator of fluid volume. It is released by the adrenal cortex in response to an increased plasma renin level and acts on the kidney to conserve sodium and water and increase potassium excretion.

< **SECTION ONE:**   Fluid disturbances

Hypovolemia

Depletion of ECF volume is termed "hypovolemia." It occurs because of abnormal skin, GI, or renal losses; bleeding; decreased intake; or movement of fluid into a nonequilibrating third space. Depending on the type of fluid lost, hypovolemia may be accompanied by acid-base, osmolar, or electrolyte imbalances. Severe ECF volume depletion can lead to hypovolemic shock. Compensatory mechanisms in hypovolemia include increased sympathetic nervous system stimulation (increased heart rate, increased inotropy—cardiac contraction, increased vascular resistance), increased thirst, increased release of ADH, and increased release of aldosterone. Prolonged hypovolemia may lead to the development of acute renal failure (see "Acute Renal Failure," p. 173).

ASSESSMENT

Signs and symptoms: Dizziness, weakness, fatigue, syncope, anorexia, nausea, vomiting, thirst, confusion, constipation.

Physical assessment: Decreased BP, especially when standing (orthostatic hypotension); increased HR; decreased urine output; poor skin turgor; dry, furrowed tongue; sunken eyeballs; flat neck veins; increased temperature; and acute weight loss, except with third spacing (see Table 3-13).

TABLE 3-13
Weight loss an an indicator of ECF deficit in the adult

Acute weight loss	Severity of deficit
2-5%	Mild
5-10%	Moderate
10-15%	Severe
15-20%	Fatal

Hemodynamic measurements: Decreased CVP, decreased pulmonary artery pressure (PAP), decreased cardiac output (CO), decreased mean arterial pressure (MAP), increased systemic vascular resistance (SVR).

History and risk factors

1. *Abnormal GI losses:* Vomiting, NG suctioning, diarrhea, intestinal drainage.
2. *Abnormal skin losses:* Exessive diaphoresis secondary to fever or exercise; burns.
3. *Abnormal renal losses:* Diuretic therapy, diabetes insipidus, renal disease (polyuric forms), adrenal insufficiency, osmotic diuresis (e.g., uncontrolled diabetes mellitus, postdye study).
4. *Third spacing or plasma-to-interstitial fluid shift:* Peritonitis, intestinal obstruction, burns, ascites.
5. *Hemorrhage*
6. *Altered intake:* Coma, fluid deprivation.

DIAGNOSTIC STUDIES

1. *BUN*: May be elevated due to dehydration, decreased renal perfusion, or decreased renal function.
2. *Hematocrit*: Elevated with dehydration; decreased in the presence of bleeding.
3. *Serum electrolytes:* Variable, depending on type of fluid lost. Hypokalemia often occurs with abnormal GI or renal losses. Hyperkalemia occurs with adrenal insufficiency. Hypernatremia may be seen with increased insensible or sweat losses and diabetes insipidus. Hyponatremia occurs in most types of hypovolemia due to increased thirst and ADH release, which lead to increased water intake and retention, thus diluting the serum sodium. See individual electrolyte imbalances, pp. 222-237.
4. *Serum total CO_2 (also known as CO_2 content)*: Decreased with metabolic acidosis and increased with metabolic alkalosis (see ''ABG values,'' below).
5. *ABG values*: Metabolic acidosis (pH <7.35 and HCO_3^- <22 mEq/L) may occur with lower GI losses, shock, or diabetic ketoacidosis. Metabolic alkalosis (pH >7.45 and HCO_3^- >26 mEq/L) may occur with upper GI losses and diuretic therapy.
6. *Urine specific gravity:* Increased due to the kidneys' attempt to save water; may be fixed at approximately 1.010 in the presence of renal disease.
7. *Urine sodium*: Demonstrates the kidneys' ability to conserve sodium in response to an increased aldosterone level. In the absence of renal disease, osmotic diuresis, or diuretic therapy, it should be <10 mEq/L.
8. *Serum osmolality*: Variable, depending on the type of fluid lost and the body's ability to compensate with thirst and anti-diuretic hormone.

MEDICAL MANAGEMENT

1. **Restoration of normal fluid volume and correction of acid-base and electrolyte disturbances:** The type of fluid replacement depends on the type of fluid lost and severity of the deficit, serum electrolytes, serum osmolality, and acid-base status.
   - *Dextrose and water solutions:* Provide free water only and will be distributed evenly through both the ICF and ECF.
   - *Isotonic normal saline:* Expands ECF only; does not enter ICF.
   - *Blood and albumin:* Expand only the intravascular portion of the ECF.

- *Mixed normal saline/electrolyte solutions:* Provide additional electrolytes (e.g., potassium and calcium) and a buffer (lactate or acetate).
2. **Restoration of tissue perfusion** in hypovolemic shock: Treatment includes rapid volume replacement and plasma expanders (e.g., albumin) to prevent capillary stasis and maintain adequate BP. Vasopressors are used only when response to volume replacement is inadequate.
3. **Treatment of underlying cause**

NURSING DIAGNOSES AND INTERVENTIONS

Fluid volume deficit related to decreased circulating volume secondary to abnormal loss of ECF or reduced intake

---

Desired outcomes. Patient attains adequate intake of fluid and electrolytes as evidenced by urine output $\geq$30 ml/hour, stable weights, specific gravity 1.010-1.030, no clinical evidence of hypovolemia (furrowed tongue, etc.), BP within patient's normal range, CVP 2-6 mm Hg, PAP 20-30/8-15 mm Hg, CO 4-7 L/min, MAP 70-105 mm Hg, HR 60-100 bpm, and SVR 900-1200 dynes/sec cm^{-5}. Serum sodium is 137-147 mEq/L and hematocrit and BUN are within patient's normal range.

---

1. Monitor I&O hourly. Initially, intake should exceed output during therapy. Alert MD to urine output <30 ml/hour for two consecutive hours. Measure urine specific gravity q8h. Expect it to decrease with therapy.
2. Monitor VS and hemodynamic pressures for signs of continued hypovolemia. Be alert to decreased BP, CVP, PAP, CO, MAP; and increased heart rate and SVR.
3. Weigh patient daily. Daily weights are the single most important indicator of fluid status because acute weight changes are indicative of fluid changes. For example, a 2 kg loss of weight equals a 2 L fluid loss. Weigh patient at the same time of day (preferably before breakfast) on a balanced scale, with patient wearing approximately the same clothing. Document type of scale used (i.e., standing, bed, chair).
4. Administer PO and IV fluids as prescribed. Document response to fluid therapy. Monitor for signs and symptoms of fluid overload or too rapid fluid administration: crackles (rales), SOB, tachypnea, tachycardia, increased CVP, increased PA pressures, neck vein distention, and edema.
5. Monitor patient for hidden fluid losses. For example, measure and document abdominal girth or limb size, if indicated.
6. Notify MD of decreases in hematocrit that may signal bleeding. Remember that hematocrit will decrease in the dehydrated patient as he or she becomes rehydrated. Decreases in hematocrit associated with rehydration may be accompanied by decreases in serum sodium and BUN.
7. Place shock patient in a supine position with the legs elevated to increase venous return. Avoid Trendelenburg, because this position causes abdominal viscera to press on the diaphragm, thereby impairing ventilation.

Alteration in tissue perfusion: Cerebral and peripheral, related to decreased circulation secondary to hypovolemia

Desired outcome: Patient has adequate perfusion as evidenced by alertness, warm and dry skin, BP within patient's normal range, HR <100 bpm, and capillary refill <3 seconds.

1. Monitor for signs of decreased cerebral perfusion: vertigo, syncope, confusion, restlessness, anxiety, agitation, excitability, weakness, nausea, and cool and clammy skin. Alert MD to worsening symptoms. Document response to fluid therapy.
2. Protect patients who are confused, dizzy, or weak. Keep siderails up and bed in lowest position with wheels locked. Assist with ambulation in step-down units. Raise patient to sitting or standing positions slowly. Monitor for indicators of orthostatic hypotension: decreased BP, increased heart rate, dizziness, and diaphoresis. If symptoms occur, return patient to supine position.
3. To avoid unnecessary vasodilation, treat fevers promptly.
4. Reassure patient and significant others that sensorium changes will improve with therapy.
5. Evaluate capillary refill, noting whether it is brisk (<3 seconds) or delayed (>4 seconds). Notify MD if refill is delayed.
6. Palpate peripheral pulses bilaterally in arms and legs (radial, brachial, dorsalis pedis, and posterior tibial). Use a Doppler if unable to palpate pulses. Rate pulses on a 0-4+ scale (see inside cover page). Notify MD if pulses are absent or barely palpable.

< N O T E :   Abnormal pulses also may be caused by a local vascular disorder.

For additional nursing diagnoses, see specific medical disorder, electrolyte imbalance, or acid-base disturbance.

REHABILITATION AND PATIENT-FAMILY TEACHING CONCEPTS

Give patient and significant others verbal and written instructions for the following:
1. Signs and symptoms of hypovolemia.
2. Importance of maintaining adequate intake, especially in the elderly, who are more likely to develop dehydration.
3. Medications: name, purpose, dosage, frequency, precautions, and potential side effects.

Hypervolemia

Expansion of ECF volume is termed "hypervolemia." It occurs whenever there is (a) excessive retention of sodium and water due to a chronic renal stimulus to save sodium and water; (b) abnormal renal function, with reduced excretion of sodium and water; (c) excessive administration of IV fluids; or (d) interstitial-to-plasma fluid shift. Hypervolemia can lead to heart failure and pulmonary edema (see "Congestive Heart Failure/Pulmonary Edema," p. 85), especially in the patient with cardiovascular dysfunction.

ASSESSMENT

Signs and symptoms: SOB, orthopnea.

Physical assessment: Edema, weight gain, increased BP (decreased BP as the heart fails), bounding pulses, ascites, crackles (rales), rhonchi, wheezes, distended neck veins, moist skin, tachycardia, gallop rhythm.

Hemodynamic measurements: Increased CVP, PAP, and MAP.

History and risk factors

1. Retention of sodium and water: Heart failure, cirrhosis, nephrotic syndrome, excessive administration of glucocorticosteroids.
2. Abnormal renal function: Acute or chronic renal failure with oliguria.
3. Excessive administration of IV fluids.
4. Interstitial-to-plasma fluid shift: Remobilization of fluid after treatment of burns, excessive administration of hypertonic solutions (e.g., mannitol, hypertonic saline) or colloid oncotic solutions (e.g., albumin).

DIAGNOSTIC TESTS

Laboratory findings are variable and usually nonspecific.

1. *Hematocrit:* Decreased due to hemodilution.
2. *BUN:* Increased in renal failure.
3. *ABG values:* May reveal hypoxemia (decreased Pao_2) and alkalosis (increased pH and decreased $Paco_2$) in the presence of pulmonary edema.
4. *Serum sodium and serum osmolality:* Will be decreased if hypervolemia occurs as a result of excessive retention of water (e.g., in chronic renal failure).
5. *Urinary sodium:* Elevated if the kidney is attempting to excrete excess sodium. Urinary sodium will not be elevated in conditions with secondary hyperaldosteronism (e.g., congestive heart failure, cirrhosis, nephrotic syndrome) because hypervolemia occurs secondary to a chronic stimulus to the release of aldosterone.
6. *Urine specific gravity:* Decreased if the kidney is attempting to excrete excess volume. May be fixed at 1.010 in acute renal failure.
7. *Chest x-ray:* May reveal signs of pulmonary vascular congestion.

MEDICAL MANAGEMENT

The goal of therapy is to treat the precipitating problem and return ECF to normal. Treatment may include the following:

1. **Restriction of sodium and water:** See Table 3-14 for a list of foods high in sodium.

TABLE 3-14
Foods that are high in sodium content

Bouillon	Olives
Celery	Pickles
Cheeses	Preserved meat
Dried fruits	Salad dressings and prepared sauces
Frozen, canned, or packaged foods	Sauerkraut
Monosodium glutamate (MSG)	Snack foods (e.g., crackers, chips, pretzels)
Mustard	Soy sauce

2. **Diuretics**
3. **Dialysis or continuous arterial-venous hemofiltration:** In renal failure or life-threatening fluid overload (see "Dialytic Therapy," p. 199 and "Continuous Arteriovenous Hemofiltration," p. 207).

< N O T E : Also see specific discussions under "Adult Respiratory Distress Syndrome," p. 18, "Acute Renal Failure," p. 173, and "Burns," p. 455.

NURSING DIAGNOSES AND INTERVENTIONS

Fluid volume excess: Edema (peripheral and pulmonary) related to surplus of circulating fluid secondary to expanded ECF volume

---

Desired outcomes: Patient is normovolemic as evidenced by adequate urinary output of at least 30-60 ml/hr, specific gravity of approximately 1.010-1.020, stable weights, and absence of edema. BP is within patient's normal range, CVP is 2-6 mm Hg, PAP is 20-30/8-15 mm Hg, MAP is 70-105 mm Hg, CO is 4-7 L/min, and HR is 60-100 bpm.

---

1. Monitor I&O hourly. With the exception of oliguric renal failure, urine output should be >30-60 ml/hour. Measure urine specific gravity q shift. If patient is diuresing, specific gravity should be <1.010-1.020.
2. Observe for and document presence of edema: pretibial, sacral, periorbital; note pitting.
3. Weigh patient daily. Daily weights are the single most important indicator of fluid status. For example, a 2 kg acute weight gain is indicative of a 2 L fluid gain. Weigh patient at the same time each day (preferably before breakfast) on a balanced scale, with patient wearing approximately the same clothing. Document type of scale used (i.e., standing, bed, chair).
4. Limit sodium intake as prescribed by MD (see Table 3-14). Consider use of salt substitutes.

< N O T E : Some salt substitutes contain potassium and may be contraindicated in patients with renal failure or in patients receiving potassium-sparing diuretics (e.g., spironolactone, triamterene).

5. Limit fluids as prescribed. Offer a portion of allotted fluids as ice chips to minimize patient's thirst. Teach patient and significant others the importance of fluid restriction and how to measure fluid volume.
6. Provide oral hygiene at frequent intervals to keep oral mucous membrane moist and intact.
7. Document response to diuretic therapy. Many diuretics (e.g., furosemide, thiazides) cause hypokalemia. Observe for indicators of hypokalemia: muscle weakness, dysrhythmias (especially PVCs and EKG changes—flattened T wave, presence of U waves). See "Hypokalemia," p. 226. Potassium-sparing diuretics (e.g., spironolactone, triamterene) may cause hyperkalemia, weakness, EKG changes (e.g., peaked T wave, prolonged PR interval, widened QRS). See "Hyperkalemia," p. 229. Notify MD of significant findings.
8. Observe for physical indicators of overcorrection and dangerous volume depletion secondary to therapy: vertigo, weakness, syncope, thirst, confusion, poor

skin turgor, flat neck veins, acute weight loss. Monitor VS and hemodynamic parameters for signs of volume depletion occurring with therapy: decreased BP, CVP, PAP, MAP, and CO; increased HR. Alert MD to significant changes or findings.

Impaired gas exchange related to decreased diffusion of oxygen secondary to pulmonary vascular congestion occurring with ECF expansion

---

Desired outcomes: Patient has adequate gas exchange as evidenced by Pao_2 $\geq$80 mm Hg, pH $\leq$7.45, and $Paco_2$ $\geq$35 mm Hg; and patient does not exhibit crackles, gallops, or other clinical indicators of pulmonary edema. PAP is $\leq$30/15 mm Hg; PAWP is $\leq$12 mm Hg; HR is <100 bpm; and RR is $\leq$20 breaths/min.

---

1. Acute pulmonary edema is a potentially life-threatening complication of hypervolemia. Monitor patient for indicators of pulmonary edema including air hunger, anxiety, cough with production of frothy sputum, crackles (rales), rhonchi, tachypnea, tachycardia, gallop rhythm, and elevation of PAP and PAWP.
2. Monitor ABGs for evidence of hypoxemia (decreaed Pao_2) and respiratory alkalosis (increased pH and decreased $Paco_2$). Increased oxygen requirements are indicative of increasing pulmonary vascular congestion.
3. Keep patient in semi-Fowler's or position of comfort to minimize dyspnea. Avoid restrictive clothing.

Potential impairment of skin and tissue integrity related to edema secondary to fluid volume excess

---

Desired outcome: Patient's skin remains free of erythema, sores, and ulcerations.

---

1. Assess and document circulation to extremities at least q shift. Note color, temperature, capillary refill, and peripheral pulses. Determine whether capillary refill is brisk (<3 seconds) or delayed (>4 seconds). Palpate peripheral pulses bilaterally in arms and legs (radial, brachial, dorsalis pedis, and posterior tibial). Use Doppler if unable to palpate pulses. Rate pulses according to a 4+ scale. Notify MD if capillary refill is delayed or pulses are absent.
2. Turn and reposition patient at least q2h to minimize tissue pressure.
3. Check tissue areas at risk (e.g., heels, sacrum, and other areas over bony prominences) with each position change.
4. Use eggcrate mattress or other device to minimize pressure.
5. Support arms and hands on pillows and elevate legs to decrease dependent edema.
6. Treat decubitus ulcers with occlusive dressings (e.g., Duoderm, Op-Site, Tegaderm) per unit protocol. Notify MD of the presence of sores, ulcers, or areas of tissue breakdown in patients who are at increased risk for infection (e.g., diabetics, immunosuppressed individuals, those with renal failure).

REHABILITATION AND PATIENT-FAMILY TEACHING CONCEPTS

Give patient and significant others verbal and written instructions for the following:
1. Signs and symptoms of hypervolemia.
2. Symptoms that necessitate MD notification after hospital discharge: SOB, chest pain, new pulse irregularity.
3. Low sodium diet, if prescribed; use of salt substitute, and avoiding foods that are high in sodium. See Table 3-14, p. 219.
4. Medications, including name, purpose, dosage, frequency, precautions, and potential side effects; signs and symptoms of hypokalemia if patient is taking diuretics.
5. Importance of fluid restriction if hypervolemia continues.
6. Importance of daily weights.

SECTION TWO: Electrolyte disturbances

Sodium imbalance: Sodium plays a vital role in maintaining concentration and volume of ECF. It is the main cation of ECF and the major determinant of ECF osmolality. Under normal conditions, ECF osmolality can be estimated by doubling the serum sodium value. Sodium imbalances usually are associated with parallel changes in osmolality. Sodium also is important in maintaining irritability and conduction of nerve and muscle tissue.

Sodium concentration is maintained *via* regulation of water intake and excretion. If serum sodium concentration is decreased (hyponatremia), the kidneys respond by excreting water. Conversely, if serum sodium concentration is increased (hypernatremia), serum osmolality increases, stimulating the thirst center and causing an increased release of ADH by the posterior pituitary gland. ADH acts on the kidneys to conserve water. The adrenal cortical hormone, aldosterone, is an important regulator of sodium and ECF volume. The release of aldosterone causes the kidney to conserve sodium and water, thereby increasing ECF volume. Because changes in serum sodium levels typically reflect changes in water balance, gains or losses of total body sodium are not necessarily reflected by the serum sodium level. Normal serum sodium is 137-147 mEq/L.

Hyponatremia

Hyponatremia (serum sodium <137 mEq/L) can occur because of a net gain of water or a loss of sodium-rich fluids that are replaced by water. Clinical indicators and treatment depend on the cause of hyponatremia and whether or not it is associated with a normal, decreased, or increased ECF volume. For more information, see "Syndrome of Inappropriate Antidiuretic Hormone," p. 347, "Acute Renal Failure," p. 173, "Burns," p. 455, and "Congestive Heart Failure," p. 85.

ASSESSMENT

Signs and symptoms

< N O T E : Neurologic symptoms usually do not occur until the serum sodium level has dropped to approximately 120-125 mEq/L.

- *Hyponatremia with decreased ECF volume:* Irritability, apprehension, dizziness, personality changes, postural hypotension, dry mucous membranes, cold and clammy skin, tremors, seizures, coma.
- *Hyponatremia with normal or increased ECF volume:* Headache, lassitude, apathy, confusion, weakness, edema, weight gain, elevated BP, hyperreflexia, muscle spasms, convulsions, coma.

Hemodynamic measurements

- *Decreased ECF volume:* Evidence of hypovolemia including decreased CVP, PAP, CO, MAP; increased SVR.
- *Increased ECF volume:* Evidence of hypervolemia including increased CVP, PAP, MAP.

History and risk factors

- *Decreased ECF volume*

1. GI losses: Diarrhea, vomiting, fistulas, NG suction.
2. Renal losses: Diuretics, salt-wasting kidney disease, adrenal insufficiency.
3. Skin losses: Burns, wound drainage.

- *Normal/increased ECF volume*

1. Syndrome of inappropriate antidiuretic hormone (SIADH): Excessive production of antidiuretic hormone.
2. Edematous states: Congestive heart failure, cirrhosis, nephrotic syndrome.
3. Excessive administration of hypotonic IV fluids.
4. Oliguric renal failure.

< N O T E : Hyperlipidemia, hyperproteinemia, and hyperglycemia may cause a pseudo-hyponatremia. Hyperlipidemia and hyperproteinemia reduce the total percentage of plasma that is water. The sodium-to-water ratio of the plasma does not change, but the plasma sodium is reduced. With hyperglycemia, the osmotic action of the elevated glucose causes a shift of water out of the cells and into the ECF, thus diluting the existing sodium. For every 100 mg/dl glucose is elevated, sodium is diluted by 1.6 mEq/L.

DIAGNOSTIC TESTS

1. *Serum sodium*: Will be <137 mEq/L.
2. *Serum osmolality*: Decreased, except in cases of pseudo-hyponatremia.
3. *Urine specific gravity:* Decreased because of the kidneys' attempt to excrete excess water. In SIADH, the urine will be inappropriately concentrated.
4. *Urine sodium*: Decreased (usually <20 mEq/L) except in SIADH and adrenal insufficiency.

MEDICAL MANAGEMENT

The goal of therapy is to get the patient out of immediate danger (i.e., return sodium to >120 mEq/L) and then gradually return sodium to a normal level and restore normal ECF volume.

- *Hyponatremia with reduced ECF volume*

1. **Replacement of sodium and fluid losses**
2. **Replacement of other electrolyte losses** (e.g., potassium, bicarbonate)
3. **IV hypertonic saline:** If serum sodium is dangerously low or the patient is very symptomatic.
4. **Hemofiltration**

- *Hyponatremia with expanded ECF volume*
1. **Removal or treatment of underlying cause**
2. **Diuretics**
3. **Fluid restriction**

< N O T E : See "Syndrome of Antidiuretic Hormone," p. 347, for specific treatment.

NURSING DIAGNOSES AND INTERVENTIONS

Potential fluid volume deficit or excess related to abnormal fluid loss, excessive intake of hypotonic solutions, or abnormal retention of water

---

Desired outcome: Patient is normovolemic as evidenced by HR 60-100 bpm, RR 12-20 breaths/min, BP within patient's normal range, CVP 2-6 mm Hg, and PAP 20-30/8-15 mm Hg.

---

1. If patient is receiving hypertonic saline, assess carefully for signs of intravascular fluid overload: tachypnea, tachycardia, SOB, crackles (rales), rhonchi, increased CVP, increased PAP, gallop rhythm, and increased BP.
2. For other interventions, see "Hypovolemia," p. 217, for **Fluid volume deficit**; see "Hypervolemia," p. 220, for **Fluid volume excess.**

Potential for injury related to altered sensorium and LOC secondary to sodium level <120-125 mEq/L

Desired outcomes: Patient does not exhibit signs of injury due to altered sensorium. Patient can verbalize orientation to person, place, and time.

---

1. Assess and document LOC, orientation, and neurologic status with each VS check. Reorient patient as necessary. Alert MD to significant changes.
2. Inform patient and significant others that altered sensorium is temporary and will improve with treatment.
3. Keep side rails up and bed in lowest position, with wheels locked.
4. Utilize reality therapy, such as clocks, calendars, and familiar objects; keep these items at the bedside within patient's visual field.
5. If seizures are expected, pad side rails and keep an airway at the bedside.

REHABILITATION AND PATIENT-FAMILY TEACHING CONCEPTS

Give patient and significant others verbal and written instructions for the following:
1. Medications, including drug name, purpose, dosage, frequency, precautions, and potential side effects. Teach signs and symptoms of hypokalemia if patient is taking diuretics and provide examples of foods that are high in potassium (see Table 3-15, p. 228).
2. Fluid restriction, if prescribed. Teach patient that a portion of fluid allotment can be taken as ice or popsicles to minimize thirst.
3. Signs and symptoms of hypovolemia if hypernatremia is related to abnormal fluid losses.

Hypernatremia

Hypernatremia (serum sodium level >147 mEq/L) may occur with water loss or sodium gain. Because sodium is the major determinant of ECF osmolality, hypernatremia always causes hypertonicity. In turn, hypertonicity causes a shift of water out of the cells, which leads to cellular dehydration and increased extracellular fluid volume.

ASSESSMENT

Signs and symptoms: Intense thirst, fatigue, restlessness, agitation, coma. Symptomatic hypernatremia occurs only in individuals who do not have access to water or who have an altered thirst mechanism (e.g., infants, the elderly, those who are comatose).

Physical assessment: Low-grade fever, flushed skin, peripheral and pulmonary edema (sodium gain); postural hypotension (water loss).

Hemodynamic measurements: Variable
- *Sodium excess:* Increased CVP and PAP.
- *Water loss:* Decreased CVP and PAP.

History and risk factors
- *Sodium gain:* IV administration of hypertonic saline or sodium bicarbonate, increased oral intake, primary aldosteronism, saltwater near drowning, drugs such as sodium polystyrene sulfonate (Kayexalate).
- *Water loss:* Increased diaphoresis, respiratory infection, diabetes insipidus, osmotic diuresis (e.g., hyperglycemia).

DIAGNOSTIC TESTS

1. *Serum sodium:* Will be >147 mEq/L.
2. *Serum osmolality:* Increased due to elevated serum sodium.
3. *Urine specific gravity:* Increased because of the kidneys' attempt to retain water; will be decreased in diabetes insipidus and osmotic diuresis (e.g., hyperglycemia).

MEDICAL MANAGEMENT

1. **IV or oral water replacement:** For water loss. If sodium is >160 mEq/L, IV D_5W or hypotonic saline is given to replace pure water deficit. See "Diabetes Insipidus," p. 340, for specific treatment.
2. **Diuretics and oral or IV water replacement:** For sodium gain.

< N O T E : Hypernatremia is corrected slowly, over approximately two days, to avoid too great a shift of water into brain cells, which could cause cerebral edema.

NURSING DIAGNOSES AND INTERVENTIONS

Potential for injury related to risk of altered sensorium and seizures secondary to cerebral edema occurring with too rapid correction of hypernatremia

---

Desired outcomes: Patient does not exhibit evidence of injury due to altered sensorium or seizures. Patient can verbalize orientation to person, place, and time.

---

1. Cerebral edema may occur if hypernatremia is corrected too rapidly. Monitor serial serum sodium levels; notify MD of rapid decreases.
2. Assess patient for indicators of cerebral edema: lethargy, headache, nausea, vomiting, increased BP, widening pulse pressure, decreased pulse rate, and seizures.
3. Assess and document LOC, orientation, and neurologic status with each VS check. Reorient patient as necessary. Alert MD to significant changes.
4. Inform patient and significant others that altered sensorium is temporary and will improve with treatment.
5. Keep side rails up and bed in lowest position, with wheels locked.
6. Utilize reality therapy, such as clocks, calendars, and familiar objects; keep these items at the bedside within patient's visual field.
7. If seizures are anticipated, pad side rails and keep an airway at the bedside.

See ''Hypovolemia,'' p. 217, for **Fluid volume deficit** (applicable to hypernatremia caused by water loss); see ''Hypervolemia,'' p. 220, for **Fluid volume excess** (applicable to hypernatremia caused by sodium gain).

REHABILITATION AND PATIENT-FAMILY TEACHING CONCEPTS

Give patient and significant others verbal and written instructions for the following:
1. Medications, including drug name, purpose, dosage, frequency, precautions, and potential side effects. Teach signs and symptoms of hypokalemia if patient is taking diuretics and review foods that are high in potassium (see Table 3-15, p. 228).
2. Signs and symptoms of hypovolemia, if hypernatremia is related to abnormal fluid loss.

Potassium imbalance: Potassium is the primary intracellular cation, and thus it plays a vital role in cell metabolism. It affects the resting potential of nerve and cardiac cells. Abnormal serum potassium levels adversely affect neuromuscular and cardiac function. A relatively small amount of potassium is located within the ECF and is maintained within a narrow range. The vast majority of the body's potassium is located within the cells. Distribution of potassium between ECF and ICF is affected by ECF pH, as well as by several hormones, including insulin, catecholamines, and aldosterone. Acute changes in serum pH are accompanied by reciprocal changes in serum potassium concentration.

The body gains potassium through foods (primarily meats, fruits, and vegetables) and medications. In addition, ECF gains potassium any time there is a breakdown of cells or movement of potassium out of the cell. An elevated serum potassium level usually does not occur unless there is a reduction in renal function. Potassium is lost from the body through the kidneys, GI tract, and skin. Potassium may be lost from ECF because of an intracellular shift. The kidneys are the primary regulators of potassium balance. Normal serum potassium is 3.5-5.5 mEq/L.

Hypokalemia

Hypokalemia occurs because of a loss of potassium from the body or a movement of potassium into the cells.

< N O T E :   Changes in serum potassium levels reflect changes in ECF potassium, not necessarily changes in total body levels.

ASSESSMENT

Signs and symptoms: Fatigue, muscle weakness, leg cramps, soft and flabby muscles, nausea, vomiting, ileus, paresthesias, enhanced digitalis effect.

Physical assessment: Decreased bowel sounds, weak and irregular pulse, decreased reflexes, and decreased muscle tone.

History and risk factors

• *Reduction in total body potassium*
1. Hyperaldosteronism.
2. Diuretics or abnormal urinary losses.
3. Increased GI losses.
4. Increased loss through diaphoresis.

< N O T E :   Poor intake may contribute to, but rarely will cause, hypokalemia.

• *Intracellular shift*
1. Increased insulin (e.g., from total parenteral nutrition).
2. Alkalosis.

DIAGNOSTIC TESTS

1. *Serum potassium*: Values will be <3.5 mEq/L.
2. *ABGs*: May show metabolic alkalosis (increased pH and HCO_3^-) because hypokalemia usually is associated with this condition.
3. *EKG*: ST-segment depression, flattened T wave, presence of U wave, ventricular dysrhythmias.

< N O T E :   Hypokalemia potentiates the effect of digitalis. EKG may reveal signs of digitalis toxicity in spite of a normal serum digitalis level.

MEDICAL MANAGEMENT

1. **Treatment of underlying cause**
2. **Replacement of potassium,** either PO (*via* increased dietary intake or medication) or IV: The usual dose is 40-80 mEq/L day in divided doses. IV potassium is necessary if hypokalemia is severe or the patient is unable to take potassium orally. IV potassium should not be administered at rates >10-20 mEq/hour or in concentrations >30-40 mEq/L, unless hypokalemia is severe, because this can result in life-threatening hyperkalemia. If potassium is administered *via* a peripheral line, the rate of administration may need to be reduced to prevent irritation of vessels. Patients receiving 10-20 mEq/hr should be on a continuous cardiac monitor. The development of peaked T waves suggests the presence of hyperkalemia and requires immediate MD notification.
3. **Potassium-sparing diuretics:** May be given in place of oral potassium supplements.

NURSING DIAGNOSES AND INTERVENTIONS

Potential alteration in cardiac output: Decreased, related to risk of ventricular dysrhythmias secondary to hypokalemia or too rapid correction of hypokalemia with resulting hyperkalemia

TABLE 3-15
Foods high in potassium

Apricots	Nuts
Artichokes	Oranges, orange juice
Avocado	Peanuts
Banana	Potatoes
Cantaloupe	Prune juice
Carrots	Pumpkin
Cauliflower	Spinach
Chocolate	Swiss chard
Dried beans, peas	Sweet potatoes
Dried fruit	Tomatoes, tomato juice, tomato sauce
Mushrooms	

Desired outcomes: EKG shows normal T-wave configuration and absence of ventricular dysrhythmias. Serum potassium levels are within normal range (3.5-5.5 mEq/L).

1. Administer potassium supplement as prescribed. Avoid giving IV potassium chloride at a rate faster than recommended, as this can lead to life-threatening hyperkalemia. Do not add potassium chloride to IV solution containers in the hanging position because this can cause layering of the medication. Instead, invert the solution container before adding the medication and mix well.

< N O T E :   IV potassium chloride can cause local irritation of veins and chemical phlebitis. Assess IV insertion site for erythema, heat, or pain. Alert MD to symptoms. Irritation may be relieved by applying an ice bag, giving mild sedation, or numbing insertion site with small amount of local anesthetic. Phlebitis may necessitate changing of IV site.

2. Administer oral and IV potassium supplements as prescribed.

< N O T E :   Oral supplements may cause GI irritation. Administer with a full glass of water or fruit juice; encourage patient to sip slowly. Alert MD to symptoms of abdominal pain, distention, nausea, or vomiting. Do not switch potassium supplements without MD prescription.

3. Encourage intake of foods high in potassium (see Table 3-15, above). Salt substitutes may be used as an inexpensive potassium supplement.
4. Monitor I&O hourly. Alert MD to urine output <30 ml/hour. Unless severe, symptomatic hypokalemia is present, potassium supplements should not be given if the patient has an inadequate urine output because hyperkalemia can develop rapidly in patients with oliguria (<15-20 ml/hour).
5. Physical indicators of abnormal potassium levels are difficult to identify in the patient who is critically ill. Monitor EKG for signs of continuing hypokalemia (ST-segment depression, flattened T wave, presence of U wave, ventricular dysrhythmias) or hyperkalemia (tall, thin T waves; prolonged PR interval; ST

depression; widened QRS; loss of P wave), which may develop during potassium replacement.

6. Monitor serum potassium levels carefully, especially in individuals at risk for developing hypokalemia, such as patients taking diuretics or receiving NG suction.

7. Administer potassium cautiously in patients receiving potassium-sparing diuretics (e.g., spironolactone or triamterene) because of the potential for the development of hyperkalemia.

8. Because hypokalemia can potentiate the effects of digitalis, monitor patients receiving digitalis for signs of increased digitalis effect: multifocal or bigeminal PVCs, paroxysmal atrial tachycardia with varying AV block, Wenckebach (type I AV) heart block.

Potential ineffective breathing patterns related to weakness or paralysis of respiratory muscles secondary to *severe* hypokalemia (<2-2.5 mEq/L)

Desired outcome: Patient has effective breathing pattern as evidenced by normal respiratory depth, pattern, and rate of 12-20 breaths/min.

---

1. If patient is exhibiting signs of worsening hypokalemia, be aware that severe hypokalemia can lead to weakness of respiratory muscles, resulting in shallow respirations and eventually, apnea and respiratory arrest. Assess character, rate, and depth of respirations. Alert MD promptly if respirations become rapid and shallow.

2. Keep manual resuscitator at patient's bedside if severe hypokalemia is suspected.

3. Reposition patient q2h to prevent stasis of secretions; suction airway as needed.

REHABILITATION AND PATIENT-FAMILY TEACHING CONCEPTS

Give patient and significant others verbal and written instructions for the following:

1. Medications, including name, purpose, dosage, frequency, precautions, and potential side effects. Teach patient the importance of taking prescribed potassium supplements if taking diuretics or digitalis. Review the indicators of digitalis toxicity.

2. Indicators of hypokalemia and hyperkalemia.

3. Foods that are high in potassium (see Table 3-15, p. 228); use of salt substitute to supplement potassium, if appropriate.

Hyperkalemia

Hyperkalemia (serum potassium level >5.5 mEq/L) occurs because of an increased intake of potassium, a decreased urinary excretion of potassium, or movement of potassium out of the cells.

< N O T E : Changes in serum potassium levels reflect changes in ECF potassium, not necessarily changes in total body levels.

ASSESSMENT

Signs and symptoms: Irritability, anxiety, abdominal cramping, diarrhea, weakness (especially of lower extremities), paresthesias.

Physical assessment: Irregular pulse; cardiac standstill may occur at levels >8.5 mEq/L.

History and risk factors

- *Inappropriately high intake of potassium:* Usually, IV potassium delivery.
- *Decreased excretion of potassium*

1. Renal disease.
2. Potassium-sparing diuretics.

- *Movement of potassium out of the cells*

1. Acidosis.
2. Insulin deficiency.
3. Tissue catabolism: For example, with fever, sepsis, trauma, surgery.

DIAGNOSTIC TESTS

1. *Serum potassium*: Will be >5.5 mEq/L.
2. *ABGs*: May show metabolic acidosis (decreased pH and HCO_3^-) because hyperkalemia often occurs with acidosis.
3. *Diagnostic EKG*: Progressive changes include tall, thin T waves; prolonged PR interval; ST depression; widened QRS; loss of P wave. Eventually, QRS becomes widened further and cardiac arrest occurs.

MEDICAL MANAGEMENT

The goal is to treat the underlying cause and return the serum potassium level to normal.

- *Subacute*

1. **Cation exchange resins (e.g., Kayexalate):** Given either orally or *via* retention enema to exchange sodium for potassium in the gut. May be combined with sorbitol to induce diarrhea and increase potassium loss in the bowels.

- *Acute*

1. **IV calcium gluconate:** To counteract the neuromuscular and cardiac effects of hypokalemia. Serum potassium levels will remain elevated.
2. **IV glucose and insulin:** To shift potassium into the cells. This reduces serum potassium temporarily (approximately 6 hours).
3. **Sodium bicarbonate:** To shift potassium into the cells. Reduces serum potassium temporarily.

< N O T E :   The effects of calcium, glucose and insulin, and sodium bicarbonate are temporary. Usually, it is necessary to follow these medications with a therapy that removes potassium from the body, for example, dialysis or administration of cation exchange resins.

4. **Dialysis:** To remove potassium from the body.

NURSING DIAGNOSES AND INTERVENTIONS

Potential alterations in cardiac output: Decreased, related to risk of ventricular dysrhythmias secondary to severe hyperkalemia or too rapid correction of hyperkalemia with resulting hypokalemia

Desired outcomes: EKG shows no evidence of ventricular dysrhythmias related to hypokalemia (U wave, PVCs) or hyperkalemia (peaked T wave). Serum potassium levels are within normal range (3.5-5.5 mEq/L).

1. Monitor I&O. Alert MD to urine output <30 ml/hr. Oliguria increases the risk for developing hyperkalemia.
2. Monitor for indicators of hyperkalemia (e.g., irritability, anxiety, abdominal cramping, diarrhea, weakness of lower extremities, paresthesias, irregular pulse). Also be alert to indicators of hypokalemia (e.g., fatigue, muscle weakness, leg cramps, nausea, vomiting, decreased bowel sounds, paresthesias, weak and irregular pulse) following treatment. Assess for hidden sources of potassium: medications (e.g., potassium penicillin G); banked blood; salt substitute; GI bleeding; or conditions causing increased catabolism, such as infection or trauma.
3. Monitor serum potassium levels, especially in patients at risk of developing hyperkalemia, such as individuals with renal failure. Notify MD of levels above or below normal range.
4. Physical indicators of abnormal potassium levels are difficult to identify in the patient who is critically ill. Monitor EKG for signs of hypokalemia (ST-segment depression, flattened T waves, presence of U wave, ventricular dysrhythmias), which may develop secondary to therapy, or continuing hyperkalemia (tall, thin T waves; prolonged PR interval; ST depression; widened QRS; loss of P wave). Notify MD *stat* if EKG changes occur.
5. Administer calcium gluconate as prescribed, giving it cautiously in patients receiving digitalis because digitalis toxicity can occur. Do not add calcium gluconate to solutions containing sodium bicarbonate because precipitates may form. For more information about calcium administration, see "Hypocalcemia," p. 233.
6. If administering cation exchange resins by enema, encourage patient to retain the solution for at least 30-60 minutes to ensure therapeutic effects.

REHABILITATION AND PATIENT-FAMILY TEACHING CONCEPTS

Give patient and significant others verbal and written instructions for the following:
1. Medications, including name, purpose, dosage, frequency, precautions, and potential side effects.
2. Indicators of both hypokalemia and hyperkalemia. Alert patient to the following signs and symptoms that necessitate immediate medical attention: weakness, pulse irregularities, and fever or other indicator of infection. Teach patient and significant others how to measure pulse rate and detect irregularities.
3. Foods high in potassium, which should be avoided. See Table 3-15, p. 228. Remind patient that salt substitute and "Lite" salt also should be avoided.
4. Importance of preventing recurrent hyperkalemia; review potential causes.

Calcium imbalance: Calcium, the body's most abundant ion, primarily is combined with phosphorus to form the mineral salts of the bones and teeth. In addition, calcium is an ingredient in the cement that holds cells together, exerts a sedative effect on nerve cells, and has important intracellular functions, including development of the cardiac action potential and contraction of muscles. Only 1%

of the body's calcium is contained within ECF, yet this concentration is regulated carefully by the hormones parathormone and calcitonin. Parathormone is released by the parathyroid gland in response to a low serum calcium level. It increases resorption of bone (movement of calcium and phosphorus out of the bone); activates vitamin D, which increases the absorption of calcium from the GI tract; and stimulates the kidneys to conserve calcium and excrete phosphorus. Calcitonin is produced by the thyroid gland when serum calcium levels are elevated. It inhibits bone resorption.

Approximately half of plasma calcium is free, ionized calcium. The remaining half is bound, primarily to albumin. Only the ionized calcium is physiologically important. The percentage of calcium that is ionized is affected by plasma pH and albumin level. Patients with alkalosis, for example, may show signs of hypocalcemia because of increased calcium and bicarbonate binding. Changes in plasma albumin level will affect total serum calcium level without changing the level of free calcium.

Hypocalcemia

Symptomatic hypocalcemia may occur because of a reduction of total body calcium or a reduction of the percentage of calcium that is ionized. Total calcium levels may be decreased due to increased calcium loss, reduced intake secondary to altered intestinal absorption, or altered regulation (e.g., hypoparathyroidism). Elevated phosphorus levels and decreased magnesium levels may precipitate hypocalcemia.

ASSESSMENT

Signs and symptoms: Numbness with tingling of fingers and circumoral region, hyperactive reflexes, muscle cramps, tetany, convulsions. In chronic hypocalcemia, fractures may be present due to bone porosity.

Physical assessment
- *Positive Trousseau's sign:* Ischemia-induced carpopedal spasm. It is elicited by applying a BP cuff to the upper arm and inflating it past systolic BP for 2 minutes.
- *Positive Chvostek's sign:* Unilateral contraction of facial and eyelid muscles. It is elicited by irritating the facial nerve by percussing the face just in front of the ear.

EKG changes: Prolonged QT interval caused by elongation of ST segment.

History and risk factors
- *Decreased ionized calcium*
1. Alkalosis.
2. Administration of citrated blood. Citrate added to the blood to prevent clotting may bind with calcium, causing hypocalcemia.
3. Hemodilution (e.g., occurring with volume replacement with normal saline after hemorrhage).

- *Increased calcium loss in body fluids:* For example, with diuretics.
- *Decreased intestinal absorption*
1. Decreased intake.
2. Impaired vitamin D metabolism.
3. Chronic diarrhea.
4. Post-gastrectomy.

- *Hypoparathyroidism*
- *Hyperphosphatemia:* For example, in renal failure.
- *Hypomagnesemia*

DIAGNOSTIC TESTS

1. *Total serum calcium level:* Will be <8.5 mg/dl. Serum calcium levels should be evaluated with serum albumin. For every 1.0 gram/dl drop in the serum albumin level, there is a 0.8-1.0 mg/dl drop in total calcium level.
2. *Ionized serum calcium:* Will be <4.5 mg/dl.
3. *Parathormone:* Decreased levels occur in hypoparathyroidism; increased levels may occur with other causes of hypocalcemia. Normal range = 150-350 pg/ml (varies among laboratories).
4. *Magnesium and phosphorus levels:* May be checked to identify potential causes of hypocalcemia.

MEDICAL MANAGEMENT

1. **Treatment of underlying cause**
2. **Calcium replacement:** Hypocalcemia is treated with PO or IV calcium. Tetany is treated with 10-20 ml of 10% calcium gluconate IV or a continuous drip of 100 ml of 10% calcium gluconate in 1000 ml D_5W, infused over at least 4 hours.
3. **Vitamin D therapy (e.g., dihydrotachysterol, calcitriol):** To increase calcium absorption from the GI tract.
4. **Aluminum hydroxide antacids:** To reduce elevated phosphorus level prior to treating hypocalcemia.

NURSING DIAGNOSES AND INTERVENTIONS

Potential for injury related to risk of tetany and seizures secondary to severe hypocalcemia

---

Desired outcomes: Patient does not exhibit evidence of injury caused by complications of severe hypocalcemia. Serum calcium levels are within normal range (8.5-10.5 mg/dl).

---

1. Monitor patient for evidence of worsening hypocalcemia: numbness and tingling of fingers and circumoral region, hyperactive reflexes, and muscle cramps. Notify MD promptly if these symptoms develop because they occur prior to overt tetany. In addition, notify MD if patient has positive Trousseau's or Chvostek's signs, as they also signal latent tetany.
2. Administer IV calcium with caution. IV calcium should not be given faster than 1 ml/minute because rapid administration can cause hypotension. Observe IV insertion site for evidence of infiltration because calcium will slough tissue. Concentrated calcium solutions should be administered through a central line. Do not add calcium to solutions containing sodium bicarbonate or sodium phosphate because dangerous precipitates will form.

< N O T E :   Digitalis toxicity may develop in patients taking digitalis because calcium potentiates its effects. Monitor patient for signs and symptoms of hypercalcemia: lethargy, confusion, irritability, nausea, and vomiting.

3. For patients with chronic hypocalcemia, administer oral calcium supplements and vitamin D preparations as prescribed. Administer oral calcium 30 minutes before meals and/or at bedtime for maximal absorption. Administer aluminum hydroxide antacids immediately after meals.
4. Encourage intake of foods high in calcium: milk products, meats, leafy green vegetables.
5. Notify MD if response to calcium therapy is ineffective. Tetany that does not respond to IV calcium may be caused by hypomagnesemia.
6. Keep symptomatic patients on seizure precautions; decrease environmental stimuli.
7. Avoid hyperventilation in patients in whom hypocalcemia is suspected. Metabolic alkalosis may precipitate tetany due to increased calcium-bicarbonate binding.

Alteration in cardiac output: Decreased, related to decreased cardiac contractility secondary to hypocalcemia or digitalis toxicity occurring with calcium replacement therapy

---

Desired outcome: Patient's cardiac output is adequate as evidenced by PAP 20-30/8-15 mm Hg, CVP ≤6 mm Hg, HR ≤100, BP within patient's normal range, and absence of the clinical signs of heart failure or pulmonary edema (crackles, SOB, etc).

---

1. Monitor EKG for signs of worsening hypocalcemia (prolonged QT interval) or digitalis toxicity with calcium replacement: multifocal or bigeminal PVCs, paroxysmal atrial tachycardia with varying AV block, Wenckebach (Type I AV) heart block.
2. Hypocalcemia may decrease cardiac contractility. Monitor patient for signs of heart failure or pulmonary edema: crackles (rales), rhonchi, SOB, decreased BP, increased HR, increased PAP, or increased CVP.

Potential impaired gas exchange related to decreased availability of oxygen secondary to laryngeal spasm occurring with severe hypocalcemia

---

Desired outcome: Patient exhibits respiratory depth, pattern, and rate (12-20 breaths/min) within normal range and is asymptomatic of laryngeal spasm: laryngeal stridor, dyspnea, or crowing.

---

1. Assess patient's respiratory rate, character, and rhythm. Be alert to laryngeal stridor, dyspnea, and crowing, which occur with laryngeal spasm, a life-threatening complication of hypocalcemia.
2. Keep an emergency tracheostomy tray at the bedside of symptomatic patients.

REHABILITATION AND PATIENT-FAMILY TEACHING CONCEPTS

Give patient and significant others verbal and written instructions for the following:
1. Medications, including drug name, purpose, dosage, frequency, precautions, and potential side effects.
2. Indicators of hypercalcemia and hypocalcemia. Review the symptoms that necessitate immediate medical attention: numbness and tingling of fingers and circumoral region and muscle cramps.
3. Foods that are high in calcium.

< N O T E : Many foods that are high in calcium, such as milk products, also are high in phosphorus and may need to be limited in patients with renal failure. In renal failure, a program of phosphorus control and calcium supplementation may be necessary.

Hypercalcemia

Symptomatic hypercalcemia can occur because of an increase in total serum calcium or an increase in the percentage of free, ionized calcium. If hypercalcemia is accompanied by a normal or elevated serum phosphorus level, calcium phosphate crystals may precipitate in the serum and deposit throughout the body. Soft tissue calcifications usually occur when the product (i.e., calcium × phosphorus) of the serum calcium and serum phosphorus exceeds 70 mg/dl.

ASSESSMENT

Signs and symptoms: Lethargy, weakness, anorexia, nausea, vomiting, polyuria, itching, bone pain, fractures, flank pain (secondary to renal calculi), depression, confusion, paresthesias, personality changes, stupor, coma.

EKG findings: Shortening of ST segment and QT interval. PR interval is sometimes prolonged. Ventricular dysrhythmias can occur with severe hypercalcemia.

History and risk factors
1. *Increased intake of calcium:* For example, excessive administration during cardiopulmonary arrest.
2. *Increased intestinal absorption:* For example, with vitamin D overdose or hyperparathyroidism.
3. *Increased release of calcium from bone:* Occurs with hyperparathyroidism, malignancies, prolonged immobilization, Paget's disease.
4. *Decreased urinary excretion:* For example, renal failure, medications (e.g., thiazide diuretics).
5. *Increased ionized calcium:* Acidosis.

DIAGNOSTIC TESTS

1. *Total serum calcium level:* Will be greater than 10.5 mg/dl. Serum calcium level should be evaluated with serum albumin level. For every 1.0 g/dl drop in serum albumin level, there will be a 0.8-1.0 mg/dl drop in total calcium.
2. *Ionized calcium:* Will be >5.5 mg/dl.
3. *Parathormone:* Increased levels occur in primary or secondary hyperparathyroidism.
4. *X-ray findings:* May reveal presence of osteoporosis, bone cavitation, or urinary calculi.

MEDICAL MANAGEMENT

1. **Treatment of underlying cause:** For example, antitumor chemotherapy for malignancy or partial parathyroidectomy for hyperparathyroidism.
2. **IV normal saline:** Administered rapidly to increase urinary calcium excretion. Furosemide is administered to prevent fluid overload.
3. **IV phosphates:** To cause a reciprocal drop in serum calcium.
4. **Low-calcium diet and cortisone:** To reduce intestinal absorption of calcium. Steroids compete with vitamin D, thereby reducing intestinal absorption of calcium.
5. **Decreased bone resorption.** Accomplished *via* increased activity level, indomethacin, or mithramycin. Mithramycin, a cytotoxic antibiotic, acts directly on bone to reduce decalcification and is used primarily to treat hypercalcemia associated with neoplastic disease. Compressional loads (e.g., weight bearing) stimulate bone deposition, thus increased activity decreases bone resorption.
6. **Calcitonin:** To reduce bone resorption, increase bone deposition of calcium and phosphorus, and increase urinary calcium and phosphate excretion.
7. **Sodium bicarbonate:** To treat acidosis and reduce the percentage of calcium that is ionized.

NURSING DIAGNOSES AND INTERVENTIONS

Potential for injury related to neuromuscular and sensorium changes secondary to hypercalcemia

---

Desired outcomes: Patient does not exhibit evidence of injury due to neuromuscular or sensorium changes. Patient verbalizes orientation to person, place, and time. Serum calcium levels are within normal range (8.5-10.5 mg/dl).

---

1. Monitor patient for worsening hypercalcemia. Assess and document LOC; patient's orientation to person, place, and time; and neurologic status with each VS check.
2. Personality changes, hallucinations, paranoia, and memory loss may occur with hypercalcemia. Inform patient and significant others that altered sensorium is temporary and will improve with treatment. Utilize reality therapy: clocks, calendars, and familiar objects; keep them at the bedside within patient's visual field.
3. Hypercalcemia causes neuromuscular depression with poor coordination, weakness, and altered gait. Provide a safe environment. Keep side rails up and bed in lowest position with wheels locked. Assist patient with ambulation if it is allowed.
4. Because hypercalcemia potentiates the effects of digitalis, monitor patient taking digitalis for signs and symptoms of digitalis toxicity: anorexia, nausea, vomiting, irregular pulse. EKG changes may include multifocal or bigeminal PVCs, paroxysmal atrial tachycardia with varying AV block, Wenckebach (Type I AV) heart block.
5. Monitor serum electrolyte values for changes in serum calcium (normal range is 8.5-10.5 mg/dl); potassium (normal range is 3.5-5.5 mEq/L); and phosphorus (normal range is 2.5-4.5 mg/dl) secondary to therapy. Notify MD of abnormal values.

6. Encourage increased mobility to reduce bone resorption. Ideally, patient should be out of bed and up in a chair at least 6 hours/day.

Alteration in pattern of urinary elimination: Dysuria, urgency, frequency, and polyuria secondary to administration of diuretics, calcium stone formation, or changes in renal function occurring with hypercalcemia

---

Desired outcome: Patient exhibits voiding pattern and urine characteristics that are normal for patient.

---

1. Monitor I&O hourly. Alert MD to unusual changes in urine volume, for example, oliguria alternating with polyuria, which may signal urinary tract obstruction, or continuous polyuria, which may be indicative of nephrogenic diabetes insipidus.
2. Because hypercalcemia can impair renal function, monitor patient's renal function carefully: urine output, BUN, creatinine. For more information, see "Acute Renal Failure," p. 173.
3. Provide patient with a low-calcium diet and avoid use of calcium-containing medications (e.g., antacids such as Tums). Encourage intake of fruits (e.g., cranberries, prunes, or plums) that leave an acid ash in the urine. An acidic urine reduces the risk of calcium stone formation.
4. Assess patient for indicators of kidney stone formation: intermittent pain, nausea, vomiting, hematuria.
5. Hypercalcemia leads to an increase in calcium in the urine, which inhibits the kidneys' ability to concentrate urine. This leads to polyuria and potential volume depletion. Be alert to polyuria. Also monitor for signs of volume depletion when giving diuretics: decreased BP, CVP, PAP; increased HR.

REHABILITATION AND PATIENT-FAMILY TEACHING CONCEPTS

Give patient and significant others verbal and written instructions for the following:
1. Medications, including drug name, purpose, dosage, frequency, precautions, and potential side effects.
2. Signs and symptoms of hypercalcemia.
3. Foods and OTC medications (e.g., antacids) that are high in calcium.
4. If stone formation is a concern, foods that leave an acid ash. Review signs and symptoms of nephrolithiasis.
5. After hospital discharge, the importance of increased fluid intake (up to 3 liters in nonrestricted patients) to minimize risk of stone formation.

SELECTED REFERENCES

Ayus JC, et al: Changing concepts in treatment of severe symptomatic hyponatremia. *Am J Med* June 1985; 78: 897-901.

Bass M: Common complications of immunosuppression in the renal transplant patient. *Am Neph Nurs Assoc J* Aug 1986; 13(4).

Borg N (ed): *Core Curriculum for Critical Care Nursing.* W.B. Saunders, 1981.

Bretan PN, McAninch JW, Federle MD, et al:

Computerized tomographic staging of renal trauma. *J Urol* 1986; 136: 561-565.

Carbone V, Bonato J: Nursing implications in the care of the chronic hemodialysis patient in the critical care setting. *Heart Lung* Nov 1985 14 (6): 570-577.

Cardona VD (ed): *Trauma Nursing.* Medical Economics Books, 1985.

Cass AS, et al: Renal trauma found during laparotomy for intra-abdominal injury. *J Trauma* 1985; 25: 997-1000.

Cass AS, et al: Clinical indications for radiographic evaluation of blunt renal disease. *J Urol* 1986: 136: 370-371.

Cogan M, Garovoy M: *Introduction to Dialysis*. Churchill Livingstone, 1985.

Fang, LST: *Manual of Clinical Nephrology*. McGraw Hill, 1983.

Flamenbaum W, Hamburger RJ: *Nephrology— An Approach to the Patient with Renal Disease*. Lippincott, 1982.

Freeman LM, Bizek KS: A fluid challenge protocol. *Crit Car Nurs* Jan/Feb 1984; 4(1): 46-48.

Golper TA: In depth review: Continuous arteriovenous hemofiltration in acute renal failure. *Am J Kidney Dis* Dec 1985; VI (6): 373-386.

Guerriero WG, Devine CJ: *Urologic Injuries*. Appleton-Century-Crofts, 1984.

Harwood C, Cook C: Cyclosporine in transplantation. *Heart Lung,* Nov 1985; 14(6): 529-540.

Horne MM, Jansen PR: Renal-Urinary Disorders. In: *Manual of Nursing Therapeutics.* Swearingen PL (ed). Addison-Wesley, 1986.

Kaplan AA: Predilution versus postdilution for continuous arteriovenous hemofiltration. *Trans Am Soc Artif Ind Org* 1985; 31: 28-32.

King G: Continuous arterio-venous hemofiltration: A nursing perspective. *Am Nephr Nurs Assoc J,* June 1986; 13(3): 151-154.

Lancaster LE: *The Patient with End Stage Renal Disease,* 2nd ed. Wiley, 1984.

Lauer A, et al: Continuous arteriovenous hemofiltration in the critically ill patient. *Ann Intern Med,* 1983; 99: 455-460.

Locke S, et al: Continuous arteriovenous hem-
ofiltration: An alternative to standard hemodialysis in unstable patients. *Am Nephr Nurs Assoc J,* April 1985; 12(2): 127-131.

Metheny NM, Snively WD: *Nurses Handbook of Fluid Balance,* 4th ed. Lippincott, 1983.

Morris PJ: *Kidney Transplantation Principles and Practice*. Grune & Stratton, 1984.

Nurses' Clinical Library: *Renal and Urologic Disorders*. Springhouse, 1984.

Raskin, B: Fluid and Electrolyte Disturbances. In: *Manual of Nursing Therapeutics*. Swearingen, PL (ed). Addison-Wesley, 1986.

Rice V: Magnesium, calcium, and phosphate imbalances: Their clinical significance. *Crit Car Nurs* May/June 1983; 3: 90-109.

Rolmer JC, et al: Nursing management of continuous arteriovenous hemofiltration for acute renal failure. *Focus on Crit Care,* Oct 1986; 13(5): 21-30.

Rose BD: *Clinical Physiology of Acid-Base and Electrolyte Disorders*. McGraw-Hill, 1984.

Rose BD: *Pathophysiology of Renal Disease*. McGraw-Hill, 1981.

Sommers MS: Blunt renal trauma. *Crit Care Nurs*. In press.

Urrows ST: Physiology of body fluids. *Nurs Clin N Am* Sept 1980; 15(3): 537-547.

Weiskittel P, Sommers MS: Care of the patient with lower urinary tract trauma. *Crit Care Nurs*. In press.

Wenkelman C: Hemofiltration: A new technique in critical care nursing. *Heart Lung,* May 1985; 14(3): 265-276.

Williams PL: Continuous ultrafiltration: A new ICU procedure for the treatment of fluid overload. *Crit Care Nurs,* July/Aug 1984: 44-48.

Zuidema GD, Rutherford RD, Ballinger WF: *The Management of Trauma*. Saunders, 1985.

4
NEUROLOGIC
DYSFUNCTIONS

Myasthenia gravis

Guillain-Barré syndrome

Cerebral aneurysm and subarachnoid hemorrhage

Head injury

Care of the patient following intracranial surgery

Meningitis

Acute spinal cord injuries

Status epilepticus

Drug overdose

Delirium tremens

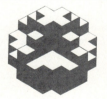

Myasthenia gravis

Myasthenia gravis (MG) is an autoimmune disorder that manifests as weakness and abnormal fatigability of the voluntary striated skeletal muscles. The abnormality occurs at the neuromuscular junction on the postsynaptic membrane, where individuals with MG exhibit a marked reduction in the number of acetylcholine receptors (AChR). Acetylcholine (ACh), a neurotransmitter, is synthesized and stored in the terminal expansion of motor nerve axons. Neurotransmission involves the release of ACh into the synaptic cleft and the attachment of ACh to AChR on the postsynaptic membrane. In turn, this interaction activates the muscle action potential, which is responsible for muscle contraction. This process takes only milliseconds and is terminated by the removal of ACh from the neuromuscular junction, in part by the action of acetylcholinesterase, which catalyzes the breakdown of ACh, deactivating it. In approximately 85-90% of MG patients, an anti-AChR antibody is present, which is believed to cause structural damage to the postsynaptic AChR, inhibit receptor site synthesis, and cause receptor site blockade. If production of new receptor sites is insufficient, failure of neuromuscular transmission eventually occurs.

MG is associated with an increased rate of occurrence of other autoimmune disorders, including rheumatoid arthritis, scleroderma, thyrotoxicosis, systemic lupus erythematosus, and pernicious anemia. Studies have shown that the thymus gland, which plays a role in the development of the immune system, undergoes pathologic changes in 75% of individuals with MG. MG affects women (usually between 15-35 years of age) three times more often than men (usually after age 40). The course of the disease is dependent on the muscle groups involved and the degree of their involvement. Remissions and exacerbations can occur.

ASSESSMENT

General signs and symptoms: Weakness and abnormal fatigability of skeletal muscles that worsen as effort is sustained and the day progresses.

Ocular form: Limited to the eyes and can be mild in nature. This form usually responds poorly to drug therapy but may remit spontaneously. Eye signs include ptosis, diplopia, and inability to maintain upward gaze.

Generalized forms

1. **Mild:** Slow onset, usually begins with eye signs and spreads to bulbar (cranial) nerves and skeletal muscles but spares the respiratory muscles. The mild form of MG may remit; however, if it progresses to a moderate or severe form, remission is less likely. If progression occurs, it usually begins within two years of the onset of symptoms.
   - *Eye signs:* Ptosis, diplopia, inability to control extraocular muscles.
   - *Bulbar signs:* Difficulty in chewing, dysphagia, dysarthria, inability to close mouth, nasal regurgitation of fluids, mushy-nasal tone to voice, neck muscle weakness with head bob, inability to raise chin off chest.
   - *Limbs:* Girdle weakness.
2. **Moderate:** Onset slow to moderate with early eye involvement. All muscle groups are involved to varying degrees.
   - *Eye and bulbar signs:* See "Mild," above. This type of MG is associated with severe bulbar signs and symptoms.
   - *Skeletal muscle involvement:* Decreased strength in all extremities; inability to maintain position without support.
   - *Respiratory muscle involvement:* Diaphragmatic and intercostal weakness,

dyspnea, ineffective cough, accumulation of secretions, and potential for respiratory arrest.

3. **Severe or acute, fulminating:** Rapid onset with severe bulbar and skeletal weakness. Respiratory muscle involvement occurs early. Incidence of myasthenic or cholinergic crisis (see below) is high in this type of MG. Response to treatment is poor and there is a high mortality rate, usually due to respiratory failure, respiratory infections, or aspiration of food or fluids. See signs and symptoms of "mild" and "moderate" forms, above.

Myasthenic and cholinergic crises: Patients with any of the generalized forms of MG may experience crisis, either myasthenic or cholinergic. Crisis may occur rapidly or incipiently, ultimately resulting in respiratory failure, which necessitates intubation or tracheostomy with mechanical ventilation. Crisis is a dramatic and frightening occurrence for the patient with MG. This individual is acutely aware of how she or he feels and tends to be very knowledgeable about the disease. It is important for the nurse to listen to and observe the patient closely because a subjective complaint of increasing anxiety, apprehension, or insomnia may herald the onset of crisis.

While RR and ABGs can be normal, the patient may be experiencing subtle decreases in chest expansion and air movement due to muscle weakness. These changes may be accompanied by increasing dysphagia, dysarthria, dysphonia, and an accumulation of oropharyngeal secretions, which increases the risk of aspiration.

- *Myasthenic crisis:* Results from the need for more medication, either because of tolerance to the medication or an exacerbation of the disease due to infection, trauma, surgery, temperature extremes, stress, endocrine imbalance, or intake of medications with neuromuscular blocking properties such as sedatives, tranquilizers, narcotics, or antibiotics (e.g., neomycin, kanamycin, gentamicin, streptomycin, tetracycline).
  —*Signs and symptoms:* Increasing muscle weakness in spite of normal or increasing drug dosage, increasing anxiety and apprehension, severe ocular and bulbar weakness, and respiratory muscle weakness that occurs rapidly and can lead to respiratory arrest.
- *Cholinergic crisis:* Results from an overdose of anticholinesterase medication, which blocks the acetylcholine receptor sites, causing a neuromuscular depolarizing block.
  —*Signs and symptoms:* Increasing muscle weakness, increasing anxiety and apprehension, fasciculations (twitching) around the eyes and mouth, diarrhea and cramping, sweating, pupillary constriction, sialorrhea (excessive salivation), and difficulty in breathing and swallowing.

DIAGNOSTIC TESTS

1. *Tensilon test:* Tensilon (edrophonium chloride) is a short-acting anticholinesterase agent that delays hydrolysis of ACh, permitting the ACh released by the nerve to act repeatedly over a longer period of time. In the patient with MG, weakness and muscle fatigue will improve within 30-60 seconds of IV Tensilon injection (2-10 mg) and last up to 5 minutes.
   This test also identifies the type of crisis. In myasthenic crisis, the weakness improves with Tensilon, while in cholinergic crisis the symptoms worsen.
2. *Neostigmine bromide (Prostigmin bromide) test:* In the individual with MG,

weakness and muscle fatigue will improve within 15 minutes, peak at 30 minutes, and last up to 2 hours after IM injection of neostigmine (1-2 mg).

3. *Electromyography (EMG):* Muscle action potentials are recorded from selected skeletal muscles. The amplitude of the evoked muscle action potentials falls rapidly in individuals with MG.

4. *Mediastinoscopy:* To evaluate for the presence of thymic abnormalities, which are present in 75% of patients with MG. Of this group, 85% have thymic hyperplasia, while 15% have gross or microscopic thymomas.

5. *CT scan of the thymus gland:* To evaluate for the presence of thymic abnormality (see above).

6. *Thyroid studies*: To evalute for hyperthyroidism. Frequently, thyroid abnormalities are present in young women with MG. MG also is associated with a condition known as Hashimoto's thyroiditis, an autoimmune disorder.

7. *Other laboratory studies:* Serum creatine phosphokinase (CPK), erythrocyte sedimentation rate (ESR), and antinuclear antibody levels are studied because of the frequent occurrence of other immunologic disorders with MG.

MEDICAL MANAGEMENT AND SURGICAL INTERVENTIONS

1. **Emergency interventions for myasthenic or cholinergic crisis:** Include identification of the type of crisis (see "Tensilon test," p. 241), intubation, ventilation, suction, oxygen, IV insertion, and medications. To treat myasthenic crisis, the patient is given neostigmine bromide to treat the muscle weakness and then is hospitalized until the precipitating factor(s) are identified and treated. In cholinergic crisis, the anticholinesterase medications (i.e., neostigmine bromide or pyridostigmine bromide [Mestinon bromide]) are *withheld* and the patient may be given atropine sulfate or pralidoxime chloride (Protopam chloride) to reactivate cholinesterase at the neuromuscular junction.

2. **Pharmacotherapy during noncrisis periods**
   - *Anticholinesterase agents:* For example, pyridostigmine bromide (Mestinon), neostigmine bromide (Prostigmin bromide), ambenonium chloride (Mytelase). These drugs inhibit the hydrolysis of ACh by acetylcholinesterase at the neuromuscular junction. Generally, pyridostigmine is the drug of choice because it is longer acting and has fewer side effects. The patient usually is started on one tablet q3h during the day and the dose is adjusted as required. Sustained-release preparations usually are given at bedtime to maintain patient's strength throughout the night and early morning hours.
   - *Adrenal corticosteroids:* With their use, clinical improvement has been shown in 70-100% of patients with MG. Although mechanism of action of steroids has not been established, studies have shown that they exert certain direct influences on neuromuscular transmission. In addition, they suppress the action of the immune system at many levels by decreasing the size of the thymus gland and lymphatic tissue, decreasing circulating lymphocyte population, and decreasing antireceptor reactivity of peripheral lymphocytes. Treatment must be continued indefinitely. Indications for their use include weakness that is uncontrolled by anticholinesterase drugs or surgery and patients who refuse surgery. Steroids produce favorable results in patients with all degrees of muscle involvement from ocular to severe respiratory impairment. Steroids are used alone or in conjunction with anticholinesterase drugs.
   - *Immunosuppressive drugs:* Cytotoxic drugs such as azathioprine (Imuran) and

cyclophosphamide (Cytoxan) may be used alone or in combination with other therapies in situations in which there is a poor response to steroids. Side effects can be serious and include toxic hepatitis, thrombocytopenia, leukopenia, infections, nausea, vomiting, and alopecia. Leukemia and lymphoma also can occur.

3. **Thymectomy:** May lead to clinical improvement, especially in patients with hyperplasia of thymic tissue. Two approaches are used: the transcervical approach or the thoracotomy approach with sternal splitting. Usually, best results are seen with a combination of surgery and medication in patients under 50-60 years of age with recent onset of moderate, generalized MG. Plasmapheresis sometimes is used prior to surgery to increase strength and allow for a decrease in medication dosage.

4. **Plasmapheresis:** Involves a complete exchange of plasma with the removal of abnormal circulating antibodies that interfere with the acetylcholine receptors.
   - *Potential complications:* Coagulation abnormalities; hypovolemia, hypocalcemia, hypokalemia, and other electrolyte imbalances; decreased ability to fight infection; rebound increase in antireceptor antibodies; and increase in weakness during and after treatment due to removal of plasma-bound drugs.

5. **Radiotherapy:** For severe cases of MG when patient is unresponsive to other therapies. Total body and splenic irradiation have been utilized.

6. **Respiratory support:** Endotracheal tube or tracheostomy with mechanical ventilation may be necessary, depending on the degree of involvement of the respiratory muscles.

7. **Nutritional support:** If patient's dysphagia is severe, IV fluids or tube feedings *via* NG or gastrostomy tube may be needed.

NURSING DIAGNOSES AND INTERVENTIONS

Impaired gas exchange related to decreases in chest expansion and air movement secondary to weakness and abnormal fatigability of pharyngeal, diaphragmatic, intercostal, and accessory muscles of respiration

---

Desired outcomes: Patient has adequate gas exchange as evidenced by orientation to person, place, and time; $Pao_2 \geq 80$ mm Hg; and $Paco_2 \leq 45$ mm Hg. RR is ≤ 20 breaths min with normal depth and pattern (eupnea), vital capacity is $\geq 75-85\%$ of predicted value, and tidal volume is ≥ 1000 ml.

---

1. Assess patient for indicators of altered respiratory function: diminished or adventitious breath sounds; changes in rate, rhythm, and depth of respirations; changes in skin color; nasal flaring or intercostal or suprasternal retractions; and restlessness, irritability, confusion, or somnolence.

2. Monitor ventilatory capability *via* pulmonary function tests. Vital capacity $<75\%$ of predicted value, tidal volume <1000 ml, and respiratory rate $>34/$ min are signals of the need for assisted ventilation.

3. Monitor ABG results. Falling Pao_2 (<60 mm Hg) and rising $Paco_2$ (>50 mm Hg), coupled with changes in vital capacity, tidal volume, and increasing respiratory rate, indicate the need for endotracheal intubation, tracheostomy, or mechanical ventilation to support respiration. As indicated, prepare patient for this procedure.

< N O T E :   If patient already is being ventilated mechanically, ventilator set-tings will vary, depending on patient size and ABG results. Check ventilator set-tings at set intervals and suggest changes as patient's needs change.

4. Provide pulmonary toilet q2h and prn. In addition, turn client after each phys-iotherapy session to facilitate lung expansion, decrease risk of atelectasis, and prevent consolidation of secretions.

Ineffective airway clearance related to inability to cough secondary to weakness and abnormal fatigability of diaphragmatic, intercostal, pharyngeal, and accessory muscles of respiration

---

Desired outcomes: Patient's airway is clear as evidenced by auscultation of normal breath sounds and absence of adventitious breath sounds. Patient is asymptomatic of atelectasis and URI as evidenced by normothermia, BP within patient's normal range, HR $\leq$100 bpm, and RR $\leq$20 breaths/min with normal depth and pattern (eupnea).

---

1. Assess effectiveness of patient's cough and the quality, amount, and color of sputum. Alert MD to significant findings, including patient's inability to raise secretions; secretions that are tenacious, thick, or voluminous; or change in secretion color (i.e., to green, tan, brown, bloody).
2. Suction patient as indicated, using hyperinflation before and after procedure with 100% oxygen.

< N O T E :   If patient has a tracheostomy, always suction the trachea and mouth before deflating tracheostomy cuff to prevent aspiration of secretions. This is especially important with MG patients because of their increase in secretions (sialorrhea).

3. If the patient has a tracheostomy and is receiving oral or enteric feedings, inflate the tracheostomy cuff and elevate HOB prior to each feeding to prevent aspi-ration of food. Place patient in semi- to high-Fowler's position at all times to facilitate chest excursion and decrease risk of aspiration.
4. Assess VS for indicators of atelectasis and URI, such as temperature elevation and increased HR, RR, and BP. Notify MD of significant findings.
5. Increase activity as allowed and tolerated to minimize stasis of secretions and facilitate expansion of the lung.
6. Protect patient from URI by using sterile technique when suctioning and dis-couraging visits by individuals known to have infections.
7. If indicated, obtain sputum specimen for culture; report results.
8. If prescribed, administer or assist with IPPB treatments.

Impaired swallowing related to decreased or absent gag reflex, decreased strength or excursion of muscles involved in mastication, facial paralysis, or mechanical obstruction (tracheostomy)

Desired outcomes: Patient demonstrates capability for safe and effective swallow-ing as evidenced by presence of gag reflex and adequate strength and excursion of muscles involved in mastication. Patient has RR of 12-20 breaths/min with normal pattern and depth (eupnea) and does not exhibit restlessness, adventitious breath sounds, or other clinical indicators of aspiration.

---

1. Assess patient for the presence of the gag reflex, ability to swallow, and strength and excursion of muscles involved in mastication.
2. If patient cannot swallow, confer with MD regarding alternate method of nutritional support such as IV fluids or nasogastric or gastrostomy feedings.
3. Following return of patient's gag reflex and ability to swallow, begin oral feedings cautiously.
   - When reinstating oral intake, begin with ice chips, which help stimulate the swallowing reflex, and progress to semi-solids (e.g., oatmeal, jello) and then to solids.
   - Elevate HOB ≥70 degrees to facilitate gravity flow through the pylorus and minimize the potential for regurgitation and aspiration.
   - Provide small feedings at frequent intervals (e.g., q4h).
   - Avoid cold foods and beverages, which cause bloating and upward pressure on the diaphragm and may impede respiratory excursion.
   - Keep suction equipment at the bedside; suction excess secretions as necessary after each feeding. Provide materials for oral hygiene after every meal.
4. If patient begins oral feedings with a tracheostomy tube in place, elevate HOB ≥70 degrees to facilitate movement of food through the pylorus and minimize the potential for regurgitation and aspiration. Inflate tracheostomy tube cuff for 30 minutes before and after feeding to prevent aspiration in the event that the patient vomits or regurgitates. Progress the diet slowly, as described with #3, above.
5. If patient is unable to communicate verbally, be alert to signs of respiratory distress that can occur in response to aspiration: dyspnea or change in rate and depth of respirations, restlessness or agitation, pallor, and presence of adventitious breath sounds. If these signs occur, discontinue feeding immediately; ensure that HOB is elevated; and provide oxygen *via* nasal cannula, mask, or endotracheal tube. If a tracheostomy tube is in place, suction through the tube to remove food or secretions, which may be obstructing the airway. As prescribed, obtain specimen for ABG analysis or arrange for a chest x-ray.

Sensory-perceptual alterations related to diplopia or ptosis secondary to ocular involvement with myasthenia gravis

---

Desired outcome: Patient relates that vision is adequate.

---

1. Assess for and document signs of weakness of the ocular muscles (i.e., diplopia, ptosis, or incomplete closure of the eye).
2. As indicated, provide assistance with ADL and ambulation to protect patient from injury.
3. Provide an eyepatch or frosted lens for the patient with diplopia; alternate the patch or lens to the opposite eye q2-3h during patient's awake hours.

4. Provide eyelid crutches for the patient with ptosis or loosely tape eyelids open, *only* when providing direct care.
5. Administer artificial tears in each eye at least q4-6h to lubricate and protect corneal tissue.

Knowledge deficit: Thymectomy procedure, including preoperative and postoperative care

---

Desired outcome: Patient verbalizes understanding of the surgical procedure, including preoperative and postoperative care.

---

1. Assess patient's knowledge of thymectomy and its relationship to myasthenia gravis. Provide explanations as indicated.
2. Describe the preoperative routine both verbally and with written material. Discuss preoperative medications, application of antiembolic hose, the potential for postoperative discomfort, and the availability of analgesia. Advise patient that the medication regimen may change after surgery, as removal of the thymic tissue may result in improvement in the patient's condition. If the patient will have a thoracotomy approach, explain that chest tubes will be present after surgery, and that with a transcervical approach, a portable wound drainage system (e.g., Hemovac) will be present to collect wound drainage.
3. During the preoperative period, teach coughing and deep-breathing techniques that will be employed after surgery for expanding the lungs and mobilizing secretions into the upper airway.
4. Explain that plasmapheresis may be done preoperatively to improve the patient's clinical state. See **Knowledge deficit:** Purpose and procedure for plasmapheresis, below.
5. Explain that pulmonary function and ABG studies will be done preoperatively to provide baseline data that will be used to evaluate respiratory status, and postoperatively to assist in determining the patient's readiness for extubation.
6. Prepare patient for the possibility of tracheostomy with assisted ventilation for the pre- and postoperative period to prevent respiratory problems that can occur as a result of the stresses of surgery or the risk of myasthenic or cholinergic crisis.
7. Preoperatively, devise a communication system that utilizes aids such as a magic slate, hand signals, call bell, or word board, as patient may require a ventilator postoperatively. (A communication system already may be in use if the patient is on a ventilator.)
8. Explain that the results of a thymectomy are variable and may not be apparent for several months to years.

Knowledge deficit: Purpose and procedure for plasmapheresis

Desired outcome: Patient verbalizes knowledge of the purpose and procedure for plasmapheresis.

---

1. Assess patient's previous experience with and knowledge of plasmapheresis.
2. As appropriate, teach patient the following about plasmapheresis: Blood is withdrawn *via* an arterial catheter, anticoagulated, and then passed through a cell separator. The plasma portion of the blood that contains the AChR antibodies is removed. RBCs, WBCs, and platelets are mixed with saline, potassium, and plasma protein fraction and are then returned to the body, minus the plasma, *via* a venous access.
3. Advise patient that plasmapheresis generally is done to control severe symptoms until other modalities (medications, thymectomy) take effect, when other treatments have failed, or to increase patient's strength and improve general status before surgery.
4. Explain that patient should eat prior to plasmapheresis and that nutrition will be provided during the procedure.
5. Advise patient that the nurse will perform several assessment procedures before, during, and after plasmapheresis. See **Fluid volume deficit** related to temporary loss of body fluid secondary to plasmapheresis, below.
6. Advise patient that the procedure may take several hours (up to 8) and that it may be performed as often as 3-4 times per week, depending on patient's condition.
7. Explain that the patient's degree of weakness may increase during and after the procedure because of the removal of plasma-bound medications (corticosteroids and anticholinesterase agents). Reassure patient that he or she will be monitored closely during the procedure and medicated appropriately after plasmapheresis.
8. Advise patient that plasmapheresis provides only short-term improvement and has no long-term benefit. It is expensive as well, costing nearly $1500 per procedure.

Fluid volume deficit (with concomitant risk of clotting abnormalities, electrolyte disturbances, and myasthenic or cholinergic crises) related to temporary loss of body fluid secondary to plasmapheresis

Hypovolemia: Can occur secondary to rapid removal of up to 3 L of body fluid during plasmapheresis with volume replacement that is too slow during the procedure.

Desired outcomes: Patient becomes normovolemic as evidenced by BP within patient's normal range; HR 60-100 bpm; peripheral pulses >2+ on a 0-4+ scale; urine output ≥30 ml/hr; good skin turgor; stable weights; orientation to person, place, and time; and absence of thirst. Hematocrit is >37%.

---

1. Perform a baseline assessment of patient's weight, skin turgor, and VS before the procedure is begun. During plasmapheresis, monitor patient for thirst, poor skin turgor, dizziness, confusion, nausea, and flattened neck veins. Assess VS continuously for evidence of hypovolemia, including decreased BP and increased HR. Monitor hematocrit for elevation, which occurs with hypovolemia. Weigh patient after procedure. Remember that 1 liter of fluid equals 1 kg, so hypovolemia can be reflected readily in weight changes.
2. Provide fluids during plasmapheresis as prescribed, either *via* oral, enteric tube, or IV access.

3. Monitor and record I&O throughout the procedure. Be alert to oliguria (urinary ouput <30 ml/hr for two consecutive hours).
4. Protect patients who are dizzy or confused by keeping side rails up and the bed in its lowest position.

Clotting abnormalities: Can occur secondary to removal of clotting factors during plasmapheresis

---

Desired outcomes: Patient forms clots and does not exhibit prolonged bleeding. PT is 11-15 seconds, PTT is 30-40 seconds, and platelet count is 150,000-400,000 µl.

---

1. Assess PT, PTT, and platelet count prior to and after procedure. Be alert to PT and PTT greater than controls and to increased platelet count.
2. Be alert to signs of impaired clotting, such as oozing from arterial puncture, venous access, or IV sites. Monitor patient for epistaxis or other signs of hemorrhage, such as elevated pulse rate, decreasing BP, or changes in patient's mental status.
3. Apply firm, continuous (e.g., 10 minutes) pressure to the arterial puncture site once the catheter or needle is removed. A pressure dressing is recommended.
4. Instruct patient to alert staff to the presence of bleeding from puncture and other sites.

Hypokalemia: Can occur secondary to removal of potassium during the plasma exchange

---

Desired outcome: Patient has normal potassium level as evidenced by HR ≥60 bpm, normal sinus rhythm on EKG, serum potassium level 3.5-5.5 mEq/L, and absence of leg cramps and other clinical indicators of hypokalemia.

---

1. Assess serum potassium before, during, and after plasma exchange. Be alert to decreasing levels.
2. Monitor for physical signs of hypokalemia, including bradycardia, fatigue, leg cramps, nausea, and paresthesias.
3. Observe cardiac monitor for signs of cardiac dysrhythmias: ST-segment depression, flattened T wave, presence of U wave, and ventricular dysrhythmias. Report abnormal cardiac rhythms to MD.
4. During reinfusion of blood, administer potassium as prescribed to prevent hypokalemia and dangerous dysrhythmias. If prescribed, administer antiarrhythmic agents.

< C A U T I O N : Patients on prednisone or digitalis preparations are at increased risk for hypokalemia and should be monitored closely for its occurrence.

Hypocalcemia: Can occur secondary to binding of calcium to acid-citrate-dextrose (ACD), the anticoagulant used during plasmapheresis

---

Desired outcome: Patient has normal calcium level as evidenced by orientation to person, place, and time; normal QT intervals on EKG; serum calcium levels 8.5-10.5 mg/dl; and absence of paresthesias and other clinical indicators of hypocalcemia.

---

1. Assess serum calcium levels before, during, and after plasmapheresis. Be alert to decreasing levels.
2. Monitor patient for signs of hypocalcemia, such as numbness with tingling of fingers and circumoral area, hyperactive reflexes, muscle cramps, tetany, paresthesia, Chvostek's sign, irritability, emotional instability, impaired memory, and confusion.
3. Observe cardiac monitor for evidence of hypocalcemia: prolonged QT interval caused by elongation of ST segment.
4. Encourage patient to drink milk before and during the plasma exchange.
5. As prescribed, administer calcium gluconate during plasmapheresis if indicators of hypocalcemia occur.

Myasthenic crisis: Can occur secondary to removal of circulating anticholinesterase drugs during plasmapheresis

Cholinergic crisis: Can occur secondary to removal of antibodies and decreased need for anticholinesterase drugs following plasmapheresis

---

Desired outcome: Patient is asymptomatic of myasthenic or cholinergic crisis as evidenced by vital capacity $\geq$1 L, the ability to swallow effectively, and absence of diplopia and other clinical indicators of crisis.

---

1. In the event of crisis, have the following available: IV infusion apparatus, medications (edrophonium chloride [Tensilon], neostigmine bromide, atropine, and pralidoxime chloride [Protopam chloride]), manual resuscitator, oxygen, suction equipment, and intubation tray if patient is not already intubated.
2. Monitor patient for evidence of crisis, such as decreased vital capacity (<1 L), inability to swallow, ptosis, diplopia, dysarthria, dysphonia, dyspnea, muscle weakness, and nasal flaring. Stay with patient if these signs appear and notify MD promptly.

See "Renal Transplant" for the following: **Knowledge deficit:** Immunosuppressive medications and their side effects, p. 195. Also see nursing diagnoses and interventions in the following: "Management of the Adult on Mechanical Ventilation," pp. 66-70; "Providing Nutritional Support," pp. 490-505; "Caring for the Critically Ill with Life-Threatening Disorders," pp. 511-522; and "Caring for the Family of the Critically Ill," pp. 522-526.

REHABILITATION AND PATIENT-FAMILY TEACHING CONCEPTS

Give patient and significant others verbal and written instructions for the following:
1. Medications, including drug name, purpose, dosage, schedule, precautions, potential side effects, and signs of overdose (particularly of anticholinesterase agents).

2. Importance of carrying an identification card denoting the diagnosis, medications, contraindications, and physician's name and number.
3. Indicators of impending myasthenic or cholinergic crisis.
4. List of specific information on how to cope with special problems of myasthenia gravis.
   - When to expect peak effect of medications and how to time ADL based on medication effects.
   - Use of a battery-operated clock set to proper times to ensure precise timing of medications.
   - Importance of taking medications with food to minimize nausea and avoiding foods that cause hyperactivity of the GI tract, thereby decreasing absorption of the medication.
   - Avoiding OTC medications without physician approval.
   - Importance of avoiding alcohol intake for at least one hour after taking medication as it increases rate of absorption of the medication; and avoiding tonic water, which contains quinine, a substance that can increase muscle weakness.
   - Taking small, frequent meals (i.e., 6 times/day), which may be less tiring than eating 3 larger meals a day.
   - Eating meals composed of semi-solid foods, which are easier to swallow than solids or liquids.
   - Consuming room temperature or cool foods and beverages, which are easier to swallow than hot substances, which tend to increase muscle weakness.
   - If taking steroids, the importance of eating foods high in potassium (see Table 3-15, p. 228).
   - Importance of avoiding emotional and temperature extremes, which can result in increased muscle weakness.
5. Address of the local chapter of the Myasthenia Gravis Foundation. The national office of the Myasthenia Gravis Foundation is located at 15 East 26th Street, New York, New York 10010.

Guillain-Barré syndrome

Guillain-Barré syndrome (G-BS) is an acute or subacute postinfectious polyneuritis. The frequency of G-BS following an infection, along with its occurrence in conjunction with diseases of lymphoid tissue (e.g., Hodgkin's disease), suggests that it is an autoimmune disorder.

G-BS mainly affects the Schwann cell, which synthesizes and maintains the peripheral nerve myelin sheath. The result is the segmental loss of myelin along the peripheral nerve axon. Cellular inflammatory infiltrates consisting of T- and B-lymphocytes, macrophages, and neutrophils appear in the areas of myelin loss. Studies suggest that the macrophages penetrate the basement membrane and strip apparently normal myelin from intact axons, causing the characteristic signs and symptoms of G-BS. The ventral (motor) root axons of the anterior horn cells, which innervate voluntary skeletal muscles, are primarily involved. Dorsal (sensory) root axons of the posterior horn also are affected, but to a lesser degree. Recovery of neurologic function is dependent on proliferation of Schwann cells and remyelination of axons. Recovery can be expected in 85-95% of cases, with minor residual deficits occurring in less than half of affected patients.

ASSESSMENT

General signs and symptoms: Ascending flaccid motor paralysis is the classic presenting sign and is associated with the early loss of deep tendon reflexes (DTRs). Weakness, which usually precedes the paralysis, is symmetrical and generally begins in distal muscle groups and ascends to involve more proximal muscles. Muscles of respiration (intercostals and diaphragm) frequently are involved and approximately half of all patients will require ventilation. Complaints of distal paresthesias are common. In more serious or prolonged cases, proprioceptive and vibratory dysfunctions are present. In addition, loss of pain and temperature sensations in a glove and stocking distribution has been reported. Sensory complaints usually appear first, with muscle weakness developing rapidly over 24-72 hours. Fifty percent of patients reach the peak of dysfunction within 2 weeks. By 4 weeks, 90% will have reached peak of dysfunction.

- *Autonomic nervous system involvement* (occurs in most G-BS patients): Sinus tachycardia, bradycardia, orthostatic hypotension, hypertension, excessive diaphoresis, bowel and bladder retention, loss of sphincter control, increased pulmonary secretions, and cardiac dysrhythmias (a common cause of death).
- *Involvement of cranial nerves III, IV, and VI:* Ptosis, diplopia, pupillary dilation.
- *Involvement of cranial nerve V:* Paresis or paralysis of muscles of mastication, decreased facial sensations, and loss of corneal reflex.
- *Involvement of cranial nerve VII:* Paresis or paralysis of facial muscles, facial droop, loss of taste on the anterior two-thirds of the tongue, loss of secretion of submandibular, sublingual, and lacrimal glands.
- *Involvement of cranial nerve VIII:* Vertigo, nystagmus.
- *Involvement of cranial nerves IX and X:* Paresis or paralysis of soft palate, pharynx, and larynx; dysphagia, dysarthria, and hoarseness; and loss of gag reflex.
- *Involvement of cranial nerve XI:* Paresis or paralysis of sternocleidomastoid and trapezius muscles with inability to turn head or shrug shoulders.
- *Involvement of cranial nerve XII:* Paresis or paralysis of the tongue.

Physical assessment: Symmetric motor weakness, decreased or absent DTR's, hypotonia or flaccidity of affected muscles, presence of respiratory abnormalities (i.e., nasal flaring, hypoventilation), facial paralysis.

History and risk factors: Respiratory or gastrointestinal illness 4 weeks prior to onset of the neurologic symptoms, in which a viral agent, such as parainfluenza 2, herpes zoster, measles, mumps, rubella, or varicella is present (50% of cases); recent vaccination (15% of cases), for example, for swine influenza; recent surgical procedure (5% of cases).

DIAGNOSTIC TESTS

The diagnosis for G-BS is based on clinical presentation, history of antecedent illness, and cerebrospinal fluid (CSF) findings.

1. *Lumbar puncture (LP) and CSF analysis:* CSF analysis usually shows an elevated protein, without any increase in WBCs. This is referred to as the "albuminocytologic dissociation." This dissociation usually is noted during the course of G-BS and is helpful in differentiating G-BS from other CNS disorders, such as infection. CSF protein, normally between 15-45 mg/100 ml, may peak 4-6 weeks after onset of G-BS to levels of several hundred mg/ml. This

elevation may persist for months. CSF pressure, which is normally between 0-15 mm Hg (90-180 mm H_2O), may be elevated in severe cases.

2. *Electrodiagnostic studies:* Electromyography (EMG) and nerve conduction velocity (NCV) demonstrate profound slowing of motor conduction velocities and conduction blocks due to the demyelination of peripheral nerves. Although these changes may not appear initially, they will become apparent several weeks into the illness.

3. *CBC:* Moderate leukocytosis may occur early in disease, possibly due to the inflammatory process associated with demyelination in G-BS, but will return to normal as the disease runs its course.

4. *Pulmonary function studies:* May be done during initial diagnostic evaluation. Vital capacity (VC) of <1 L indicates a possible need for assisted ventilation.

5. *ABG studies:* Performed if VC drops below 1 L or if patient demonstrates dyspnea, confusion, restlessness, nasal flaring, use of accessory muscles of respiration, or breathlessness (noted during a count by the patient from 1-10). A decrease in PaO_2 >10-15 mm Hg or increase in $PaCO_2$ of 10-15 mm Hg greater than baseline or normal value signals the need for immediate intubation or tracheostomy.

MEDICAL MANAGEMENT

1. **Respiratory support:** Endotracheal intubation or tracheostomy with assisted mechanical ventilation, as necessary.

2. **Pharmacotherapy**
   - *Corticosteroids:* May slow or halt demyelinating process and decrease inflammation along the peripheral nerves. Although their use is controversial, prednisone and adrenocorticotropic hormone (ACTH) have been used with varied results.
   - *Immunosuppressive agents:* Mechanisms of action are not known, but it is believed that they may suppress the immunoinflammatory response that causes the demyelination of the peripheral nerve myelin sheath. Cyclophosphamide and azathioprine have been used with varied results.

3. **Plasmapheresis:** Involves a complete exchange of plasma with the removal of abnormal circulating antibodies that affect the peripheral nerve myelin sheath. Removal of these auto-antibodies may lessen the duration and severity of G-BS.

4. **Maintenance and monitoring of cardiovascular function:** As necessary, cardiac monitoring may be initiated for dysrhythmias, arterial pressure monitoring may be used to evaluate hypertension or hypotension, and antihypertensive agents or vasopressors may be administered to maintain BP within normal levels.

5. **Management of bowel and bladder dysfunction:** Nasogastric suction and parenteral infusion may be started for patients with paralytic ileus; an in-dwelling urinary catheter may be inserted for patients with urinary retention.

6. **Nutritional management:** Parenteral feedings are given until return of peristalsis. Tube feedings or gastrostomy feedings are used for patients with severe dysphagia. With recovery of gag reflex and swallowing ability, the diet will progress to semisolid and solid foods, which are more readily swallowed than liquids.

7. **Management of motor dysfunction:** Active and passive ROM exercises are

performed at frequent intervals during all phases of G-BS. However, they must not be done strenuously during the acute phase, as this may exacerbate weakness and possibly accelerate the demyelinating process. Activity must be balanced with caloric intake to prevent muscle wasting. As the patient's condition stabilizes, physical and occupational therapy personnel should be involved in the planning of the rehabilitation process. The primary goal is maintenance of the patient's mobility and independence.

NURSING DIAGNOSES AND INTERVENTIONS

Impaired gas exchange related to decreased lung expansion secondary to weakness or paralysis of intercostal and diaphragmatic muscles

---

Desired outcomes: Patient has adequate gas exchange as evidenced by orientation to person, place, and time; HR $\leq$100 bpm; BP within patient's normal range; Pao_2 $\geq$80 mm Hg; and $Paco_2$ $\leq$45 mm Hg. RR is 12-20 breaths/min with normal pattern and depth (eupnea), vital capacity is $\geq$1 L, tidal volume is $\geq$75% of predicted value, patient is normothermic, and clinical indicators of respiratory dysfunction, including adventitious breath sounds and restlessness, are absent.

---

1. Monitor patient's respiratory status and results of diagnostic tests for evidence of distress or other abnormalities. Be alert to and report the following to the MD: adventitious (crackles, rhonchi), decreased, or absent breath sounds; temperature $\geq$37.8° C (100° F); increased HR and BP; tidal volume or vital capacity decreased from baseline; a decrease in Pao_2 or increase in $Paco_2$ $\geq$10-15 mm Hg from baseline or normal values; abnormal respiratory rate or rhythm; increasing restlessness or anxiety; and confusion.
2. In the presence of the above indicators, be prepared to assist with patient intubation or tracheotomy.
3. Prepare patient for the likelihood of these interventions; explain that they will be temporary measures.
4. Maintain mechanical ventilation *via* endotracheal or tracheostomy as indicated; check ventilator settings at regular intervals to ensure that they are within prescribed limits.
5. Continue to monitor ABG results. Improvement is indicated by an increase in Pao_2 (optimally to $\geq$80 mm Hg) and a decrease in $Paco_2$ (optimally to $\leq$45 mm Hg). Notify MD of continued abnormalities.

Ineffective airway clearance related to inability to cough or swallow secondary to increasing paralysis of respiratory, pharyngeal, and facial muscles and absence of gag reflex

---

Desired outcomes: Patient's airway is clear as evidenced by auscultation of normal breath sounds and absence of adventitious breath sounds. Patient is asymptomatic of URI and atelectasis as evidenced by normothermia, HR $\leq$100 bpm, BP within normal range, RR 12-20 breaths/min with normal pattern and depth (eupnea), negative cultures, WBC count $\leq$11,000 μl, and secretions that are thin and clear.

1. Assess neurologic function qh, or as often as needed. Ascending motor and sensory dysfunctions usually occur rapidly (over 24-72 hours) and can lead to life-threatening respiratory arrest.

2. Monitor patient for the following: adventitious (crackles, rhonchi), decreased, or absent breath sounds; temperature $\geq 37.8°$ C ($100°$ F); increased HR and BP; tidal volume or vital capacity decreased from baseline; a decrease in PaO_2 or increase in $PaCO_2$; abnormal respiratory rate or rhythm; and increasing restlessness or anxiety.

3. Using sterile technique, suction the airway as needed, as determined by auscultation findings. As the paresis or paralysis subsides (usually after 2-4 weeks, the usual time of the peak of the dysfunction), cranial nerve function will begin to return (i.e., gag reflex, swallowing, and coughing). Evaluate patient's ability to cough, whether or not he or she is being ventilated. Assess for the presence or absence of breath sounds and for the presence of adventitious sounds to determine effectiveness of patient's cough.

4. Assess color, consistency, amount, and odor of pulmonary secretions. Culture sputum specimens as prescribed.

5. Monitor CBC results for elevation of WBC count.

6. Administer antibiotics as prescribed.

7. Deliver oxygen and humidification as prescribed.

8. Maintain mechanical ventilation as prescribed; confirm that ventilator settings are within prescribed limits.

9. Unless contraindicated, maintain adequate hydration (up to 2-3 L/day) to minimize thickening of pulmonary secretions.

10. Turn and reposition patient at least q2h to prevent stasis of secretions.

11. Protect patient from exposure to individuals with infection, particularly URI.

Impaired physical mobility related to sensorimotor deficits secondary to ascending flaccid paralysis and paresthesias

---

Desired outcomes: Patient is asymptomatic of contracture formation as evidenced by full range of motion of all joints. Skin remains intact.

---

1. Assess neurologic function qh or as often as indicated. Ascending motor and sensory dysfunction usually occurs rapidly, over 24-72 hours. During the stage of G-BS crisis when neurologic dysfunction is progressing, assess motor and sensory levels starting with the lower extremities and working upward to determine level of deficit.

   - Assess muscle symmetry by using a side-to-side comparison.
   - Assess muscle strength: *For lower extremities,* have patient pull heel of foot toward the buttocks as you provide resistance by holding onto the foot. *For upper extremities,* have patient extend and flex the wrists and arms against your resistance.
   - Assess DTRs of the Achilles, patellae, biceps, triceps, and brachioradialis. Normal response is +2; report decreased (+1) or absent (0) response.
   - Assess for the presence of paresthesias, including the location, degree, and whether or not it is ascending.

- Assess for the presence or absence of position sense by moving patient's big toe or thumb up and down while patient's eyes are closed. Also note presence or absence of vibratory sense by placing a vibrating tuning fork over bony prominences.
- Assess for the presence or absence of response to light touch or pinprick by starting at the feet and working upward to determine the level of dysfunction.

< N O T E :   Sensory symptoms are usually milder than motor complaints, with vibration and position sensations affected most often. When light touch, pinprick, and temperature sensations are affected, they are most often found in a stocking-glove distribution. Patients frequently experience muscle tenderness and sensitivity to pressure.

- Assess for cranial nerve dysfunction. See descriptions, pp. 251 and 257.
2. Record and report sensorimotor deficit, including degree of involvement.
3. Turn and reposition patient in correct anatomic alignment q2h or more often if requested by patient. Support patient's position with pillows and other positioning aids.
4. To maintain patient's muscle function and prevent contractures, ensure that active or passive ROM exercises are performed q2h during all phases of G-BS. Involve significant others in the exercises, if appropriate.

< C A U T I O N :   During the acute phase of G-BS, avoid strenuous movements, which may exacerbate the demyelinating process.

5. Obtain a physical therapy referral and begin the rehabilitation planning process during the early stages of the disorder.
6. As indicated, apply splints to hands-arms and feet-legs to help prevent contracture; alternate splints so that they are on two hours and off two hours.
7. Apply antiembolic stockings as prescribed to help promote tissue perfusion and minimize the risk of thrombophlebitis, deep-vein thrombosis, and pulmonary emboli.
8. Utilize a sheepskin or air mattress to help maintain skin integrity. A circle bed, Roto Rest kinetic treatment table, Clinitron bed, Kin Air, or Mediscus Air bed may be used to manage the respiratory, autonomic, and musculoskeletal problems that occur with G-BS. See appendicized section, "Caring for the Critically Ill on Prolonged Bed Rest," pp. 506-511, for interventions related to maintaining skin integrity.

Potential for injury related to risk of autonomic nervous system dysfunction (autonomic dysreflexia) secondary to untoward precipitating event

---

Desired outcome: Patient is asymptomatic of autonomic dysreflexia as evidenced by normal T-wave configuration on EKG, HR ≥60 bpm, BP within patient's normal range, cool and dry skin, patient's normal strength, and absence of headache and chest and abdominal tightness.

---

1. Assess for signs of autonomic dysreflexia: cardiac dysrhythmias; bradycardia (HR <60 bpm); elevated and sustained BP (e.g., ≥250-300/150 mm Hg), possibly for several days; facial flushing; increased sweating, possibly due to loss

of thermal regulation; extreme generalized warmth; profound weakness; and complaints of severe headache or tightening in the chest and abdomen.

2. Place patient on cardiac monitor as prescribed.

< N O T E : Because of the risk of fatal cardiac dysrhythmias with G-BS, it is recommended that patients be monitored for the first 10-14 days of hospitalization.

3. Monitor patient carefully during activities that are known to precipitate autonomic dysreflexia: position changes, vigorous coughing, straining with bowel movements.

4. Be aware of and implement measures to prevent factors that may precipitate autonomic dysreflexia:
   - *Bladder stimuli:* Urinary tract infection, cystoscopy, urinary catheter insertion, clogged urinary catheter, urinary calculi.
   - *Bowel stimuli:* Fecal impaction, rectal examination, enemas, suppositories.
   - *Sensory stimuli:* Pressure caused by tight clothing, dressings, bedcovers, thigh straps on urinary drainage bags; prolonged pressure on skin surface or over bony prominences; temperature changes, such as exposure to a cool breeze or draft.

5. If indicators of autonomic dysreflexia are present, implement the following:
   - Elevate HOB or place patient in a sitting position to promote decrease in BP.
   - Monitor BP and HR q3-5min until patient stabilizes.
   - Determine and remove offending stimulus.
     —For example, if patient's bladder is distended, catheterize cautiously, using sufficient lubricant.
     —If patient has an in-dwelling urinary catheter, check for obstruction such as granulation in catheter or kinking of tubing. As indicated, irrigate catheter, using no more than 30 ml normal saline.
     —If urinary tract infection is suspected, obtain a urine specimen for culture and sensitivity once crisis stage has passed.
     —Check for fecal impaction. Perform the rectal examination gently, using an ointment containing a local anesthetic (e.g., Nupercaine).
     —Check for sensory stimuli and loosen clothing, bed covers, or other constricting fabric as indicated.

6. Notify MD if symptoms do not abate, especially the elevated BP, because the consequences are life-threatening: seizures, subarachnoid or intracerebral hemorrhage, fatal cerebrovascular accident.

7. As prescribed, administer antihypertensive agent and monitor its effectiveness.

Alteration in cardiac output: Decreased, related to ''artificial hypovolemia'' secondary to reduced peripheral vascular tone occurring with overactive sympathetic nervous system

< N O T E : These patients experience a decreased cardiac output due to the ''artificial hypovolemia'' created by an enlarged vascular space containing normal volume. It is similar to the vascular response seen in anaphylactic or septic shock.

Desired outcome: Patient exhibits adequate cardiac output as evidenced by BP within patient's normal range; HR 60-100 bpm; urinary output ≥30 ml/hr; peripheral pulses >2+ on a 0-4+ scale; orientation to person, place, and time; PAWP

6-12 mm Hg; SVR 900-1200 dynes/sec/cm^{-5}; CO 4-7 L/min; and normal sinus rhythm on EKG.

1. Monitor patient for indicators of decreased cardiac output: drop in systolic BP >20 mm Hg from baseline, systolic BP <80 mm Hg, or a continuing drop in systolic BP of 5-10 mm Hg with every assessment; HR >100 beats/min; irregular HR; restlessness, confusion, and dizziness; warm and flushed skin; peripheral edema; and decreasing urinary output (<30 ml/hr for two consecutive hours). Monitor hemodynamic pressures, particularly PAWP, CO, and SVR.
2. Continuously assess cardiac rate and rhythm per cardiac monitor; report changes in rate and rhythm.
3. As prescribed, administer fluids to treat the hypotension.
4. As prescribed, administer vasopressor (e.g., epinephrine) to counteract peripheral vasodilatation. Monitor for therapeutic effects.

Potential sensory-perceptual alterations related to sensorimotor dysfunction secondary to cranial nerve involvement with G-BS

Desired outcome: Patient relates the presence of normal vision and exhibits the gag reflex, ability to masticate, normoreflexive pupils and corneas, intact corneas, and full ROM of head and shoulders.

1. Assess cranial nerve function. Patients with G-BS commonly exhibit deficits in the following cranial nerves: III, IV, V, VI, VII, IX, X, XI, and XII.
2. Evaluate cranial nerves III, IV, and V by checking for extraocular eye movements, pupillary light reflex, degree of ptosis, and for the presence of diplopia.
   • If patient experiences a deficit, place objects where patient can see them. Assist patient with ADLs as indicated.
   • Cover one eye with a patch or frosted lens if patient is experiencing diplopia; alternate patch or lens q2-3h during patient's waking hours.
   • Use eyelid crutches for patients with ptosis.
3. Evaluate cranial nerves V and VII by checking patient's facial sensation and movement, ability to masticate, and the corneal reflex.
   • In the presence of a deficit, assess patient for corneal irritation or abrasion. Apply artificial tear drops or ointments as prescribed. Secure the eyelid in a closed position if corneal reflex is diminished or absent.
4. Evaluate cranial nerves IX, X, and XII by checking for pharyngeal sensation and movement (swallowing), the presence or absence of the gag reflex, and control of the tongue.
   • If a deficit is found, provide suctioning during oral hygiene. Do not feed patient an oral diet until the gag reflex returns.
5. Assess cranial nerve XI by checking patient's ability to shrug the shoulders and turn head from side to side.
   • If a deficit is found, position patient's head in a position of comfort and proper anatomic alignment.

Alteration in bowel elimination related to decreased intake secondary to NPO status with hypoperistalsis or paralytic ileus

---

Desired outcome: Patient has bowel elimination pattern normal for patient.

---

1. Assess patient's gastrointestinal status, noting absence or presence and quality of the following: bowel sounds, abdominal distention, nausea, vomiting, and abdominal discomfort. In the presence of hypoperistalsis or paralytic ileus, patient will exhibit high-pitched, tinkling sounds that will be heard early in obstruction or ileus; or a decrease or absence of sounds occurring with complete obstruction or paralytic ileus.
2. If patient is having bowel movements, determine the amount, consistency, and frequency. Question patient about his or her usual pattern of bowel elimination.
3. Begin bowel training program based on patient's needs and status of dietary intake. Examples include the following:
   - Provide a high-roughage diet if patient is able to chew and swallow without difficulty; give patient prune juice every evening.
   - Establish a regular time for elimination (e.g., 30 minutes after meals) and have a bedpan readily available.
   - Facilitate patient's normal bowel habits: ensure privacy; provide warm oral fluids with each attempt at defecation.
   - Administer stool softeners (e.g., docusate sodium) or bulk-building additives such as psyllium.
   - Administer prescribed medicated suppositories.

   < C A U T I O N : Care must be taken to avoid stimulation of autonomic dysreflexia by using generous amounts of anesthetic ointment and ensuring gentle insertion when giving suppository or enema.

   - Provide 2-3 L/day of fluid to prevent dehydration and constipation.

   < N O T E : This may be contraindicated for patient with impaired renal or cardiac status.

Knowledge deficit: Purpose and procedure for plasmapheresis

Desired outcome: Patient verbalizes knowledge of the purpose and procedure for plasmapheresis.

---

1. Assess patient's previous experience with and knowledge of plasmapheresis.
2. As appropriate, teach patient the following about plasmapheresis: Blood is withdrawn *via* an arterial catheter, anticoagulated, and then passed through a cell separator. The plasma portion of the blood that may contain the autoantibody whose target is the peripheral nerve myelin sheath is removed. RBCs, WBCs, and platelets are mixed with saline, potassium, and plasma protein fraction and are then returned to the body, minus the plasma, *via* a venous access.
3. Advise patient that plasmapheresis *may* lessen the duration and severity of the symptoms of G-BS.

   < N O T E : Benefits of plasmapheresis with G-BS have not been determined definitively. Although plasmapheresis is still in the experimental stage with this

disorder, some studies have shown a rapid but temporary improvement in symptoms.

4. Explain that patient should eat prior to plasmapheresis and that nutrition will be provided during the procedure.
5. Advise patient that the nurse will perform several assessment procedures before, during, and after plasmapheresis. See **Impaired physical mobility**, p. 254, for neuroassessment parameters. Also see **Fluid volume deficit,** p. 247, in "Myasthenia Gravis" for the following complications: hypovolemia, clotting abnormalities, hypokalemia, and hypocalcemia.
6. Advise patient that the procedure may take several hours (up to 8) and that it may be performed as often as 3-4 times per week, depending on patient's condition.
7. Advise patient that plasmapheresis provides only short-term improvement and has no long-term benefit. It is expensive, as well, costing nearly $1500 per procedure.

See "Renal Transplant" for the following: **Knowledge deficit:** Immunosuppressive medications and their side effects, p. 195. See "Myasthenia Gravis" for the following: **Impaired swallowing** related to decreased or absent gag reflex, decreased strength or excursion of muscles involved in mastication, facial paralysis, or mechanical obstruction (tracheostomy), p. 244. For other nursing diagnoses and interventions, see the following as appropriate: "Management of the Adult on Mechanical Ventilation," pp. 66-70; "Providing Nutritional Support," pp. 490-505; "Caring for the Critically Ill on Prolonged Bed Rest," pp. 506-511; "Caring for the Critically Ill with Life-Threatening Disorders," pp. 511-522; and "Caring for the Family of the Critically Ill," pp. 522-526.

REHABILITATION AND PATIENT-FAMILY TEACHING CONCEPTS

Recovery from GB-S is expected for 85-95% of patients, with less than half of patients experiencing minor residual symptoms. The recovery phase may be protracted, up to as long as 2 years. Rehabilitation planning, which should begin at the time of diagnosis, will vary for each patient and family. The entire health team, including physicians; nurses; respiratory, physical, and occupational therapists; social workers; community health nurses; support groups; clergy; and psychologists should be involved in the rehabilitation process. In addition, patient should be given the address of local G-BS support groups.

Cerebral aneurysm and subarachnoid hemorrhage

An aneurysm is a localized dilatation of an arterial lumen caused by weakness in the vessel wall. Ninety percent of cerebral aneurysms are saccular or berry (congenital), while fusiform, septic, miliary, dissecting, and traumatic aneurysms comprise the other ten percent. Saccular aneurysms are believed to result from a congenital hypoplasia of the muscle (medial) layer in the arterial wall, in combination with hypertension and atherosclerosis. Ninety percent of berry aneurysms occur at the bifurcation of the blood vessels comprising the Circle of Willis. The remainder occur in the posterior cerebral circulation, often at the bifurcation of the basilar and vertebral arteries.

Most aneurysms are silent until they rupture, although nearly half of the affected population experience some warning sign or symptom as a result of expansion of the lesion and compression of cerebral tissue. When rupture occurs, the patient hemorrhages into the subarachnoid space (SAS). If the patient survives the initial effects of subarachnoid hemorrhage (SAH), which include destruction of brain tissue by the force of arterial blood, intracerebral hemorrhage, and sharply increased ICP, he or she also must survive two of the common causes of morbidity and mortality—rebleeding and cerebral arterial vasospasm. The risk of rerupture with rebleeding from an aneurysm is greatest in the first 24-48 hours following the initial bleed, but may occur as long as 6 months later. In addition, the patient is at risk for rebleeding between 7-14 days post-SAH, when the normal process of hemolysis of the aneurysmal clot should occur.

Cerebral vasospasm, the constriction of the arterial smooth muscle layer of the major cerebral arteries, causes a dramatic decrease in cerebral blood flow, which in turn leads to cerebral ischemia and progressive neurologic deficit. It can be seen on angiography 3-4 days post-SAH, peaks between 7-10 days, and resolves in approximately 3 weeks. The pathogenesis of cerebral vasospasm is poorly understood but seems to be directly related to the amount of blood in the SAS post-SAH. The greater the volume of blood, the more pronounced the vasospasm.

In addition to rebleeding and vasospasm, the patient with a ruptured cerebral aneurysm and SAH also is at risk for diabetes insipidus (see p. 340) or syndrome of inappropriate antidiuretic hormone (SIADH, see p. 347) as a result of compression, irritation, or destruction of the posterior portion of the pituitary gland or the hypothalamus. In addition, acute or chronic hydrocephalus may develop as a result of the irritative or destructive effects of blood in the SAS. The SAH may damage the arachnoid villi or block CSF reabsorption pathways. The patient also may experience permanent neurologic deficit, the degree of which depends on the effects of the initial rupture and SAH, location of the SAH, and development of any complications.

ASSESSMENT

Signs and symptoms before and after rupture depend on the size, site, and amount of bleeding.

Warning signs and symptoms (pre-bleed): Headaches (possibly localized); generalized, transient weakness; fatigue; occasional ptosis due to third cranial nerve palsy.

Early indicators (after initial bleed): Meningeal signs (due to presence of blood in the SAS) include headache, nuchal rigidity, fever, photophobia, lethargy, nausea, and vomiting. Patients report that the headache is the worst they've ever experienced, a sensation of a "bullet going off in the head."

Increased ICP: (Caused by SAH or intracerebral hemorrhage and the subsequent cerebral edema): Sudden severe headache, nausea and vomiting, papilledema, dysphasia, seizures.

Indicators of herniation secondary to increased ICP: Alterations in LOC ranging from alert to profoundly comatose, with no response to any stimuli; VS changes (vary with level of ICP); bradycardia; increasing systolic BP with a widening pulse pressure; irregular respiratory patterns (e.g., Cheyne-Stokes, ataxic, apneustic, central neurogenic hyperventilation); and hemisensory changes and hemiparesis or hemiplegia due to involvement of hemispheric sensory and motor pathways. In addition, patient may have pupillary dilatation caused by involvement of the third cranial nerve; dysconjugate gaze and inability to move one eye beyond midposition due to involvement of the third, fourth, and sixth cranial nerves. Involvement of other cranial nerves depends on the severity of neurologic insult.

< N O T E :   See "Head Injury," p. 270, for additional detail on herniation syndromes.

Altered hypothalamic regulatory mechanism: Vomiting, increased diaphoresis, increased serum glucose, glycosuria, and proteinuria.

Physical assessment: Pathologic reflexes due to the presence of blood in the SAS.
- *Kernig's sign*: Resistance to full extension of the leg at the knee when the hip is flexed.
- *Brudzinski's sign*: Flexion of the hip and knee during passive neck flexion.

Funduscopic assessment: May reveal retinal hemorrhage(s) at the side of the optic disk. Hemorrhage is caused by blood from the SAS being forced along the optic nerve sheath under high pressure. The patient may complain of blurred vision or blind spots (scotomata).

International grading system: Purpose is to permit objective and continuing evaluation of the patient's admitting symptoms and their progression. Grading is done according to symptom presentation and LOC.
- *Grade 1:* Asymptomatic or minimal headache
  Slight nuchal rigidity
  Alert with no neurologic deficit
- *Grade 2:* Mild to severe headache
  Nuchal rigidity
  Possible cranial nerve palsies, of which third (oculomotor) is the most common; ptosis
  Alert with minimal neurologic deficit
- *Grade 3:* Drowsy, confused
  Definite change (decrease) in LOC
  May have mild focal neurologic deficits
- *Grade 4:* Stupor, semicomatose
  Mild to severe hemiparesis
  Possible early posturing (decerebrate or decorticate)
- *Grade 5:* Profound coma
  Posturing
  Moribund appearance

DIAGNOSTIC TESTS

1. *Lumbar puncture (LP) and cerebrospinal fluid (CSF) analysis:* To confirm presence of blood in the CSF, which signals that SAH has occurred. CSF pressure, which normally is 0-15 mm Hg (90-180 mm H_2O), may be as high as 250 mm H_2O, with the pressure proportionate to the degree of bleeding. Protein may be increased as much as 80-130 mg/dl (normal is 15-50 mg/dl). WBC count may be greater than the normal of 10/mm; and CSF glucose may be low (<40 mg/dl) in the presence of SAH.
2. *Skull x-ray:* May show calcification or local erosion of bone seen in the region

of the internal carotid artery or at the base of the skull due to pressure of enlarging cerebral aneurysm.

3. *CT scan:* To identify presence of aneurysm and subarachnoid or intracerebral hemorrhage; and size, site, and amount of bleeding. Scan also may reveal the presence of hydrocephalus due to blocked CSF reabsorption pathways. If the aneurysm is small, it may not appear on the scan.

4. *Cerebral angiography:* To confirm diagnosis of ruptured aneurysm and SAH. It is used to show size, location, vessels involved, and presence of other aneurysms as well as to determine accessibility of the aneurysm and presence of hematoma, vasospasm, and hydrocephalus. A four-vessel study involving both carotids and vertebrals is recommended due to the 20% chance of an existing second aneurysm. Very small aneurysms can be missed on angiogram, as are those that do not fill with contrast material due to the presence of vasospasm or a blood clot within the aneurysm.

5. *Magnetic resonance imaging (MRI):* To reveal very small aneurysms that are not visualized with CT or angiography.

6. *ABG analysis:* To detect hypoxemia and hypercarbia and determine appropriate respiratory therapy.

MEDICAL MANAGEMENT AND SURGICAL INTERVENTIONS

1. **Respiratory support:** To maintain airway and provide intubation and ventilation as necessary. Serial ABG tests are performed to identify hypoxemia (Pao_2 <80 mm Hg) and hypercarbia ($Paco_2$ >45 mm Hg). Hypercarbia is a potent cerebral vasodilator, which can increase ICP in patients who are already at risk.

2. **Complete bedrest with restriction of activities:** Patients are kept in a quiet, dark environment under constant supervision. ADLs are completed by nursing staff. Active ROM and isometric exercises are restricted during acute and preoperative stages to prevent increased ICP. Passive ROM is prescribed to prevent formation of thrombi with subsequent pulmonary emboli.

3. **ICP monitoring:** See this section under ''Head Injury,'' p. 274.

4. **HOB elevation:** To help facilitate venous outflow from the intracranial cavity and lower ICP. A 15-45 degree angle usually is prescribed.

5. **Fluid and electrolyte management:** Fluids are limited to 1500-1800 ml/24 hrs to prevent overhydration with subsequent cerebral edema and further increases in ICP. Electrolytes are replaced as indicated by patient's clinical picture and laboratory values. Accurate I&O measurement is essential.

6. **Nutrition therapy:** Adequate nutritional intake is maintained *via* parenteral nutrition or lipid emulsions, enteral feedings, and oral intake as indicated by patient's neurologic status.

7. **Pharmacotherapy**
   - *Sedatives:* Phenobarbital is the drug of choice for reducing restlessness and irritability, which can increase BP and ICP.
   - *Antipyretics:* Acetaminophen is used to control fever, which increases cerebral metabolic activity. It may be administered along with hypothermia blanket and chlorpromazine to decrease temperature and control shivering. Usually, aspirin is avoided because of its propensity for affecting the clotting cascade.
   - *Analgesics:* Acetaminophen for mild pain and codeine sulfate for more severe

pain. Although codeine will not depress neurologic indicators, it can cause constipation so it should be administered with stool softeners to prevent straining.

- *Stool softeners:* Docusate sodium (Colace) is the drug of choice for preventing straining, which can increase ICP.
- *Corticosteroids:* Dexamethasone (Decadron) is the drug most commonly used for its anti-inflammatory actions in relieving cerebral edema and decreasing ICP. There is some disagreement as to its effectiveness. It must be administered cautiously and the patient monitored carefully for side effects, including GI tract irritation. Antacids are administered concurrently and histamine H_2 antagonists may be given to inhibit gastric secretions.
- *Antihypertensives:* Hydralazine hydrochloride (Apresoline), methyldopa (Aldomet), or reserpine is administered to reduce BP in patients with persistent hypertension. They may be used in combination with a thiazide diuretic.
- *Osmotic diuretics:* Mannitol, urea (Ureaphil), and glycerol may be used to reduce ICP and treat cerebral edema *via* diuresis and a slightly hypovolemic state. All must be used with caution due to the risk of electrolyte imbalances and other serious side effects and adverse reactions.
- *Loop diuretics:* Furosemide (Lasix) is being used by some physicians because it seems to decrease cerebral edema without causing the rise in intracranial blood volume that is seen with mannitol.
- *Anticonvulsants:* Phenytoin and phenobarbital may be used to control or prevent seizures.
- *Antifibrinolytics:* Epsilon aminocaproic acid (EACA-Amicar) may be used to prevent lysis of the aneurysmal clot, which occurs normally between 7-14 days postrupture. It delays the spontaneous breakdown of the clot and provides time for further stabilization of the patient in preparation for surgery. Amicar usually is administered *via* continuous infusion for the patient with SAH. The length of therapy is determined by patient's status, readiness for surgery, and physician preference.

8. **Experimental treatments for cerebral vasospasm:** The following are experimental treatments. To date no completely effective method has been found.
- *Craniotomy:* Performed within 48 hours to evacuate the blood clot that is present after SAH in an attempt to prevent vasospasm.
- *Hemodilution:* To improve cerebral blood flow by decreasing blood viscosity.
- *Hypervolemic-hypertensive therapy:* To reduce the neurologic deficit caused by vasospasm by increasing blood volume and arterial pressure.

< N O T E : While this method has been proven to be an effective treatment for vasospasm, it carries great risks and the patient's BP, ICP, and neurologic status must be monitored closely. If used preoperatively (rare), this therapy may precipitate a rise in ICP with rerupture and rebleeding from the aneurysm. When used postoperatively, the patient may experience cerebral edema with cerebral ischemia and subsequent neurologic deficit.

- *Theophylline:* To dilate smooth muscle and increase cerebral perfusion.
- *Isoproterenol:* To dilate smooth muscle, increase cardiac output, and increase cerebral perfusion.
- *Mannitol:* To decrease cerebral edema and ICP and increase cerebral perfusion.

- *Plasma protein fraction, colloids, or whole blood:* To expand volume, increase BP, and thus increase cerebral perfusion.
- *Nitroprusside sodium:* To relax smooth muscle and dilate cerebral vessels.
- *Nifedipine:* To inhibit calcium influx across the cell membrane of vascular smooth muscles, thereby decreasing peripheral vascular resistance and BP and causing vasodilatation.
- *Barbiturate coma:* To decrease metabolic needs of the brain until the vasospasm subsides and blood flow improves (used rarely). For more detail, see discussion, p. 275, with "Head Injury."

9. **Placement of a shunt for treatment of hydrocephalus:** Twenty to twenty-five percent of patients with subarachnoid hemorrhage from a ruptured cerebral aneurysm develop hydrocephalus. A shunt is placed to drain CSF and thereby prevent enlargement of the ventricles with compression of cerebral tissue and increased ICP. The procedure involves the placement of one end of a small catheter into a ventricle, with the other end draining into a body cavity or space (i.e., subarachnoid space, cistern, peritoneum, vena cava, pleura). Major complications include infection and malfunction. If the shunt has a valve for the purpose of controlling drainage or preventing reflux of CSF, the surgeon may request that the valve be pumped periodically to ensure proper functioning. Usually, the valve is located behind or above the ear and is the approximate diameter of a fingertip. Pumping involves gentle, serial compressions of the tissue over the shunt. If the valve is working properly, the emptying and refilling of the valve will be felt with palpation.

10. **Surgical interventions:** Surgical treatment is based on the patient's clinical status and neurosurgeon's preference. Surgical timing is a continuing source of controversy. Some surgeons operate on patients with Grade 1 or 2 symptoms within a few days of the initial SAH. By doing so, their intent is to avoid rebleeding, an often fatal complication. Others prefer to wait more than 2 weeks until the peak time for vasospasm (7-10 days post-SAH) has passed. Use of antifibrinolytic and antihypertensive agents reduces the risk of rebleeding during the presurgical period. Patients in Grades 3-5 generally are considered poor surgical risks, especially in the period immediately following SAH. If these patients are unstable clinically, the trend is to treat them medically until they show improvement and stabilize. Surgery is considered for any patient with a large intracranial clot that causes a life-threatening intracranial shift. It is delayed for patients with cerebral vasospasm until the vasospasm subsides.

    Repair of a cerebral aneurysm requires a craniotomy with either clipping or ligation of the neck of the aneurysm, coagulation of the aneurysm, or encasement of the aneursymal sac in surgical gauze or plastic. The method of repair depends on the size, site, and number of perforating arteries, as well as the patient's clinical condition and surgeon preference.

NURSING DIAGNOSES AND INTERVENTIONS

Potential for injury related to risk of increased intracranial pressure (IICP) and herniation secondary to cerebral edema, cerebral hypoxia, hypercarbia, rebleeding, and cerebral vasospasm

Desired outcome: Patient is asymptomatic of IICP and herniation as evidenced by ICP 0-15 mm Hg; orientation to person, place, and time; equal and normoreactive pupils; BP within patient's normal range; HR 60-100 bpm; RR 12-20 breaths/min with normal depth and pattern (eupnea); bilaterally equal motor function, with extremity strength and tone normal for patient; and absence of headache, papilledema, nystagmus, and nausea.

1. Assess qh for the following indicators of IICP and herniation: decreasing LOC, increasing restlessness, confusion, irritability, disorientation, increasing sensorimotor deficits, increasing headache, increasing nuchal rigidity, papilledema, vomiting, seizures, dysphasia, pupil inequality, sluggish or absent pupillary light reflex, abnormal ocular movement (nystagmus, dysconjugate gaze), increasing systolic BP with widening pulse pressure, slow and bounding pulse, and an abnormal respiratory pattern (e.g., Cheyne-Stokes, ataxic, apneustic, central neurogenic hyperventilation).

2. Assess for and treat conditions that can cause increasing restlessness with concomitant IICP: distended bladder, constipation, hypoxemia, headache, fear, anxiety.

3. Implement measures that help prevent IICP and herniation:
   - Maintain complete bedrest.
   - Keep HOB elevated 15-45 degrees or as prescribed to promote cerebral venous outflow.
   - Avoid hyperflexion, hyperextension, or hyperrotation of the neck to decrease the risk of jugular vein compression, which can impede venous outflow, thereby increasing ICP.
   - Instruct patient to avoid activities that use isometric muscle contractions (pulling or pushing siderails and pushing against the footboard). These activities raise systolic BP, which increases ICP.
   - Caution patient about straining with bowel movements as this causes an increase in intrathoracic pressure, which increases ICP.
   - Instruct patient to exhale through the mouth when moving in bed or having a bowel movement.
   - Instruct patient to avoid coughing as it increases intrathoracic pressure and ICP. Teach patient to open mouth when sneezing to minimize the increase in ICP.
   - Maintain a quiet, relaxing environment; decrease external stimuli in the room, such as the lights or noise. Limit visitors if appropriate and encourage them to talk quietly with patient and try to keep conversations as nonstressful for the patient as possible.
   - Complete ADLs (feeding, bathing, dressing, toileting) for patient.
   - Maintain a patent airway and adequate ventilation to prevent cerebral hypoxia, which with hypoxemia and hypercarbia can cause dramatic cerebral vasodilatation, with an increase in cerebral edema and ICP.
   - Monitor ABG values for evidence of hypoxemia (Pao_2 <80 mm Hg) or hypercarbia ($Paco_2$ >45 mm Hg), which can lead to IICP. Administer oxygen *via* nasal cannula, mask, endotracheal tube, or tracheostomy as prescribed.

- Avoid vigorous, prolonged suctioning if patient is intubated, as this can precipitate hypoxemia, hypercarbia, and anxiety, which in turn can increase ICP.
- When suctioning patient, hyperventilate patient as prescribed to increase Pao_2 and decrease $Paco_2$, which will help prevent cerebral vasodilatation.
- Limit fluids intake to 1000-1800 ml/24 hrs as prescribed.
- Monitor and record I&O accurately.

4. Administer antihypertensive medication as prescribed to keep BP at desired levels.
5. Administer stool softeners as prescribed to prevent constipation, which can lead to straining and IICP with herniation.
6. As prescribed, administer antitussives to prevent coughing and antiemetics to prevent or treat vomiting. Both coughing and vomiting can increase intrathoracic pressure and ICP.
7. If ICP monitoring is utilized, assess for IICP (ICP $\geq$15 mm Hg or elevated above patient's baseline) and notify MD promptly (see discussion in "Head Injury," p. 274).
8. If IICP occurs suddenly, hyperinflate patient with a manual resuscitator at a rate of $\geq$50 breaths/min to decrease $Paco_2$.
9. As prescribed for acutely increased ICP, administer bolus of mannitol (i.e., 1.5-2 g/kg, as a 15-25% solution infused over 30-60 minutes). Because of this relatively high dose and rapid infusion rate, monitor renal status before and during administration, and evaluate fluid and electrolyte status (see detailed discussion, pp. 214-237), body weight, and total output before and after the infusion. Notify MD if cerebral spinal fluid pressure is not reduced within 15 minutes of starting the infusion.

Potential fluid volume excess: Cerebral, related to risk of rebleeding from cerebral aneurysm secondary to normal hemolytic response

---

Desired outcomes: Patient is asymptomatic of rebleeding from ruptured cerebral aneurysm as evidenced by orientation to person, place, and time; equal and normoreactive pupils; BP within patient's normal range; HR 60-100 bpm; RR 12-20 breaths/min with normal depth and pattern (eupnea); bilaterally equal motor function, with extremity strength and tone normal for patient; and absence of headache, papilledema, nystagmus, and nausea. ICP is 0-15 mm Hg.

---

1. Assess for signs and symptoms of IICP with herniation, which can signal that rerupture with rebleeding from cerebral aneurysm has occurred. See **Potential for injury** related to risk of increased intracranial pressure (IICP), p. 264.
2. Administer antifibrinolytic agent (i.e., epsilon aminocaproic acid) as prescribed to prevent the normal hemolytic response and stabilize the blood clot around the ruptured aneurysm.
3. Monitor administration of epsilon aminocaproic acid. Utilize an infusion controller or pump to ensure accurate infusion. Initial loading dose of 5 grams is followed with 1-1½ grams/hour, not to exceed 24-36 grams in 24 hours. Mix with D_5W, normal saline, or lactated Ringer's solution.
   - Be aware that rapid administration may induce hypotension, bradycardia, or cardiac dysrhythmias.

- Monitor for and report the following side effects: nausea, cramps, diarrhea, dizziness, tinnitus, headache, skin rash, malaise, nasal stuffiness, postural hypotension.
- Be alert to clotting or thrombosis, which can be precipitated by this medication. Assess for indicators of thrombophlebitis: calf erythema, warmth, tenderness, or increase in size; or positive Homan's sign. Provide antiembolic hose as prescribed.
- Assess for indicators of pulmonary emboli: chest pain, dyspnea, fever, tachycardia, cyanosis, falling BP, restlessness, agitation.
- Monitor and report blood levels of epsilon aminocaproic acid *via* use of chromatography, which is available in some institutions.
- Notify MD promptly of significant findings.

Potential alteration in tissue perfusion: Cerebral, related to risk of cerebral vasospasm secondary to ruptured cerebral aneurysm

---

Desired outcomes: Patient is asymptomatic of cerebral vasospasm as evidenced by orientation to person, place, and time; equal and normoreactive pupils; BP within patient's normal range; HR 60-100 bpm; RR 12-20 breaths/min with normal depth and pattern (eupnea); bilaterally equal motor function, with extremity strength and tone normal for patient; and absence of headache, papilledema, nystagmus, and nausea. ICP is 0-15 mm Hg.

---

1. Assess for indicators of IICP with herniation (see **Potential for injury** related to risk of increased intracranial pressure (IICP), p. 264), which may occur abruptly in a patient who may be awake and alert. Cerebral vasospasm generally affects the major cerebral vessels in the hemisphere or at the site of the ruptured aneurysm and can cause a focal neurologic deficit with or without a major or sudden loss of consciousness.

< N O T E : Vasospasm also may be characterized by a gradual onset of confusion and deteriorating LOC associated with focal motor deficits. A headache that worsens over time and increasing BP may precede the onset of cerebral vasospasm.

2. In the presence of the above indicators, prepare patient for cerebral angiography or CT scan with contrast medium, the only methods for confirming presence of vasospasm and ruling out rebleeding.
3. Administer the prescribed medications (i.e., mannitol, nitroprusside sodium, nifedipine) and intravenous fluids (e.g., colloids or whole blood to increase volume, BP, and subsequently cerebral perfusion) for treating cerebral vasospasm.
4. Continue to treat the IICP (see **Potential for injury** related to risk of increased intracranial pressure, p. 264).

Potential fluid volume excess: Cerebral, related to risk of hydrocephalus secondary to rupture of cerebral aneurysm

---

Desired outcomes: Patient is asymptomatic of hydrocephalus as evidenced by orientation to person, place, and time; equal and normoreactive pupils; BP within patient's normal range; HR 60-100 bpm; RR 12-20 breaths/min with normal depth and pattern (eupnea); bilaterally equal motor function, with extremity strength and tone normal for patient; clear vision; and absence of headache, papilledema, nystagmus, and nausea. ICP is 0-15 mm Hg.

< N O T E : Hydrocephalus occurs when reabsorption of CSF is decreased or prevented due to damage to the arachnoid villi (the pathway to venous circulation) by the presence of blood in the subarachnoid space.

1. Assess for indicators of IICP (see **Potential for injury** related to risk of increased intracranial pressure, p. 264), which may occur more slowly than signs and symptoms that would be seen with rebleeding or vasospasm. In particular, be alert to the following: increased headache, increasing sleepiness, problems with recent memory, confusion, difficulty in being aroused, nausea and vomiting, blurred vision, and diplopia.
2. If hydrocephalus is suspected, prepare patient for CT scan, which will demonstrate increasing size of the ventricles in the presence of hydrocephalus.
3. If hydrocephalus has been diagnosed, prepare patient for insertion of a ventricular shunt to drain excess CSF fluid from the ventricular system. CSF may be shunted to several areas: the cisterna magna *via* a ventriculo-cisternal shunt, the peritoneal cavity *via* a ventriculo-peritoneal shunt (the most common), or less commonly, to the right atrium *via* a ventriculo-atrial shunt.
   - After the shunting, assess patient for indicators of IICP caused either by the disease itself or malfunction of the shunt.
   - Position patient on side opposite the insertion site, either flat or with head elevated slightly (as prescribed) to prevent pressure on shunt mechanism.
   - Assess VS; orientation to time, place, person; LOC; pupillary light reflex; and motor function.
   - Monitor I&O and limit fluids as prescribed.
   - Avoid severe head and neck rotation, flexion, or hyperextension to prevent kinking, compression, or twisting of the shunt catheter, which would impede the flow of CSF.
   - If the shunt has a valve for controlling drainage or preventing reflux of CSF, pump the valve to ensure proper functioning, according to surgeon directive (see description, p. 264).
   - Assess for indicators of meningitis (see p. 289), peritonitis (see p. 388), or septicemia (see p. 433) due to presence of shunt mechanism.

Alteration in bowel elimination: Constipation related to prolonged immobility, decreased fluid intake, inadequate intake of fiber, and restriction against Valsalva maneuver for straining

---

Desired outcome: Patient has bowel movements within his or her normal pattern.

---

1. Obtain data regarding patient's normal bowel elimination pattern, including date of most recent bowel movement.
2. Assess for indicators of constipation, including abdominal distention, cramping,

and complaints of fullness or pressure in the abdomen or rectum. Auscultate for bowel sounds.

3. Advise patient to defecate whenever the need arises but to refrain from straining, as this can increase ICP dramatically, thus increasing the risk of rerupturing and rebleeding from the aneurysm. Instruct patient to exhale slowly when defecating, as this will help prevent a sudden increase in ICP.

4. Assist patient into a semi- or high-Fowler's position to facilitate bowel elimination, unless this position is contraindicated. Use of a bedside commode is recommended over a bedpan, as the physical and emotional stress of getting on a bedpan may increase ICP more than moving with assistance to a commode.

5. Teach patient to select foods high in fiber to facilitate bowel elimination.

6. Unless contraindicated, offer patient a warm drink to stimulate peristalsis. Record amount on I&O record.

7. Administer stool softeners as prescribed.

8. Be aware that stimulation of the rectal sphincter and rectum *via* use of rectal thermometers, suppositories, enemas, or digital evacuation of an impaction are contraindicated in this patient. This type of stimulus may cause patient to perform a Valsalva-type maneuver, which in turn may increase intrathoracic and intracranial pressures, resulting in the potential for rerupture and rebleeding from the aneurysm.

See "Meningitis" for the following: **Alteration in comfort:** Headache, photophobia, and fever, p. 291. See "Status Epilepticus" for the following: **Potential for injury** related to risk of oral and musculoskeletal trauma secondary to seizure activity, p. 314. See "Diabetes Insipidus" for the following: **Fluid volume deficit** related to decreased circulating volume secondary to polyuria, p. 342. See "Syndrome of Inappropriate Antidiuretic Hormone" for the following: **Fluid volume excess** related to retention secondary to increased level of serum ADH with increased water reabsorption from the kidneys, p. 348. As appropriate, see other nursing diagnoses and interventions in the following: "Management of the Adult on Mechanical Ventilation," pp. 66-70; "Providing Nutritional Support," pp. 490-505; "Caring for the Critically Ill on Prolonged Bed Rest," pp. 506-511; "Caring for the Critically Ill with Life-Threatening Disorders," pp. 511-522; and "Caring for the Family of the Critically Ill," pp. 522-526.

REHABILITATION AND PATIENT-FAMILY TEACHING CONCEPTS

Give patient and significant others verbal and written instructions for the following:

1. Referrals to physical, speech, and occupational therapists, depending on presence and degree of patient's deficits.

2. Medications, including drug name, purpose, dosage, schedule, precautions, and potential side effects.

3. Wound care; signs and symptoms of infection.

4. Care of ventricular shunt, if present, including description of signs and symptoms of shunt infection (e.g., fever, localized redness, tenderness, and swelling found directly over the site or along the entire course of the shunt). Depending on the type of shunt inserted, provide patient and family with specific instructions for shunt care and steps to take should the shunt malfunction. In some

cases, these instructions will be provided by the manufacturer of the shunt system.

5. Signs and symptoms of rerupture and rebleeding, which can occur up to 6 months after initial rupture.

6. Guidelines for activity restrictions, which will depend on patient's neurologic deficits. For example, is patient has sensory-perceptual alterations, safety will be a concern. If patient has motor deficit (i.e., hemiparesis or hemiplegia), he or she may require an assistive device such as a wheelchair, cane, or walker.

7. As needed, referral to social service agencies for assistance with financial concerns resulting from the illness.

8. Referral to community nursing or VNA for professional nursing assistance at home.

Head injury

The most common causes of head injury are automobile and motorcycle accidents, followed by falls, violence (e.g., gunshot or stab wounds), and sports-related injuries such as those occurring with boxing and football. The outcome of the injury is determined by the extent of damage at the time of impact and the time interval between injury and initiation of treatment. *Primary injury* occurs with impact and includes contusion, concussion, laceration, and fracture. *Secondary injury* often follows the primary injury and is categorized as (1) intracranial events that include hematomas, intracranial hypertension, and CNS infection; and (2) extracranial events including hypotension, hypoxia, and hypercarbia. Secondary events contribute further to the primary injury and result in poorer recovery and a higher risk of mortality.

Herniation syndrome: Herniation occurs when there is a sudden increase in intracranial pressure (ICP), causing a displacement of the brain from a compartment of high pressure (supratentorial) to one of lower pressure (infratentorial). Deterioration occurs in a rostral-caudal progression. *Cingulate herniation* occurs when the hemisphere expands and shifts laterally, forcing the cingulate gyrus under the falx cerebri, which in turn compresses and displaces the internal cerebral vein. In addition, there may be compression of the ipsilateral anterior cerebral artery and surrounding tissue, resulting in cerebral ischemia and edema. *Central or transtentorial herniation* occurs when the hemispheres, basal nuclei, and diencephalon are displaced through the tentorial notch, thereby compressing the midbrain, and thus affecting the pons and medulla. This type of herniation is seen commonly with lesions in the frontal, parietal, and occipital lobes. *Uncal herniation* occurs when expanding lesions at the temporal fossa shift the tip of the temporal lobe (uncus) toward the midline and protrude over the incisural edge of the tentorium. This then flattens the adjacent midbrain, pushing it against the opposite incisural edge. The expanding lesion compresses the third nerve and posterior cerebral artery on the same side. Astute nursing assessment for early indicators of herniation can be critical in preventing irreversible damage. See Table 4-1, p. 272, for more information on these types of herniation.

ASSESSMENT

Depressed skull fracture: Signs and symptoms are determined by the amount of brain damage or involvement. The injury may result in cerebral edema; decreased LOC, hemiparesis, convulsions, and headache may occur.

Basilar skull fracture: Raccoon's eyes (periorbital ecchymosis), Battle's sign (mastoidal ecchymosis), otorrhea, rhinorrhea, and anosmia (impairment of the sense of smell) all may be present.

Epidural hematoma: Brief loss of consciousness followed by a lucid period; severe vomiting, headache, rapid deterioration with decreased LOC, ipsilateral dilated pupil, contralateral hemiparesis, and seizures may occur.

Subdural hematoma: Altered LOC, headache, personality changes, ipsilateral dilated pupil, contralateral weakness.

Subarachnoid hemorrhage: Restlessness, severe headache, nuchal rigidity, elevated temperature, positive Kernig's sign (loss of ability to extend leg when thigh is flexed on abdomen).

Concussion: Transient loss of consciousness, memory loss, nausea, vomiting, dizziness, headache.

Contusion: Loss of consciousness; speech, sensory, or motor disturbances, depending on site involved; anterograde or retrograde memory loss.

Cingulate herniation: Paralysis or weakness of one or both legs resulting from compression of the anterior cerebral artery.

Central or transtentorial herniation: Change in LOC is one of the earliest signs. Motor responses may begin with a contralateral hemiparesis that worsens to abnormal flexion or extention posturing and eventually to flaccidity. Bilateral Babinski's sign may be present. The respiratory pattern may progress from deep sighs and yawns, to Cheyne-Stokes respirations, to sustained and irregular hyperventilation, to shallow, rapid, and irregular respirations. Initially the pupils are small and reactive to light, with a small range of contraction. Later they become midpositioned, fixed, and irregular. Oculocephalic and oculovestibular responses progress from conjugate to absent. Motor responses may begin with a contralateral hemiparesis that worsens to abnormal posturing, and eventually to flaccidity. Bilateral Babinski's sign may be present.

Uncal herniation: The ipsilateral pupil is moderately dilated, with sluggish constriction that may last for hours before other signs occur. Deterioration may be rapid, leading to a fixed and dilated ipsilateral pupil. Without prompt treatment, the contralateral pupil becomes fixed and dilated. Ipsilateral hemiplegia is followed by bilateral signs and eventually to abnormal posturing. Alterations in LOC may be very subtle (i.e., restlessness, irritability, confusion) at first and progress to a change in the response to painful stimuli, to abnormal posturing, to absence of all responses. The respiratory pattern seen in the late stage is that of regular, sustained hyperventilation.

< N O T E : See Table 4-1 for assessment of central and uncal herniations.

Other signs and symptoms

- *Increased intracranial pressure (IICP):* Headache, vomiting, papilledema, alterations in LOC (i.e., irritability, restlessness, confusion progressing to coma), pupillary changes, motor or sensory changes, and alterations in respiratory pattern (i.e., Cheyne-Stokes).
- *Abnormal flexion (decorticate) posturing:* Abnormal flexion of the arms, wrists, and fingers in response to noxious stimulation. Extension, internal rotation, and plantarflexion are seen in the lower extremities. This type of posturing is seen with hemispheric dysfunction.
- *Abnormal extension (decerebrate) posturing:* Abnormal extension and hyperpronation of the arms and extension and plantarflexion of the lower extremi-

TABLE 4-1
Assessment of central and uncal herniations

	Central herniation			
	Diencephalic (early)	Diencephalic (late)	Midbrain/upper pons	Lower pons/upper medulla
Respiratory pattern	deep sighs, yawning	Cheyne-Stokes	hyperventilation that is sustained and regular	shallow, rapid, irregular
Pupils: size/reaction	small; react to bright light; small range of contraction	small; react to bright light; small range of contraction	midpositioned; irregularly shaped; fixed reaction to light	midpositioned; fixed
Oculocephalic/Oculo-vestibular responses (Dolls' head maneuver/Ice water caloric)	full conjugate or slightly roving eye movements; full conjugate lateral; ipsilateral response to ice water ear irrigation	same as early; nystagmus absent	impaired; may be dysconjugate	no response
Motor responses at rest	contralateral paresis, which may worsen bilateral Babinski's	motionlessness	abnormal extension posturing	flaccidity
to stimulus	bilateral Babinski's	abnormal flexion posturing	rigidity	bilateral Babinski's

Uncal herniation

	Early third nerve	Late third nerve
Respiratory pattern	normal	hyperventilation that is regular and sustained
Pupils: size/reaction	moderate dilation; ipsilateral to primary lesion; sluggish constriction; brisk contralateral pupillary reaction	widely dilated and fixed ipsilateral pupil
Oculocephalic/Oculovestibular responses (Dolls' head maneuver/ice water caloric)	present or dysconjugate, full conjugate, slow ipsilateral eye movement or dysconjugate due to contralateral eye not moving medially	impaired or absent full lateral movement with contralateral eye; absence of medial movement with ipsilateral eye
Motor response to stimulus	contralateral extensor plantar reflex	ipsilateral hemiplegia; abnormal posturing; absence of all responses

SOURCE : Plum F., Posner J., 1980.

ties in response to noxious stimulation. Opisthotonos (severe muscle spasm causing the back to arch, the head to hyperextend, the feet to plantarflex, and the arms and hands to flex at the joints) may be present. This type of posturing is seen with dysfunction of the brain stem.

DIAGNOSTIC TESTS

1. *Complete neurologic examination:* Single most important diagnostic tool.
2. *Spinal x-rays:* Detect spinal injuries, especially cervical.
3. *CT scan:* Identifies type, location, and extent of injury.
4. *Magnetic resonance imaging (MRI):* Identifies type, location, and extent of injury. Although not used in critically ill patients, it may be used in follow-up.
5. *Skull x-ray:* Detects skull fractures, shift of calcified pineal gland, or changes in the sella turcica.
6. *Angiography:* Visualizes cerebral circulation if CT scan is unavailable.
7. *EEG:* Determines presence of brain death or locates area of irritability. Subclinical (electrical) seizure activity may be present in a comatose patient.
8. *Lumbar puncture (LP):* Performed only if meningitis is suspected. Because of the risk of herniation, it is not done if papilledema (early indicator of optic nerve compression due to increased ICP) is present on opthalmoscopic exam.
9. *Evoked response potentials:* Evaluate the integrity of anatomic pathways and their connections and may aid in predicting outcome. The test is an electrical manifestation of the brain's response to an external stimulus—either auditory, visual, or somatosensory.
10. *Serum electrolytes:* Rule out hyponatremia, hypernatremia, or any other imbalance as cause of symptoms.

MEDICAL MANAGEMENT AND SURGICAL INTERVENTIONS

Medical interventions are aimed primarily at controlling intracranial pressure, preventing secondary injuries and medical complications, and removing mass lesions, if present.

1. **Maintaining airway, respirations, and therapeutic oxygen levels**
   - *Mechanical ventilation:* To attain a state of hyperventilation. Because CO_2 is a potent vasodilator, which causes an increase in cerebral blood flow, the goal is vasoconstriction *via* hyperventilation. Vasoconstriction lowers ICP by lowering intravascular blood volume. Pa_{CO_2} is maintained between 25-30 mm Hg.
   - Oxygen: Pa_{O_2} is maintained at ≥ 80 mm Hg to prevent cerebral tissue anoxia, which can cause secondary injuries such as hypoxia or intracranial hypertension.
   - *Positive end expiratory pressure (PEEP):* To increase arterial oxygen levels.

   $<$ N O T E : ICP monitoring is highly recommended with PEEP because PEEP increases intrathoracic pressure, which further increases ICP.

2. **Monitoring intracranial pressure (ICP):** The goal is to maintain cerebral perfusion pressure (CPP) between 60-80 mm Hg. CPP equals mean systemic arterial pressure $\left(\text{MSAP} \dfrac{[\text{systolic} + 2 \text{ diastolic}]}{3} \right)$ minus mean ICP (CPP = MSAP − ICP). CPP <30 mm Hg is incompatible with life.

< N O T E :   See Table 4-2, p. 276, for types of intracranial monitoring.

3. **Maintaining blood pressure within acceptable range:** Both hypertension and hypotension have the potential of increasing cerebral edema. Hypotension results in decreased delivery of oxygen to brain tissue, causing a reduction in pH, which increases $Paco_2$ and leads to cerebral vasodilatation. IV fluids and vasopressors may be given to maintain BP and thus prevent this cycle from occurring. Arterial and hemodynamic monitoring are initiated to evaluate status on an ongoing basis.

4. **Maintaining fluid and electrolyte balance:** Because delivery of D_5W alone could lead to cerebral edema, a combination of D_5W and saline is delivered intravenously at a two-thirds maintenance (approximately 1000-1500 ml/day). The patient is put on strict I&O, weight is measured daily to detect hydration imbalance, and an NG tube is inserted for gastric decompression and prevention of vomiting and aspiration. Supplementation of electrolytes is done in response to lab results.

5. **Nutritional support:** Usually, hyperalimentation and intralipids are delivered until bowel sounds are heard and the GI system returns to normal functioning; then tube feedings are begun until patient can tolerate an oral diet.

6. **Maintaining normothermia:** Hyperthermia increases metabolic demand, which may increase blood flow to a compromised brain and result in cerebral edema. As necessary, antipyretics such as aspirin or acetaminophen are given in an attempt to keep patient's temperature within acceptable range. If antipyretics are ineffective, a cooling blanket is used. In addition, if an infecting organism is present, antibiotics are prescribed to treat it. Tranquilizers such as chlorpromazine may be given to control shivering, which can increase ICP.

7. **Preventing and controlling seizures:** Antiepilepsy drugs may be given prophylactically to prevent seizure activity, which can increase cerebral blood flow (see "Status Epilepticus," p. 313).

8. **Proper head positioning:** Usually, the HOB is elevated 30 degrees to facilitate venous drainage. The head is kept in a neutral position with the neck stabilized with sand bags or pillows. In addition, the neck must be kept free of constricting objects such as tracheostomy ties and oxygen tubing, which could lead to cerebral hypoxia.

9. **Pharmacotherapy**
   - *Hyperosmotics* (e.g., mannitol 20%, 0.5-1.5 g/kg per bolus): To draw water from the cells into the intravascular system, reducing intracellular volume to prevent cerebral edema.
   - *Diuretics and glucocorticoids:* To decrease cerebral edema, which could increase ICP.

< N O T E :   There is much controversy about the effectiveness of glucocorticoids in reducing cerebral edema in head injury.

   - *Pancuronium:* To decrease the skeletal muscle response that is seen with abnormal flexion and extension posturing, thereby reducing the risk of intracranial hypertension. Pancuronium requires intubation and mechanical ventilation.

10. **Barbiturate coma:** To reduce cerebral metabolic rate in the presence of uncontrolled intracranial hypertension. A loading dose of pentobarbital 3-10 mg/

TABLE 4-2
Types of intracranial monitoring

Type	Placement	Advantages/uses	Disadvantages
Intraventricular cannula	lateral ventricle in nondominant hemisphere through burr hole	CSF measurement CSF drainage drug administration compliance testing	rapid CSF drainage can result in collapsed ventricles or subdural hematoma cannula tip may catch on ventricular wall risk of intracerebral bleeding and infection may become plugged with debris possible difficult insertion due to shifting or collapse of ventricle compliance testing may be unreliable
Subarachnoid screw	subarachnoid space through twist drill hole	pressure monitoring less risk of infection than cannula useful with small ventricles does not penetrate brain	no CSF drainage some risk of infection risk of hemorrhage or hematoma during insertion brain may herniate into bolt, making recording unreliable
Epidural sensor	epidural space burr hole fiber optic sensor	lowest risk of infection easy to insert dura not penetrated	no direct measurement of CSF no CSF drainage inability to recalibrate to zero cannot measure compliance

kg is given slowly *via* IV push, with a maintenance dose of 1-3 mg/kg/h to maintain serum barbiturate levels at 3-5 mg %. Because of the depressant effects of barbiturates, patients require intubation and controlled ventilation, an arterial line, and hemodynamic and intracranial monitoring. Patients are in a deep coma and require total nursing care for all of their needs. Vasopressors may be needed to maintain systolic BP at ≥80 mm Hg, which will help maintain CPP at 60-80 mm Hg.

11. **Treatment of complications** as they arise: For example, diabetes insipidus (see p. 340), syndrome of inappropriate antidiuretic hormone (see p. 347), adult respiratory distress sydrome (see p. 18), pulmonary edema (see p. 86), gastrointestinal bleeding (see p. 394), anemia, and disseminated intravascular coagulation (see p. 418) may occur.

12. **Surgical interventions:** Epidural and subdural hematomas are evacuated *via* a burr hole and craniotomy, respectively. Intracerebral hematomas also are evacuated, depending on the site, neurologic findings, and presence of a midline shift indicative of increased ICP and the possibility of herniation. Depressed skull fractures may require elevation, debridement, and repair of dural or venous sinus tears. Penetrating wounds require debridement and surgical repair. Scalp lacerations may necessitate debridement and suturing.

NURSING DIAGNOSES AND INTERVENTIONS

Potential for impaired gas exchange related to risk of cerebral hypoxia secondary to aspiration pneumonia, neurogenic pulmonary edema, chest injury, imposed inactivity, or decreased ventilatory drive occurring with pressure on respiratory center

---

Desired outcomes: Patient has adequate gas exchange as evidenced by orientation to person, place, and time; Pa_{O_2} ≥80 mm Hg; RR 12-20 breaths/min with normal depth and pattern (eupnea); and absence of adventitious breath sounds. Pa_{CO_2} values remain between 25-30 mm Hg.

---

1. Assess patient's respiratory rate, depth, and rhythm. Auscultate lung fields for breath sounds q1-2h and prn. Monitor for respiratory patterns described under assessment data, pp. 270-271.

2. Assess patient for signs of hypoxia, including confusion, agitation, restlessness, and irritability. Remember that cyanosis is a late indicator of hypoxia.

3. Ensure a patent airway *via* proper positioning of neck and frequent assessment of the need for suctioning. Ensure hyperoxygenation of patient before and after each suction attempt to prevent dangerous, suction-induced hypoxia.

4. Monitor ABG values; report significant findings or changes to MD. Be alert to levels indicative of hypoxemia (Pa_{O_2} <80 mm Hg) and to Pa_{CO_2} ≥25-30 mm Hg, as higher levels may increase cerebral blood flow and hence, ICP.

5. Ensure that oxygen is delivered within prescribed limits.

6. Assist with turning q2h, within limits of patient's injury, to promote lung drainage and expansion and alveolar perfusion. Unless contraindicated, raise HOB 30 degrees to enhance gas exchange.

7. Encourage deep breathing at frequent intervals to promote oxygenation. Avoid coughing exercises for patients at risk of increased ICP.

8. Maintain intubation or tracheostomy and perform chest physiotherapy as directed by MD or ICU protocol.

Potential for infection (CNS) related to vulnerability secondary to direct access to the brain in the presence of skull fracture, penetrating wounds, craniotomy, or intracranial monitoring

---

Desired outcome: Patient is free of infection as evidenced by normothermia, WBC count ≤11,000 μl, negative cultures, HR ≤100 bpm, BP within patient's normal range, and absence of agitation, purulent drainage, and other clinical indicators of infection.

---

1. Assess VS at frequent intervals for indicators of CNS infection. Be alert to elevated temperature and increased HR and BP.
2. Monitor patient for signs of systemic infection, including discomfort, malaise, agitation, and restlessness.
3. Inspect cranial wounds for the presence of erythema, tenderness, swelling, and purulent drainage. Obtain prescription for culture as indicated.
4. Avoid nasal or ear packing to collect CSF drainage. Apply a sterile dressing, instead, to collect drainage. Record amount, color, and character of drainage.
5. Caution patient against coughing, sneezing, nose blowing, or other Valsalva-type maneuvers, as these activities can damage the dura further. Avoid nasal suctioning and use of nasogastric tubes. Use orogastric tubes, instead.
6. Ensure timely administration of prescribed antibiotics.
7. Apply basic principles for care of invasive device used with ICP monitoring:
   • Use good handwashing technique before caring for patient.
   • If patient is not comatose, encourage him or her not to touch device; apply restraints if necessary.
   • Maintain aseptic technique during care of device, following protocol established by agency or MD.

Alteration in tissue perfusion: Cerebral, related to impaired blood flow secondary to hypotension, intracranial hypertension, or infections that can occur with secondary head injury

---

Desired outcomes: Patient has adequate cerebral perfusion as evidenced by equal and normoreactive pupils; orientation to person, place, and time; adequate and bilaterally equal strength and tone in the upper and lower extremities; RR 12-20 breaths/min with normal depth and pattern (eupnea); HR 60-100 bpm; ICP 0-15 mm Hg; cerebral perfusion pressure 60-80 mm Hg; and absence of headache, vomiting, and other clinical indicators of increased ICP.

---

1. Assess neurologic status at least hourly. Monitor pupils, LOC, and motor activity; and perform cranial nerve assessments. A decrease in LOC is an early indicator of increased ICP and impending herniation. Changes in the size and reaction of the pupils, a decrease in motor function (i.e., hemiplegia, abnormal flexion posturing), and cranial nerve palsies all are indicative of impending herniation.

2. Monitor VS at frequent intervals. Be alert to changes in respiratory pattern (e.g., Cheyne-Stokes), fluctuations in BP and pulse, widening pulse pressure, and slow HR.

3. Monitor patient for indicators of increased ICP, including headache, vomiting, papilledema, decreasing LOC, alterations in vision (e.g., diplopia), sensorimotor dysfunction, pupillary changes, seizures.

4. Monitor hemodynamic status to evaluate cerebral perfusion pressure and ensure that it is 60-80 mm Hg. Be alert to decrease in mean systolic arterial blood pressure (<80 mm Hg) or increase in mean arterial pressure. Perform ongoing assessment of ICP, recording pressure at least hourly. Notify MD if pressure changes significantly (e.g., >15 mm Hg, depending on patient status or MD preference). Perform ongoing calibration and zeroing of transducer to ensure accuracy of readings.

5. Maintain a patent airway and ensure precise delivery of oxygen to promote optimal cerebral perfusion.

6. Facilitate cerebral venous drainage by maintaining HOB at a 30 degree elevation.

7. To help prevent fluid volume excess, which could add to cerebral edema, ensure precise delivery of IV fluids at consistent rates. Usual protocol is two-thirds maintenance, or 1000-1500 ml/day.

8. Ensure timely administration of medications that are prescribed for the prevention of sudden increase or decrease in BP, HR, RR.

9. Treat elevations in ICP immediately:
   - Make sure HOB is elevated 30 degrees.
   - Loosen constrictive objects around neck that may be impeding blood flow.
   - If patient has recently been repositioned, return patient to original position as he or she might not be tolerating new position.
   - Ensure that head is maintained in a neutral position *via* use of sand bags.
   - Assess for factors that may be contributing to patient's increased ICP: distended bladder or abdomen, fear, anxiety.
   - Evaluate activities (e.g., suctioning, bathing, dressing changes) that can increase pressure; reorganize care plan accordingly.
   - Hyperoxygenate patient before and after suctioning, according to ICU protocol.

Ineffective thermoregulation related to fluctuations secondary to injury to or pressure on hypothalamus

---

Desired outcome: Patient remains normothermic.

---

1. Monitor for signs of hyperthermia: temperature >38.33° C (101° F), pallor, absence of perspiration, torso that is warm to the touch.

2. As prescribed, obtain blood, urine, and sputum cultures for ruling out underlying infection.

3. Be alert to signs of meningitis: fever, chills, nuchal rigidity, Kernig's sign, Brudzinski's sign. For more information, see "Meningitis," p. 287.

4. Assess wounds for evidence of infection, including erythema, tenderness, purulent drainage.

5. If patient is hyperthermic, remove excess clothing and administer tepid baths, hypothermic blanket, or ice bags to axilla or groin.
6. As prescribed, administer antipyretics such as aspirin or acetaminophen.
7. As prescribed, administer chlorpromazine to treat or prevent shivering, which can cause further increases in ICP.

Potential impairment of physical mobility related to prolonged inactivity secondary to head injury, spasticity, or decreased LOC

Desired outcome: Upon recovery, patient has full range of motion without verbal or nonverbal indicators of pain.

---

1. Begin performing passive ROM exercises q4h on all extremities immediately upon patient's admission. Monitor ICP during exercise, being alert to dangerous elevations.
2. Teach passive ROM exercises to significant others. Encourage their participation in patient exercise as often as they are able.
3. Reposition patient q2h within restrictions of the head injury, using logrolling technique as indicated.
4. Ensure proper anatomic position and alignment. Support alignment with pillows, trochanter rolls, wrapped sand bags.
5. For patient who has spasticity, use foot cradles to keep linen off the feet. To maintain dorsiflexion, provide patient with shoes that are cut off at the toes, with the shoes ending just proximal to the head of the patient's metatarsals. Because there is no contact of the balls of the feet with a hard surface, the risk of spasticity will be minimized.
6. For patients without spasticity, use foot supports to prevent plantarflexion and external hip rotation.
7. To maintain anatomic position of the hands, provide spastic patient with a splint or cone that is secured with an elastic band. Either device will limit spasticity by pressing on the muscles, while the elastic band will stimulate the extensor muscles, thereby promoting finger extension. Flaccid patients, however, can be helped to maintain functional grasp *via* placement of a rolled washcloth within patient's grasp.
8. Consult with physical therapy regarding use of splints or other supportive devices.

Potential alteration in tissue integrity: Corneal, related to inability to blink secondary to altered LOC or cranial nerve damage

---

Desired outcome: Patient's corneas remain intact.

---

1. Assess for indicators of corneal irritation: red and itching eyes, ocular pain, sensation of a foreign object in eye, scleral edema, and blurred vision.
2. Avoid exposing patient's eyes to irritants such as baby powder or talc.

3. Lubricate patient's eyes q2h with isotonic solution, either eye drops or ointment.

4. If corneal irritation or edema is present, apply eye patches or warm, sterile compresses over closed eyes. Because the patient may open his or her eyes with the patches in place, do not tape the patches as the patch material may cause further irritation. Caution patient against rubbing eyes; restrain patient's hands if he or she is incoherent.

5. Facilitate an ophthalmic consultation as indicated.

See "Cerebral Aneurysm and Subarachnoid Hemorrhage" for the following: **Potential for injury** related to risk of increased intracranial pressure, p. 264. As appropriate, see nursing diagnoses and interventions in "Care of the Patient following Intracranial Surgery," p. 286; and in "Meningitis," p. 290. See "Status Epilepticus" for the following: **Potential for injury** related to risk of oral and musculoskeletal trauma secondary to seizure activity, p. 314. Also see nursing diagnoses and interventions in the following: "Management of the Adult on Mechanical Ventilation," pp. 66-70, and "Management of the Adult with Hemodynamic Monitoring," pp. 168-170. The head injury patient is at risk for diabetes insipidus and syndrome of inappropriate antidiuretic hormone. See "Diabetes Insipidus" for the following: **Fluid volume deficit** related to decreased circulating volume secondary to polyuria, p. 342. See "Syndrome of Inappropriate Antidiuretic Hormone" for the following: **Fluid volume excess** related to retention secondary to increased level of serum ADH with increased water reabsorption from the kidneys, p. 348. Also see the following as appropriate: "Providing Nutritional Support," pp. 490-505; "Caring for the Critically Ill on Prolonged Bed Rest," pp. 506-511; "Caring for the Critically Ill with Life-Threatening Disorders," pp. 511-522; and "Caring for the Family of the Critically Ill," pp. 522-526.

REHABILITATION AND PATIENT-FAMILY TEACHING CONCEPTS

Rehabilitation needs differ from one individual to the next, depending on the degree of neurologic deficit. Give patient and significant others verbal and written instructions for the following, as appropriate:

1. Referrals to community resources: VNA, community support groups, psychotherapy, vocational rehabilitation agencies, physical therapy, speech therapy, occupational therapy, cognitive retraining specialists, and rehabilitation or head injury rehabilitation centers.

2. First aid measures for seizures (see "Status Epilepticus," p. 312).

3. Importance of follow-up care with MD and support services.

4. Medications, including drug name, purpose, dosage, schedule, precautions, and potential side effects.

5. If patient had a concussion or contusion, a description of problems that may occur at home that necessitate prompt medical attention: confusion, sleepiness, motor deficits, alteration in LOC, visual problems. Provide emergency phone numbers.

6. Address of National Head Injury Foundation: 18A Vernon Street, Framingham, MA 01701.

Care of the patient following intracranial surgery

Cranial surgery is performed for the following reasons: removal of a space-occupying lesion such as a tumor, hematoma, or abscess; repair of a vascular abnormality such as aneurysm or arteriovenous malformation (AVM); drainage of cerebrospinal fluid (CSF) from the ventricular system; correction of depressed skull fracture; biopsy of tissue to confirm a diagnosis and facilitate treatment; control of seizures; and reduction of pain.

The surgical approach selected by the neurosurgeon depends primarily on the location of the pathology. The *supratentorial* approach most often is used to remove or correct problems in the frontal, temporal, or occipital lobes as well as the diencephalic area (pituitary, hypothalamus). Lesions of the cerebellum and brain stem usually are removed via the *infratentorial* approach. The *transphenoidal* approach gains access to the pituitary gland to remove a tumor, control bone pain associated with metastatic cancer, or attempt to arrest the progression of diabetic retinopathy in the patient with diabetes mellitus. Following intracranial surgery, the major goals of treatment are to maintain cerebral function through control of ICP; recognize, prevent, or treat complications; provide supportive care until the patient can resume ADLs; and prepare and plan for rehabilitation.

COMPLICATIONS FOLLOWING INTRACRANIAL SURGERY

1. **Increased intracranial pressure (IICP) with herniation:** Caused by cerebral edema, hemorrhage, infection, surgical trauma. Some cerebral edema is expected following intracranial surgery and usually peaks about 72 hours postoperatively. For more information on herniation, see ''Head Injury,'' p. 270.

2. **Intracranial bleeding:** May be intracerebral, intracerebellar, subarachnoid, subdural, extradural, or intraventricular. Bleeding may be caused by the lengthy and extensive surgical procedure, prolonged anesthesia, preexisting medical problems, or medications.

3. **Hydrocephalus:** May appear preoperatively or occur postoperatively as an acute or chronic complication. Usually it is caused by a slowing or complete stoppage of the flow of CSF through the ventricular system secondary to edema, bleeding, scarring, or obstruction.

4. **Cerebrovascular accident (CVA):** Can occur intraoperatively or postoperatively as the result of fluctuations in blood pressure that lead to cerebral ischemia and infarction. CVA secondary to cerebral arterial vasospasm may be seen following subarachnoid hemorrhage. Air embolism is a possible cause of CVA for the patient undergoing infratentorial surgery in the sitting position.

5. **Seizures:** Generalized or partial seizures can occur as a result of surgical trauma, irritation of cerebral tissue by the presence of blood, cerebral edema, cerebral hypoxia, hypoglycemia, preexisting seizure disorder, or inadequate anticonvulsant levels.

6. **CNS infection:** Meningitis, encephalitis, ventriculitis, or wound infection can occur as a result of blood remaining in the subarachnoid space (aseptic meningitis) or contamination before, during, or after surgery. A gunshot wound to the brain may introduce organisms at the time of injury. Following surgery, the presence of moist, bloody head dressings (a positive culture medium) or break in sterile technique during a dressing change may lead to CNS infection. (See ''Meningitis,'' p. 287.)

7. **Diabetes insipidus (DI) and syndrome of inappropriate antidiuretic hormone (SIADH):** The result of a disturbance in the hypothalamus or posterior lobe of the pituitary gland. Antidiuretic hormone (ADH) is produced within the supraoptic nuclei of the hypothalamus and stored in the posterior pituitary. This disturbance may result from edema, manipulation, or partial or total removal of the gland. DI is the result of a decrease or loss of production of ADH, which leads to excessive urinary output with a potential for serious fluid and electrolyte problems (see "Diabetes Insipidus," p. 340). SIADH, a less common problem, is the result of an increase in the release of ADH leading to reabsorption of large amounts of water *via* the renal tubules with concurrent loss of large amounts of sodium. Like DI, SIADH also can cause serious fluid and electrolyte problems (see "Syndrome of Inappropriate Antidiuretic Hormone," p. 347).

8. **Cardiac dysrhythmias:** May occur as a result of cerebral hypoxia or ischemia, manipulation of the brain stem, or the irritating effects of blood in the CSF (see "Dysrhythmias and Conduction Disturbances," p. 95).

9. **Hyperthermia:** May be caused by injury or irritation of the hypothalamic temperature regulating centers or presence of blood in the CSF, or it may be an indicator of wound infection, atelectasis, pneumonia, or urinary tract infection. Regardless of the cause, an elevated temperature is detrimental because it increases metabolic needs of the brain, potentially leading to increased blood flow to the area with concomitant cerebral edema.

10. **CSF leak:** Caused by a channel between the subarachnoid space (SAS) and the outside as a result of a tear or rupture of the dura mater. A CSF leak may be present preoperatively following a skull fracture or may occur during surgery. CSF leakage from the ear is called otorrhea; from the nose it is called rhinorrhea. The leakage of CSF is indicative of an open pathway to the SAS, which carries a serious risk of infection.

11. **Loss of the corneal reflex:** May be caused by surgical trauma to motor pathways from the frontal lobe or trauma or edema of the brain stem cranial nerve nuclei. It can result in corneal abrasion, ulceration, and blindness if it is not recognized and treated promptly.

12. **Periocular edema:** Can occur following supratentorial surgery with manipulaton of the scalp or frontal bones of the cranium or retraction of the frontal lobes.

POSTOPERATIVE NEUROLOGIC DEFICITS

Some neurologic deficit(s) may be present preoperatively and should be noted and documented. Deficits that occur after surgery may be due to surgical trauma or the presence of cerebral edema, which will interfere with normal brain function. With time, these deficits may improve. The following are some of the neurologic deficits that may be present in the patient following intracranial surgery.

1. *Diminished level of consciousness (LOC):* The degree of improvement in LOC will depend on the amount of preoperative damage to cerebral tissue. Generally, LOC improves as anesthesia wears off, cerebral edema subsides, and ICP decreases.

2. *Communicative and cognitive deficits:* The ability to communicate and understand postoperatively will depend on the degree of preoperative dysfunction,

site of the lesion, extensiveness of the surgical procedure, and degree of post-operative cerebral edema.

- *Broca's (expressive, motor, non-fluent) dysphasia:* Describes an individual who can comprehend the situation and follow commands appropriately but cannot articulate wishes and needs.
- *Wernicke's (receptive, sensory, fluent) dysphasia:* Describes an individual who does not understand the situation and cannot follow commands appropriately.

3. *Motor and sensory deficits:* Motor deficits (weakness or paralysis) are caused by injury or edema to the primary motor cortex and cortico-spinal (pyramidal) tracts. Generally, improvement will be seen as cerebral edema subsides. Early physical therapy is necessary in order to prevent long-term disabilities, such as foot or wrist drop, contractures, and hip rotation. Sensory deficits are caused by injury or edema to the primary sensory cortex or the sensory-associated areas of the parietal lobe. In addition, damage to the spinothalamic tracts will cause sensory deficits. Examples of sensory deficits include the inability to distinguish objects according to size, shape, weight, texture, and consistency and the inability to distinguish changes in temperature, touch, pressure, and position. As with motor deficits, improvement in sensory perception will occur as cerebral edema subsides.

4. *Cranial nerve impairment:* The degree and presence of cranial nerve deficit will depend on the site of the lesion, preoperative deficit, degree of postoperative cerebral edema, and the surgical approach. Infratentorial surgery for lesions in the posterior fossa (brain stem and cerebellum) may involve significant cranial nerve manipulation and trauma with considerable postoperative cranial nerve deficit. Deficit(s) may improve with decreasing cerebral edema or may be permanent. Assessment of cranial nerve dysfunction is an important nursing function.

- *Cranial nerve II:* Controls the visual system. Damage may result in decreased or absent visual acuity or a loss of vision in a particular field such as homonymous hemianopia (same-sided visual field cut) or bitemporal hemianopia (loss of outer visual fields in each eye), which can occur with a lesion involving the pituitary gland with involvement of the optic chiasm.
- *Cranial nerves III, IV, and VI:* Control ocular muscles. Weakness or paralysis with diplopia may be the result of damage to these cranial nerves. Ptosis may occur with damage to cranial nerve III.
- *Cranial nerves V and VII:* Control facial muscles and facial sensation and are responsible for the corneal reflex. Diminished or absent corneal reflex may result in corneal abrasion, ulceration, or blindness.
- *Cranial nerves VII, IX, X, and XII:* Control the muscles and sensations (e.g., gag reflex) involved in eating, swallowing, and phonation.

5. *Respiratory complications:* Respiratory complications in the patient following intracranial surgery can be particularly serious because any increase in $Paco_2$ resulting in hypercarbia will lead to cerebral vasodilatation with a subsequent increase in intracranial volume, and thus IICP. Respiratory complications include the following:

- Partial or complete airway obstruction due to accumulation of secretions and improper positioning.
- Neurogenic pulmonary edema due to a sudden increase in ICP.

- Cerebral edema causing compression of brain stem respiratory centers.
- Atelectasis and pneumonia.
- Pulmonary embolus.

6. *Gastrointestinal bleeding (Cushing's ulcer) and paralytic ileus:* The develop-ment of GI bleeding is associated with cerebral trauma and the postoperative neurosurgical patient. Although the etiology is unclear, it is believed that stress from the trauma or surgery can lead to continued vagal stimulation, which in turn leads to a hyperacidic state that causes gastric erosion, ulceration, and ultimately hemorrhage. Gastric erosion, ulceration, and hemorrhage also can be precipitated by medications, especially the corticosteroids. Paralytic ileus is common following abdominal surgery but also may occur after neurologic sur-gery. Decreased or absent peristalsis may be the result of prolonged anesthesia, immobility, trauma, electrolyte deficiencies, and mechanical obstruction.

7. *Thrombophlebitis, deep vein thrombosis (DVT), and pulmonary embolus:* All of these complications are related to or the result of prolonged bed rest and im-mobility following intracranial surgery. Other factors, such as pre-existing co-agulopathies and blood dyscrasias, may influence the development of these complications postoperatively.

MEDICAL MANAGEMENT FOLLOWING INTRACRANIAL SURGERY

1. **Respiratory support:** Oxygen supplements, intubation, and mechanical venti-lation are provided as indicated.
2. **Activity restrictions:** Will depend on patient's LOC and general condition.
3. **Positioning:** For most patients, HOB is elevated 30 degrees to promote venous drainage, thereby reducing ICP.
   - In posterior fossa surgery (infratentorial approach), the supporting muscles of the neck are altered. This necessitates turning the patient with the neck in alignment with the head and support of the head, neck, and shoulders in the process.
   - Following craniectomy, during which a bone flap is removed, the patient should not be positioned on the side on which bone has been removed. Label patient's head dressing, chart, and bed with this information.
   - After procedures in which a large intracranial space has been left due to ex-tensive surgery, patient should not be positioned on operative side immedi-ately postoperatively as this may cause a sudden shift in intracranial contents, with subsequent hemorrhage or herniation.
4. **Pharmacotherapy:** The following may be prescribed postoperatively:
   - *Corticosteroids (e.g., dexamethasone):* To decrease cerebral edema.

< N O T E :   Use is controversial as there is disagreement as to their effective-ness.

   - *Osmotic diuretics (e.g., mannitol, urea):* To control cerebral edema causing IICP.
   - *Anticonvulsants (e.g., phenytoin, phenobarbital):* To prevent seizures in the immediate postoperative period caused by cerebral edema and irritation due to surgical manipulation of the brain. Anticonvulsants may be continued pro-phylactically for a period of one or two years following surgery.
   - *Antibiotics:* To prevent or treat postoperative infection.
   - *Antipyretics:* For prompt treatment of elevated temperature, which if left un-

treated can increase metabolic activity, causing increased use of oxygen and glucose supplies.

- *Analgesics:* To treat or control pain due to headache. Drugs of choice are acetaminophen alone or with codeine sulfate.
- *Antacids (e.g., Maalox):* To prevent the formation of gastric ulceration occurring from steroid use or as a result of the stress of surgery.
- *Histamine H_2 receptor antagonists (e.g., cimetidine):* To suppress gastric secretions to prevent or facilitate healing of Cushing's ulcer.

5. **Fluid and electrolyte management:** To prevent or treat increasing cerebral edema. Usually, fluids are limited to 1500-1800 ml/day, depending on patient's body size and overall condition.

6. **Nutritional support:** The method and type of nutritional support are determined by the patient's condition and may include any of the following: oral feedings, enteral feedings, supplements, or parenteral nutrition (i.e., TPN, fat emulsion therapy).

7. **Physical medicine consults:** To evaluate patient for physical, occupational, and speech therapy and begin planning for rehabilitation.

NURSING DIAGNOSES AND INTERVENTIONS

Potential for injury related to risk of development of gastric (Cushing's ulcer) secondary to hyperacidic state

---

Desired outcomes: Patient's gastric pH tests >5 and patient is asymptomatic of Cushing's ulcer and GI bleeding as evidenced by gastric secretions and stool negative for blood, HR ≤ 100 bpm, BP within patient's normal range, and absence of midepigastric discomfort. Hematocrit tests 37%-47% (female) or 40%-54% (male) and hemoglobin tests 14-18 g/dl (male) or 12-16 g/dl (women).

---

1. Monitor for indicators of GI bleeding or ulceration: midepigastric discomfort, occult or frank blood in stool or gastric secretions, decreasing BP, increasing HR. If these indicators are present, notify MD, who probably will prescribe the insertion of an NG tube.
2. Monitor hematocrit or hemoglobin results daily; report decreasing values.
3. Test NG drainage pH q4h. Administer H_2 receptor antagonists or antacids as prescribed to maintain pH >5.
4. Implement measures to prevent ulceration and hemorrhage:
   - As prescribed, administer antacids to prevent gastric ulceration and histamine H_2 receptor antagonists to suppress gastric secretions and promote healing.
   - Administer steroids, aspirin, phenytoin, and other medications that irritate gastric mucosa with a meal or snack.
   - Limit patient's intake of acidic or spicy foods as well as caffeine-containing substances such as coffee, cola, and chocolate.

See "Cerebral Aneurysm and Subarachnoid Hemorrhage" for the following: **Potential for injury** related to risk of IICP secondary to cerebral edema, p. 264; **Potential alteration in tissue perfusion:** Cerebral, related to risk of cerebral vasospasm, p. 267; **Potential fluid volume excess:** Cerebral, related to risk of hydrocephalus, p. 267; and **Alteration in bowel elimination:** Constipation, related to prolonged immobility, decreased fluid intake, inadequate intake of fiber, and restriction against Valsalva maneuver for straining, p. 268. See "Head Injury" for the following: **Potential for infection (CNS)** related to vulnerability secondary to direct access to the brain in the presence of skull fracture, penetrating wounds, craniotomy, or intracranial monitoring, p. 278; **Ineffective thermoregulation** related to fluctuations secondary to injury to or pressure on the hypothalamus, p. 279; **Potential impairment of physical mobility** related to prolonged inactivity secondary to head injury, spasticity, or decreased LOC, p. 280; **Potential alteration in tissue integrity:** Corneal, related to inability to blink secondary to altered LOC or cranial nerve damage, p. 280. See "Meningitis" for the following: **Alteration in comfort:** Headache, photophobia, and fever, p. 291. See "Status Epilepticus" for the following: **Potential for injury** related to risk of oral and musculoskeletal trauma secondary to seizure activity, p. 314. See "Diabetes Insipidus" for the following: **Fluid volume deficit** related to decreased circulating volume secondary to polyuria, p. 342. See "Syndrome of Inappropriate Antidiuretic Hormone" for the following: **Fluid volume excess** related to retention secondary to increased level of serum ADH with increased water reabsorption from the kidneys, p. 348. In addition, see the appendix for the following: "Providing Nutritional Support," pp. 490-505; "Caring for the Critically Ill on Prolonged Bed Rest," pp. 506-511; "Caring for the Critically Ill with Life-Threatening Disorders," pp. 511-522; and "Caring for the Family of the Critically Ill," pp. 522-526.

REHABILITATION AND PATIENT-FAMILY TEACHING CONCEPTS:

Give patient and significant others verbal and written instructions for the following:
1. Referrals to physical, speech, and occupational therapists, depending on presence and degree of deficit. Patient's condition may necessitate transfer to a rehabilitation center.
2. Medications, including drug name, purpose, dosage, schedule, precautions, and potential side effects.
3. Wound care; signs and symptoms of infection.
4. Referral to social services, as needed, for assistance with financial concerns resulting from the illness.
5. Referral to community nursing or Visiting Nurse Association for professional nursing services at home.

Meningitis

Meningitis is inflammation of the brain and spinal cord, which can involve all three meningeal membranes (dura mater, arachnoid, and pia mater). There are several types of meningitis, including bacterial, fungal, parasitic, and spirochetal.

Bacterial meningitis: The most common form, it can occur as a complication of a bacteremia (e.g., endocarditis, pneumonia), otitis media, sinusitis, penetrating head wound, skull fracture, brain abscess, or neurosurgery. *Hemophilus influenzae* is the leading cause of bacterial meningitis. Meningococcal meningitis, caused by *Neiserria meningitidis,* is the next leading cause, followed by pneumococcal meningitis, which is caused by *Streptococcus pneumoniae.* Prompt recognition and treatment of the offending organism yields the best prognosis. Overall mortality rate is 10-40%.

Tuberculous meningitis: *Mycobacterium tuberculosis* causes the majority of cases. Although this type of meningitis occurs most often in the first 5 years of life, it can occur with pulmonary tuberculosis in the adult population. Because interventions exist for detection, prophylaxis, and treatment, it can be prevented. The infection reaches the CNS *via* the bloodstream and can be fatal in 1-8 weeks if untreated. With prompt diagnosis and treatment, mortality rate is 10-20%. Patients in a comatose state when treatment is initiated have a mortality rate between 50-70%. Residual physical and mental deficits (e.g., visual and auditory impairment, motor deficit) occur in 10-30% of cases.

Viral meningitis: A complication of a systemic viral infection. Enteroviruses are the cause of 50-80% of viral meningitis. Mumps is the second most common cause, followed by herpes simplex virus, which usually is seen in young, sexually active adults. The other viruses are lymphocytic choriomeningitis virus, varicella, and arbovirus. Prognosis is good.

Fungal meningitis: Less common than bacterial meningitis. The most common fungal infections of the CNS are caused by *Cryptococcus neoformans* (a complication of AIDS), *Coccidiodes immitis, Blastomyces dermatitidis,* and *Histoplasma capsulatum.* Fungal meningitis develops slowly, with signs and symptoms similar to those of tuberculous meningitis.

Spirochetal: Lyme disease is caused by a tick-borne spirochete and is believed to consist of 3 stages (see assessment data below). The disease peaks in late summer and early fall. Highly endemic areas are southeastern Connecticut, Long Island, Cape Cod, New York's Westchester County, and central New Jersey.

ASSESSMENT

Bacterial meningitis: Fever, stiff neck and back, headache, lethargy, vomiting, Kernig's sign, and Brudzinski's sign (see p. 261).

- *Hemophilus influenzae:* Often a complication of otitis media, sinusitis, or a respiratory infection. Clinical signs that distinguish it from meningococcal or pneumococcal meningitis are the early development of deafness within 24-36 hours of onset. In addition, morbilliform and petechial rashes may be present. Common complications include sterile subdural effusions and thrombosis of cerebral veins. Prognosis is poor if appropriate therapy is not initiated promptly or if the patient continues to seize and remain in coma for any length of time.

- *Meningococcal meningitis:* Often a complication of bacteremia, metastatic infection, or immunologic reactions. Fever, skin and conjunctival petechiae, morbilliform rash that resembles a viral exanthem, and aggressive behavior are typical clinical findings. Although complications are rare, they can include dysfunction of cranial nerves VI, VII, and VIII; as well as aphasia, ventriculitis, subdural empyema, cerebral venous thrombosis, and disseminated intravascular coagulation (DIC). Acute fulminant meningococcemia carries a poor prognosis because of the complication of DIC.

- *Pneumococcal meninigitis:* Risk is higher in individuals who have sickle cell disease, have undergone a splenectomy, or are immunocompromised. Clinical manifestations include fever and headache; coma and seizures may be present initially or shortly after onset. Although neurologic complications are uncommon, subdural empyema, ventriculitis, cerebral vein thrombosis, hemiplegia, hydrocephalus, severe leukopenia or thrombocytopenia, and memory problems can occur.

Tuberculous meningitis: Low-grade fever, general malaise, mild headache that progresses in intensity over a 1-2 week period. Nuchal rigidity develops slowly and can become severe; marked opisthotonus is possible. Other signs include Kernig's sign; Brudzinski's sign; cranial nerve palsy involving the VI, VIII, and IV nerves that initially is unilateral but becomes bilateral; change in LOC that can progress to coma; and seizures (focal more common in adults). In addition, signs of increased ICP may be present. Complications include hydrocephalus, cerebral arteritis that can result in hemiplegia, and spread of infection to other body systems.

Viral meningitis: Clinical signs vary according to the age group involved; often, patients are asymptomatic. This nonspecific clinical syndrome is characterized by a headache that is more severe than usual, fever, nuchal rigidity, drowsiness, malaise, occasional nausea, vomiting, and photophobia. Usually, Kernig's and Brudzinski's signs are absent.

Fungal meningitis: Fever, headache, nausea, personality changes, and dysfunction of cranial nerves III and VI.

Spirochetal (Lyme disease)
- *Stage one:* Headache, stiff neck, lethargy, irritability, changes in mental status, and characteristic skin rash (erythema chronicum migrans).
- *Stage two:* Headache, nausea, vomiting, malaise, and irritability (occurring one month after onset of the infection).
- *Stage three:* Arthritis.

DIAGNOSTIC TESTS

1. *Lumbar puncture (LP):* Analyzes cerebrospinal fluid (CSF). An LP should not be performed if focal signs are seen on examination or papilledema is present on fundoscopic exam as these signs may signal an expanding lesion or increased ICP. See Table 4-3 for typical findings.
2. *Counterimmunoelectrophoresis (CIE):* Detects bacterial antigens in the CSF.
3. *Latex agglutination:* Detects microbial antigens in the CSF.
4. *Blood, urine, and sputum cultures:* Help identify the infecting organisms.
5. *CBC:* Assesses for presence of infection.
6. *CT scan with contrast:* To rule out hydrocephalus and detect exudate in the nonventricular CSF spaces.

TABLE 4-3
CSF findings typical of meningitis

	White cell count	Glucose	Protein
Normal	0-5 mm^3 lymphs	40-80 mg/dl	15-50 mg/dl
Bacterial	Predominantly polys	<40 mg/dl	>100 mg/dl
Viral	Predominantly lymphs (may see polys initially)	Normal	Slightly elevated
Tuberculous	Predominantly lymphs	<40 mg/dl or 50% of blood sugar drawn simultaneously	100-500 mg/dl; may increase gradually with progression of the disease
Fungal	Predominantly lymphs	Slightly decreased	Elevated

MEDICAL MANAGEMENT

The goal is prompt diagnosis and treatment to prevent complications and death (mortality rate is high).

1. **Bacterial meningitis**
   - *Hemophilus influenzae:* Chloramphenicol 25 mg/kg IV q6h, or ampicillin 50 mg/kg IV q4h × 10 days.
   - *Neisseria meningitidis:* Penicillin G 50,000 units/kg IV q4h for 10 days.
   - *Streptococcus pneumoniae:* See *Neisseria meningitidis.*
2. **Viral meningitis:** No pharmacologic treatment.
3. **Fungal meninigitis:** Amphotericin B; dosage depends on the offending organism.
4. **Tuberculous meningitis:** Isoniazid 8-10 mg/kg/day (usually 300-600 mg); rifampin 600 mg/day. *For severely ill patients:* ethambutol 25 mg/kg/day × 1-2 months or streptomycin 1 g/day IM × 6-8 weeks and then biweekly. Pyridoxine 50 mg/day is given to prevent peripheral neuropathy.
5. **Lyme disease:** Penicillin G ≥20 million units/day IV in divided doses × 10 days. If the patient is allergic to penicillin, tetracycline 500 mg PO qid × 30 days is given.
6. **Nutritional support:** Usually, total parenteral nutrition (TPN) with intralipids is given until bowel sounds are heard and the GI system returns to normal functioning. Then, tube feedings are begun until the patient can tolerate an oral diet.
7. **Seizure control:** Antiepilepsy drugs are given to control seizure activity.
8. **Maintenance of normothermia:** Hyperthermia increases metabolic demand, which increases cerebral blood flow, which in turn can increase ICP. As necessary, antipyretics such as ASA and acetaminophen are given in an attempt to keep patient's temperature within established limits.
9. **Isolation:** According to hospital and CDC guidelines.
   - Bacterial (etiology unknown), *Hemophilus influenzae, Neisseria meningitidis* (known or suspected): Respiratory isolation for 24 hours after start of effective therapy. After 24 hours of therapy, the patient no longer is considered infectious by the airborne route because of the sensitivity of the organisms to antibiotics, thereby rapidly diminishing infectivity of the patient.

NURSING DIAGNOSES AND INTERVENTIONS

Potential for injury related to risk of increased ICP secondary to herniation or cerebral edema

---

Desired outcomes: Patient verbalizes knowledge of the importance of avoiding Valsalva-like activities. Patient's ICP remains within normal range as evidenced by orientation to person, place, and time; bilaterally equal and normoreactive pupils; bilaterally equal strength and tone of extremities; absence of cranial nerve palsies; RR 12-20 breaths/min with normal depth and pattern (eupnea); HR 60-100 bpm; BP within patient's normal range; and absence of headache, vomiting, papilledema, and other clinical indicators of increased ICP.

---

1. Assess neurologic status at least hourly. Monitor pupils, LOC, and motor activity; and perform cranial nerve assessments. A decrease in LOC is an early

indicator of increased ICP and impending herniation. Changes in pupillary size and reaction, a decrease in motor function (i.e., hemiplegia, abnormal posturing) and cranial nerve palsies also may be signs of impending herniation.

2. Monitor patient for physical indicators of increased ICP, including headache, vomiting, and papilledema.

3. Monitor VS at frequent intervals. Be alert to changes in respiratory pattern (e.g., Cheyne-Stokes respirations), fluctuations in BP and pulse, widening pulse pressure, and slow pulse rate.

4. Maintain a patent airway and deliver oxygen as precribed to promote optimal cerebral perfusion. Be sure patient's neck is free of constricting objects, such as tracheostomy ties and oxygen tubing.

5. Avoid overhydration, which would add to cerebral edema, by ensuring precise delivery of IV fluids at consistent, prescribed rates.

6. Ensure timely delivery of medications that are prescribed for the prevention of sudden increases or decreases in BP, HR, or RR.

7. Teach patient the importance of avoiding activities that increase intracranial pressure: coughing, straining, bending over.

Alteration in comfort: Headache, photophobia, and fever related to meningeal irritation

---

Desired outcome: Patient verbalizes that a reduction in or relief of pain has occurred and does not exhibit nonverbal signs of discomfort.

---

1. Maintain a quiet environment for patient. Overstimulation may increase BP, which can aggravate patient's headache.

2. Plan and group patient care so that it is administered within a pattern that allows for uninterrupted periods (at least 90 minutes) of rest.

3. Organize visiting hours so that patient can have uninterrupted periods of rest.

4. Darken patient's room to minimize the discomfort of photophobia. Provide blindfolds if darkening the room is not possible.

5. Monitor temperature q2h and prn. Administer tepid baths or cooling blanket to keep temperature within prescribed limits.

6. Administer analgesics, antipyretics, and antibiotics as prescribed.

Potential for infection related to risk of cross-contamination secondary to communicable nature of bacterial and aseptic meningitis

---

Desired outcome: Other patients, staff members, and patient's significant others do not exhibit evidence of having acquired meningitis (see assessment and diagnostic test data).

For patient with bacterial meningitis

1. Bacterial meningitis is transmitted *via* airborne droplets as well as *via* contact with oral secretions. Provide patient with a private room for 24 hours after start of effective therapy.

2. Enforce respiratory isolation for 24 hours after start of effective therapy.
- Ensure masks are worn for those in close contact with patient.
- As with touching *any* patient secretion or excretion, ensure that gloves are worn when in contact with oral secretions.
- Ensure careful handwashing technique after contact with patient and potentially contaminated articles and before coming into contact with another patient.

For patient with aseptic (nonbacterial or viral meningitis)

3. Viral meningitis can be transmitted either *via* stool or oral secretions.
- Ensure that gowns are worn if soiling of clothing is likely.
- Ensure that gloves are worn for touching infective material.
- Enforce strict handwashing after touching patient or articles that may be contaminated and before caring for another patient.

See "Status Epilepticus" for the following: **Potential for injury** related to risk of oral and musculoskeletal trauma secondary to seizure activity, p. 314. Because these patients are at risk for SIADH, see "Syndrome of Inappropriate Antidiuretic Hormone" for the following: **Fluid volume excess** related to retention secondary to increased level of serum ADH with increased water reabsorption from the kidneys, p. 348. Also see appropriate nursing diagnoses and interventions, in "Sepsis," pp. 438-442, as these patients are at risk for septic shock. As indicated, see other nursing diagnoses and interventions in the following: "Providing Nutritional Support," pp. 490-505; "Caring for the Critically Ill on Prolonged Bed Rest," pp. 506-511; "Caring for the Critically Ill with Life-Threatening Disorders," pp. 511-522; and "Caring for the Family of the Critically Ill," pp. 522-526.

REHABILITATION AND PATIENT-FAMILY TEACHING CONCEPTS

Rehabilitation and teaching needs will differ from one patient to the next, depending on the degree of neurologic deficit. Give patient and significant others verbal and written instructions for the following, as appropriate:

1. Referrals to community resources (e.g., VNA, community support groups, physical therapy, occupational therapy, and rehabilitation center).

2. First aid measures for seizures. If patient has recurring seizures, provide address of Epilepsy Foundation of America: 4351 Garden City Drive, Suite 406, Landover, Maryland 20785.

3. Importance of follow-up care with MD and support services. In the event that emergency care may be needed, provide phone numbers of appropriate emergency personnel.

4. Medications, including drug name, dosage, purpose, schedule, precautions, and potential side effects.

5. Prophylaxis for family and significant others exposed to *Hemophilus influenzae:*
- *Pediatric:* rifampin 10-20 mg/kg/24 hr $\times$ 4 days.
- *Adults:* rifampin 600 mg/day $\times$ 4 days.

Neiserria meningitidis:
- *Children <1 year:* rifampin 5 mg/kg/24 hr $\times$ 4 days.
- *Children 1-12:* rifampin 10 mg/kg/24 hr $\times$ 4 days.
- *Adults:* rifampin 600 mg q12h $\times$ 4 doses.

Acute spinal cord injury

In general, a spinal cord injury (SCI) results from concussion, contusion, laceration, hemorrhage, or impairment of blood supply. This trauma to the spinal cord may be secondarily increased by the ischemia and subsequent edema that occur. Most often, SCI is caused by a motor vehicle accident, sports-related incident, or act of violence. Of the 15,000-20,000 new SCIs per year, half of the involved population are rendered paraplegic and the other half quadriplegic. Although life expectancy is good postinjury, morbidity and mortality most often are the result of infection. Renal disease (infection, calculi, septicemia) and pulmonary disease (e.g., pneumonia) account for 30-40% of all deaths.

SCI is classified in several ways: according to *type and etiology* such as open (gunshot or stab wound) or closed (motor vehicle accident, falls, sports-related incident); *site* (level of the spinal cord involved); *mechanism* such as flexion (e.g., occurring as a result of sudden deceleration in a head-on collision, backward fall down a flight of stairs, or diving into a swimming pool) or extension, (e.g., whiplash or fall involving hyperextension of the neck); *stability* (integrity of the supporting structures such as ligaments or bony facets); and whether it is *complete versus incomplete* (complete meaning the absence of all voluntary motor, sensory, and vasomotor function below the level of injury; and incomplete meaning presence of some percentage of voluntary motor or sensory function below the level of injury).

Fractures involving the vertebral bodies: These fractures may or may not cause SCI. Conversely, severe SCI may occur without evidence of damage to the vertebrae. With more severe fractures such as the "burst" fracture (fragmentation of a vertebral body with penetration of the spinal cord) there is almost always paralysis. The penetration of the spinal cord with bony fragments will cause hemorrhage, infection, and leakage of CSF.

Spinal shock: Immediately following SCI, most patients experience a period of spinal shock, which is the loss of all reflex activity below the level of injury as a result of a complete neurovascular shutdown. It may last minutes or be prolonged over days and weeks. Generally, the duration is 1-6 weeks, although periods of 6 months to a year have been reported. Generally, the more quickly the individual shows signs of return to function, the better the prognosis.

ASSESSMENT

Acute indicators (spinal shock): Flaccid paralysis of all skeletal muscles; absence of DTRs, cutaneous sensation, proprioception (position sense), visceral and somatic sensation, and penile reflex; urinary and fecal retention; unstable BP; hypotension; anhidrosis (absence of sweating).

< N O T E :   While spinal shock is seen in SCIs at *any* level, the loss of central control of peripheral vascular tone is seen most dramatically in high cervical spine injuries, with interruption of the sympathetic nervous system. This loss of sympathetic innervation causes venous pooling in the extremities and splanchnic vasculature, which decreases venous return to the heart, resulting in low cardiac output and low tissue perfusion pressure. This causes the patient to be bradycardic and hypotensive. With spinal cord injuries lower than the mid-thoracic area, the patient will experience a phase of spinal shock, with loss of sympathetic innervation to vasculature below the level of the lesion; however, the effects of that loss are not as dramatic. The patient will be susceptible to bradycardia and hypotension in relation to position change but this will not be a serious problem.

Indicators of the recovery phase of spinal shock: As spinal shock subsides, the patient may experience the following: (1) flexor spasms evoked by cutaneous stimulation; (2) reflex emptying of the bowel and bladder; (3) extensor or flexor rigidity; (4) hyperreflexic DTRs; and (5) reflex priapism or ejaculation in the male, evoked by cutaneous stimulation.

Levels of cord injury

- *C4 and above:* Loss of all muscle function, including muscles of respiration. With complete cord transection, the patient will expire, probably at the scene of the accident, unless immediately ventilated.
- *C4-5:* Same as above, but with sparing of the phrenic nerve. This means that the patient probably will require assisted ventilation, owing to weak or absent intercostal muscle function. Patient will be quadriplegic.
- *C6-8:* Quadriplegic but will retain function of respiratory muscles and may have some movement of neck, shoulders, chest, and upper arms.
- *T1-3:* Will have neck, shoulder, chest, arm, hand, and respiratory function; will experience difficulty maintaining a sitting position.
- *T4-10:* Same as above, but with more stability of trunk muscles. The lower the lesion, the greater the independence. The patient will be paraplegic.

< N O T E : 80% of individuals with lesions at or above T6 (quadriplegics/high paraplegics) will experience episodes of autonomic dysreflexia (AD). See discussion on the next page.

- *T11-L2:* Will have use of upper extremities, neck, and shoulders. Chest and trunk muscles will provide stability and patient will have some muscle function of upper thigh. At this level there may be loss of voluntary bowel and bladder control but the patient will have reflex emptying of the bowel. Men may experience difficulty getting and maintaining an erection and may have decreased seminal emission.
- *L3-S1:* Will have muscle function of all muscle groups in the upper body and most of the muscle function in the lower extremities. There will be loss of voluntary bowel and bladder function with reflex emptying. Men may experience decreased or lack of ability to have an erection, with decreased seminal emission.
- *S2-4:* Will have function of all muscle groups but may have some lower extremity weakness. There may be flaccidity of bowel and bladder, as well as loss of the ability to have a reflex erection.

Cord syndromes

1. *Anterior cord syndrome:* This syndrome involves injury to the anterior portion of the spinal cord supplied by the anterior spinal artery and may be associated with acute traumatic herniation of an intervertebral disc. Surgical decompression is necessary and the prognosis varies with each patient and depends on the degree of structural damage and edema.
   —*Signs and symptoms:* Varying degrees of paralysis occur below the level of the injury, along with diminution of pain and temperature sensations. Patient will retain senses of touch, motion, position, and vibration.
2. *Central cord syndrome:* Generally seen with hyperextension injuries or interruption of blood supply to the cervical spinal cord. Usually it is seen in the elderly, often with some evidence of vertebral injury on radiography. In this syndrome,

motor and sensory deficits are less severe in the lower extremities than in the upper extremities due to the central arrangement of cervical fibers in the spinal cord. In many cases, the most peripheral sacral and some lumbar fibers are spared. Incomplete injuries carry a relatively good prognosis. Steroids are used to decrease edema and many patients are able to ambulate with an assistive device and may regain bowel and bladder function. The regaining of useful function in the hands carries a less favorable prognosis.

—*Signs and symptoms:* Motor and sensory deficits usually are severe in the upper extremities and profound in the hands and fingers. With sparing of sacral and some lumbar fibers, there will be some motor and sensory function in the perineum, genitalia, and lower extremities.

3. *Lateral cord (Brown-Séquard) syndrome:* Results from a horizontal hemisection of the spinal cord, for example from a gunshot or stab wound. Patients usually present with bilateral motor and sensory impairment, with a relative difference in function from one side to the other. Prognosis is usually good for recovery of upper and lower extremity function.

—*Signs and symptoms:* Ipsilateral weakness and decrease in light touch, vibratory, and position senses, with contralateral hypalgesia. Usually there are bilateral motor and sensory deficits but motor activity will be better on one side and sensory activity will be better on the other.

4. *Horner's syndrome:* Seen following an incomplete (partial transection) injury in the cervical region of the spinal cord. The lesion affects either the preganglionic sympathetic trunk or the postganglionic sympathetic neurons of the superior cervical ganglion. It usually affects the ipsilateral side of the face.

—*Signs and symptoms:* Ipsilateral miosis, enophthalmos (backward displacement of the eye in its socket), ptosis, and anhidrosis.

Autonomic dysreflexia (AD): Life-threatening response of the autonomic nervous system to a stimulus, creating an exaggerated sympathetic nervous system response. This response can occur during the acute phase of SCI or it may not appear until several years postinjury. It affects individuals with lesions at or above T6. If AD is not identified promptly, treated, and reversed, the potential consequences include seizures, subarachnoid hemorrhage, and fatal cerebrovascular accident.

• *Causes:* Stimuli to the *bladder* (most common) such as distention, infection, calculi, cystoscopy; *bowel* such as fecal impaction, rectal exam, suppository insertion; or *skin* such as tight clothing or sheets, temperature extremes, sores, or areas of broken skin.

• *Signs and symptoms:* Classic triad includes a throbbing headache, cutaneous vasodilation, and sweating, which occur above the level of the lesion. The patient also may exhibit the following: hypertension (BP >250-300/150 mm Hg), nasal congestion, flushed skin (above the level of the lesion), blurred vision, nausea, and bradycardia. Below the level of the lesion there will be pilomotor erection (goose bumps), pallor, chills, and vasoconstriction.

DIAGNOSTIC TESTS

1. *Spinal x-rays:* AP and lateral films are done to detect fractures or dislocations of vertebral bodies, assess for narrowing of the spinal canal, and check for hematomas. Additional views or tomograms may be necessary to view some levels of the spinal cord, particularly in obese and heavily muscled patients.

< C A U T I O N : This stage in the evaluation of the patient with a possible SCI is extremely dangerous, as any sudden or incorrect movement of the injured area could cause further trauma to the spinal cord.

2. *CT scan:* Same purpose as above; may reveal soft tissue injury.
3. *Magnetic resonance imaging (MRI):* Same purpose as above; will define internal organ structures, detect tissue changes such as edema or infarction, and evaluate blood flow patterns and blood vessel integrity.
4. *Myelography:* To identify site of spinal canal blockage, which can occur owing to fractures, dislocations, or herniation or protrusion of an intervertebral disc. Radiopaque dye is injected into the spinal subarachnoid space through a lumbar or cervical puncture.
   * *Pretest:* Have patient or family member sign a consent form. Question patient or significant others regarding patient's sensitivity to iodine, shellfish, or contrast material. Ensure that patient is NPO for 4-6 hours.
   * *Posttest:* If a water-soluble dye was used (e.g., metrizamide), elevate HOB for at least 8 hours to prevent dye from irritating cerebral meninges. Seizures are a complication of this dye substance. If an oil-based dye (e.g., Pantopaque) was used, it will be removed *via* the puncture site immediately after the test or during surgery if it is scheduled after the test. Keep patient flat for 6-8 hours after dye removal.
5. *Pulmonary fluoroscopy:* To evaluate the degree of diaphragmatic movement in an individual with a high cervical injury. If the injury is at C4 or below, the diaphragm will move up and down with inspiration; however, if the injury is at a slightly higher level, the innervation of the diaphragm may be partial, causing paradoxical respiratory movements that will lead to an ineffective breathing pattern. If this occurs, the patient will require assisted ventilation.
6. *Hemoglobin and hematocrit:* To detect blood loss due to hemorrhage caused by internal injury.
7. *Urinalysis:* To detect the presence of bacteria or blood, which are indicative of contused kidneys or ruptured bladder.
8. *ABG values and pulmonary function studies:* To assess effectiveness of respirations and to detect the need for oxygen, tracheostomy, and mechanical ventilation.
9. *Cystogram:* To assess bladder capacity and function.

MEDICAL MANAGEMENT AND SURGICAL INTERVENTIONS

1. **Immobilization of the injured site** with or without surgical intervention
   * *Cervical spine injury:* Skeletal traction from 20-40 pounds is used to immobilize and reduce the fracture or dislocation. Traction may be achieved *via* Vinke, Gardner-Wells, Trippi-Wells, or Crutchfield tongs, which are inserted through the outer table of the skull. These tongs are attached to ropes and pulleys with weights to achieve bony reduction and proper alignment. Most likely, the patient will be placed on a Stryker or Foster frame, a Roto-Rest kinetic treatment table, or circle bed. The patient also may be immobilized with a halo device and a plaster or fiberglass jacket for skeletal fixation of the head and neck. This device allows for earlier mobilization and rehabilitation.

< C A U T I O N :   A circle bed must be used cautiously with the SCI patient. If the patient is turned too quickly, orthostatic hypotension due to venous pooling may occur, with potentially serious or fatal complications.

Surgical intervention during the immediate postinjury phase is controversial. Surgery may be performed if (1) the neurologic deficit is progressing; (2) there are compound fractures; (3) the injury involves a penetrating wound of the spine; (4) there are bone fragments in the spinal canal; or (5) there is acute anterior spinal cord trauma. Surgeries may include decompression laminectomy, closed or open reduction of the fracture, or spinal fusion for stabilization.

- *Thoracic spine injury:* May require surgical stabilization *via* Harrington rods or laminectomy with spinal fusion, utilizing bone taken from the iliac crest.
- *Lumbar spine injury:* May necessitate surgical stabilization with laminectomy and spinal fusion. If the injury is stable, it may be treated with closed reduction. Some patients with lumbar spine injury may be immobilized with a halo device with femoral distraction. This device may be connected to traction with weights for reduction and stabilization prior to surgery.

2. **Respiratory management:** The need for assisted ventilation is based on level of injury, ABG values, pulmonary function tests, pulmonary fluoroscopy, and physical assessment data. Initially, the patient may be intubated, and later, tracheotomized. Individuals with high cervical injury who survive the initial injury but have paralysis of the muscles of respiration may require permanent tracheostomy with mechanical ventilation. Some of these individuals may be candidates for phrenic nerve stimulation, which if successful can give the patient periodic independence from the ventilator. Phrenic nerve stimulation is performed only at specialized spinal cord trauma centers.

3. **Aggressive pulmonary care:** To prevent, detect, and treat atelectasis, pulmonary infection, and respiratory failure, as pulmonary problems are a major source of morbidity and mortality in the SCI patient. Chest physiotherapy, intubation, and ventilation are instituted as indicated.

4. **Nasogastric tube placement:** To decompress the stomach, prevent aspiration of gastric contents, and decrease the risk of paralytic ileus (often seen within 72 hours of injury in patients with lesions higher than T6).

5. **Urinary catheterization:** Insertion of an in-dwelling or intermittent catheter to decompress an atonic bladder in the immediate postinjury phase (spinal shock). With the return of the reflex arc after spinal shock subsides, patients with lesions above T12 generally will develop a reflex neurogenic bladder that fills and empties automatically. Patients with lesions at or below T12 generally will have an atonic, areflexic neurogenic bladder that overfills, distending the bladder and causing overflow incontinence.

6. **Pharmacotherapy**
- *Corticosteroids* (e.g., dexamethasone): To decrease the inflammatory response at the site of injury. Use of corticosteroids is controversial and their efficacy has not been substantiated.
- *Osmotic diuretics* (e.g., mannitol, urea): To decrease edema at the site of injury.
- *Antacids:* To prevent gastric ulceration, which may occur post-SCI due to hyperacidity of gastric secretions and increased production of gastric acid.

The risk of ulceration with hemorrhage is further increased if steroids are used.

- *Histamine H_2 receptor antagonists* (e.g., cimetidine, ranitidine): To suppress secretion of gastric acid and to prevent or treat ulcers in the patient with increased production of gastric acid and an increased susceptibility to gastric ulceration and perforation.
- *Stool softeners* (e.g., docusate sodium): To begin bowel retraining program and prevent fecal impaction with distention of the bowel, which could stimulate an episode of autonomic dysreflexia.
- *Hyperosmolar laxatives* (e.g., glycerin suppository): To prevent fecal impaction and facilitate movement of the bowels on a regular basis (part of a bowel program).
- *Irritant or stimulant laxatives* (e.g., bisacodyl): To stimulate bowel movements as part of a bowel training program.
- *Analgesics* (e.g., acetaminophen or acetaminophen with codeine). To decrease pain associated with the injury or surgery.
- *Sedatives:* To decrease anxiety due to the injury, hospitalization, or fear of the prognosis.
- *Antihypertensives* (e.g., hydralazine hydrochloride, methyldopa, nitroprusside sodium): To treat the severe hypertension seen in autonomic dysreflexia.
- *Vasopressors* (e.g., epinephrine): To treat the hypotension that may occur in the immediate postinjury stage due to loss of vasomotor control below the level of injury, with resultant vasodilation and a relative hypovolemia.

< N O T E :   Orthostatic hypotension may become a permanent problem, especially in patients with cervical and high thoracic injuries. Caregivers must be taught to move the patient slowly into the upright position to avoid a sudden drop in BP, which can cause cerebral hypoxia and loss of consciousness. Abdominal binders and ace bandages or thigh-high antiembolic stockings also may aid in preventing orthostatic hypotension.

- *Antibiotics:* To prevent or treat wound, respiratory, or urinary tract infection.
- *Anticoagulants* (heparin sodium): To prevent thrombophlebitis, deep-vein thrombosis, and pulmonary emboli.

< N O T E :   SCI patients are at high risk for development of vascular complications because they are immobilized, have lost vasoconstrictive capabilities below the level of injury, and cannot constrict the muscles in the lower extremities to facilitate venous flow. Patients who are not candidates for anticoagulation may have an inferior vena cava umbrella or Greenfield filter inserted to trap emboli traveling from the lower extremities to the lungs.

NURSING DIAGNOSES AND INTERVENTIONS

Impaired gas exchange related to hypoventilation secondary to paresis or paralysis of the muscles of respiration (diaphragm, intercostals) occurring with high cervical spine injury or ascending cord edema

---

Desired outcomes: Patient has adequate gas exchange as evidenced by orientation to person, place, and time; Pao_2 $\geq$80 mm Hg; and $Paco_2$ $\leq$45 mm Hg. RR is 12-20 with normal depth and pattern (eupnea), HR is 60-100 bpm, BP is stable and within patient's normal range, and vital capacity is ≥ 1 L. Motor and sensory losses remain at the same spinal cord level as the initial findings.

< N O T E : Patients with cervical injuries usually are intubated prior to arrival in the ICU. However, with some high thoracic or low cervical lesions, patients who ventilate independently in the emergency room may arrive in ICU without assisted ventilation. Such a patient may be at risk for an increasingly higher level of cord damage owing to hemorrhage and edema, which can result in a higher level of dysfunction and a change in respiratory status requiring assisted ventilation.

1. Assess for signs of respiratory dysfunction: shallow or slow respirations, vital capacity <1 liter, changes in sensorium, anxiety, restlessness, tachycardia, and pallor.
2. Monitor ABG studies; report abnormalities. Be particularly alert to Pao_2 <60 mm Hg and $Paco_2$ >50 mm Hg, as these findings are indicative of the need for assisted ventilation.
3. Monitor patient for evidence of ascending cord edema: increasing difficulty with swallowing secretions or coughing, presence of respiratory stridor with retraction of accessory muscles of respiration, bradycardia, fluctuating BP, and increased motor and sensory loss at a higher level than the initial findings.
4. Before attempting oral intubation with neck flexion, ensure that cervical x-rays have confirmed the absence of cervical involvement. If patient exhibits evidence of respiratory distress and cervical involvement has not been ruled out, do not hyperextend the neck for resuscitation; but rather, utilize either nasal intubation or the jaw-thrust method to prevent further cervical cord injury.
5. If patient has undergone immobilization *via* placement of cranial tongs or traction with a halo apparatus, monitor patient's respiratory status q1-2h for the first 24-48 hours and then q4h if patient's condition is stable. Be alert to absent or adventitious breath sounds and inspect chest movement to ensure that the plaster or fiberglass vest is not restricting diaphragmatic movement.
6. If intubation *via* endotracheal tube or tracheostomy becomes necessary, explain the procedure to patient and signficant others.
7. See section "Management of the Adult on Mechanical Ventilation," p. 61, for interventions related to mechanical ventilation.

Potential for ineffective airway clearance related to decreased or absent cough reflex secondary to cervical or high thoracic spine injury

---

Desired outcome: Patient has a clear airway as evidenced by auscultation of normal breath sounds and absence of adventitious breath sounds.

---

1. Monitor patient's respiratory status and be alert to the following indicators of ineffective airway clearance: adventitious breath sounds (i.e., crackles, rhonchi), decreased or absent breath sounds (bronchial, bronchovesicular, vesicular), increased HR (>100 bpm) and BP (>10 mm Hg over patient's normal), decreased tidal volume (<75-85% of predicted value) or vital capacity (<1 L), shallow or rapid respirations (>20 breaths/min), pallor, cyanosis, increased restlessness, and anxiety.

2. Monitor and report abnormal ABG (i.e., decreased Pao_2 or increased $Paco_2$) and chest x-ray results.
3. Suction patient as often as needed, as indicated by auscultation findings.
4. If indicated by the assessment findings, prepare patient for intubation or tracheostomy with mechanical ventilation. See section "Management of the Adult on Mechanical Ventilation," p. 61, for more information.
5. If patient does not require intubation with mechanical ventilation, implement the following measures to improve airway clearance:
   - Place patient in a semi-Fowler's position unless it is contraindicated (e.g., patient in cervical tongs with traction).
   - Turn patient from side to side at least q2h to help mobilize secretions.
   - Keep room humidified to help loosen secretions.
   - Unless contraindicated keep patient hydrated with at least 2-3 L/day of fluid.
   - If patient has respiratory muscle control, teach coughing and deep-breathing exercises, which should be performed at least q2h.
   - If patient's cough is ineffective, implement the following method known as "quad coughing": Place palm of hand under patient's diaphragm and push up on the abdominal muscles as patient exhales.

Potential for injury related to risk of autonomic dysreflexia (AD) secondary to abnormal response of the autonomic nervous system to a stimulus

---

Desired outcomes: Patient is asymptomatic of AD as evidenced by dry skin above the level of injury, BP within patient's normal range, HR 60-100 bpm, and absence of headache and other clinical indicators of AD. EKG demonstrates normal sinus rhythm.

---

1. Assess for the classic triad of AD: throbbing headache, cutaneous vasodilation, and sweating above the level of injury. In addition, extremely elevated BP (e.g., $\geq$250-300/150 mm Hg), nasal stuffiness, flushed skin (above the level of the injury), blurred vision, nausea, and bradycardia also can occur. Be alert to the following signs of AD that occur below the level of injury: pilomotor erection, pallor, chills, and vasoconstriction.
2. Assess for cardiac dysrhythmias, optimally *via* cardiac monitor during initial postinjury stage (2 weeks).
3. Be aware of and implement measures to prevent factors that may precipitate AD: *bladder stimuli* (i.e., distention, calculi, infection, cystoscopy); *bowel stimuli* (i.e., fecal impaction, rectal exam, suppository insertion); *skin stimuli* (i.e., pressure from tight clothing or sheets, temperature extremes, sores, or areas of broken skin).
4. If indicators of AD are present, implement the following:
   - Elevate HOB or place patient in a sitting position. This will decrease BP by promoting cerebral venous return.
   - Monitor BP and HR q3-5min until patient stabilizes.
   - Determine and remove offending stimulus.
     —For example, if patient's bladder is distended, catheterize cautiously, using sufficient lubricant that contains local anesthetic.

—If patient has an in-dwelling urinary catheter, check for obstruction such as granulation in catheter or kinking of tubing. As indicated, irrigate catheter, using no more than 30 ml normal saline.

—If urinary tract infection is suspected, obtain a urine specimen for culture and sensitivity once crisis stage has passed.

—Check for fecal impaction. Perform the rectal examination gently, using an ointment containing a local anesthetic (e.g., Nupercaine).

—Check for sensory stimuli and loosen clothing, bed covers, or other constricting fabric as indicated.

5. Notify MD if symptoms do not abate, especially the elevated BP, because the consequences are life-threatening: seizures, subarachnoid or intracerebral hemorrhage, fatal cerebrovascular accident.

6. As prescribed, administer antihypertensive agent and monitor its effectiveness.

7. Remain calm and supportive of patient and signficant others during these episodes.

8. Upon resolution of the immediate crisis, answer patient's and significant others' questions regarding cause of the AD. Provide patient and family teaching regarding signs and symptoms and methods of treatment of AD. This is particularly critical for the SCI patient who has sustained injury above T6, who is at risk for AD for life.

Potential alteration in cardiac output: Decreased, related to relative hypovolemia secondary to enlarged vascular space occurring with neurogenic shock

---

Desired outcome: Patient has adequate cardiac output as evidenced by orientation to person, place, and time; systolic BP ≥90 mm Hg (or within patient's normal range); HR 60-100 bpm; RAP 4-6 mm Hg; RVP 25/0-5 mm Hg; PAP 20-30/8-15 mm Hg; PAWP 6-12 mm Hg; SVR 900-1200 dynes/sec/cm^{-5}; normal amplitude of peripheral pulses (>2+ on a 0-4+ scale); and urinary output ≥30 ml/hr.

< N O T E : In neurogenic shock, blood volume is normal but the vascular space is enlarged, causing peripheral pooling, decreased venous return, and decreased cardiac output.

1. Monitor patient for indicators of decreased cardiac output: drop in systolic BP >20 mm Hg, systolic BP <90 mm Hg, or a continuous drop of 5-10 mm Hg with each assessment; HR >100 bpm; irregular HR; lightheadedness; fainting; confusion; dizziness; flushed skin; diminished amplitude of peripheral pulses; or a change in BP, HR, mental status, and color associated with a change in position. Monitor I&O and be alert to urine output <30 ml/hr for two consecutive hours. Also assess hemodynamic measurements. In the presence of neurogenic shock, anticipate decreased RAP, RVP, PAP, PAWP, and SVR. For detail, see Table 2-14, "Hemodynamic Profile of Shock," p. 133.

2. Implement measures to prevent episodes of decreased cardiac output due to orthostatic hypotension:
   • Change patient's position slowly.
   • Perform ROM exercises q2h to prevent venous pooling.
   • Apply elastic antiembolic hose as prescribed to promote venous return.

- Avoid placing pillows under patient's knees, gatching the bed, or allowing patient to cross the legs or sit with legs in a dependent position.
- Collaborate with physical therapy in progressing patient from a supine to upright position, utilizing a tilt table.

3. As prescribed, administer fluids to control mild hypotension.
4. Administer and monitor for therapeutic effects of vasopressors.

Potential for injury related to risk of development of Cushing's ulcer secondary to increased production of gastric acid

---

Desired outcomes: Patient's gastric pH tests >5 and patient is asymptomatic of Cushing's ulcer as evidenced by gastric aspirate and stools negative for blood, BP within patient's normal range, HR ≤100 bpm, and absence of midepigastric or referred shoulder pain. Hematocrit is 40%-54% (male) or 37%-47% (female), hemoglobin is 14-18 g/dl (male) or 12-16 g/dl (female), and RBC count is 45-60 million μl (male) or 40-55 million μl (female).

< N O T E : After return of bowel sounds, any major trauma victim is at high risk for development of gastric ulcers due to increased production of gastric acid. Although ulceration can occur at any time in the SCI patient, it is most likely to occur within 3 weeks of the injury.

1. Assess for indicators of GI ulceration or hemorrhage: midepigastric pain (dull, gnawing, burning ache) if patient has sensation; and hematemesis, melena, constipation, anemia, pallor, decreased BP, increased HR, and complaints of shoulder pain.
2. Test gastric aspirate and stools for blood q8h. Promptly report presence of blood to MD.
3. Monitor CBC for signs of anemia: decreases in Hgb, Hct, and RBCs.
4. As prescribed, implement measures to treat or prevent ulceration and hemorrhage:
   - Monitor gastric pH q2h; administer antacids q2-4h or as prescribed to maintain gastric pH >5.
   - Administer histamine H_2 antagonists to suppress secretion of gastric acids, decrease irritating effects of gastric secretions, and facilitate healing.
   - Insert NG tube and attach to suction to remove gastric contents.
   - Perform iced-saline lavage.
   - Prepare patient for surgery as indicated.
5. For the patient with GI ulceration and hemorrhage, bowel perforation is an added risk. Be alert to the following indicators: pallor, shock state, abdominal distention, vomiting of coffee-ground material, absent bowel sounds, elevated WBC count (>11,000 μl), and presence of ambient air on abdominal x-ray. In some cases, the only indicators will be tachycardia and shoulder pain. Bowel perforation is an emergency situation, requiring immediate surgical intervention.

Potential alteration in tissue perfusion: Peripheral and cardiopulmonary, related to risk of thrombophlebitis, deep-vein thrombosis (DVT), and pulmonary emboli secondary to venous stasis occurring with decreased vasomotor tone and immobility

Desired outcome: Patient is asymptomatic of thrombophlebitis, DVT, and pulmonary emboli as evidenced by absence of heat, swelling, discomfort, and erythema in the calves and thighs; HR ≤100 bpm; RR ≤20 breaths/min with normal pattern and depth (eupnea); BP within patient's normal range; PaO_2 ≥80 mm Hg; and absence of chest or shoulder pain.

1. Assess for indicators of thrombophlebitis and DVT: unusual heat and erythema of calf or thigh, increased circumference of calf or thigh, tenderness or pain in extremity (depending on patient's level of injury and whether injury is complete or incomplete), positive Homan's sign.

2. Assess for indicators of pulmonary emboli: sudden chest or shoulder pain, tachycardia, dyspnea, tachypnea, hypotension, pallor, cyanosis, cough with hemoptysis, restlessness, increasing anxiety, low PaO_2.

3. Implement measures to prevent development of thrombophlebitis, DVT, and pulmonary emboli:
   - Change patient's position at least q2h to prevent venous pooling.
   - Perform ROM exercises on all extremities q1-2h to promote venous return and prevent venous stasis.
   - Avoid use of knee gatch or pillows under the knees, which can compromise circulation.
   - If patient is out of bed and in a chair, do not allow patient to cross legs at the knee or sit with legs dependent for longer than ½-1 hour. For the patient experiencing some return of spinal reflex arcs below the level of the injury with spasticity of lower extremities, caution patient to alert nurse should legs become crossed.
   - Apply antiembolic hose as prescribed.
   - Maintain adequate hydration of at least 2-3 L/day, unless contraindicated, to prevent dehydration and concomitant increase in blood viscosity, which can promote thrombus formation.
   - Administer prophylactic low-dose heparin as prescribed.

4. If the patient exhibits signs of thrombophlebitis or DVT, implement the following:
   - Notify MD.
   - Maintain bed rest unless otherwise directed.
   - Maintain rest of affected extremity, keeping extremity in a neutral or elevated position, as prescribed.
   - Discourage activities that promote vasoconstriction, such as smoking.
   - Administer anticoagulants and antiplatelet aggregating agents as prescribed.

< N O T E :   SCI patients who are not candidates for anticoagulation may require surgical intervention (intracaval filter) to prevent pulmonary emboli due to thrombophlebitis or DVT.

   - Apply warm, moist heat as prescribed.

< N O T E :   Use of heat is not prescribed by some MDs due to concern that heat causes vasodilation, which may mobilize a thrombus.

5. If patient exhibits evidence of pulmonary emboli, perform the following, in addition to the interventions for thrombophlebitis and DVT on p. 303:
   - Elevate HOB if not contraindicated.
   - Administer oxygen.
   - As prescribed, administer vasopressors (for hypotension) and analgesics (for pain).
   - Prepare patient for diagnostic procedure (i.e., perfusion lung scan) or surgical intervention (e.g., insertion of intracaval filter).
   - Remain calm and provide support and reassurance to patient and significant others.

Potential impairment of skin and tissue integrity related to prolonged immobility secondary to immobilization device or paralysis

---

Desired outcome: Patient's skin and tissue remain intact.

---

1. Perform a complete skin assessment at least q8h. Pay close attention to skin that is particularly susceptible to breakdown (i.e., skin over bony prominences and around halo vest edges). Be alert to erythema, warmth, open or macerated tissue, and foul odors (indicative of infection with tissue necrosis).
2. Turn and reposition patient and massage susceptible skin at least q2h. Post a turning schedule and include patient in the planning and initiating of this schedule.

< C A U T I O N :   Do not turn patient without a written prescription until the injured area of the spinal cord has been stabilized. If turning is allowed prior to immobilization with tongs, halo, or surgery, use log-rolling technique only, utilizing at least 3 people to turn patient: one to support the head and neck and keep them in alignment during the procedure and two to turn the patient.

3. Keep skin clean and dry.
4. Pad halo jacket edges (e.g., with sheepskin) to minimize irritation and friction.
5. Provide pressure-relief mattress most appropriate for patient's injury.
6. For more information related to the maintenance of skin and tissue integrity, see the same nursing diagnosis, p. 508, in the appendicized section, "Caring for the Critically Ill on Prolonged Bed Rest."

Potential alteration in nutrition: Less than body requirements related to decreased oral intake secondary to anorexia, difficulty eating in prone position, fear of choking and aspiration, and inability to feed self due to paralysis of upper extremities; and decreased GI motility secondary to autonomic nervous system dysfunction

---

Desired outcome: Patient has adequate nutrition as evidenced by balanced nitrogen state per nitrogen balance studies, serum albumin 3.5-5.5 g/dl, thyroxine-binding prealbumin 200-300 µg/ml, and retinol-binding protein 40-50 µg/ml.

---

1. Perform a complete baseline assessment of patient's nutritional status. See section "Providing Nutritional Support," p. 490.

2. Assess patient's readiness for oral intake: presence of bowel sounds, passing of flatus, or bowel movement.

< N O T E :   Next to fecal impaction, paralytic ileus is the second most common GI disorder of SCI patients. It usually occurs within 72 hours of the injury and is associated with gastric distention. See **Alteration in bowel elimination,** p. 308, for more information.

3. When the patient begins an oral diet, progress slowly from liquids to solids as tolerated.

4. Monitor and record percentage of each meal eaten by patient.

5. Implement measures to maintain or improve patient's intake.
- Obtain dietary consult in order to provide patient with his or her favorite foods, as well as those that are of high nutritious value.
- Make mealtime more pleasant: provide oral hygiene before and after meals and decrease external stimuli (this will help patient concentrate on chewing and swallowing, as well, to minimize the risk of aspiration).
- Provide small, frequent feedings as they may be more readily digested, less likely to cause abdominal distention, which may compromise respiratory movement, and less fatiguing.
- If patient is in a Stryker or Foster frame, feed in a prone position to minimize the risk of aspiration. If patient is in a Halo device or has been stabilized, feed in high-Fowler's position.
- Feed patient slowly, providing small, bite-size pieces, which facilitate digestion and help prevent choking.
- Provide straws for liquids; teach patient to sip slowly.

6. Once patient has been stabilized, consult with occupational therapy for selection of assistive devices that will enable patient to feed self.

Urinary retention related to inhibition of the spinal reflex arc secondary to spinal shock following SCI

Desired outcomes: Patient has urinary output of ≥30 ml/hr and is asymptomatic of autonomic dysreflexia (AD) as evidenced by BP within patient's normal range, vision normal for patient, dry skin above the level of injury, HR ≥60 bpm, and absence of headache, nasal congestion, flushed skin above the level of injury, and nausea, as well as absence of the following findings below the level of injury: pilomotor erection (goosebumps), pallor, chills.

< C A U T I O N :   Urinary retention with stretching of the bladder muscle may trigger AD. Therefore, it is critical that retention be assessed for and treated promptly.

1. Assess for indicators of urinary retention: suprapubic distention and intake greater than output.

2. Catheterize patient on admission as prescribed. Patients usually have an indwelling catheter for the first 48-72 hours after injury, followed by intermittent catheterization in an attempt to retrain the bladder.

3. Ensure continuous patency of the drainage system to prevent reflux of urine into the bladder or blockage of flow, which could cause urinary retention or urinary tract infection, which may precipitate AD.

4. If an episode of AD is triggered by a distended bladder, obstructed catheter, kinked tubing, or urinary tract infection, implement the following:
   • Have someone notify MD.
   • If patient is not already catheterized, catheterize patient using an anesthetic jelly.
   • If the catheter is obstructed, gently instill no more than 30 ml normal saline in an attempt to open the catheter.
   • If the catheter remains obstructed, remove it and insert another, using an anesthetic lubricating agent.
   • If a urinary tract infection is the suspected triggering factor, obtain a specimen of urine for culture and sensitivity testing.
   • For other treatment interventions, see **Potential for injury** related to risk of AD, p. 300.

Reflex incontinence related to uninhibited activity of the spinal reflex arc secondary to recovery phase from spinal shock in patients with cord lesions above T12

Desired outcome: Patient does not experience urinary incontinence.

---

1. As prescribed, catheterize patient on a regularly scheduled basis, for example, q4-6h or q8-12h.
2. If episodes of urinary incontinence occur, catheterize more frequently. If more than 500 ml of urine are obtained, catheterize more often and reduce fluid intake.
3. Measure the amount of residual urine and attempt to increase the length of time between catheterizations, as indicated by decreased amounts (i.e., <50-100 ml urine).
4. Monitor and record I&O. Encourage a consistent intake of fluids, evenly distributed throughout the day, to prevent overdistention, which can cause incontinence and increase the risk for AD.
5. Decrease fluid intake prior to bedtime to prevent nighttime incontinence.
6. Discourage intake of caffeine-containing beverages and foods (e.g., colas, chocolate, coffee, tea), as they have a diuretic effect and may stimulate increased urine production, bladder spasms, and reflex incontinence.
7. Teach patient and significant others the procedure for intermittent catheterization. Alert them to the indicators of UTI (restlessness, incontinence, malaise, anorexia, fever, cloudy or foul-smelling urine) and the importance of adequate fluid intake, regular urine cultures, and good handwashing and cleansing of the urinary catheter prior to catheterization. (The patient with a lesion above T12 who has a reflex neurogenic bladder eventually may be able to empty the bladder automatically and may not require catheterization.)

< C A U T I O N : UTI is one of the leading causes of morbidity and mortality in the SCI patient. The SCI patient may not be aware of the presence of urinary tract infection until he or she is severely ill due to a pyelonephritis (calculi, infection, septicemia).

Urinary retention (with overflow incontinence) related to loss of reflex activity for micturition and bladder flaccidity secondary to cord lesion at or below T12

Desired outcome: Patient has urinary output without incontinence.

---

1. As prescribed, either insert an in-dwelling urinary catheter or catheterize patient intermittently on a regularly-scheduled basis (e.g., q4-6h).
2. If intermittent catheterization is used and episodes of urinary incontinence occur, catheterize more frequently. If more than 500 ml of urine are obtained, catheterize more often and reduce fluid intake.
3. Measure the amount of residual urine and attempt to increase the length of time between catheterizations, as indicated by decreased amounts (i.e., <50-100 ml urine).
4. Monitor and record I&O. Distribute fluids evenly throughout the day to prevent overdistention, which can cause incontinence and increase the risk for AD.
5. Decrease fluid intake prior to bedtime to prevent nighttime incontinence.
6. Discourage intake of caffeine-containing beverages and foods (e.g., colas, chocolate, coffee, tea), as they have a diuretic effect and may stimulate increased urine production.
7. When patient or significant other is ready, teach bladder-emptying techniques such as straining or Credé method.

< N O T E : Even with these techniques, patients may experience dribbling of urine, which will necessitate catheterization or incontinence panties.

8. Teach patient and significant others the procedure for intermittent catheterization. Alert them to the indicators of UTI (restlessness, incontinence, malaise, anorexia, fever, cloudy or foul-smelling urine) and the importance of adequate fluid intake, regular urine cultures, and good handwashing and cleansing of the urinary catheter prior to catheterization.

< C A U T I O N : UTI is one of the leading causes of morbidity and mortality in the SCI patient. The SCI patient may not be aware of the presence of urinary tract infection until he or she is severely ill owing to a pyelonephritis (calculi, infection, septicemia).

Ineffective thermoregulation related to inability of the body to adapt to environmental temperature changes secondary to poikilothermic reaction occurring with SCI.

Desired outcome: Patient remains normothermic.

< N O T E : With SCI, the patient may become poikilothermic, meaning that the patient adapts his or her own body temperature to that of the environment and is unable to control core body temperature *via* vasodilatation to lose heat or vasoconstriction to conserve heat.

1. Monitor patient's temperature at least q4h and assess patient for signs of ineffective thermoregulation: complaints of being too warm, excessive diaphoresis,

warmth of skin above level of injury, complaints of being too cold, pilomotor erection (goosebumps), or cool skin above the level of injury.

2. Implement measures to attain normothermia:
- Regulate room temperature.
- Provide extra blankets to prevent chills.
- Protect patient from drafts.
- Provide warm food and drink if patient is chilled; provide cool drinks if patient is warm.
- Provide heating device (e.g., hot water bottles) to increase body warmth.

< C A U T I O N :   Use care to prevent thermal injury when using heating and cooling devices.

- Utilize fans or air conditioners to prevent overheating.
- Remove excess bedding to facilitate heat loss.
- Provide a tepid bath or cooling blanket to facilitate cooling.

Potential for injury related to risk of paralytic ileus with concomitant risk of autonomic dysreflexia (AD) secondary to SCI

Desired outcome: Patient is asymptomatic of paralytic ileus as evidenced by auscultation of normal bowel sounds; and asymptomatic of AD as evidenced by BP within patient's normal range, vision normal for patient, dry skin above the level of injury, HR ≥60 bpm, and absence of headache, nasal congestion, flushed skin above the level of injury, and nausea, as well as absence of the following findings below the level of injury: pilomotor erection (goosebumps), pallor, chills.

< N O T E :   Paralytic ileus occurs most often in patients with SCI at T6 and above and usually within the first 72 hours following the injury.

1. Assess for indicators of paralytic ileus: decreased or absent bowel sounds, abdominal distention, anorexia, vomiting, and altered respirations as a result of pressure on the diaphragm. Report significant findings promptly.

2. Observe closely for signs of autonomic dysreflexia, which can be triggered by the distention of the abdomen (for assessment and treatment of AD, see interventions with **Potential for injury** related to risk of AD, p. 300).

3. If indicators of paralytic ileus appear, implement the following, as prescribed:
- Restrict intake.
- Insert NG tube to decompress the stomach; attach to suction.
- Insert a rectal tube if prescribed.

< C A U T I O N :   Stimulation of the rectum by a rectal tube may precipitate an episode of AD; therefore, application of anesthetic ointment prior to insertion is recommended.

- If patient has a rectal tube in place, he or she may not have sensation in the rectal area. Therefore, special care is necessary to prevent damage to the rectal mucosa and anal sphincter. Remove the tube as soon as possible.

Alteration in bowel elimination: Constipation or fecal impaction related to hypotonic or atonic bowel secondary to spinal shock

Desired outcome: Patient has bowel elimination of soft and formed stools every 2-3 days or within patient's preinjury pattern.

1. Monitor patient for indicators of constipation (nausea, abdominal distention, malaise) and fecal impaction (nausea, vomiting, increasing abdominal distention, palpable colonic mass, or presence of hard fecal mass on digital exam).
2. Until bowel sounds are present and paralytic ileus has resolved, maintain patient on NPO status with NG suction.
3. Perform a gentle digital exam to determine presence of fecal impaction and check for rectal reflexes.
4. Prior to return of rectal reflex arc, it may be necessary to remove feces from the rectum manually. If a fecal impaction is present in an atonic bowel, a small enema may be necessary.

< C A U T I O N : Be aware that overdistention of the bowel or stimulation of the anal sphincter due to impaction, rectal exam, or enema may precipitate AD. Use generous amounts of anesthetic lubricant when performing rectal exam or administering an enema.

Alteration in bowel elimination: Constipation related to inability to defecate secondary to lack of voluntary control of the anal sphincter and lack of sensation of a fecal mass following return of reflex arc

Desired outcome: Patient has bowel elimination of soft and formed stools every 2-3 days or within patient's preinjury pattern.

1. Obtain history of patient's preinjury bowel elimination pattern.
2. Assist patient with selection of menu items that are high in fiber.
3. Unless contraindicated, maintain a minimum daily fluid intake of 2-3 L/day of fluid.
4. Administer stool softeners (i.e., docusate sodium) daily.
5. If possible, avoid enemas for long-term bowel management, as the SCI patient cannot retain the enema solution. However, if the patient becomes impacted, a gentle small-volume cleansing enema, followed by manual removal of fecal material, may be necessary.
6. Assess patient's readiness for bowel retraining program, including neurologic status and current bowel patterns, noting frequency, amount, and consistency. Usually, bowel retraining is initiated when the patient is neurologically stable and can resume a sitting position.
7. Because use of a bedpan may impair the patient's ability to evacuate the bowel, provide a bedside commode, if allowed.
   * Provide ample time each day for bowel elimination. One-half hour after mealtime coincides with the gastrocolic reflex.
   * Ensure patient's privacy.
   * Stimulate the rectal sphincter with digital stimulation or insert suppository (i.e., bisacodyl) to initiate reflex peristalsis with reflex evacuation.

< C A U T I O N :   See precautions with **Potential for injury** related to risk of AD, p. 300.

- If the patient has upper extremity function, teach patient how to perform digital rectal stimulation, insertion of suppository, and abdominal massage to facilitate bowel movement.

Potential for infection related to vulnerability secondary to presence of invasive immobilization devices

Desired outcome: Patient is free of infection at insertion site for tongs or halo device as evidenced by normothermia and negative cultures and absence of erythema, swelling, warmth, purulent drainage, or tenderness at insertion site.

1. Assess insertion sites q8h for indicators of infection: erythema, swelling, warmth, purulent drainage, and increased or new tenderness. Also be alert to pin migration. If the pin appears to be loose, notify MD and instruct patient to remain still until the pin can be secured.
2. Perform pin care as prescribed. Some physicians advocate cleansing the site with half-strength normal saline and hydrogen peroxide, leaving any superficial crust intact, followed by application of an antibiotic ointment. Others advocate cleansing with hydrogen peroxide and no antibiotic ointment. Some physicians prescribe the application of sterile dressings around the pins, while others prefer to leave the area open to air. Use sterile applicators and follow aseptic technique during the procedure.

Sensory-perceptual alterations related to visual impairment secondary to presence of immobilization device or use of therapeutic bed

Desired outcome: Patient expresses satisfaction with visual capabilities.

1. Assess for factors that limit the patient's visual capabilities: presence of tongs, cervical traction, halo device; and use of Stryker or Foster frame, Roto Rest kinetic treatment table, or circle bed.
2. Provide for increased visualization of patient's surroundings:
   - Obtain prism glasses for patient who must remain supine or is unable to turn his or her head owing to halo traction device. If prism glasses are unavailable, provide a hand mirror for patient with upper extremity function.
   - Position mirrors to increase the amount of area that can be visualized from patient's position.
   - Approach patient and converse within patient's visual field.
   - Keep clocks, calendars, and other personal objects within patient's visual field.

Altered sexuality pattern related to loss of aspects of sexual functioning secondary to SCI

Desired outcomes: Over time, patient expresses acceptance of changes in sexual function and verbalizes knowledge of alternate methods of sexual expression with his or her partner.

1. Assess patient's level of sexual function or loss from a neurologic and psychologic perspective. The general rule for men is that the higher the lesion, the greater the chance of maintaining the ability to have an erection, but with less chance for ejaculation. For women, ovulation may stop for several months due to stress following the injury. However, ovulation usually returns and the woman can become pregnant and have a normal pregnancy. Both men and women with high lesions may experience feelings of excitement similar to a preinjury orgasm.

2. Evaluate your own feelings about sexuality. If you are uncomfortable discussing this subject with the patient, arrange for a knowledgable staff member to speak with patient about his or her concerns.

3. Elicit patient's knowledge, concerns, and questions about his or her sexual function following the spinal cord injury.

4. It is normal for males to experience a reflex erection upon resolution of the spinal shock, particularly for individuals with lesions in the cervical and thoracic areas. Reassure patient that this is normal, and therefore, nothing to be embarrassed about.

5. Expect acting-out behavior related to the patient's sexuality. This is a normal response to the patient's concern regarding his or her sexual prognosis.

6. Provide accurate information regarding expected sexual function in an open, interested manner, based on your assessment of the patient's readiness for information.

7. Facilitate communication between the patient and his or her partner.

8. Refer patient and his or her partner to a sex therapist or other knowledgable rehabilitation professional upon resolution of the critical stages of SCI.

For other nursing diagnoses and interventions, see the following as appropriate: "Management of the Adult on Mechanical Ventilation," pp. 66-70; "Providing Nutritional Support," pp. 490-505; "Caring for the Critically Ill on Prolonged Bed Rest," pp. 506-511; "Caring for the Critically Ill with Life-Threatening Disorders," pp. 511-522; and "Caring for the Family of the Critically Ill," pp. 522-526.

REHABILITATION AND PATIENT-FAMILY TEACHING CONCEPTS

Give patient and significant others verbal and written instructions for the following:

1. Referrals to rehabilitation center, depending on patient's level of injury and rehabilitation potential.

2. Reviews of exercises and assistive devices provided by occupational and physical therapists.

3. Medications, including drug name, purpose, dosage, schedule, precautions, and potential side effects.

4. Signs and symptoms of autonomic dysreflexia, triggering mechanisms, and emergency personnel to contact should it occur. Suggest that patient carry a

Medic-Alert identification card or bracelet to alert emergency personnel to the syndrome should it occur outside the health care setting.

5. Bowel and bladder retraining programs specific to patient.

6. Referrals to social service agency for assistance with financial concerns resulting from the injury.

7. Referrals to community nursing or VNA for professional assistance at home.

8. Indicators of respiratory (SOB, productive cough, bloody sputum, temperature elevation); urinary (cloudy and foul-smelling urine, difficulty with intermittent catheterization, bloody urine); gastrointestinal (nausea, vomiting, incontinence, recurring impaction, blood in vomitus or stool, persistent shoulder pain); circulatory (pain, swelling, redness in lower extremities); and skin (persistent irritation, rash, or area of breakdown) problems that necessitate medical attention.

9. Referrals for follow-up counseling regarding sexual function and expression.

10. Addresses and phone numbers for the following:

National Spinal Cord Injury Association
369 Elliot Street
Newton Upper Falls, MA 02164
Spinal Cord Injury Hot Line: 800-638-1733

American Spinal Injury Association
250 East Superior Street
Room 619
Chicago, Il 60611

Status epilepticus

Status epilepticus is a state of recurring seizures of at least 20 minutes in duration in which the patient does not return to full consciousness from the postictal state before experiencing another seizure. The two major types of status epilepticus are convulsive and nonconvulsive. *Nonconvulsive status* includes absence (petit mal), simple partial (focal), and complex partial (psychomotor or temporal lobe) seizures. *Convulsive status* (generalized tonic-clonic seizures) is the more common type and is considered a life-threatening medical emergency because of the hypoxia and neuronal metabolic exhaustion that occur. Neuronal death is possible.

A common cause of status epilepticus in individuals with epilepsy is noncompliance with medications or a drop in serum levels caused by alcohol abuse or infection. Other causes for individuals with and without preexisting epilepsy include acute metabolic disturbances (hypoglycemia, hyponatremia, hypocalcemia), cerebrovascular accident, central nervous system (CNS) infection (meningitis, encephalitis), CNS trauma or tumors, and alcohol or drug abuse. Prompt treatment is vital in preventing complications such as cardiac dysrhythmias, hyperthermia, aspiration, hypertension, hypotension, anoxia, hyperglycemia, hypoglycemia, dehydration, myoglobinuria, and oral or musculoskeletal injuries. Mortality rate in status epilepticus is 10-12%.

ASSESSMENT

Absence status: Characterized by some alteration in LOC, ranging from a dreamy state to stupor. Automatisms (lip smacking, chewing, swallowing) or mild clonic movements such as fluttering of the eyelids may be present. Clinically, absence status is difficult to differentiate from complex partial status (see below).

Complex partial status: Rare, manifesting as a prolonged confused state or a series of complex partial seizures without return to normal consciousness between seizures. Automatisms and speech difficulty may be present. Once this period of status passes, confusion and sleepiness may ensue.

Simple partial status: The second most common form of status epilepticus, commonly manifested as focal motor status. Usually, consciousness remains intact and motor activity is localized to one area of the body, such as the face or hand. It may last for hours or days.

Convulsive status: The most common form of status epilepticus, it is characterized by generalized tonic-clonic seizures without return to full consciousness.

Ictal coma: If the patient arrives to the critical care area in a coma, subclinical (electrical) seizure activity may be present. Assessment for minor myoclonic jerks, such as fluttering of the eyelids or eye movements, or focal motor activity is imperative.

History and risk factors: Epilepsy, drug or alcohol abuse, recent head injury, infection, headaches. If the patient is taking antiepilepsy medications, record the following: drug name, dosage, time last taken, length of time drug has been taken, and any recent medication changes. Determine whether patient is taking any other medications, including name, dose, and time last taken.

DIAGNOSTIC TESTS

1. *Serum drug screen:* Rules out drug or alcohol intoxication.
2. *Serum electrolytes, BUN, glucose, CBC:* Rule out electrolyte imbalance or metabolic disturbance as the cause of status epilepticus.
3. *Antiepilepsy serum drug level:* To determine the amount of drug in patient's system.
4. *ABG analysis:* To obtain baseline levels and determine state of oxygenation.
5. *EKG:* Evaluates cardiovascular status, especially during administration of drugs such as phenytoin that may lead to hypotension and dysrhythmias.
6. *EEG:* Performed during the seizure and can differentiate between absence or complex partial status.
7. *CT scan:* To rule out presence of a brain lesion.

MEDICAL MANAGEMENT

1. **Maintenance of alveolar ventilation and other vital functions:** Cardiopulmonary function and VS are assessed closely. Oral airway, oxygen, and if necessary, intubation and respiratory support, are initiated.
2. **Prevention of Wernicke-Korsakoff syndrome:** 100 mg IV thiamine and 50 ml of 50% glucose are administered if alcoholism or hypoglycemia is suspected.
3. **Administration of fast-acting anticonvulsant:** Up to 20 mg IV diazepam is given to achieve high serum and brain concentrations. It is not used as a long-acting anticonvulsant.
   - Do not infuse faster than 2 mg/min due to respiratory depression that can occur with faster infusion rate.
   - Monitor respiratory status continuously during administration.
4. **Administration of long-acting anticonvulsant:** IV phenytoin. Usual loading dose is 18 mg/kg.

- Do not infuse faster than 50 mg/min, as hypotension or dysrhythmias can develop.
- Flush line with normal saline only. Microcrystallization occurs when used with dextrose, and also may occur when used in saline as a continuous drip.
- Monitor VS closely.

5. **Diazepam per continuous drip:** If seizures continue.
   - Usual dosage is 100 mg in 500 ml D_5W.
   - Usual delivery is 10-15 mg/hr.
   - Monitor respiratory status continuously.
6. **Administration of IV phenobarbital:** If patient is allergic to phenytoin.
   - Usual dosage is 10-20 mg/kg.
   - Do not give simultaneously with diazepam as both are sedatives and can cause respiratory depression and hypotension.
7. **Paraldehyde, lidocaine, general anesthesia, or neuromuscular blockade:** To stop the seizure activity if interventions 3-6 are ineffective. Neuromuscular blockade will stop the movements but not the electrical activity.
8. **Nutritional support:** Enteral or parenteral nutrition may be necessary, depending on the duration of the status epilepticus and patient's underlying nutritional state.

NURSING DIAGNOSES AND INTERVENTIONS

Potential for injury related to risk of oral and musculoskeletal trauma secondary to seizure activity

---

Desired outcome: Patient's oral cavity and musculoskeletal system do not exhibit evidence of trauma following the seizure.

---

1. Pad the side rails, keep side rails up at all times, maintain bed in its lowest position, and keep an oral airway at the bedside.
2. Perform protective measures during the seizures.
   - Put something soft such as a pillow under patient's head.
   - Move sharp or potentially dangerous objects away from patient.
   - Loosen any tight clothing.
   - Avoid restraining patient, as the force of the tonic-clonic movements could traumatize the patient.
   - Avoid forcing airway into patient's mouth when jaws are clenched. Force could break teeth, causing patient to swallow or aspirate them.
   - Avoid use of tongue blade, which could splinter.
   - Stay with patient; assess and record seizure type and duration. Record any automatic behavior (e.g., lip smacking, chewing movements), motor activity, incontinence, tongue biting, and postictal state.
3. After seizure, reorient and reassure patient.

Impaired gas exchange related to hypoventilation and bradypnea secondary to depressant effect of seizures on respiratory center and increased need for oxygen secondary to continuous seizure activity

Desired outcome: Patient has adequate gas exchange as evidenced by Pao_2 $\geq$80 mm Hg, $Paco_2$ 35-45 mm Hg, pH 7.35-7.45, and RR 12-20 breaths/min with normal depth and pattern (eupnea).

1. Assess patient's respiratory status, including rate, depth, rhythm, and color. Be alert to use of accessory muscles of respiration, rapid or labored respirations, and cyanosis (a late sign of dysfunction).
2. Position an oral airway to help maintain ventilation. To prevent injury, avoid forcing airway into mouth.
3. Keep patient turned to the side to allow secretions to drain; suction as necessary.
4. Monitor ABGs to assess oxygenation. Be alert to hypoxemia (Pao_2 <80 mm Hg) and respiratory acidosis ($Paco_2$ >45 mm Hg and pH <7.35).
5. Keep intubation equipment readily available for airway and ventilation assistance.
6. Administer oxygen as indicated per nasal cannula, mask, or manual resuscitator.
7. Administer antiepilepsy medications within prescribed parameters to avoid further depression of respiratory center.

Alteration in tissue perfusion: Cerebral and cardiopulmonary, related to decreased blood flow to and increased metabolic demands on the cells secondary to continuous seizure activity

Desired outcome: Patient has adequate cerebral and cardiopulmonary perfusion as evidenced by orientation to person, place, and time; normal sinus rhythm on EKG; BP within patient's normal range; RR 12-20 breaths/min with normal depth and pattern (eupnea); and absence of headache, papilledema, and other clinical indicators of increased ICP.

1. Maintain airway and ventilation to ensure maximum delivery of oxygen to the brain cells.
2. Monitor VS q2-4 minutes. Respiratory depression, decreased BP, and dysrhythmias can occur with rapid infusion of diazepam and phenytoin. Blood pressure must be maintained within normal limits for optimal brain perfusion.
3. Monitor cardiac status *via* cardiac monitor. Be alert to dysrhythmias.
4. Ensure safe administration of antiepileptic drugs: diazepam at 2 mg/minute or phenytoin at 50 mg/minute.
5. Perform baseline and serial neurologic assessments to assess for presence of focal findings suggestive of an expanding lesion. See ''Head Injury,'' p. 271, for signs and symptoms of increased intracranial pressure (IICP).

Noncompliance with prescribed medication regimen related to misunderstanding physician's instructions, not understanding importance of following medication schedule, running out of medication, or stopping medication intentionally owing to frustration or denial of the disease

Desired outcome: Patient verbalizes understanding of the rationale and importance of taking the medication as prescribed, as well as the consequence of noncompliance.

1. Determine patient's reason for noncompliance.
2. Assess patient's understanding of epilepsy and its treatment.
3. Ensure that patient is aware that stopping the antiepilepsy medication can result in serious problems, including status epilepticus. Explain that if patient plans to stop the medication for any reason, he or she should do so with physician guidance so that it can be done as safely as possible, although the risk of status epilepticus would remain.
4. Evaluate the effect epilepsy has on patient's lifestyle.
5. Once the problem has been identified, work with the patient to find a solution. For example, if the patient is experiencing a side effect from the medication, such as gastric upset, suggest that patient try taking the medication after meals. If the gastric upset is a result of increasing the medication, advise patient to increase the dose more slowly.
6. Refer patient to regional epilepsy support groups and the Epilepsy Foundation of America (EFA), including regional affiliate and national headquarters.
7. As appropriate, refer patient to nurse specialist or social worker at regional center for individual counseling.

Knowledge deficit: Disease process, treatment, and necessary lifestyle changes for epilepsy

Desired outcome: Patient verbalizes understanding of epilepsy, including the etiology, pathophysiology, and seizure classification, as well as its treatment and necessary lifestyle changes.

1. Assess patient's understanding of epilepsy.
2. As indicated, teach patient about the disease, its etiology, pathophysiology, and seizure classification.
3. Ask patient to describe the seizure(s) in detail, including warning signals (aura) that occur at the beginning of the seizure. Explain to patient that this aura or warning is the beginning of the seizure and patient should lie down or get into a safe position to prevent injury.
4. Assess patient's knowledge of the antiepilepsy medication, including its name, purpose, schedule, dosage, precautions, and side effects. Teach patient the importance of maintaining a constant blood level of the medication by taking the medication every day as prescribed. Explain that if the medication is missed or taken erratically, he or she cannot attain the blood level that is necessary for preventing seizure breakthrough. If a dose of medication is missed, instruct patient to notify his or her physician.
5. Advise patient that a normal life is possible.
6. Teach patient that sleep deprivation can precipitate SE and that each individual must know his or her own limits. However, having epilepsy does not mean that it is necessary to get more sleep than do individuals who do not have epilepsy.

7. Teach patient and signficant others the safety interventions that should be made during a seizure (see **Potential for injury** related to risk of oral and musculoskeletal trauma, p. 314). In addition, explain the importance of easing patient to the floor and turning patient into a side-lying position.

8. Inform patient of the state driving regulations for individuals with epilepsy.

9. Teach patient the importance of avoiding dangerous machinery and heights if his or her seizures are not being controlled adequately by medications.

Ineffective individual coping related to frustration secondary to unpredictable nature of the disease

---

Desired outcome: Patient verbalizes feelings, identifies strengths and ineffective coping behaviors, and demonstrates a responsible role in his or her own care.

---

1. Assess patient's knowledge of the disease and its treatment. See **Knowledge deficit**, on the preceding page.

2. Encourage patient to express feelings of frustration so that you can evaluate areas of major concern.

3. Involve patient in decisions regarding care so that he or she has more of a sense of control over the disease. For example, encourage patient to participate in the decision for scheduling the medications.

4. Help patient set realistic goals for employment and living arrangements. Refer patient to regional or local Epilepsy Foundation of America (EFA) as appropriate.

5. To involve patient in self-care, encourage him or her to educate others in what to do should the patient have a seizure.

6. Encourage patient's involvement in support groups, where patient may learn coping strategies from other individuals with the same disorder.

7. For more interventions, see the same nursing diagnosis in the appendicized section, ''Caring for the Critically Ill with Life-Threatening Disorders,'' p. 516.

For other nursing diagnoses and interventions, see the following as appropriate: ''Management of the Adult on Mechanical Ventilation,'' pp. 66-70; ''Caring for the Critically Ill with Life-Threatening Disorders,'' pp. 511-522; and ''Caring for the Family of the Critically Ill,'' pp. 522-526.

REHABILITATION AND PATIENT-FAMILY TEACHING CONCEPTS

Give patient and significant others verbal and written instructions for the following:

1. Review of the disease process, causes, and classification of seizure type.

2. Medications, including drug name, purpose, dosage, schedule, precautions, side effects, and procedure to follow if a dose is missed.

3. Importance of follow-up care. Provide telephone numbers of MD or nurse specialist for questions or emergencies that may occur after hospital discharge.

4. Importance of periodic blood work for evaluation of antiepilepsy medication blood levels.

5. Safety interventions during seizures.

6. State driving regulations for individuals with epilepsy.

7. Importance of obtaining a Medic-Alert bracelet to inform emergency personnel of the disorder and medications that are being taken.
8. Referrals for counseling, support groups, or vocational rehabilitation.
9. Referrals to regional epilepsy center and EFA affiliate. In addition, provide the following address: Epilepsy Foundation of America, 4351 Garden City Drive, Suite 406, Landover, Maryland 20785.

Drug overdose

Drug overdose is a problem that is widespread, affecting all ages, races, and socioeconomic levels. The primary effects of drug overdose are seen on the neurologic, cardiovascular, and respiratory systems. Oftentimes, the drug can be identified by history, family or friends, and physical findings. Prognosis varies, depending on the rapidity of treatment and the amount and type of drug ingested.

ASSESSMENT

1. **Amphetamines** (amphetamine, dextroamphetamine, methamphetamine)
   - *Indicators of acute intoxication:* Anxiety, hyperactivity, irritability, repeated compulsive movements, tooth grinding, aggressive or violent behavior, paranoia, psychoses, hallucinations, vomiting, diarrhea, seizures.
   - *Physical assessment:* Rapid HR, dilated pupils, and signs of malnutrition. The presence of needle marks, scars from abscesses, thrombophlebitis, and elevated temperature may alert the examiner to IV use of these drugs.
   - *Life-threatening effects:* Cardiac dysrhythmias, seizures, respiratory arrest, coma.
   - *Drug half-life:* As long as one week.
   - *Lethal dose for adult:* 1.5 grams/kg.
2. **Barbiturates** (amobarbital, secobarbital, pentobarbital, phenobarbital, butabarbital)
   - *Indicators of acute intoxication.* Decreased mental alertness (change in LOC), respiratory depression leading to apnea, flaccid extremities, seizures.
   - *Physical assessment:* Bradycardia (HR ≤60 bpm), decreased BP, decreased or absent deep tendon reflexes (DTRs), hypothermia, nystagmus, reactive pupils, absent oculocephalic reflex (Doll's eyes), cool and dry skin.
   - *Life-threatening effects:* Increasing CNS depression leading to coma; respiratory depression leading to apnea, cardiovascular collapse, and death.
   - *Drug half-life:* Varies from 8 hours to as along as 6 days, according to the drug used.
   - *Lethal dose:* Varies from patient to patient, depending on patient's drug history and whether or not alcohol or other drugs are involved.
   - *Level of barbiturate intoxication:* See Table 4-4. This grading system may be helpful in determining patient's prognosis and treatment plan.
3. **Cocaine**
   - *Indicators of acute intoxication:* Delirium, aggressive behavior, paranoia, agitation, hallucinations, tremors, seizures.
   - *Physical assessment:* Elevated temperature progressing to malignant hyperthermia, increased HR, elevated BP, tachypnea, dilated pupils, abnormal respiratory patterns (e.g., Cheyne-Stokes) leading to apnea and respiratory failure, status epilepticus. In addition, patient may present with needle marks or

T A B L E   4 - 4
Classification of barbiturate intoxication

Group 0   Asleep, arousable, will follow commands and answer questions.
Group I   Unconscious, unarousable, withdraws from noxious stimuli appropriately,
            DTRs present, corneal reflex may be absent.
Group II   Unconscious, unarousable, no appropriate response to noxious stimuli, DTRs
            present, no cardiorespiratory depression.
Group III   Unconscious, no response to stimuli, DTRs and other reflexes absent, no car-
            diorespiratory depression.
Group IV   Unconscious, unresponsive, DTRs absent, respiratory failure, hypotension,
            cardiovascular collapse.

< N O T E :   If the individual with barbiturate overdose receives medical attention before
experiencing cardiorespiratory collapse with CNS damage, he or she may recover completely.

tracks from injection of cocaine, a perforated nasal septum from prolonged
inhalation of the substance, and a single long fingernail for scooping the cocaine for inhalation.
- *Life-threatening effects:* Cardiovascular collapse. Sometimes the agent used to
  cut the cocaine (e.g., lidocaine) causes the cardiovascular collapse that can
  lead to death. Lidocaine can cause hypotension, CNS depression, and seizures, which may precipitate status epilepticus and death.
- *Half-life:* 60 minutes.

4. **Nonbarbiturate CNS depressants:** Benzodiazepines (diazepam, chlordiazepox-
   ide), chloral hydrate, ethchlorvynol, glutethimide, methaqualone. The indicators
   of overdose with these drugs are similar to those of barbiturates, with a few
   specific exceptions listed below.
   - *Benzodiazepines* (e.g., Valium, Librium): Ataxia, hypotonia, hypotension,
     prolonged sleep, respiratory depression, coma.
   - *Chloral hydrate* (Noctec, Somnos): Miosis. The toxic dose is approximately
     10 grams, although death has occurred with as little as 4 grams.
   - *Ethchlorvynol* (Placidyl): Prolonged, deep coma; nystagmus; pancytopenia.
   - *Glutethimide* (Doriden): Dilated pupils, depressed or absent corneal and pu-
     pillary reflexes, diminished or absent peristalsis, muscle spasms, seizure. Al-
     though lethal dose is reported to be 10-20 grams, individuals have died with
     as little as 5 grams and survived after 35 grams.

5. **Opiates:** Codeine sulfate, morphine sulfate, meperidine hydrochloride, heroin,
   hydromorphone hydrochloride, opium, oxycodone hydrochloride, oxymorphone
   hydrochloride, methadone hydrochloride.
   - *Indicators of acute intoxication:* Depressed mental status, somnolence, sei-
     zures, pulmonary edema, cardiogenic shock.
   - *Physical assessment:* Cool and moist skin; flaccid skeletal muscles; pupils that
     are equal, pinpoint, and reactive; hypothermia, bradycardia, decreased BP,
     hypoventilation, cyanotic skin and mucous membranes. The individual may
     have needle marks or tracks.
   - *Life-threatening effects:* Usually occurs with IV administration of overdose
     resulting in apnea, circulatory collapse, generalized seizures, and cardiopul-
     monary arrest, which causes death.

6. *Tricyclic antidepressants:* Amitriptyline hydrochloride (Elavil), doxepin hydrochloride (Sinequan), imipramine hydrochloride (Presamine, Tofranil), trimipramine maleate (Surmontil).
   - *Indicators of acute intoxication:* Hyperpyrexia, pupillary dilation, hypertension, tachycardia.
   - *Physical assessment:* Increased BP and HR; dry skin and mucous membranes, dilated pupils.
   - *Life-threatening effects:* Coma, seizures, cardiac dysrhythmias, cardiac conduction defects.
7. *Alcohol*
   - *Indicators of acute intoxication:* Confusion, aggressive behavior, memory lapses.
   - *Pre-delirium indicators.* Nausea, vomiting, irritability, tremulousness.
   - *Findings after abrupt withdrawal:* Delirium tremens (see p. 324).

Nursing history: Indicators of suicide attempt (i.e., note, previous attempts); circumstances surrounding the overdose; whether or not patient is under psychiatric care; patient's family situation; medical illness; education and employment status; known abuser.

< N O T E :   If a suicide attempt is suspected, facilitate a referral to psychiatric liaison and social services, as appropriate.

DIAGNOSTIC TESTS

1. *Toxicology screen (serum and urine):* To detect and identify the presence and type of drug.
2. *Serum alcohol:* To detect presence and amount of alcohol in the blood.
3. *Hematologic studies:* CBC to rule out infection and check platelet count in suspected ASA overdose; and electrolytes, blood sugar, liver function studies, BUN, and creatinine to evaluate for the presence of metabolic dysfunction. Hepatitis screen is done because of the high rate of serum hepatitis in the IV drug user population.
4. *Serology:* To assess for sexually-transmitted diseases.
5. *Human immunodeficiency virus (HIV):* To check for AIDS owing to the high rate of this disorder among the IV drug abuser population. (Check institutional policies regarding confidentiality.)
6. *Lumbar puncture:* To rule out neuroinfectious diseases as a cause of the comatose state. It is done only in the *absence* of papilledema, which would signal presence of increased ICP.
7. *CT scan:* To rule out intracranial pathology.
8. *EKG:* To evaluate for cardiac dysrhythmias.
9. *Chest x-ray:* To obtain baseline data on the pulmonary system; rule out aspiration pneumonia, which can occur with barbiturates, nonbarbiturate CNS depressants, cocaine, and amphetamines; and assess for pulmonary edema, which can occur with opiates.
10. *ABG analysis:* To obtain baseline data for respiratory management.
11. *EEG:* To evaluate brain wave activity.

< N O T E :   An isoelectric (flat) reading, which may be mistaken for brain death, may be seen in extreme barbiturate overdose.

MEDICAL MANAGEMENT

The following interventions are directed toward treatment of the comatose state.

1. **Respiratory management:** To maintain airway, respirations, and therapeutic oxygen levels. As indicated, pulmonary edema and aspiration pneumonia are treated, as well. See "Acute Pneumonia," p. 7 and "Congestive Heart Failure/ Pulmonary Edema," p. 86 for management.

2. **Cardiovascular management:** To maintain adequate systemic circulation. Modalities of therapy will depend on the symptoms that result from the specific drug taken. Hemodynamic monitoring may be necessary. See "Management of the Adult with Hemodynamic Monitoring," p. 167, as appropriate.

3. **Fluids and electrolytes:** Type and amount will depend on the state of hydration, presence of medical complications (e.g., pulmonary edema), cardiovascular status, and type of drug used by patient. For detail, refer to specific medical disorders throughout the text.

4. **Nutrition:** Usually the patient is given parenteral nutrition or intralipids until bowel sounds return and the GI system returns to normal. Then enteral feedings are begun until the patient can tolerate an oral diet.

5. **Pharmacotherapy**
   - *Antihypertensives:* For treatment of hypertension seen with overdose of cocaine, amphetamines, and tricyclic antidepressants.
   - *Vasopressors:* To treat hypotension seen in overdose of opiates, barbiturates, and nonbarbiturate CNS depressants.
   - *Antiarrhythmics:* To treat cardiac dysrhythmias that may occur with overdose of any drug.
   - *Antipyretics:* ASA or acetaminophen as indicated for fever.
   - *Anticonvulsants:* To treat seizures and status epilepticus. For detail, see "Status Epilepticus," p. 313.
   - *Narcotic antagonists:* For example, naloxone hydrochloride (Narcon), to reverse the neurologic and respiratory depressant effects of narcotics.
   - *Antibiotics:* To treat the complications of aspiration pneumonia, cellulitis, septicemia, and endocarditis.
   - *L-tryptophan:* Amino acid that promotes sleep.

6. **Maintenance of normothermia:** If antipyretics are ineffective, a cooling blanket may be used to control hyperthermia. Tranquilizers such as chlorpromazine may be given to control shivering.

7. **Treatment of complications:** The following may occur: aspiration pneumonia (see "Acute Pneumonia," p. 7), pulmonary edema (see "Congestive Heart Failure/Pulmonary Edema," p. 86), septicemia (see "Sepsis," p. 433), bacterial endocarditis (see "Acute Infective Endocarditis," p. 110), shock (see "Cardiogenic Shock," p. 133), hepatitis (see "Hepatic Failure," p. 364), hypertensive crisis (See "Hypertensive Crisis," p. 122), cardiac dysrhythmias (see "Dysrhythmias and Conduction Disturbances," p. 95), status epilepticus (See "Status Epilepticus," p. 312), malignant hyperthermia, malnutrition (See "Providing Nutritional Support," p. 490), and perforated nasal septum.

NURSING DIAGNOSES AND INTERVENTIONS

Fluid volume deficit (with concomitant electrolyte imbalance) related to decreased intake secondary to decreased LOC; or decreased circulating volume secondary to vomiting or diaphoresis

Desired outcomes: Patient is normovolemic as evidenced by urine output ≥30 ml/ hr, BP within patient's normal range, stable weights, urine specific gravity 1.010- 1.030, HR ≤100 bpm, CVP 2-6 mm Hg, PAWP 6-12 mm Hg, and absence of thirst and other clinical indicators of dehydration. Serum potassium is 3.5-5.5 mEq/ L, serum osmolality is 275-300 mOsm/kg, urine osmolality is 300-1090 mOsm/kg, BUN is 10-20 mg/dl, serum creatinine is 0.7-1.5 mg/dl, urine sodium is 40-180 mEq/24 hrs (diet dependent), hematocrit is 37%-47% (female) or 40%-54% (male), and serum protein is 6.0-8.3 g/dl.

1. Monitor hydration status on an ongoing basis. Be alert to continuing dehydra- tion as evidenced by poor skin turgor, dry mucous membranes, complaints of thirst, weight loss >0.5 kg/day, urine specific gravity >1.030, weak pulse with tachycardia, and postural hypotension.
2. Assess for indicators of electrolyte imbalance, in particular presence of hypo- kalemia. Be alert to irregular pulse, cardiac dysrhythmias, and serum potassium level <3.5 mEq/L.
3. Monitor I&O hourly; assess for output elevated out of proportion to intake, bearing in mind the insensible losses.
4. Monitor lab values, including serum electrolytes, and serum and urine osmolal- ity. Be alert to BUN elevated out of proportion to the serum creatinine (indi- cator of dehydration rather than renal disease), high urine specific gravity, low urine sodium, and rising hematocrit and serum protein concentration.
5. Maintain fluid intake as prescribed; administer prescribed electrolyte supple- ments.

Sensory-perceptual alterations related to disorientation, agitation, and hallucina- tions secondary to drug overdose and withdrawal symptoms

Desired outcome: Patient verbalizes orientation to person, place, and time.

1. At frequent intervals, assess patient's orientation to person, place, and time. Reorient as necessary.
2. Orient patient to the unit and explain all procedures before performing them. Include significant others in orientation process.
3. Do not leave patient alone if he or she is agitated or confused.
4. Maintain a calm, quiet environment to minimize patient's sensory overload. Dim lights when possible.
5. Administer antianxiety agents as prescribed.
6. If patient is hallucinating, intervene in the following ways:
   • Be reassuring. Explain that hallucinations may be very real to patient but that they are not real, they are caused by the substance patient consumed, and will go away eventually.
   • As appropriate, try to involve family and significant others, as patient may have more trust in them.
   • Explain that restraints are necessary to prevent harm to patient and others. Reassure patient that restraints will be kept on only as long as they are

needed. As indicated, suggest to patient that you may release one restraint at a time as patient's condition improves.

- Tell patient that you will check on him or her at frequent intervals (e.g., q5-10min), or that you will stay at patient's side.

Potential impaired gas exchange or ineffective airway clearance related to hypoventilation, suppression of cough reflex, and decreased diffusion of oxygen secondary to respiratory depressant effects of drugs, accumulation of pulmonary secretions, and pulmonary edema occurring with drug use or overdose

---

Desired outcome: Patient has adequate respiratory function as evidenced by Pao_2 ≥80 mm Hg; $Paco_2$ 35-45 mm Hg; pH 7.35-7.45; RR 12-20 breaths/min with normal depth and pattern (eupnea); clear sputum; presence of normal breath sounds; and absence of adventitious breath sounds, restlessness, and other clinical indicators of respiratory dysfunction.

---

1. Assess respiratory function hourly and prn. Be alert to alterations, including rapid, shallow, irregular, or slow respirations; dyspnea; use of accessory muscles of respiration; decreased or absent breath sounds; adventitious breath sounds (e.g., crackles, rhonchi); restlessness and confusion; and cyanosis (a late sign).
2. Monitor ABG values for evidence of hypoxemia (Pao_2 <80 mm Hg) and respiratory acidosis ($Paco_2$ >45 mm Hg and pH <7.35).
3. Assess amount, color, and consistency of sputum. Be alert to frothy pink sputum, which is a sign of pulmonary edema, and to greenish-yellow sputum, which can occur with pneumonia.
4. Turn patient q2h. Teach patient to deep breathe and cough hourly, if awake. Instruct alert patient to use incentive spirometer q2h.
5. If patient is not intubated, raise HOB 30 degrees to facilitate gas exchange.
6. If patient is intubated monitor for the presence of rhonchi and crackles (rales) and suction as needed. See section "Management of the Adult on Mechanical Ventilation," p. 61.
7. Administer oxygen and perform chest physiotherapy as prescribed.
8. Administer prescribed medications (e.g., antibiotics, antipyretics, diuretics).
9. Increase activity as allowed and tolerated to mobilize and prevent stasis of secretions.

Ineffective thermoregulation related to fluctuations secondary to sympathetic response occurring with cocaine overdose

---

Desired outcome: Patient remains normothermic.

---

1. Monitor for signs of hyperthermia: temperature >38.3° C (>101° F), pallor, absence of perspiration, and torso that is warm to the touch.
2. As prescribed, obtain blood, urine, and sputum cultures to rule out underlying infection.

3. If patient is hyperthermic, remove excess clothing and administer tepid baths, a cooling blanket, or ice bags to the axillae and groin.
4. Administer antipyretics as prescribed.

See "Head Injury" for the following: **Potential alteration in tissue integrity: Corneal,** related to inability to blink secondary to altered LOC, p. 280. See "Status Epilepticus" for the following: **Potential for injury** related to risk of oral and musculoskeletal trauma secondary to seizure activity, p. 314. Also see "Providing Nutritional Support," pp. 490-505; "Caring for the Critically Ill with Life-Threatening Disorders," pp. 511-522; and "Caring for the Family of the Critically Ill," pp. 522-526.

REHABILITATION AND PATIENT-FAMILY TEACHING CONCEPTS

Give patient and significant others verbal and written instructions for the following:
1. Referrals to community resources as appropriate: VNA, physical therapy, occupational therapy, cognitive retraining specialists, Narcotics Anonymous, halfway houses, drug treatment centers, individual and family counseling, and employee assistance programs.
2. Importance of follow-up care with MD and support services for primary drug problem and its complications.
3. Appropriate diet and vitamin and mineral supplements to treat malnutrition.

Delirium tremens

Delirium tremens (DTs) is an acute psychophysiologic response to the sudden cessation of alcohol consumption in an individual who is an ethanol abuser or one who has been drinking excessively for a prolonged period. The onset can occur within 3 days of the alcohol cessation or as long as 4 weeks later. DTs can be an isolated medical emergency or it can occur concurrently with other illnesses such as pneumonia, pancreatitis, and alcohol hepatitis. The mortality rate is 5-15% for uncomplicated DTs and as high as 25% when associated with other disorders. Death is attributed to dehydration, oversedation, excessive psychomotor agitation, infection, fat emboli, hyperpyrexia, hypertension, and dysrhythmias associated with hypokalemia.

ASSESSMENT

Indicators of mild alcohol withdrawal: Tremors, irritability, disorientation, insomnia, anxiety, sensory hyperactivity, diaphoresis, hyperreflexia, vomiting, diarrhea, tachycardia, tachypnea, hypertension, hyperthermia (slight).

Indicators of DTs: (Most evident 48-60 hours after cessation of alcohol) diaphoresis, tremors, insomnia, hypertension, global confusion, urinary incontinence, and seizures. In addition, patient may have visual, auditory, tactile, and (rarely) olfactory hallucinations.

Physical assessment: Poor skin turgor, dry mucous membranes, increased HR (>100 bpm), rectal temperature >38° C (100.2° F), increased RR (>20 breaths/min), hepatomegaly, splenomegaly, peripheral edema, ascites, increased BP, dilated pupils, hyperreflexia, altered mental state.

DIAGNOSTIC TESTS

1. *Serum alcohol level:* To determine blood level of alcohol.

< N O T E : In the chronic alcoholic, tolerance is increased so a high level may be expected. However, test results may be very low or negative at the onset of DTs.

2. *Toxicology screen:* To rule out presence of drugs.
3. *CBC:* To rule out anemia, infection, and liver dysfunction.
4. *Liver function tests:* To rule out hepatic disease.
5. *Electrolytes, BUN, creatinine, blood sugar:* To rule out dehydration, renal disease, or hypoglycemia.

< C A U T I O N : Alcohol causes depletion of liver glycogen stores and impairment of gluconeogenesis, resulting in hypoglycemia.

6. *T_3, T_4, TSH:* To rule out thyroid storm.
7. *CT scan:* To rule out intracranial pathology.
8. *Lumbar puncture:* To rule out meningitis, as symptoms are similar to those of DTs.

MEDICAL MANAGEMENT

1. Bedrest with mechanical restraint: Protects patient and others from injury due to patient's severely agitated state.

< N O T E : If patient is seizing, do not restrain, as it may cause injury.

2. Nutritional support: Depending on patient's nutritional state, may involve enteral feedings or parenteral nutrition and intralipids.
3. Rehydration: Most patients experience a fluid deficit and require fluid replacement of 4-10 liters in the first 24 hours, with careful replacement thereafter, calculated by I&O and estimated insensible losses.
4. Electrolyte replacement: Potassium, sodium, chloride, glucose, and magnesium, as well as glucose, may be replaced, depending on laboratory values.
5. Pharmacotherapy
   - *Tranquilizers or antianxiety medications:* For example, benzodiazepines, which may be given IV or PO.
   - *Anticonvulsants:* To treat seizures and status epilepticus (see "Status Epilepticus," p. 312).
   - *Thiamine:* 100 mg IV given on admission prior to glucose administration to prevent Wernicke-Korsakoff syndrome and then 100 mg PO daily.
   - *Multivitamins and minerals (C and B-complex):* To treat malnutrition and dehydration.
   - *Antipyretics:* ASA or acetaminophen to treat fever.
6. Treatment of Wernicke-Korsakoff syndrome: Wernicke's encephalopathy, which is seen in chronic alcoholics, is a thiamine deficiency disease manifested by confusion, memory loss, ataxia, nystagmus, extraocular movement dysfunctions, stupor, and coma. Korsakoff's psychosis is manifested by poor memory, disorientation, and confabulation. Thiamine is administered to treat this syndrome, although a significant response may not be seen.

< C A U T I O N : If glucose is administered before thiamine in a thiamine-deficient individual, it may precipitate Wernicke's encephalopathy.

NURSING DIAGNOSES AND INTERVENTIONS

Fluid volume deficit (with concomitant electrolyte imbalance) related to decreased circulating volume secondary to vomiting, diaphoresis, or prolonged dehydration

---

Desired outcomes: Patient is normovolemic as evidenced by urine output ≥ 30 ml/hr, urine specific gravity 1.010-1.030, stable weights, balanced I&O (considering insensible losses), CVP 2-6 mm Hg, PAWP 6-12 mm Hg, BP within patient's normal range, HR 60-100 bpm, and absence of thirst and other clinical indicators of dehydration. Serum potassium is 3.5-5.5 mEq/L.

---

1. Monitor hydration status on an ongoing basis. Be alert to continuing dehydration, as evidenced by poor skin turgor, dry mucous membranes, complaints of thirst, weight loss >0.5 kg/day, and urine specific gravity >1.035.
2. Assess for indicators of electrolyte imbalance, in particular those of hypokalemia. Be alert to irregular pulse, cardiac dysrhythmias, and serum potassium level <3.5 mEq/L. For detail and treatment, see "Hypokalemia," p. 226.
3. Monitor I&O hourly.
4. Maintain IV fluid intake as prescribed, typically 6 L/first 24 hours, which is titrated according to daily I&O. Encourage oral intake if patient can take oral fluids.
5. Because of the rapid and large infusions of IV fluids, monitor patient for evidence of fluid volume excess: dyspnea, crackles (rales), peripheral edema, change in mental status.
6. Administer prescribed electrolyte supplements. Assess patient and lab values for evidence of improvement. Refer to appropriate section(s) in "Fluid and Electrolyte Disturbances," pp. 214-237, for detail.

Sleep pattern disturbance related to confusion and agitation secondary to DTs; and deprivation of REM sleep secondary to alcohol ingestion

---

Desired outcomes: Patient verbalizes that adequate rest and sleep are being attained. Patient rests undisturbed for 90-120 minute periods.

---

1. As prescribed, administer antianxiety medication. Assess for its effects, including oversedation, which also can interrupt sleep patterns.
2. Provide a calm and quiet environment for patient, minimizing environmental stimuli as much as possible. For example, dim the lights and limit visitors so that patient can sleep.
3. Group nursing care activities so that patient can have periods of uninterrupted sleep or rest, optimally 90-120 minutes at a time.

Impaired gas exchange related to decreased diffusion of oxygen secondary to shallow breathing pattern and accumulation of pulmonary secretions occurring with chronic alcoholism (i.e., due to pneumonia or pulmonary edema) and the possibility of oversedation during treatment

Desired outcome: Patient has adequate gas exchange as evidenced by PaO_2 ≥80 mm Hg; RR 12-20 breaths/min of normal pattern and depth (eupnea); orientation to person, place, and time; presence of normal breath sounds; and absence of adventitious breath sounds and other clinical indicators of respiratory dysfunction.

1. Assess respiratory function hourly and prn. Be alert to alterations including rapid, shallow, irregular, or slow respirations; dysnpea; use of accessory muscles of respiration; decreased or absent breath sounds; adventitious breath sounds (e.g., crackles, rhonchi); restlessness and confusion; and cyanosis (a late sign).
2. Monitor ABG values for evidence of hypoxemia.
3. Assess amount, color, and consistency of sputum. Patients with pneumonia may have thick, yellow-green sputum; patients with pulmonary edema may have large amounts of pink and frothy sputum.
4. Turn patient q2h to help prevent stasis of secretions. Teach patient to deep breathe and cough hourly. Instruct patient in use of incentive spirometer, if he or she is capable of following directions for use.
5. Raise HOB 30 degrees to facilitate gas exchange.
6. If patient is intubated, monitor for presence of rhonchi and crackles (rales) and suction as needed.
7. Administer oxygen and perform chest physiotherapy as prescribed.
8. Administer antibiotics as prescribed.
9. Increase activity as allowed and tolerated to mobilize secretions.

See "Drug Overdose" for the following: **Sensory-perceptual alterations** related to disorientation, agitation, and hallucinations, p. 322. See "Status Epilepticus" for the following: **Potential for injury** related to risk of oral and musculoskeletal trauma secondary to seizure activity, p. 314. As appropriate, see nursing diagnoses and interventions in the following: "Providing Nutritional Support," pp. 490-505; "Caring for the Critically Ill with Life-Threatening Disorders," pp. 511-522; and "Caring for the Family of the Critically Ill," pp. 522-526.

REHABILITATION AND PATIENT-FAMILY TEACHING CONCEPTS

Give patient and significant others verbal and written instructions for the following:
1. Referrals to community agencies, Alcoholics Anonymous, Al-Anon, Al-a-teen, detoxication centers, halfway houses, outpatient psychiatric care, as appropriate.
2. Medications, including drug name, purpose, dosage, schedule, side effects, and precautions. Explain that certain foods and drugs (e.g., cough medicine, mouthwash) contain alcohol and should be avoided.
3. Importance of follow-up care with MD and support services for medical problems, including malnutrition.
4. Appropriate diet and vitamin and mineral supplements to promote optimal nutrition status.

SELECTED REFERENCES

Bell J, Hannon K: Pathophysiology involved in autonomic dysreflexia. *J Neuro Nurs* 1986; 18 (2): 86-88.

Bolan F, Barza M: Acute Bacterial Meningitis in Children and Adults. *Med Clin N Am* 1985; 69(2): 231-239.

Browne T, Feldman R: *Epilepsy Diagnosis and Management*. Little, Brown, 1983.

Centers for Disease Control 1981-1986: Guidelines for Isolation Precautions. In: *Guidelines for Prevention and Control of Nosocomial Infections*. US Department of Health and Human Services.

Cloward RB: Acute cervical spine injuries. *Clin Symp* 1980; 32(1).

Delgado-Esculta A, Bajorek J: Status epilepticus: Mechanisms of brain damage and rational management. *Epilepsia* 1982; 23 (Suppl. 1): 529-541.

Delgado-Esculta, et al: Management of status epilepticus. *New Eng J Med* 1982; 306 (22): 1337-1340.

Hickey JV: *The Clinical Practice of Neurological and Neurosurgical Nursing*. Lippincott, 1981.

Ingersoll GL: Abdominal pathology in spinal cord injured persons. *J Neuro Nurs* 1985; 17(6): 343-348.

Jeannett B, Teasdale G: *Management of Head Injuries*. FA Davis, 1981.

Kess R: Suddenly in crisis: Unpredictable myasthenia. *Am J Nurs* 1984; 87(8) 994-998.

Koski CL: Guillain-Barre syndrome. *Neurol Clin* 1984; 2(2): 355-36.

LeFrock J, Smith B: Gram-negative bacillary meningitis. *Med Clin N Am* 1985; 69(2): 243-251.

Leppik I: Status epilepticus. *Clin Ther* 1985; 7(2): 272-278.

Molavi A, LeFrock J: Tuberculous meningitis. *Med Clin N Am* 1985; 69(2): 315-328.

Mitchell PH: Intracranial hypertension: Implications of research for nursing care. *J Neurosurg Nurs,* 1980; 12: 145-153.

Noroian EL: Myathenia gravis: A nursing perspective. *J Neuro Nurs;* 18(2): 74-80.

Persaud DH: Assessing sexual functions of the adult with traumatic quadriplegia. *J Neuro Nurs* 1986; 18(1): 11-12.

Plum F, Posner J: *Diagnosis of Stupor and Coma, 3rd edition*. FA Davis, 1980.

Porter R: *Epilepsy: 100 Elementary Principles*. Saunders, 1984.

Ratzan K: Viral meningitis. *Med Clin N Am* 1985; 69(2): 399-411.

Redelman K: Neurological Injuries. *Crit Care Qu* 1979; 2(1).

Rudy EB: *Advanced Neurological and Neurosurgical Nursing*. Mosby, 1984.

Swift CM: Neurologic Disorders. In: *Manual of Nursing Therapeutics: Applying Nursing Diagnoses to Medical Disorders*. Swearingen PL (ed). Addison-Wesley, 1986.

Taylor JW, Ballinger S: Neurological Dysfunctions and Nursing Interventions. McGraw-Hill, 1980.

Tindall GT, Fleisher AS: Head injury. *Hosp Med,* 1976; 12: 89-110.

Weinstein L: Bacterial meningitis. *Med Clin N Am* 1985; 69(2): 219-229.

5
ENDOCRINOLOGIC
DYSFUNCTIONS

Diabetic ketoacidosis

Hyperosmolar hyperglycemic nonketotic coma

Diabetes insipidus

Syndrome of inappropriate antidiuretic hormone

Addisonian crisis

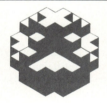

Diabetic ketoacidosis

Diabetic ketoacidosis (DKA) is a life-threatening condition resulting from insulin deficiency or an inability of the cells to utilize available insulin. Because insulin facilitates the use of glucose by body tissues, a deficiency of this hormone leads to decreased cellular uptake of plasma glucose as well as an increased release of glucose from the liver. In addition, increased glucagon is released from the pancreas, promoting the conversion of glycogen to glucose in the liver. The result of these three actions is plasma hyperglycemia with intracellular starvation. Plasma hyperglycemia produces an osmotic diuresis, with concomitant loss of sodium and potassium, and can lead to severe dehydration and hypovolemic shock. Thromboembolism can occur owing to dehydration with increased blood viscosity and platelet aggregation and adhesiveness. Cerebrovascular accident can occur as a result of decreased cerebral perfusion or thromboemboli.

When cells are unable to use glucose, the body is forced to break down fats and protein to produce the energy necessary for cell function. Protein depletion decreases the body's ability to fight disease, while the plasma hyperglycemia encourages bacterial growth, making individuals with DKA extremely susceptible to infection. Fat breakdown increases the amount of plasma ketones and leads to ketoacidosis. In addition, dehydration decreases tissue perfusion, resulting in lactic acidosis. The lowered pH stimulates the respiratory center, producing the deep, rapid respirations known as Kussmaul respirations. The large amount of ketones lends a fruity or acetone odor to the breath. If not treated promptly, the acidosis and dehydration depress consciousness to the point of coma. Left untreated, death may result from hypovolemia or central nervous system depression.

ASSESSMENT

Signs and symptoms: Polyuria, polydipsia, polyphagia, weight loss, fatigue, nausea, vomiting, and abdominal pain.

Physical assessment: Dry, flushed skin; dry mucous membranes; poor skin turgor; hypotension; tachycardia; altered LOC (irritability, lethargy, coma); fruity odor to the breath.

History and risk factors: Type I (insulin-dependent) diabetes mellitus; recent psychologic, emotional, or physical stressors such as surgery, trauma, pregnancy, or infection (most episodes of DKA are precipitated by infection); insufficient exogenous insulin replacement; undiagnosed diabetes mellitus; heredity.

EKG and hemodynamic findings: EKG may show dysrhythmias associated with hyperkalemia: peaked T waves, widened QRS, prolonged P-R intervals, flattened to absent P wave. As hyperkalemia worsens, these signs are progressive, in the order given, and may lead to asystole. CVP may be <2 mm Hg and PAWP <6 mm Hg. After treatment, hypokalemia is possible as manifested by the following EKG findings: flat or inverted T waves, depressed ST-segments, or increased ventricular dysrhythmias.

< N O T E : For more assessment information, see Table 5-2, p. 338, Comparison of DKA to HHNC (hyperosmolar hyperglycemic nonketotic coma).

DIAGNOSTIC TESTS

See Table 5-2, p. 338.

MEDICAL MANAGEMENT

1. **Rehydration:** Usually, normal saline or 0.45% saline is administered until plasma glucose falls to between 200-300 mg/dl. After that, dextrose-containing solutions usually are given to prevent rebound hypoglycemia. Initially, IV fluids are administered rapidly (i.e., 200-300 ml/hr).

2. **Rapid-acting insulin:** Usually given IV for rapid action and because poor tissue perfusion caused by dehydration makes SC route less effective. The initial dose may vary between 10-25 units or 0.3 u/kg. Then the patient is maintained on 5-10 units per hour or 0.1 u/kg/hr as a continuous infusion. Dosage is adjusted, based on serial glucose levels.

3. **Restoration of electrolyte balance:** Sodium is replaced with IV normal saline. Potassium must be monitored and replaced carefully because potassium returns to the intracellular compartment following correction of acidosis and the patient is then at risk of becoming hypokalemic. Use of phosphorus replacement is controversial. Recent studies suggest that there is no difference in the outcome of patients who receive phosphorus replacement than those who do not.

4. **IV bicarbonate:** For pH <7.1. Its use is limited because acidosis will be corrected by insulin therapy. Excessive use of sodium bicarbonate can produce alkalosis and respiratory depression.

5. **Insertion of nasogastric tube:** Prevents gastric aspiration, particularly in comatose patients.

6. **Treatment of underlying cause:** For example, infection is treated with appropriate antibiotics.

NURSING DIAGNOSES AND INTERVENTIONS

Fluid volume deficit (with concomitant electrolyte disturbance) related to decreased circulating volume secondary to hyperglycemia and osmotic diuresis

---

Desired outcomes: Patient becomes normovolemic as evidenced by BP ≥110/70 mm Hg (or within patient's normal range), MAP ≥70 mm Hg, HR 60-100 bpm, CVP 2-6 mm Hg, PAWP 6-12 mm Hg, and urinary output ≥30 ml/hr. EKG exhibits normal sinus rhythm, serum potassium is 3.5-5.5 mEq/L, serum sodium is 137-147 mEq/L, and serum glucose is 100-150 mg/dl.

---

1. Monitor VS q15min until stable for 1 hour. Notify MD promptly of the following: HR >120 bpm or BP <90/60 or decreased ≥20 mm Hg from baseline, MAP decreased ≥10 mm Hg from baseline, CVP <2 mm Hg, and PAWP <6 mm Hg.

2. Monitor patient for physical indicators of dehydration, such as tachycardia, orthostatic hypotension, cyanosis, poor skin turgor, dry mucous membranes, and sunken and soft eyeballs.

3. Measure I&O accurately. Decreasing urinary output may signal diminishing intravascular fluid volume or impending renal failure. Report to MD urine output <30 ml/hr for 2 consecutive hours.

4. Administer IV fluids as prescribed to ensure adequate rehydration. Be alert to indicators of fluid overload, which can occur secondary to the rapid infusion of fluids: jugular vein distention, dyspnea, crackles (rales), CVP >6 mm Hg.

5. Administer insulin as prescribed to prevent worsening hyperglycemia and cor-

rect existing hyperglycemia. Be aware that insulin, when added to IV solutions, may be absorbed by the container and plastic tubing. Before initiating treatment, flush the tubing with 50-100 ml of the insulin-containing IV solution to ensure that maximum absorption by the container and tubing has occurred before patient use.

6. Monitor lab results for abnormalities. With insulin therapy, the serum glucose should decline steadily until it stabilizes between 150-300 mg/dl. A too-rapid return to normal levels may produce fluid shifts and cerebral edema. Notify MD if serum glucose drops to <100 mg/dl and discontinue insulin drip until MD gives further instructions. Serum potassium should decline until it reaches normal. Promptly report to MD serum potassium levels <3.5 mEq/L. Serum sodium levels will increase gradually with appropriate IV saline replacement.

7. Observe for clinical manifestations of electrolyte imbalance as follows:
   • *Hyperkalemia:* Lethargy, nausea, hyperactive bowel sounds with diarrhea, numbness or tingling in extremities, muscle weakness.
   • *Hypokalemia:* Muscle weakness, hypotension, anorexia, drowsiness, hypoactive bowel sounds.
   • *Hyponatremia:* Headache, malaise, muscle weakness, abdominal cramps, nausea, seizures, coma.
   • *Hypoglycemia:* Headache, impaired mentation, dizziness, nausea, pallor, tremors, agitation, tachycardia, diaphoresis.
   • *Metabolic acidosis:* Lassitude, nausea, vomiting, Kussmaul's respirations, lethargy progressing to coma.
   • *Hypophosphatemia:* Muscle weakness, progressive encephalopathy possibly leading to coma.
   • *Hypomagnesemia:* Anorexia, nausea, vomiting, lethargy, weakness, personality changes, tetany, tremor or muscle fasciculations, seizures, confusion progressing to coma.
   • *Hypochloremia:* Hypertonicity of muscles, tetany, depressed respirations.

8. Monitor patient continuously on cardiac monitor. Observe for EKG changes typical of hyperkalemia or hypokalemia (see "EKG and hemodynamic findings," p. 330).

9. To prevent accidental injury caused by altered mentation occurring with cellular dehydration or electrolyte imbalance, institute safety measures, such as padded side rails; bed in lowest position with side rails up when not at patient's side; and bite block, oral airway, and supplemental oxygen at the bedside. Apply soft restraints as necessary to prevent falls. Reorient and reassure patient as needed.

Potential for infection related to susceptibility secondary to protein depletion and hyperglycemia

---

Desired outcome: Patient is free of infection as evidenced by normothermia, HR ≤100 bpm, BP within patient's normal range, WBC count <11,000 µl, and negative cultures.

---

1. Monitor patient for evidence of infection (see Table 5-1, on the next page). Monitor lab results for increased WBC count and culture purulent drainage as prescribed.

TABLE 5-1
Infectious processes necessitating medical intervention

Classification	Indicators
Upper respiratory infection	Fever, chills, cough productive of sputum, crackles (rales), rhonchi, dyspnea.
Urinary tract infection	Burning or pain with urination, cloudy or malodorous urine, fever, chills, tachycardia, diaphoresis, nausea, vomiting, abdominal pain.
Systemic sepsis	Fever, chills, tachycardia, diaphoresis, nausea, vomiting, hypothermia (gram-negative sepsis), flushed skin, hypotension.
Localized (IV sites)	Erythema, swelling, purulent drainage, warmth.

2. Ensure good handwashing technique when caring for patient.
3. Because patient is at increased risk of bacterial infection, use of invasive lines should be limited. Peripheral IV sites should be rotated q48-72 hours, depending on agency policy. Central lines should be discontinued as soon as feasible, and when in place should be handled carefully. Schedule dressing changes according to agency policy and inspect the site(s) for signs of local infection, including erythema, swelling, or purulent drainage. Document the presence of any of these indicators and notify MD.
4. Provide good skin care to maintain skin integrity. Use eggcrate mattress on the bed to help prevent skin breakdown. Air circulation beds are recommended for severe skin breakdown.
5. Use meticulous aseptic technique when caring for or inserting in-dwelling catheters to minimize the risk of bacterial entry *via* these sites.

< N O T E :   Because of the increased risk of infection, limit use of in-dwelling urethral catheters to patients who are unable to void in a bedpan or when continuous assessment of urine output is essential.

6. To help prevent pulmonary infection, provide incentive spirometry and encourage its use, along with deep-breathing and coughing exercises, qh while patient is awake.

Potential for injury related to confusion, obtundation, coma, or seizures secondary to cerebral edema or dehydration

Desired outcome: Patient verbalizes orientation to person, place, and time; RR is 12-20 breaths/min with normal depth and pattern (eupnea); adventitious breath sounds are absent; normal breath sounds are auscultated over patient's airways; and patient's oral cavity and musculoskeletal system remain intact and free of injury.

1. Reduce the likelihood of falls for confused patients by maintaining bed in lowest position, siderails up at all times, and using soft restraints as necessary.
2. Monitor respiratory status, especially airway patency, at frequent intervals.

Keep oral airway, manual resuscitator and mask, and supplemental oxygen at the bedside.

3. Insert NG tube in comatose patients, as prescribed, to decrease the likelihood of aspiration.

4. Elevate HOB to 45 degrees to minimize the risk of aspiration.

5. Initiate seizure precautions. For details, see **Potential for injury** related to risk of oral or musculoskeletal injury secondary to seizure activity, p. 314, in "Status Epilepticus."

Potential alteration in tissue perfusion: Peripheral, related to risk of thromboembolism secondary to increased viscosity of blood, increased platelet aggregation and adhesiveness, and patient immobility

---

Desired outcomes: Patient has adequate perfusion as evidenced by peripheral pulses >2+ on a 0-4+ scale, brisk capillary refill (<3 seconds), warm skin, and absence of swelling, bluish discoloration, erythema, and discomfort in the calves and thighs. Hematocrit is 40%-54% (male) or 37%-47% (female) and BUN is ≤20 mg/dl.

---

1. Monitor hematocrit results. With proper fluid replacement, results should return to normal within 24-48 hours. Assess for a falling BUN value as an indicator of improved tissue perfusion and renal function.

2. Assess peripheral pulses q2-4h. Report any decrease in amplitude or absence of pulse(s) to MD immediately.

3. Be alert to indicators of deep vein thrombosis such as erythema, pain, tenderness, warmth, swelling, or bluish discoloration or prominence of superficial veins in the extremities, especially the lower extremities. Arterial thrombosis may produce cyanosis with delayed capillary refill, mottling, and coolness of the extremity. Report significant findings to MD immediately.

4. Perform ROM exercises to all extremities q4h to increase blood flow to the tissues.

5. Apply antiembolic hose, ace wraps, or pneumatic alternating pressure stockings to the lower extremities as prescribed to aid in the prevention of thrombosis.

Also see nursing diagnoses and interventions in the following: "Caring for the Critically Ill on Prolonged Bed Rest," pp. 505-511; "Caring for the Critically Ill with Life-Threatening Disorders," pp. 511-522; and "Caring for the Family of the Critically Ill," pp. 522-526.

REHABILITATION AND PATIENT-FAMILY TEACHING CONCEPTS

Patients in intensive care units often experience heightened anxiety, and at times, denial of the severity of the disease, which blocks learning. Use simple terms and incorporate patient teaching frequently into patient care routines. Give patient and significant others verbal and written instructions for the following:

1. Causes, prevention, and treatment of DKA. As needed, explain the disease

process of diabetes mellitus and DKA and the common early symptoms of worsening hyperglycemia including polyuria, polydipsia, polyphagia, dry and flushed skin, and increased irritability. Stress the importance of maintaining regular diet, exercise, and medication regimen for optimal control of serum glucose levels and prevention of adverse physical effects of diabetes mellitus, such as peripheral neuropathies and increased atherosclerosis.

2. Importance of testing urine sugar and acetone or blood glucose levels qid: before meals and at bedtime. Explain that urine sugar and acetone levels $>2+/N$ or blood glucose >200 mg/dl should be reported to MD so that insulin dose can be increased. As indicated, review testing procedure with patient.

3. Medications, including drug name, dosage, route, and potential side effects. Teach patient that insulin must be taken every day and that lifetime insulin therapy is necessary to achieve control of blood glucose. Explain that insulin is administered 2-4 times a day as prescribed and that it may require adjustment during periods of illness or stress.

4. Indicators of *insulin excess* (hypoglycemia) such as dizziness, impaired mentation, irritability, pallor, tremors; and indicators of *insulin deficiency* (hyperglycemia) such as increased polyuria and polydipsia, dry and flushed skin. Teach patient the importance of receiving prompt treatment if any of these indicators occurs.

5. Importance of dietary changes as prescribed by MD. Typically, patient is put on a fixed calorie ADA diet composed of 60% carbohydrates, 20% fats, and 20% proteins. Explain that the fats should be polyunsaturated and the proteins chosen from low-fat sources. Teach patient the importance of eating 3 meals a day at regularly scheduled times and a bedtime snack.

6. Causes for adjustments in insulin dosage: (1) increased or decreased food intake; (2) any physical (e.g., exercise) or emotional stress. Teach patient that exercise and emotional stress increase release of glucose from the liver, which may increase insulin demand. Instruct patient to monitor blood glucose levels closely during periods of increased emotional stress and periods of increased or decreased exercise and to adjust insulin dose accordingly.

7. Susceptibility to infection: Explain that individuals with diabetes are more susceptible to infection and that preventive measures such as good hygiene and meticulous, daily foot care are necessary to prevent infection. Stress the importance of avoiding exposure to communicable diseases and that the following indicators of infection necessitate prompt medical treatment: fever, chills, increased HR, diaphoresis, nausea, and vomiting. In addition, teach patient and significant others to be alert to wounds or cuts that do not heal, burning or pain with urination, and a productive cough.

8. Necessity of continued medical follow-up; confirm time and date of next medical appointment.

9. Procedure for obtaining Medic-Alert bracelet or card identifying patient's diagnosis.

10. Address of American Diabetes Association for pamphlets and magazines related to the disease, its complications, and appropriate treatment:
American Diabetes Association, Inc.
18 East 48th Street
New York, New York 10017

Hyperosmolar hyperglycemic nonketotic coma

Hyperosmolar hyperglycemic nonketotic coma (HHNC) is a life-threatening emergency resulting from a relative or actual insulin deficiency that causes severe hyperglycemia. Usually, patients are elderly with undiagnosed or inadequately treated non-insulin dependent diabetes mellitus (NIDDM, or type II diabetes). Usually, HHNC is precipitated by a stressor, such as trauma or infection, that increases insulin demand. It is believed that enough insulin is present to prevent lipolysis and the formation of ketone bodies, thereby preventing acidosis, but not enough to prevent hyperglycemia. Without adequate insulin to facilitate utilization by most body cells, glucose molecules accumulate in the bloodstream, causing serum hyperosmolality with resultant osmotic diuresis and simultaneous loss of electrolytes, most notably potassium, sodium, and phosphate. Patients may lose up to 25% of their total body water. Owing to increasing serum hyperosmolality and extracellular fluid loss, fluids are pulled from individual body cells, causing intracellular dehydration and body cell shrinkage. Neurologic deficits (i.e., slowed mentation, confusion, seizures, or coma) can occur as a result. Although loss of extracellular fluid stimulates aldosterone release, which will help the body retain sodium and prevent further loss of potassium, the aldosterone cannot halt severe dehydration. As extracellular volume decreases, the blood becomes more viscous and flow is impeded. Thomboemboli are common owing to increased blood viscosity, enhanced platelet aggregation and adhesiveness, and immobility. Cardiac workload is increased and may lead to myocardial infarction. Renal blood flow is decreased, potentially resulting in renal impairment or failure. Cerebrovascular accident may result from thromboemboli or decreased cerebral perfusion. These severe complications, in addition to the initial precipitating disorder, contribute to a mortality rate in excess of 50%.

Unlike DKA, in which acidosis produces severe symptoms requiring prompt hospitalization, symptoms of HHNC develop slowly and frequently are nonspecific. The cardinal symptoms of polyuria and polydipsia are the first to appear, but they may be ignored by elderly patients or their families. Neurologic deficits may be mistaken for signs of impending CVA or senility. Owing to the similarity of these symptoms to other disease processes common to this age group, proper diagnosis and treatment may be delayed, allowing progression of pathophysiologic processes.

ASSESSMENT

Signs and symptoms: Polyuria, polydipsia, weakness, orthostatic hypotension, lethargy, confusion progressing to coma.

Physical assessment: Poor skin turgor, dry mucous membranes, tachycardia, tachypnea with shallow respirations.

History and risk factors: NIDDM (type II diabetes); increased insulin demand due to stressors such as trauma, infection, myocardial infarction (MI); high-caloric enteral or parenteral feedings in a compromised patient; use of diabetogenic drugs (e.g., glucocorticoids, phenytoin, some diuretics, sympathomimetics, thyroid preparations).

EKG and hemodynamic findings: Evidence of hypokalemia (increased PVCs, depressed T waves); and CVP >3 mm Hg below patient's baseline, PAD pressure >4 mm Hg below patient's baseline, and PAWP >4 mm Hg below patient's baseline.

< N O T E :   Because these patients usually are older than 50 years of age and have preexisting cardiac or pulmonary disorders, hemodynamic parameters often

cannot be evaluated based on normal values, but rather on what is normal or optimal for each individual patient. CVP, PAWP, and PAD pressures should therefore be evaluated in terms of deviations from patient's baseline and concurrent clinical status.

< N O T E : See Table 5-2, p. 338, for a comparison of DKA to HHNC

DIAGNOSTIC TESTS

1. *Serum osmolality:* Will be >350 mOsm/kg. A quick bedside calculation of serum osmolality can be obtained by using this formula:

$$2(Na + K) + \frac{BUN(mg/dl)}{2.8} + \frac{glucose\ (mg/dl)}{18} = mOsm/L$$

For example: Na^+ = 140; K^+ = 4.5; BUN = 20, glucose = 120.

$$2\ (140 + 4.5) + \frac{20}{2.8} + \frac{120}{18} = 289 + 7 + 6.7 = 302.7$$

2. See Table 5-2, p. 338, for a discussion of other diagnostic tests.

MEDICAL MANAGEMENT

1. **Replacement of electrolytes and extracellular fluid volume:** Most often, 0.45% saline or normal saline is used; potassium or phosphate supplements may be added, based on laboratory values. IV fluids will be changed to 5% dextrose in normal saline or 5% dextrose in 0.45% saline to prevent hypoglycemia as blood glucose decreases.
2. **Rapid-acting insulin:** Usually administered in low doses. Because of poor tissue perfusion in these patients, the IV route is preferred. In the majority of cases, continuous drips are used and titrated, based on serum glucose levels.
3. **Insertion of pulmonary artery flow-directed catheter:** To assess fluid status on a continuous basis.
4. **Treatment of underlying cause:** The most frequent cause is infection, which is treated with appropriate antibiotics.

NURSING DIAGNOSES AND INTERVENTIONS

See ''Diabetic Ketoacidosis'' for the following: **Fluid volume deficit** (with concomitant electrolyte disturbance) related to decreased circulating volume secondary to hyperglycemia and osmotic diuresis, p. 331; **Potential for infection** related to susceptibility secondary to protein depletion and hyperglycemia, p. 332; and **Potential for injury** related to confusion, obtundation, coma, or seizures secondary to cerebral edema or dehydration, p. 333; and **Potential alteration in tissue perfusion:** Peripheral related to risk of thromboembolism, p. 334. For other nursing diagnoses and interventions, see the following as appropriate: ''Caring for the Critically Ill with Life-Threatening Disorders,'' pp. 511-522; and ''Caring for the Family of the Critically Ill,'' pp. 522-526.

REHABILITATION AND PATIENT-FAMILY TEACHING CONCEPTS

Patients in intensive care units often experience heightened anxiety, and at times, denial of the severity of the disease that blocks learning. Use simple terms and

TABLE 5-2
Comparison of DKA to HHNC

	DKA	HHNC
Diabetes type:	Usually IDDM (type I)	Usually NIDDM (type II)
Typical age group	Any age	Usually over 50
Signs and symptoms	Polyuria, polydipsia, polyphagia, weakness, orthostatic hypotension, lethargy, changes in LOC, fatigue, nausea, vomiting, abdominal pain.	Same as DKA
Physical assessment	Dry, flushed skin; poor skin turgor; dry mucous membranes; decreased BP; tachycardia; altered LOC (irritability, lethargy, coma); Kussmaul's respirations; fruity odor to the breath.	Same as DKA, but no Kussmaul's respirations or fruity odor to the breath. Instead, patient will have tachypnea with shallow respirations.
History and risk factors	Undiagnosed type I diabetes mellitus; recent stressors such as surgery, trauma, infection, MI; insufficient exogenous insulin.	Undiagnosed type II diabetes mellitus; recent stressors such as surgery, trauma, pancreatitis, MI, infection; high-caloric enteral or parenteral feedings in a compromised patient; use of diabetogenic drugs (e.g., phenytoin, thiazide diuretics, thyroid preparations, mannitol, corticosteroids, sympathomimetics); dialysis; major burns treated with high concentrations of sugar.
Monitoring parameters	*EKG:* Dysrhythmias associated with hyperkalemia: peaked T waves, widened QRS, prolonged P-R interval, flattened or absent P wave. As hyperkalemia worsens, these signs progress in the order given and may lead to asystole. Hypokalemia (<3.0 mEq/L) may produce depressed ST segments, flat or inverted T waves, or increased ventricular dysrhythmias.	EKG evidence of hypokalemia as listed with DKA. *Hemodynamic measurements:* CVP >3 mm Hg below patient's baseline; PADP and PAWP >4 mm Hg below patient's baseline.

Diagnostic tests	*Serum glucose:* 200-800 mg/dl — 800-2000 mg/dl
	Serum ketones: elevated — normal or slightly elevated
	Urine glucose: positive — positive
	Urine acetone: positive — negative
	Serum osmolality: 300-350 mOsm/L — >350 mOsm/L
	Serum pH: <7.38 — normal or mildly acidotic due to lactic acidosis (pH 7.30-7.42)
	Serum sodium: <137 mEq/L — elevated, normal, or low
	Serum hematocrit: elevated due to osmotic diuresis with hemoconcentration — elevated due to hemoconcentration
	BUN: elevated >20 mg/dl — elevated
	Serum creatinine: >1.5 mg/dl — elevated
	Serum potassium: normal or elevated above 5.5 mEq/L initially and then decreased — normal or <3.5 mEq/L
	Serum phosphorus, magnesium, chloride: decreased — decreased
Onset:	Hours to days — Hours to days; can be longer.
Mortality rate:	<10% — >50% due to age group and complications such as CVA, thrombosis, pancreatitis.

incorporate patient teaching frequently into patient care routines. Give patient and significant others verbal and written instructions for the following:

1. Causes, prevention, and treatment of HHNC. Allow patient to verbalize fears and feelings about the diagnosis; correct any misconceptions. As needed, explain the disease process of diabetes mellitus and HHNC and the common early symptoms of worsening diabetes, including polyuria, polydipsia, polyphagia, dry and flushed skin, and increased irritability.

2. Importance of testing urine sugar and acetone or blood glucose levels qid: before meals and at bedtime. Explain that urine sugar and acetone levels $>2+/N$ or blood glucose >200 mg/dl should be reported to MD so that insulin dose can be increased. As indicated, review testing procedure with patient.

3. Importance of dietary changes as prescribed by MD. Typically, patient with NIDDM (type II diabetes) is obese and will be on a reduced-calorie diet with fixed amounts of carbohydrates, fat, and protein. Explain that the fats should be polyunsaturated and the proteins chosen from low-fat sources. Teach patient the importance of eating 3 meals a day at regularly scheduled times and a bedtime snack. Explain that increased or decreased food intake will necessitate an adjustment in insulin dosage. Provide a referral to a dietician as needed.

4. Importance of taking oral hypoglycemic agents as prescribed. In addition, explain that exogenous insulin may be required during periods of physical and emotional stress and that blood glucose levels should be monitored closely during these times.

5. For patient with NIDDM, that regular exercise is beneficial in maintaining blood glucose levels by increasing insulin effectiveness and reducing serum triglyceride and cholesterol levels, thus also decreasing the risk of atherosclerosis. Aerobic exercises such as walking or swimming are most effective in lowering blood glucose levels.

6. Necessity of preventive measures for infection, such as good hygiene and meticulous, daily foot care. Stress the importance of avoiding exposure to communicable diseases and that the following indicators of infection necessitate prompt medical treatment: fever, chills, tachycardia, diaphoresis, and nausea and vomiting. In addition, teach patient and significant others to be alert to wounds or cuts that do not heal, burning or pain with urination, and cough that is productive of sputum.

7. Procedures for obtaining Medic-Alert bracelet or card identifying patient's diagnosis.

8. Necessity for continued medical follow-up; confirm date and time of next medical appointment.

9. In addition, provide booklets or pamphlets from the American Diabetes Association or pharmaceutical companies about diabetes and appropriate treatment.

Diabetes insipidus

Diabetes insipidus (DI) is caused by a deficiency in the synthesis or release of antidiuretic hormone (ADH) from the posterior pituitary gland (neurogenic) or a decrease in kidney responsiveness to ADH (nephrogenic), resulting in decreased water reabsorption by the renal tubules. Regardless of the etiology of DI, the patient will excrete large amounts of free water, resulting in profound diuresis of extremely dilute urine. As a result of the loss of free water, extracellular fluid volume decreases and plasma osmolality and serum sodium rise. Severe extracellular and intracellular dehydration, hypotension, and hypovolemic shock can occur. As plasma osmolality increases, so does blood viscosity, which increases the risk of thromboemboli. Decreased cerebral perfusion, cerebral dehydration, and hypernatremia produce neurologic symptoms ranging from confusion, restlessness, and irritability to seizures and coma.

DI can be permanent or temporary, depending on the severity, type, and location of the injury. Onset can be sudden and dramatic with inflammatory disease or some types of trauma, or gradual with tumor, infiltrative disease, and other types of trauma. With gradual onset there are three phases. The first phase immediately follows the injury and is characterized by increasing polyuria and polydipsia that lasts for approximately 4-5 days. During the second phase, symptoms subside for approximately 6 days, coinciding with the release of stored ADH from the posterior pituitary gland. In phase three there is almost always permanent polyuria and polydipsia.

ASSESSMENT

Signs and symptoms: Polyuria with dilute urine; polydipsia.

< N O T E :   As much as 5-40 liters of urine may be excreted per day.

Physical assessment: Often unremarkable. If fluid intake is inadequate, patients may show signs of dehydration such as poor skin turgor and dry mucous membranes.

History and risk factors: Head injury, especially to the base of the brain; meningitis or encephalitis; brain tumors, especially in the hypothalamus or pituitary region; neoplasms such as leukemia or breast cancer; surgery in the area of the pituitary gland; intracranial hemorrhage; any disorder that causes an increase in intracranial pressure (ICP); and cerebral hypoxia or anoxic brain death.

Monitoring parameters

- *Urine output:* >200 ml/hour for two consecutive hours, or >500 ml/hour in the presence of any of the above risk factors.
- *CVP:* <2 mm Hg.
- *PAWP:* <6 mm Hg.

DIAGNOSTIC TESTS

1. *Urine osmolality:* Decreased to <200 mOsm/kg in the presence of disease.
2. *Specific gravity:* Less than 1.007.
3. *Serum osmolality:* Increased to >300 mOsm/kg.
4. *Serum sodium:* Increased to >147 mEq/L.
5. *Plasma ADH:* Decreased.
6. *Water deprivation test:* Preliminary measurements of weight, serum and urine osmolality, and urine specific gravity are obtained. Fluid intake is prohibited and the above parameters are measured hourly until urine specific gravity exceeds 1.020 and urine osmolality exceeds 800 mOsm/kg (a negative result) or when 5% of body weight is lost or urine specific gravity does not increase for 3 consecutive hours (a positive result). In order for a definite diagnosis of DI to be made, it is necessary also to perform the vasopressin test, explained on p. 342.

< C A U T I O N :   The water deprivation test can take up to 16 hours to com-

plete and may produce hypernatremia, severe dehydration, and hypovolemic shock. Patients must be monitored continuously throughout the test.

7. *Vasopressin test:* Vasopressin (exogenous ADH) is administered SC. Urine specimens are collected q15min for 2 hours and evaluated for quantity and osmolality. With complete neurogenic DI, urine osmolality will remain <200 mOsm/kg.

< C A U T I O N : This test can induce congestive heart failure secondary to fluid overload in susceptible individuals.

MEDICAL MANAGEMENT

1. **Rehydration:** Hypotonic IV solutions are frequently used to replace free water lost in the urine. Fluid replacement is very rapid until hemodynamic status becomes stabilized, at which time it is then based on urine output.

2. **Exogenous vasopressin (Pitressin):** Several preparations are available; dosage is adjusted to patient response. Side effects include hypertension because of vasoconstrictive effects on peripheral vessels, angina or MI due to constriction of coronary vessels, abdominal or uterine cramping, increased peristalsis of the GI tract, and water intoxication. For more information, see Table 5-3, p. 344.

3. **Chlorpropamide:** Stimulates ADH release and kidney response to ADH in nephrogenic DI.

4. **Thiazide diuretics combined with restriction of sodium:** Enhance water reabsorption in nephrogenic DI.

5. **Transsphenoidal hypophysectomy:** Treatment of choice for pituitary tumors because it produces immediate results, has a low mortality rate, and can treat tumors that are resistant to radiation therapy. It can involve removal of the tumor itself, leaving the gland intact, or removal of all or part of the pituitary gland, depending on the size and location of the tumor.

   To enter the sella turcica through the sphenoid process, the upper lip is elevated and an incision is made in the gingiva above the maxilla. Because of the site of the incision, patients are at high risk for postoperative infection, particularly of the brain. To minimize this possibility, antibiotic nasal sprays are used preoperatively; nasal packing that is impregnated with an antibiotic ointment is kept in place for 24-72 hours after surgery. Complications include pituitary hemorrhage, frontal lobe damage, and hormonal deficiencies following removal of the gland. Tumors most often occur in the anterior pituitary gland, therefore most postoperative hormone deficiencies are caused by a lack of anterior pituitary hormones. In addition, the patient may have increased ICP due to edema or bleeding in the sella turcica and will return from surgery with two black eyes.

NURSING DIAGNOSES AND INTERVENTIONS

Fluid volume deficit related to decreased circulating volume secondary to polyuria

---

Desired outcomes: Patient is normovolemic as evidenced by BP 110-120/70-80 mm Hg (or within patient's normal value), CVP ≥2 mm Hg, PAWP ≥6 mm Hg, HR 60-100 bpm, intake equal to output plus insensible losses, urine specific gravity

1.010-1.030, and stable weights. Serum sodium is 137-147 mEq/L, serum osmolality is 275-300 mOsm/kg, and urine osmolality is 300-900 mOsm/24 hours.

---

1. Keep careful I&O records. Urine output >200 ml/hour for 2 consecutive hours, or 500 ml/hour, in the presence of risk factors (see p. 341), should be reported to MD promptly.
2. Provide adequate fluids. Keep water pitcher full and within easy reach of patient.
3. For unconscious patients or those who cannot maintain adequate fluid intake orally, administer IV fluids as prescribed. Usually, a hypotonic solution is administered as follows: 1 ml IV fluid for each 1 ml of urine output.
4. Administer vasopressin and antidiuretics as prescribed; observe for and document effects.
5. Weigh patient daily, at the same time and using the same scale and garments to prevent error. Report weight loss >1 kg/day to MD.
6. Monitor for signs of continuing fluid volume deficit: poor skin turgor; dry mucous membranes; rapid and thready pulse; and systolic BP, CVP, or PAWP below patient's baseline.
7. Monitor lab studies, including serum sodium, serum and urine osmolality, and urine specific gravity; report significant findings to MD.

Potential for injury related to risk of undesirable side effects secondary to administration of exogenous vasopressin

---

Desired outcomes: Patient's HR is 60-100 bpm; BP is 110-120/70-80 mm Hg (or within patient's normal range); CVP is 2-6 mm Hg; PAWP is 6-12 mm Hg; RR is 12-20 breaths/min with normal depth and pattern (eupnea); and patient verbalizes orientation to person, place, and time and denies the presence of chest or abdominal pain, nausea, or headache. Serum sodium is 137-147 mEq/L.

---

1. Monitor VS carefully. Report increase in HR >20 over baseline or decrease in systolic BP >20 less than baseline.
2. Instruct patient to notify nurse promptly if chest pain or difficulty in breathing occurs; notify MD accordingly. Keep vasodilators, such as nitroglycerine, at bedside for easy, rapid administration.
3. Monitor carefully for signs of water intoxication: changes in LOC, headache, nausea, abdominal pain, seizures, CVP or PAWP increased over baseline, and decreased serum sodium.
4. Initiate seizure precautions, if indicated: siderails up and padded, airway and supplemental oxygen at the bedside.

Potential for injury related to risk of increased ICP secondary to edema or intracranial bleeding following transsphenoidal hypophysectomy

---

Desired outcomes: Patient verbalizes orientation to person, place, and time; has RR 12-20 breaths/min with a normal pattern and depth (eupnea); and displays equal

T A B L E 5 - 3
Vasopressin preparations

Generic name	Brand name	Onset	Duration	Usual dose	Advantages/ Disadvantages	Comments
Nasal						
Vasopressin	Pitressin	within 1 hr	4-8 hrs	5-10 U bid-tid	Action decreased by nasal congestion/discharge or atrophy of nasal mucosa.	Administer by spray, cotton pledget, or dropper.
Desmopressin acetate	DDAVP	within 1 hr	8-20 hrs	0.1-0.4 ml qd in 1-3 doses (10-40 μg)	See above.	See above. Store in refrigerator at 4° C (39.2° F)
Lypressin	Diapid	within 1 hr	3-8 hrs	7-14 μg qid	See above	See above. Store at <40° C (100° F).
Subcutaneous						
Vasopressin	Pitressin	½-1 hr	2-8 hrs	0.25-0.5 ml (5-10 U) q3-4h prn increased thirst or increased urine output		
Desmopressin acetate	DDAVP, Stimate	within ½ hr	1½-4 hrs	0.5 ml-1ml (2 μg-4μg) qd in 2 divided doses		Keep refrigerated at 4° C.

Intramuscular						
Vasopressin tannate in oil	Pitressin tannate in oil	within 1-2 hrs	36-48 hrs	0.3-1 ml (1.5-5 U) q2-3 days for increased thirst or increased urine output	Longer duration of action/slower absorption than SC route. Response cumulative over 2-3 days.	Store at 13-18° C (55-65° F). Shake well before withdrawing from vial. Can warm solution by immersing vial in warm water.
Vasopressin tannate	Pitressin	½-1 hr	2-8 hrs	0.25-0.5 ml (5-10 U) q3-4h for increased thirst or increased urine output		
Intravenous						
Desmopressin acetate	DDAVP	within ½ hr	1½-4 hrs	0.5-1.0 ml (2-4 µg) qd in 2 divided doses	Not for home use.	Keep refrigerated at 4° C. Dilute in 10-50 ml 0.9% NaCl and infuse over 15-30 min.

and normoreactive pupils and bilaterally equal motor strength and tone that are normal for patient. Patient verbalizes understanding of the importance of avoiding Valsalva-type activities.

1. Elevate HOB 30 degrees to minimize ICP.
2. Perform neurochecks at frequent intervals to assess for signs of increased ICP, including changes in LOC, respiratory rate or rhythm, and pupillary reflexes.
3. Teach patient to avoid coughing, sneezing, straining, bending, or other Valsalva-type activities, as they can increase stress on the operative site, increase ICP, and cause CSF leak. Explain to patient that if coughing or sneezing becomes necessary, it should be done with the mouth open to minimize the increase in ICP. As appropriate, administer cathartics, stool softeners or antiemetics to minimize straining and nausea.
4. For more information see "Care of the Patient Following Intracranial Surgery," p. 282.

Potential for infection related to vulnerability secondary to incisional opening into sella turcica

Desired outcome: Patient is normothermic; verbalizes orientation to person, place, and time; and does not display evidence of cerebrospinal fluid (CSF) leakage or nuchal rigidity.

1. Inspect nasal packing at frequent intervals for frank bleeding or evidence of CSF (*non*sanguineous) leak. Because a CSF leak would signal a serious breach in cranial integrity, elevate the HOB to minimize the chance of bacterial migration into the brain. Promptly report significant findings to MD.
2. Be alert to indicators of infection, including elevated temperature, nuchal rigidity, and altered LOC.
3. To prevent injury to operative site, which could lead to infection, teach patient to avoid brushing teeth until instructed to do so by MD. Provide mouthwash and cotton swabs for oral hygiene.
4. For more information, see "Care of the Patient Following Intracranial Surgery," p. 282.

See "Diabetic Ketoacidosis" for the following: **Potential for injury** related to confusion, obtundation, coma, or seizures secondary to cerebral edema or dehydration, p. 333; and **Potential alteration in tissue perfusion:** Peripheral, related to risk of thromboembolism, p. 334. Also see the following as appropriate: "Caring for the Critically Ill with Life-Threatening Disorders," pp. 511-522; and "Caring for the Family of the Critically Ill," pp. 522-526.

REHABILITATION AND PATIENT-FAMILY TEACHING CONCEPTS

Give patient and significant others written and verbal instructions for the following:

1. Obtaining a Medic-Alert bracelet and ID card for those patients with permanent diabetes insipidus.
2. Appropriate administration of exogenous vasopressin and its side effects.
3. Indicators that necessitate medical attention, including signs and symptoms of dehydration and water intoxication.
4. Importance of continued medical follow-up; confirm date and time of next medical appointment.

Following transsphenoidal hypophysectomy

5. Necessity for lifetime exogenous hormone replacement if the anterior posterior gland was removed or damaged.
6. If the entire pituitary gland was removed, the indicators of hormone replacement excess or deficiency
   - *Adrenal hormone excess:* weight gain, moon face, easy bruising, fatigue, polyuria, polydipsia.
   - *Adrenal hormone deficiency:* weight loss, easy fatigability, abdominal pain, excess pigmentation.
   - *Thyroid hormone excess:* heat intolerance, irritability, tachycardia, weight loss, diaphoresis.
   - *Thyroid hormone deficiency:* bradycardia, cold intolerance, weight gain, slowed mentation.
   - *Androgen replacement deficiency:* some degree of sexual dysfunction, ranging from menstrual irregularities to infertility and impotence.
7. For patients with permanent need for hormone replacement, the method for obtaining a Medic-Alert bracelet and ID card outlining diagnosis and appropriate treatment in the event of an emergency.

Syndrome of inappropriate antidiuretic hormone

Syndrome of inappropriate antidiuretic hormone (SIADH) is caused by excessive release of ADH, resulting in severe water retention. The action of ADH is that of increasing reabsorption of water in the late-distal tubules and collecting ducts of the kidney. Normally, ADH secretion is stimulated by one of three mechanisms: (1) increased plasma osmolality causes movement of fluid out of specialized cells (osmolreceptors) located in the hypothalamus, decreasing the size of the cells and increasing the rate of electrical discharge; (2) decreased plasma volume is sensed by stretch receptors located in the left atrium and pulmonary vasculature; or (3) decreased blood pressure is sensed by pressure receptors located in the carotid arteries and aorta. See "History and risk factors," p. 348, for other potential causes of ADH secretion.

In the presence of excessive ADH, water that normally would be excreted is reabsorbed into the circulation, resulting in water retention and eventually, water intoxication. Because the retained water expands extracellular fluid volume, serum osmolality decreases and serum sodium levels decrease due to dilutional effects. Decreased serum osmolality causes movement of water into the cells. This action in the brain can result in cerebral edema, which produces neurologic deficits. With further water retention, the glomerular filtration rate rises and more sodium is filtered out into the urine. In addition, the increase in extracellular fluid volume depresses aldosterone secretion, adding further to renal excretion of sodium. Without prompt treatment, water intoxication, cerebral edema, and severe hyponatremia may lead to death.

ASSESSMENT

Signs and symptoms: Decreased urine output with concentrated urine. Signs of water intoxication may appear, including altered LOC, fatigue, headache, diarrhea, anorexia, and seizures.

< N O T E :   Because of the loss of sodium, edema will not accompany the fluid volume excess.

Physical assessment: Weight gain without edema, elevated BP.

History and risk factors: Oat cell carcinoma of the lung; carcinoma of the pancreas, duodenum, prostate, or thymus gland; and some forms of leukemia, any of which may secrete a biologically active form of ADH. ADH secretion also can be stimulated by fear, pain, or stress, although the exact mechanism by which this occurs is unknown. Other causes include head trauma, brain tumors, intracerebral hemorrhage, meningitis or encephalitis, positive pressure ventilation (stimulates pressure receptors in the carotid sinus and aortic arch), and use of medications such as chlorpropamide, acetaminophen, morphine, amitriptyline, thiazide diuretics, and cancer chemotherapy drugs.

Monitoring parameters: CVP >6 mm Hg; PAWP >12 mm Hg in the absence of underlying cardiac or pulmonary disease; and urine output <30 ml/hr in the presence of adequate fluid intake.

DIAGNOSTIC TESTS

1. *Serum sodium:* Decreased to <137 mEq/L.
2. *Plasma osmolality:* Decreased to <275 mOsm/kg.
3. *Urine osmolality:* Elevated disproportionately in relation to plasma osmolality.
4. *Urine sodium:* Increased to >200 mEq/L.
5. *Urine specific gravity:* Greater than 1.030.
6. *Plasma ADH:* Elevated.

MEDICAL MANAGEMENT AND SURGICAL INTERVENTIONS

1. **Fluid restriction:** Based on urine output plus insensible losses.
2. **Hypertonic (3%) sodium chloride and IV furosemide (e.g., Lasix):** To replace serum sodium and promote excretion of water for patients with severe hyponatremia or seizures.
3. **Lithium or demeclocycline:** Inhibits action of ADH on the distal renal tubules to promote water excretion.
4. **Thoracotomy:** To excise cancerous lesions of the lung.
5. **Craniotomy:** To excise brain tumors or evacuate subdural or subarachnoid hematomas.
6. **Transsphenoidal hypophysectomy:** For discussion, see "Diabetes Insipidus," p. 342. Diabetes insipidus is the most common complication because of damage to the pituitary gland during surgery.

NURSING DIAGNOSES AND INTERVENTIONS

Fluid volume excess related to retention secondary to increased level of serum ADH with increased water reabsorption from the kidneys

Desired outcomes: Patient is normovolemic as evidenced by orientation to person, place, and time; intake that approximates output plus insensible losses; stable weights; CVP 2-6 mm Hg; PAWP 6-12 mm Hg; BP within patient's normal range; urine specific gravity 1.010-1.030; and HR 60-100 bpm. Serum sodium is 137-147 mEq/L, urine osmolality is 300-1090 mOsm/kg, and serum osmolality is 275-300 mOsm/kg.

1. Assess LOC, VS, hemodynamic measurements, and I&O hourly; measure weight daily. Be alert to decreasing LOC; elevated BP, CVP, and PAWP; urine output <30 ml/hr; and weight gain. Promptly report significant findings or changes to MD.
2. Monitor lab results, including serum sodium, urine and serum osmolality, and urine specific gravity. Be alert to decreased serum sodium and plasma osmolality, urine osmolality elevated disproportionately in relation to plasma osmolality, and increased urine sodium. Report significant findings to MD.
3. Maintain fluid restriction as prescribed. Explain necessity of this treatment to patient and significant others.
4. Administer demeclocycline, lithium, and furosemide as prescribed; observe and document patient's response carefully.
5. Administer hypertonic sodium chloride as prescribed. Rate of administration usually is based on serial serum sodium levels. To minimize the risk of hypernatremia, make sure that lab tests are drawn on time and results are reported to MD promptly.
6. Institute seizure precautions to prevent injury to the patient in the event of seizure. These include padded siderails, supplemental oxygen, bite block, and oral airway at the bedside, and siderails up at all times when staff is not present.

See "Diabetes Ketoacidosis" for the following: **Potential for injury** related to confusion, obtundation, coma, or seizures secondary to cerebral edema or dehydration, p. 333. If the patient has undergone a transsphenoidal hypophysectomy, see "Diabetes Insipidus" for the following: **Potential for injury** related to risk of increased ICP secondary to edema and cerebral bleeding with transsphenoidal hypophysectomy, p. 343; and **Potential for infection** related to vulnerability secondary to opening into sella turcica, p. 346.

REHABILITATION AND PATIENT-FAMILY TEACHING CONCEPTS

Give patient and significant others verbal and written information for the following:
1. Importance of fluid restriction for the prescribed period.
2. Medications, including name, dosage, route, purpose, and potential side effects.
3. Importance of obtaining daily weights as an indicator of hydration status.
4. Indicators of water intoxication, including altered LOC, fatigue, headache, nausea, vomiting, and anorexia, any or all of which should be reported promptly to MD.
5. For patient who has had a transsphenoidal hypophysectomy, see "Rehabilitation and Patient-Family Teaching Concepts," p. 347, in "Diabetes Insipidus."

Addisonian crisis

Addisonian or adrenal crisis is the severe deficiency of adrenocortical hormones caused by atrophy of the adrenal gland due either to inadequate stimulation from the pituitary gland or destruction of the adrenal glands themselves. Adrenal gland destruction is known as *primary Addison's disease* and it results in inadequate circulating levels of all of the adrenocortical hormones: glucocorticoids (cortisol is the major hormone), mineralcorticoids (primarily aldosterone), and androgens. When adrenal gland dysfunction occurs secondary to pituitary insufficiency, it is called *secondary Addison's disease,* and its usual result is a deficiency of the glucocorticoids and androgens.

Deficiency of glucocorticoids retards the mobilization of tissue protein and inhibits the ability of the liver to store glycogen, causing hypoglycemia and muscle weakness to occur. Wound healing is slowed and patients become particularly susceptible to infection. There is a loss of vascular tone in the periphery, as well as decreased vascular response to the catecholamines—epinephrine and norepinephrine. In primary Addison's disease, decreased secretion of aldosterone causes severe sodium and water loss from the kidneys and increased reabsorption of potassium. In either condition, shock can develop within hours and immediate treatment must be instituted to prevent death. In primary Addison's disease shock is a result both of hypovolemia and loss of vascular tone, while in secondary Addison's disease, the primary etiology is the absence or decrease in vascular tone and normal vascular response to stress, resulting in peripheral vasodilatation and pooling of blood.

ASSESSMENT

Signs and symptoms: Cyanosis, dyspnea, hypotension, abdominal pain, fever, tachycardia, nausea, confusion, and apprehension.

Physical assessment: Hyperpigmentation in skin creases, elbows, and knees of patients with primary Addison's disease; orthostatic hypotension; muscle weakness; poor skin turgor; sunken and soft eyeballs; loss of body hair in axilla and pubic areas due to androgen deficiency. X-ray may reveal small heart size.

History and risk factors: Long-term exogenous steroid use, bilateral adrenalectomy, fulminating infections, surgery of the pituitary gland, radiation of pituitary or adrenal glands. Addisonian crisis may be precipitated by any emotional or physiologic stressor such as trauma, surgery, or infection in susceptible individuals, as well as abrupt withdrawal of exogenous steroids in patients who have been on high doses for a long period of time.

EKG findings: Signs of hyperkalemia: peaked T waves, widening QRS, lengthened PR interval, and flattened to absent P wave. As hyperkalemia worsens, these signs are progressive in the order given and ultimately may reveal asystole.

DIAGNOSTIC TESTS

1. *Random serum cortisol levels:* Decreased.
2. *Serum cortisol levels:* Because levels normally vary throughout the day, specimens should be drawn at 8-hour intervals, starting at 8 AM. In healthy individuals, the 8 AM level will be the highest, with the lowest at midnight. Patients with Addison's disease will not demonstrate this variation and will remain low throughout the day.
3. *Serum adrenocorticotropic hormone (ACTH) levels:* Will be elevated in primary Addison's and decreased in secondary Addison's.

4. *Serum sodium levels:* Decreased to <137 mEq/L.
5. *Serum aldosterone levels:* Depressed in primary Addison's.
6. *Serum potassium levels:* Increased to >5.5 mEq/L.
7. *Fasting blood glucose:* Decreased to <80 mg/dl.
8. *IV ACTH stimulation test:* Differentiates primary from secondary Addison's. IV ACTH is infused over an 8-hour period and serial serum cortisol levels are drawn q8h for 48 hours. An increase in serum cortisol indicates secondary Addison's, while no change is diagnostic of primary Addison's.

MEDICAL MANAGEMENT

1. **IV hydrocortisone:** Maintains glucocorticoid activity, while exerting some sodium-retentive effects.
2. **IV fluids:** Usually D_5NS is administered rapidly to correct dehydration and prevent vascular collapse.
3. **Insertion of flow-directed pulmonary artery catheter:** To assess volume status on a continuous basis.
4. **IV glucose:** To correct hypoglycemia.
5. **Insulin and glucose or sodium polystyrene sulfonate (Kayexalate):** For long-term treatment of hyperkalemia.
6. **Vasopressors:** If necessary, until adequate rehydration has occurred. These patients have decreased response to alpha-stimulation, so vasopressor will be less effective than they would be in normal individuals.
7. **Treatment of underlying cause**
8. **Supplemental sodium (PO or IV):** To correct hyponatremia.

NURSING DIAGNOSES AND INTERVENTIONS

Fluid volume deficit (with concomitant electrolyte disturbance) related to decreased circulating volume secondary to impaired secretion of aldosterone causing increased sodium excretion with resultant diuresis

---

Desired outcomes: Patient is normovolemic as evidenced by BP within patient's normal range; HR 60-100 bpm; RR 12-20 breaths/min with normal pattern and depth (eupnea); CVP 2-6 mm Hg; PAWP 6-12 mm Hg; normal sinus rhythm on EKG; and orientation to person, place, and time. Serum sodium is 137-147 mEq/L and serum potassium is 3.5-5.5 mEq/L.

---

1. Monitor VS and hemodynamic measurements q15min until they have been stable for one hour. Immediately report to MD a BP <90/60 mm Hg, HR >120 bpm, CVP <2 mm Hg, and PAWP <6 mm Hg.
2. Monitor patient at frequent intervals for evidence of hypotension. Measure BP and HR with patient reclining, then sitting. A drop of ≥20 mm Hg or an increase in HR >20 bpm and lasting for more than 3 minutes after changing position is indicative of mild to moderate dehydration.
3. Administer IV fluids as prescribed to replace extracellular fluid volume. Patients may need up to 6 L/hr for the first 1-2 hours.
4. Administer mineralcorticoids as prescribed.
5. Administer sodium supplements as prescribed to correct hyponatremia and facilitate fluid retention.

6. Monitor patient continuously on cardiac monitor; observe for EKG changes typical of hyperkalemia (see "EKG findings," p. 350).
7. Evaluate HR for abnormal rate (<60 or >100 bpm).
8. Observe for clinical manifestations of electrolyte imbalance as follows:
   - *Hyperkalemia:* lethargy, nausea, hyperactive bowel sounds with diarrhea, numbness or tingling in extremities, muscle weakness.
   - *Hyponatremia:* headache, malaise, muscle weakness, abdominal cramps.
9. Monitor laboratory test results for abnormalities. With appropriate treatment, serum sodium levels should rise to normal and serum potassium levels should fall to normal. Promptly report worsening hyponatremia or hyperkalemia to MD.
10. Administer insulin and glucose or Kayexalate as prescribed to correct hyperkalemia.
11. Assess patient's LOC and respiratory status at frequent intervals. Institute safety measures as indicated: padded side rails; bed in lowest position with side rails up when not at patient's bedside; and bite block, oral airway, and supplemental oxygen at the bedside. Apply soft restraints as necessary to prevent falls. Reorient and reassure patient as needed.

Alteration in tissue perfusion: Peripheral, cardiopulmonary, and renal, related to impaired circulation secondary to loss of vascular tone and decreased vascular response to catecholamines occurring with impaired secretion of glucocorticoids

---

Desired outcome: Patient has adequate perfusion as evidenced by BP within patient's normal range, HR 60-100 bpm, peripheral pulses >2+ on a 0-4+ scale, brisk capillary refill (<3 seconds), and urine output ≥30 ml/hr.

---

1. Monitor VS and hemodynamic measurements q15min until they have been stable for one hour. Immediately report to MD a BP <90/60 mm Hg, HR >120 bpm, CVP <2 mm Hg, or PAWP <6 mm Hg.
2. Assess peripheral pulses and capillary refill hourly. Notify MD of weak or absent pulses and delayed capillary refill.
3. Monitor urine output, being alert to output <30 ml/hr for two consecutive hours. Report significant findings.
4. Administer exogenous glucocorticoids as prescribed.
5. Administer vasopressors as prescribed for treatment of hypotension.

Knowledge deficit: Adverse side effects of glucocorticoid and mineralcorticoid therapy

---

Desired outcome: Patient and significant others verbalize knowledge of the potential side effects of glucocorticoid and mineralcorticoid steroids and the precautions necessary to prevent serious dysfunction.

Glucocorticoids: Prednisone, prednisolone, and dexamethasone may cause stress ulcers (as evidenced by oral or rectal bleeding, anorexia, nausea, vomiting, and epigastric pain after meals); emotional instability (e.g., euphoria, depression, or psychotic symptoms); elevated glucose levels; and lower resistance to infection.

1. Instruct patient to take medications to mimic normal diurnal pattern of hormone levels (i.e., two-thirds of the dose in the morning and one-third of the dose in the early afternoon).
2. Teach patient to take oral medications with food to decrease gastric irritation.
3. Advise patient to weigh self at the same time every day and to report gain >2 lb/week to MD.
4. Caution patient that petechiae and easy bruising are common side effects of these drugs.
5. Instruct patients with diabetes to monitor blood glucose levels carefully and to notify MD if levels increase. Insulin dosage may need to be increased.
6. Teach patient to take precautions to avoid exposure to communicable diseases and to be alert to indicators of infection, such as elevated temperature, increased pulse rate, nausea, anorexia, diarrhea, sore throat, or productive cough. Fungal infections may produce fever, chills, malaise, and oral or vaginal monilial growth.
7. Instruct patient to notify MD immediately if oral or rectal bleeding or changes in emotional state occur.
8. Advise patient that drug dosage may have to be increased to twice the normal dose during periods of physical or emotional stress.
9. Caution patient that dosages must be decreased gradually, as prescribed, because abrupt withdrawal can precipitate Addisonian crisis.

< N O T E : Drugs that have combined glucocorticoid and mineralcorticoid actions (e.g., hydrocortisone, cortisone acetate) may produce symptoms discussed under both glucocorticoids and mineralcorticoids.

Mineralcorticoids: Deoxycorticosterone acetate, deoxycorticosterone pivalate, and fludrocortisone acetate may cause weight gain, peripheral edema, and hypertension secondary to sodium retention. In addition, they can cause hypokalemia, as manifested by muscle weakness, irregular pulse, hypotension, anorexia, and drowsiness.
1. Teach patient that a sodium-restricted diet with potassium supplements is recommended to reduce side effects listed above. See Table 2-4, p. 88, "Low Sodium Dietary Guidelines."
2. Teach patient that serum potassium levels should be monitored more frequently if diuretics or amphotericin B (frequently given for fungal infections) are being taken, as these drugs may further decrease serum potassium levels.
3. Instruct patient to weigh self daily and to report weight gain >2 lb/week to MD.
4. Advise patient that dosage may need to be increased during periods of physical and emotional stress.
5. Caution patient that dosages should be decreased gradually, as prescribed, because abrupt withdrawal may precipitate Addisonian crisis.

< N O T E : Drugs that have combined glucocorticoid and mineralcorticoid actions (e.g., hydrocortisone, cortisone acetate) may produce symptoms discussed under both glucocorticoids and mineralcorticoids.

Potential for injury related to risk of exacerbation of symptoms of Addisonian crisis secondary to increased psychologic, emotional, or physical stressors with increased hormonal demand and inadequate adrenal reserves

Desired outcome: Patient verbalizes orientation to person, place, and time; and has stable weights, urine output <80-125 ml/hr, HR 60-100 bpm, BP within patient's normal range, and serum sodium 137-147 mEq/L.

1. Monitor for signs of increasing crisis: urinary output increased from usual amount, changes in LOC, orthostatic hypotension, nausea, vomiting, and tachycardia. Report any of these findings promptly to MD.
2. Provide a quiet environment to reduce external stimuli. Put patient in a private room, if possible. Keep lights dim and minimize the use of radios or other appliances.
3. Assist patient with care and provide 90-minute periods of uninterrupted rest as often as possible. Speak softly and reassuringly to patient.
4. Limit the number of visitors and the length of time they spend with patient. Caution visitors not to discuss stress-provoking topics with patient, but rather to speak softly and reassuringly.
5. Do not allow staff or visitors with colds or contagious diseases in patient's care area.
6. Administer hormone replacements as prescribed to maintain adequate serum levels.

See "Diabetic Ketoacidosis" for the following: **Potential for infection,** p. 332; **Potential for injury** related to confusion, obtundation, coma, or seizures secondary to cerebral edema or dehydration, p. 333; and **Potential alteration in tissue perfusion:** Peripheral, related to risk of thromboembolism, p. 334. For other nursing diagnoses and interventions, see "Caring for the Critically Ill with Life-Threatening Disorders," pp. 511-522; and "Caring for the Family of the Critically Ill," pp. 522-526.

REHABILITATION AND PATIENT-FAMILY TEACHING CONCEPTS

Give patient and significant others verbal and written instructions for the following:
1. Medications, including purpose, dosage, route of administration, and potential side effects.
2. Diet instruction: Dietary sodium and potassium may need to be adjusted, based on patient's clinical condition and drug therapy (see **Knowledge deficit**, p. 352).
3. Importance of avoiding or reducing stress, both emotional and physiologic, which increases adrenal demand. Teach patient to seek medical intervention during times of increased stress (e.g., fever, infection), as medication dosages may need to be increased.
4. Indicators of excessive steroid replacement (e.g., weight gain, moon face, fatigue, polyuria, polydipsia, easy bruising) and symptoms of worsening Addison's disease (e.g., weight loss, easy fatigability that worsens throughout the day, nausea, vomiting, excessive pigmentation), which require prompt medical attention.

5. Importance of continued medical follow-up; confirm date and time of next medical appointment.

6. Procedure for obtaining a Medic-Alert bracelet or card identifying patient's diagnosis.

SELECTED REFERENCES

Alspach JG, Williams SM: *Core Curriculum for Critical Care Nursing*, 3rd ed. Saunders, 1985.

American Hospital Formulary Service: *Drug Information 86*. American Society of Hospital Pharmacists, 1986.

Burch WM: *Endocrinology for the House Officer*. Williams and Wilkins, 1984.

Christman C, Bennett J: Diabetes: New names, new test, new diet. *Nursing 87;* January 1987: 34-41.

Ganong WF: *Review of Medical Physiology*, 12th edition. Appleton-Century-Crofts, 1985.

Johanson BC, et al: *Standards of Critical Care*, 2nd ed. Mosby, 1985.

Kershner D: Endocrine Disorders. In: *Manual of Nursing Therapeutics: Applying Nursing Diagnoses to Medical Disorders*. Swearingen PL (ed). Addison-Wesley, 1986.

Mazzaferri E: *Textbook of Endocrinology*, 3rd ed. Elsevier, 1986.

Metz R, Larson EB: *Blue Book of Endocrinology*. Saunders, 1985.

Muthe NC: *Endocrinology, A Nursing Approach*. Little, Brown, 1981.

Nurses' Clinical Library: *Endocrine Disorders*. Springhouse, 1984.

6
GASTROINTESTINAL
D Y S F U N C T I O N S

Bleeding esophageal varices

Hepatic failure

Acute pancreatitis

Peritonitis

Acute gastrointestinal bleeding

Abdominal trauma

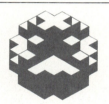

Bleeding esophageal varices

With obstruction of blood flow through the liver, portal venous pressure can rise from a normal of about 7 mm Hg to as much as 20-25 mm Hg. As a result of prolonged increased portal pressure, collateral vessels develop to divert blood from the portal circulation into the systemic circulation. Obstruction of portal flow dilates the smaller veins that normally drain blood from the lower esophagus and stomach into the portal vein. These enlarged and engorged veins that develop beneath the mucosa are known as varices. Rupture of gastroesophageal varices leads to dramatic hematemesis and to hemorrhage, which is exceedingly difficult to control. Blood loss is enhanced by thrombocytopenia and clotting disorders, which often are found in patients with hepatic disease. Portal hypertension may result in engorgement of vessels in the umbilical, retroperitoneal, and anal areas. However, collateral vessels in these sites are less likely to rupture and bleed.

Although any blockage of portal blood as it enters or leaves the liver can elevate portal venous pressure, the most common cause of portal hypertension is intrahepatic blockage of portal blood flow caused by hepatic cirrhosis. When portal venous blood is shunted from the liver by collateral vessels associated with portal hypertension, the liver shrinks in size and has an impaired ability to regenerate or perform normally. Large portosystemic shunts result in complications, including hepatic encephalopathy, septicemia, and metabolic abnormalities. In addition, acute blood loss from variceal bleeding results in hypoxic damage to liver cells and may precipitate complications of liver failure such as jaundice, ascites, and encephalopathy in individuals with cirrhosis. Mortality rate for variceal hemorrhage ranges from 35-60% and is related to the degree of hepatocellular failure.

ASSESSMENT

Signs and symptoms: Hematemesis is usually the first and most common presentation. The average amount of blood lost during a single bleeding episode is 10 units. Melena, with or without hematemesis, is another frequent occurrence. Acute gastritis, peptic ulcer disease, and Mallory-Weiss syndrome (see "Acute Gastrointestinal Bleeding," p. 394) may contribute to the usually massive blood loss, particularly among individuals with alcoholic cirrhosis. The absence of dyspepsia and epigastric tenderness help rule out peptic ulcer disease as the cause of the bleeding.

Physical assessment: Signs of hepatocellular failure such as jaundice, ascites, altered mental status, and edema are typical. Splenomegaly is commonly associated with portal hypertension. In individuals with cirrhosis, the liver may be small and firm. An enlarged and tender liver may be palpated if hepatic inflammation is present, as with viral or alcoholic hepatitis. Vascular spiders, usually above the nipple line, and palmar erythema are believed to be manifestations of circulatory abnormalities associated with cirrhosis. Large hemorrhoids may be present on rectal examination, along with stool containing occult blood or frank melena. In the presence of acute blood loss, cool, pale skin and altered mental status will be readily apparent. If aspiration of gastric contents has occurred, coarse crackles (rales) and rhonchi may be auscultated.

Vital signs and hemodynamic measurements: Usually reflect a hypovolemic state, for example, elevated HR, decreased BP, CVP, PAP, and PAWP, and increased PVR. Pulses will be weak and thready. Some patients with cirrhosis present with a hyperdynamic cardiovascular state, in which cardiac output is elevated and peripheral vascular resistance is lowered. In these patients, pulses may be bounding and the extremities will be warm and flushed. The hyperdynamic state will be more readily apparent in volume-resuscitated patients and in some patients who have undergone shunt surgery for portal decompression.

History and risk factors: Recent episode(s) of painless and often sudden hematemesis or melena, excessive ethanol ingestion (averaging >60 g/day), previously diagnosed cirrhosis, hepatitis, intra-abdominal or biliary infection, biliary disease, traumatic portal vein injury, congenital liver disease, and tumor invasion.

DIAGNOSTIC TESTS

1. *Hematologic tests:* Hematocrit and hemoglobin will be decreased because of acute blood loss and mild anemia associated with hypersplenism. Platelet and WBC counts will be decreased owing to splenic enlargement. PT and PTT are often prolonged secondary to clotting factor deficiency in patients with hepatocellular disease.

2. *Biochemical tests:* Severity of liver damage may be estimated by elevations in serum total bilirubin, decreases in serum albumin (see ''Hepatic Failure,'' p. 367), and prolongation of prothrombin time. Serum ammonia is elevated as blood is shunted from the liver by collaterals and the failing liver is unable to convert ammonia to urea. A large protein load from gastrointestinal bleeding results in greatly increased ammonia levels if hepatic failure is severe. Dietary protein and blood in the GI tract will increase serum ammonia levels. Antibiotic therapy may decrease the levels.

< N O T E : Blood specimens for serum ammonia should be placed in ice and transported to the lab immediately after collection to ensure accuracy of the test.

3. *Blood alcohol:* May be tested upon admission to help distinguish acute intoxication from encephalopathy.

4. *Occult blood tests:* To test for blood in stool or gastric secretions.

5. *Esophagoscopy:* Visualizes the esophagus and stomach directly *via* a fiberoptic esophagoscope. Varices in the esophagus and upper stomach are identified and attempts are made to identify the exact source of bleeding. Variceal bleeding may be treated by sclerotherapy during the endoscopic procedure (see Medical Management section).

< N O T E : The patient's stomach should be clear of blood and gastric contents prior to esophagoscopy. If the procedure is elective, the patient should be NPO from midnight until completion of the test.

6. *Angiographic studies:* Establish patency of the portal vein and visualize the portosystemic collateral vessels to determine cause and effective treatment for variceal bleeding.
   • The most common procedure is portal venography. The femoral artery is catheterized and contrast material is injected into the splenic artery.

< N O T E : After portal venography, the patient must be kept supine with a pressure dressing and sandbag over the puncture site for 6-8 hours. During the first few hours after the procedure, distal pulses should be checked q1-2h. Arterial thrombosis and large hematomas that compromise femoral blood flow may develop, owing to manipulation of the artery and clotting abnormalities associated with liver disease. Adequacy of urine output should be monitored closely, partic-

ularly in patients with ascites, who are especially susceptible to functional renal failure (hepato-renal syndrome) and tubular necrosis.

- Hepatic vein wedge pressure (HVWP) is measured by introducing a balloon catheter into the femoral vein and threading it into a hepatic vein branch. Normal HVWP is 5-6 mm Hg and values of about 20 mm Hg are typical for patients with cirrhosis (Sherlock, 1985).
- Direct access to the portal vein may be achieved through trans-hepatic portography. During this procedure, varices may be obliterated by injection of thrombin or gel foam into veins that supply the varices.

< N O T E : This procedure involves a direct puncture through the liver and has many of the same risks as liver biopsy. Patients returning from this procedure should be positioned on their right side and monitored closely. For more information, see ''Liver Biopsy'' in ''Hepatic Failure,'' p. 367.

7. *Barium swallow*: Used in nonemergent situations to verify the presence of gastroesophageal varices.

< N O T E : The patient should be NPO from midnight until completion of the test. Because of the constipating effects of barium, which can precipitate or enhance hepatic encephalopathy, laxatives or enemas should be given upon patient's return from the procedure.

8. *Liver biopsy*: See ''Hepatic Failure,'' p. 367.

MEDICAL MANAGEMENT AND SURGICAL INTERVENTIONS

Medical management of gastroesophageal variceal bleeding is dependent on the underlying cause of portal hypertension, severity of the bleeding episode, and previous response to therapy. Every attempt is made to stop the bleeding and preserve liver function, which is especially important for patients with cirrhosis and underlying hepatocellular disease.

1. **Fluid resuscitation:** Restoration of blood volume is achieved with combinations of lactated Ringer's (RL), D_5W, albumin, packed red cells, and fresh frozen plasma. Fresh whole blood is the optimal resuscitation fluid but is rarely available. Until blood products are available, emergency resuscitation with LR or D_5W and albumin is initiated. Saline infusions usually are avoided, as sodium is retained and contributes to ascites. Packed red cells are administered as soon as available to maintain a hematocrit of 28-30%. Fresh frozen plasma is helpful in restoring deficient clotting factors. Platelets are given only if the platelet count is markedly reduced or the patient has spontaneous bleeding from sites other than the varices. Albumin is administered if the patient continues to be hypovolemic despite a hematocrit in the 28-30% range or if the patient is hypoalbuminemic. Plasma protein fraction (PPF) usually is avoided since rapid infusion can generate hypotension.

2. **Vasopressin:** A potent vasoconstrictor that controls variceal hemorrhage by constricting the mesenteric, splenic, and hepatic arteriolar beds, thereby reducing blood flow to the portal vein and lowering portal venous pressure. Twenty units of vasopressin (Pitressin) in 100 ml D_5W are given IV over a 20-minute period. A continuous IV infusion of 0.1-0.4 units/min may be delivered for a prolonged effect. Concurrent IV infusions of nitroglycerin or nitroprusside sometimes are given to reduce vasopressin-induced coronary vasoconstriction.

3. **Nasogastric intubation:** A large-lumen NG tube may be inserted in order to aspirate blood and clots from the stomach. Lavage with iced or room temperature saline or sterile water is helpful in clearing blood from the stomach in order to estimate bleeding or prepare the patient for endoscopy. However, the effectiveness of iced lavage in reducing upper GI hemorrhage is questionable.

4. **Endoscopic sclerotherapy:** During endoscopy, varices are injected with a sclerosing solution such as sodium tetradecylsulphate to cause variceal obliteration *via* fibrosis. This treatment is used both to control acute bleeding and manage long-term bleeding *via* chronic, serial injections. Chronic sclerotherapy appears promising in preventing rebleeding in some patients, but emergency surgery is necessary if rebleeding becomes uncontrollable.

5. **Balloon tamponade:** Achieves temporary control of variceal hemorrhage by inflating esophageal and gastric balloons until the balloon pressure exceeds variceal pressure and thereby tamponades the bleeding vessels. Maximum balloon inflation pressure should not exceed 45 mm Hg. A Sengstaken-Blakemore or similar tube is used. Complications are numerous and include pharyngeal obstruction with possible asphyxia, as well as mucosal erosion with variceal rupture and exsanguination. An immediate chest x-ray is necessary after tube insertion to confirm proper placement.

6. **Surgical management:** Emergency surgery for variceal bleeding is associated with a higher operative mortality rate than elective procedures. It is desirable to control acute bleeding medically and schedule elective surgery at a later time when the patient's condition has stabilized. Portocaval shunts lower portal pressure by joining the portal vein with the vena cava. The disadvantage of this procedure is total diversion of portal blood flow to the liver and consequent disabling encephalopathy in many patients. The distal splenorenal shunt diverts blood from the problematic varices *via* the short gastric and splenic veins. Portal blood flow to the liver is preserved and the incidence of encephalopathy is greatly reduced. This procedure is much more difficult to perform and requires a high degree of surgical expertise.

7. **Beta blockade:** Recent clinical trials suggest that long-term reduction of portal hypertension may be accomplished by oral beta blocking agents (Lebrec, 1984); however, their use is controversial and remains limited.

NURSING DIAGNOSES AND INTERVENTIONS

Fluid volume deficit related to decreased circulating volume secondary to active variceal bleeding

---

Desired outcomes: Patient's variceal bleeding is resolved and circulating blood volume is restored and maintained as evidenced by MAP >70 mm Hg, HR 60-100 bpm, brisk capillary refill (<3 seconds), CVP 2-6 mm Hg, PAWP 6-12 mm Hg, CI ≥2.5 L/min/m^2, and urinary output ≥30 ml/hr. Patient verbalizes orientation to person, place, and time.

---

1. Administer prescribed fluids at rapid rate (wide open). See "Fluid resuscitation," p. 359, for types of fluids indicated. Minimize IV infusion of sodium-containing solutions, which can contribute to fluid sequestration in the abdomen (ascites) and precipitate hepatorenal syndrome in susceptible patients (see "Hepatic Failure," p. 371)

2. Monitor BP q15 min, or more frequently in the presence of active bleeding. Be alert to decreases in MAP >10 mm Hg less than baseline.

3. Monitor HR, EKG, and cardiovascular status q15 min, or more frequently in the presence of active bleeding or if using vasopressin or similar agents. Be alert to increases in HR, delayed capillary refill, and changes in LOC, which reflect hypovolemia. Be aware that an altered LOC can be caused by encephalopathy as well as hypovolemia. Anticipate vasopressin-induced reflex bradycardia; notify MD if bradycardia is severe (HR <60 bpm) or compromises tissue perfusion.

4. Measure central pressures and thermodilution CO q1-2h, or more frequently if the patient is unstable or on vasoactive agents. Be alert to low or decreasing CVP and PAWP. Assess for signs of over-aggressive fluid resuscitation, including increased CVP, PAP, and PAWP, and aggravation of variceal bleeding in some patients. Anticipate CO >8 L/min. Evaluate volume status by noting increases or decreases in PAWP values and urinary output.

5. Measure urinary output qh. Be alert to output <30 ml/hr for two consecutive hours. Anticipate decreased urinary output after intitial dose of vasopressin. Expect diuresis after vasopressin has been discontinued.

6. Monitor for physical indicators of hypovolemia, including cool extremities, capillary refill >4 seconds, absent or decreased amplitude of distal pulses, and change in LOC.

7. Measure and record all GI blood losses from hematemesis, hematochezia (red blood through rectum), and melena. Test all stools and gastric contents for occult blood.

8. Administer vasopressin as prescribed. Ensure patency of IV catheter. Monitor for serious side effects such as bradycardia, ventricular irritability, chest pain, abdominal cramping, hyponatremia, and oliguria.

9. Be alert to adverse side effects of esophageal sclerotherapy: infection, pulmonary complications (i.e., PaO_2 <80 mm Hg, basilar crackles, diminished breath sounds) and esophageal ulceration (i.e., difficulty in swallowing, pain, continued bleeding). Anticipate mild retrosternal pain and transient fever after the procedure.

10. Avoid use of in-dwelling NG tubes for routine gastric drainage, as they can irritate varices and prolong or renew bleeding.

Alteration in cardiac output: Decreased, related to risk of dysrhythmias or myocardial infarction secondary to myocardial ischemia occurring with prolonged bleeding and vasopressin-induced coronary vasoconstriction

---

Desired outcome: Patient's EKG shows normal sinus rhythm.

---

1. Monitor ABG values for evidence of hypoxemia. Be alert to and report PaO_2 <80 mm Hg.

2. Administer oxygen as indicated by ABG values.

3. Monitor hematocrit; report values <28-30/100 ml promptly.

4. Monitor patient for evidence of myocardial ischemia if hemoglobin is greatly decreased or if the patient is receiving vasopressin. Observe EKG for ventricular dysrhythmias and ST-segment changes. Instruct patient to report chest discomfort promptly.

5. Measure thermodilution CO q1-2h. Be aware that a "normal" CO may be a low value for the hyperdynamic cirrhotic patient.
6. Maintain MAP >70-80 (see **Fluid volume deficit**).
7. Minimize activity during acute bleeding episode in order to reduce myocardial oxygen demands.

Potential for ineffective airway clearance related to risk secondary to aspiration of gastric secretions, alterations in mentation (occurring with encephalopathy), or presence of balloon tamponade

---

Desired outcome: Patient's airway remains clear as evidenced by auscultation of normal breath sounds and absence of adventitious sounds.

---

1. Position patient in a side-lying position during vomiting episodes unless he or she is *fully* alert and is more comfortable in an upright position.
2. As necessary, suction oropharynx with Yankauer or similar suction device to remove blood.
3. Auscultate lung fields during and after vomiting episodes for presence of rhonchi, which can signal aspiration of gastric contents.
4. Provide oral care at frequent intervals to assist in mobilizing oropharyngeal secretions. A dilute solution of hydrogen peroxide and normal saline may be helpful in removing tenacious secretions or dried blood from the teeth and oral mucosa.
5. Implement the following interventions for patients with Sengstaken-Blakemore (S-B) or similar tubes:
   • Confer with MD regarding possibility of endotracheal intubation prior to S-B insertion.
   • Verify proper tube placement by *stat* chest x-ray.
   • Be certain that oral secretions are suctioned from above the inflated esophageal balloon *via* a proximal tube or an additional lumen in the tube for this purpose. Label proximal tube or lumen with the warning "Do Not Irrigate."
   • Ensure patency of gastric and esophageal drainage lumens. Irrigate *gastric* lumen q1-2h and as necessary, to ensure patency.
   • Be aware that proximal migration of the esophageal balloon or rupture of the gastric balloon may result in total airway obstruction. Keep a pair of scissors in an obvious place and with the patient at all times in order to cut and immediately deflate all lumens of the S-B tube should respiratory distress occur.
   • Check security of tape, tube connections, and traction initially and qh.
   • Document quantity and characteristics of gastric drainage q4h.

Potential alteration in tissue perfusion: Esophageal, related to risk of impaired circulation secondary to prolonged use of esophageal balloon tamponade

---

Desired outcomes: Esophageal balloon pressure is maintained within prescribed range (usually 20-40 mm Hg). Patient is asymptomatic of esophageal perforation as evidenced by BP within patient's normal range, HR 60-100 bpm, PAP ≥20/8,

PAWP ≥6 mm Hg, SVR ≤1200 dynes/sec/cm^{-5}, CO ≥4 L/min, and absence of sudden substernal or back pain.

1. Check the esophageal balloon pressure at least hourly. Maintain pressure within prescribed range (usually 20-40 mm Hg). Release pressure at prescribed intervals.
2. Carefully document date and time of balloon inflation and deflation. Tissue necrosis is likely if balloons are left inflated for 24-48 hours.
3. After 24 hours, assist MD in relieving traction and deflating the esophageal balloon. The tube remains in place with the gastric balloon inflated for the next 24 hours and the patient is closely monitored for rebleeding. If there is no further rebleeding, the gastric balloon is deflated and the tube removed.
4. Promptly report signs of esophageal perforation: sudden epigastric or substernal pain, back pain, shock state.

Potential for impaired swallowing related to lower esophageal pain or lower esophageal stricture secondary to sclerotherapy

Desired outcome: Patient demonstrates ability to pass food through the lower esophagus into the stomach.

1. After sclerotherapy treatments, evaluate patient for subjective complaints of difficulty in swallowing or pain when swallowing. Report signficant findings to MD.
2. Plan soft or bland diet as tolerated by patient.
3. Avoid mechanically or chemically irritating foods.
4. Caution patient that certain foods or substances (e.g., alcohol) may cause a burning sensation when swallowed due to esophageal mucosal erosion. Instruct patient to avoid mechanical or chemical irritants.

If portal hypertension is caused by cirrhosis, refer to "Hepatic Failure" for additional nursing diagnoses. For other nursing diagnoses and interventions, see "Caring for the Critically Ill with Life-Threatening Disorders," pp. 511-522, and "Caring for the Family of the Critically Ill," pp. 522-526.

REHABILITATION AND PATIENT-FAMILY TEACHING CONCEPTS

Give patient and significant others verbal and written instructions for the following:
1. Signs and symptoms of actual or impending hemorrhage, including nausea, dark stools, light-headedness, vomiting of blood, or passing of frank blood in stools.
2. Importance of seeking medical attention promptly if indicators of hemorrhage appear.
3. Importance of medical follow-up for management of variceal bleeding, either chronic sclerotherapy or shunt surgery.
4. Medications, including drug name, purpose, dosage, schedule, precautions, and potential side effects.

5. Importance of avoiding alcohol ingestion, which is caustic to the esophageal and gastric mucosa.
6. If portal hypertension is caused by cirrhosis, see same section in "Hepatic Failure."

Hepatic failure

Hepatic failure is loss of the functional capacity of the liver due to extensive hepatocellular damage. The damage may occur slowly as with cirrhosis or suddenly as with acute viral or drug-induced hepatitis. *Cirrhosis* is a chronic liver disease associated with widespread tissue necrosis, fibrosis, and nodule formation within the liver. Common causes of cirrhosis include chronic alcohol ingestion; viral hepatitis types B (HBV) and non-A, non-B (NANB) (see Table 6-1); prolonged cholestasis; and metabolic disorders. Changes in liver structure due to cirrhosis are irreversible, but compensation of liver function may be achieved if the liver is protected from further damage by cessation of alcohol or arrest of inflammatory processes. Acute (fulminant) hepatic failure is characterized by a sudden and severe liver decompensation due to massive hepatocellular necrosis. Acute hepatic failure may be caused by HB or NANB viral hepatitis or it may be the result of drug reactions, poisoning, alcoholic hepatitis, or shock, especially severe and prolonged septic shock. It is important to recognize that most cases of viral hepatitis are mild; many are undiagnosed. Less than 5% of individuals with viral hepatitis actually develop acute hepatic failure. Because preexisting liver damage generally is absent in patients with acute hepatic failure, the massive damage is potentially reversible and those who survive the acute episode usually recover completely. Individuals with alcoholic liver disease present a unique set of problems in that they may sustain an acute episode of hepatic failure superimposed upon chronic failure due to preexisting cirrhosis.

Jaundice is frequently seen with hepatic failure largely due to the inability of the failing liver to metabolize bilirubin. Metabolic encephalopathy, with varying alterations in consciousness and mental functioning, is attributed to ammonia toxicity and other metabolic derangements. In patients with cirrhosis, diversion of portal blood flow *via* large collateral vessels contributes to the encephalopathy. Bleeding tendencies are caused by inadequate vitamin K absorption, failure of the liver to synthesize clotting factors or clear activated clotting factors, and thrombocytopenia. Infections, including sepsis, are common owing to a generalized state of debilitation and failure of the liver to produce immune-related proteins and filter blood from the intestines. Often, circulatory abnormalities are present and include a hyperdynamic systemic circulation with increased cardiac output and decreased vasomotor tone. Circulatory changes in the pulmonary system include dilatation of the pulmonary vasculature and pulmonary arteriovenous shunting with ventilation-perfusion mismatch. In addition, reductions in renal circulation can result in functional renal failure (hepatorenal syndrome). Fluid retention and ascites are attributed to several factors including (1) intrahepatic vascular obstruction with transudation of fluid into the peritoneum; (2) defective albumin synthesis, resulting in decreased colloid osmotic pressure with failure to retain intravascular fluid; and (3) disturbances of various hormones including renin, aldosterone, and renal prostaglandins, resulting in sodium and water retention. Ascites and edema are associated with chronic and acute hepatic failure, although massive ascites usually is due to cirrhosis. Although prognosis with hepatic failure is difficult to evaluate, the presence of one or more of the following suggests a less-than-favorable outcome: se-

TABLE 6-1

Types and characteristics of viral hepatitis

	Hepatitis A (HAV)	Hepatitis B (HBV)	Non-A, Non-B (NANB)
Incubation	15-50 days	45-160 days	15-180 days
Transmission	Fecal-oral	Blood and body fluids (e.g., semen, saliva)	Similar to HBV
High-risk populations	Those with poor personal hygiene, poor sanitation, in institutional settings, or exposed to contaminated food or water	IV drug users; male homosexuals; medical personnel, especially in hemodialysis, surgery, emergency, critical care areas; patients and staff in institutions for the mentally retarded; immigrants or refugees from areas of high HBV endemicity	Recipients of blood and some blood products; IV drug users; male homosexuals; medical personnel
Diagnostic tests	Serum positive for IgM class antibody to hepatitis A virus (IgM anti-HAV)	Serum positive for hepatitis B surface antigen (HBsAg)	No serologic test available
Severity of acute attack	Usually mild	Mild to severe	Usually asymptomatic or mild
Chronic carrier state	No	Possible for some people	Possible for some people
Prophylaxis	Immune globulin (IG) prior to travel to high-risk areas; IG within 2 weeks after HAV exposure	Preexposure vaccination strongly encouraged for high-risk groups. For percutaneous exposure, hepatitis B immune globulin (HBIG) and vaccine series or booster recommended, depending upon source of exposure and vaccination status of exposed person	Possible IG after known percutaneous exposure

vere prolonged jaundice, persistant ascites, persistently decreased albumin, persistently prolonged prothrombin times, and severe encephalopathy.

ASSESSMENT

Signs and symptoms: Weakness, extreme fatigue, anorexia, low-grade fever, sleep disturbance. Neurologic symptoms range from mild personality changes to delirium and sometimes, deep coma. Urine may be dark owing to bilirubin, and stools may be light owing to its absence. Portal hypertension and variceal bleeding (see p. 357) may be present, usually associated with chronic failure. Men with chronic liver failure may experience impotence or diminished libido. In the later stages of hepatic failure, coma, seizures, and decerebrate rigidity are possible.

Physical assessment: Jaundice, which frequently is present with serious hepatic failure, manifests in the sclera in the early stages and as generalized, deep yellow skin with late or fulminant failure; fluid sequestration noted as edema, ascites, and weight gain; weight loss and muscle wasting in patients with chronic hepatic failure. Patient may have a fixed facial expression, slowness with speech and movement, and asterixis (flapping tremor of the hands that occurs with finger extension). Fetor hepaticus, a sweet fecal odor, may be detected on patient's breath, especially with severe failure. Small, bright red vascular spiders (spider telangiectasis, spider angioma) frequently are found on the upper trunk, face, neck, and arms of patients with cirrhosis and are notably absent in patients with acute hepatic failure. Multiple ecchymotic areas, purpura, and bleeding of the oral and nasal mucosa are manifestations of clotting abnormalities. In chronic liver disease, the liver usually is small and hard. Individuals with acute failure often have an enlarged, firm liver. The spleen is usually enlarged with chronic failure, but may not be enlarged with acute hepatic failure. Distended abdomen with shifting dullness to percussion and positive fluid wave are present due to ascites. Hydrothorax caused by transdiaphragmatic passage of ascitic fluid into the pleural cavity results in dyspnea, decreased breath sounds, and dullness to percussion on the affected (usually right) side. With severe ascites, hernias are common and the umbilicus frequently is everted. The cardiac apex may be elevated and displaced laterally due to a raised diaphragm. Usually, neck veins are distended due to increased right atrial pressure caused by increased intrapleural pressures from diaphragmatic elevation. Hormonal changes that result in gynecomastia, testicular atrophy, and scant body hair are common in males with chronic hepatic disease.

Vital signs and hemodynamic measurements: Elevated temperature due to infection, normal to bounding pulses, low to normal BP, elevated cardiac output associated with decreased peripheral vascular resistance and expanded total blood volume. In the presence of tense ascites, which increases intra-abdominal pressure, patient will exhibit impaired right ventricular filling with decreased stroke volume and decreased cardiac output. With variceal hemorrhage or late septic shock, pulses will be diminished and BP will be low, reflecting circulatory collapse.

History and risk factors: Previous hepatic or biliary disease, including cirrhosis, hepatitis, cholecystitis, and metabolic liver disease (e.g., Wilson's disease, a_1 antitrypsin deficiency); excessive alcohol ingestion; blood transfusion (non-A, non-B hepatitis is the most common transfusion-related hepatitis and is more likely to result in chronic infection than other forms); exposure to hepatotoxic agents such as halothane, MAO inhibitors, isoniazid, acetaminophen (dose >10 grams), and carbon tetrachloride. Groups at high risk for developing type-B hepatitis include immigrants, refugees, or extended travelers from China and Southeast Asia, sub-Saharan Africa, most Pacific islands, and the Amazon basin; staff in custodial institutions for the mentally retarded; male homosexuals; IV drug users; medical and dental workers with exposure to blood; and hemodialysis patients. Although the hepatitis A virus usually results in a mild infection, patients should be questioned regarding raw shellfish ingestion and possible exposure to contaminated water supplies.

DIAGNOSTIC TESTS

1. *Virologic markers:* Hepatitis A antibody (anti-HAV) is detected in the serum several weeks after the initial infection and continues to be detectable for many years after the infection. The presence of IgM anti-HAV is more helpful diag-

nostically because is implies a recent infection. The hepatitis B surface antigen (HBsAg) appears about 6 weeks after hepatitis B viral infection. The continued presence of HBsAg for >6 months is suggestive of a carrier state. Hepatitis B virus is more likely to result in severe acute and chronic infections than the type A virus. There are no serologic tests to detect the presence of non-A, non-B viruses.

2. *Serum biochemical tests*
   - *Bilirubin:* Elevated due to failure in hepatocyte metabolism and obstruction in some instances. Very high or persistently elevated levels are considered a poor prognostic sign.
   - *Alkalkine phosphatase:* Normal to mildly elevated.
   - *Transaminase (SGOT & SGPT):* Usually elevated >300 units with acute failure; normal or mildly elevated with chronic failure. SGPT is more specific for hepatocellular damage.
   - *Albumin:* Reduced, especially with ascites. Persistently low levels suggest a poor prognosis.
   - *Sodium:* Normal to low. Sodium is retained but is associated with water retention, which results in normal sodium levels or even a dilutional hyponatremia. Often, severe hyponatremia is present in the terminal stage and is associated with tense ascites and hepatorenal syndrome.
   - *Potassium:* Slightly reduced unless patient has renal insufficiency, which would result in hyperkalemia. Chronic hypokalemic acidosis is common in patients with chronic alcoholic liver disease.
   - *Glucose:* Hypoglycemia sometimes is present due to impaired gluconeogenesis and glycogen depletion in patients with severe or terminal liver disease.
   - *BUN:* May be slightly decreased due to failure of Kreb's cycle enzymes in the liver; or elevated due to bleeding or renal insufficiency.
   - *Ammonia:* Elevation is expected due to inability of the failing liver to convert ammonia to urea and shunting of intestinal blood *via* collaterals. GI hemorrhage or an increase in intestinal protein from dietary intake will increase ammonia levels (see "Variceal Bleeding," p. 358).

4. *Hematologic tests:* A mild, normocytic, normochromic anemia is expected. With acute variceal hemorrhage, a marked decrease in Hgb and Hct will be present. Decreased leukocyte and platelet counts are expected and are due in part to hypersplenism. If infection is present, the leukocyte count may increase to normal levels or be mildly elevated. Prothrombin time is prolonged and unresponsive to vitamin K therapy.

5. *Liver biopsy:* Obtains a specimen of liver for microscopic analysis and diagnosis of cirrhosis, hepatitis, or other liver disease. After local anesthesia and skin preparation, a large needle is inserted into the eighth or ninth intercostal space in the midaxillary line. It is critical that patients hold their breath at the end of expiration in order to elevate the liver maximally. Patient movement or failure to sustain expiration can result in puncture through the lung rather than liver. Type and cross-matching sometimes is done prior to the procedure in anticipation of hemorrhagic complications. Percutaneous liver biopsy is contraindicated in patients with markedly prolonged PT or very low platelet counts because of the risk of hemorrhage. In these patients a transvenous biopsy *via* the jugular and hepatic vein may be attempted instead.
   - Auscultate breath sounds immediately after the procedure and at 1-2 hour

intervals for 6-8 hours after the procedure to detect pneumothorax or hemo-thorax (unlikely but serious complications). Diminished sounds on the right side and tachypnea suggest pneumo- or hemothorax.

- Position patient on the right side for several hours after the biopsy to tam-ponade the puncture site.
- Enforce bedrest for 8-12 hours postbiopsy to minimize the risk of hemor-rhage from the puncture site.
- Monitor patient for indicators of peritonitis or intraperitoneal bleeding, which can occur as a result of puncture of blood vessels or major bile duct: severe abdominal pain, abdominal distention and rigidity, rebound tender-ness, nausea, vomiting, tachycardia, tachypnea, pallor, decreased BP, and rising temperature.

6. *EEG:* Traces the electrical impulses of the brain to detect or confirm enceph-alopathy. EEG changes occur very early, usually before behavioral or bio-chemical alterations.

7. *Psychometric testing:* Evaluates for hepatic encephalopathy. A common test is the Reitan number connection (trail-making) test. The patient's speed and ac-curacy at connecting a series of numbered circles is evaluated at intervals. A daily handwriting test is an easy check of intellectual deterioration or improve-ment.

8. *Abdominal paracentesis:* Involves the insertion of a catheter or trocar into the abdominal cavity to remove fluids. A small amount of fluid is sent for analysis of protein, electrolytes, WBCs, and culture. Larger amounts of fluid may be drained over several hours if the patient has gross ascites that interferes with cardiopulmonary functioning. This procedure can cause hypovolemia and shock as drained ascites are replaced rapidly from the blood, resulting in intra-vascular depletion. Frequent VS assessment and evaluation of urinary output are indicated. Peritoneal infection is another complication.

9. *Urinalysis:* Gross inspection will reveal dark urine with a yellow foam when shaken. Increased urobilinogen and bilirubin will be present. In the presence of ascites, 24-hour urine volume will be decreased and 24-hour sodium will be reduced (<5 mEq/day in severe cases).

10. *Liver scan*: Imaging by radioisotope, ultrasound, or CT can aid in determining size of the liver and presence of abnormal tissue, such as tumors.

MEDICAL MANAGEMENT AND SURGICAL INTERVENTIONS

1. **Correction of precipitating factors:** A patient with compensated liver disease may develop hepatic failure if any one of a number of factors disrupts hepa-tocellular functioning. GI hemorrhage or blood loss from other sources re-quires prompt detection and immediate volume resuscitation. Acute infections are treated aggressively with appropriate antibiotics. Electrolyte disturbances due to diuretics, diarrhea, or other causes must be corrected promptly. Ethanol and hepatotoxic drugs are eliminated. Sedatives and tranquilizers may contrib-ute to hepatic encephalopathy and should be discontinued. Hypoxia from any cause can aggravate hepatocellular failure and must be corrected.

2. **Fluid and electrolyte management:** Unless hyponatremia is profound, so-dium-containing foods are avoided because they contribute to ascites and pe-ripheral edema and may potentiate renal insufficiency. Hypokalemia is com-mon and must be corrected with potassium replacements as hypokalemic

alkalosis can worsen or precipitate encephalopathy. Albumin and D_5W are used for fluid resuscitation unless a low Hct signals the need for blood. Fresh frozen plasma may be used if clotting factors are deficient, but infusions of large amounts can lead to hypernatremia. Oral and IV fluid intake is restricted if ascites is present. In the unstable or comatose patient, CVP or PAP monitoring is initiated to ensure adequate tissue perfusion without fluid overload.

< N O T E : Accurate measurements and careful interpretation of hemodynamic parameters are essential because fluid balance is delicate in critically ill patients with hepatic failure and hemodynamic measurements can be difficult to interpret due to the hyperdynamic circulatory state.

3. **Bed rest:** Necessary to reduce metabolic demands placed on the liver during normal daily activity. It is strictly enforced until several days to weeks after the patient's condition has stabilized.

4. **Nutritional therapy:** A high-calorie, 80-100 gram protein diet is indicated for patients without evidence of encephalopathy to ensure tissue repair, as the liver is capable of significant regeneration under optimal circumstances. Sodium is moderately restricted, although rigid adherence to a 500 mg or less sodium-restriction diet is necessary in patients with ascites. If GI function is impaired and the patient is unable to tolerate enteral feedings, parenteral nutrition is initiated. Total caloric intake should be 2500-3000/day.

  For the patient with acute hepatic encephalopathy, protein is eliminated totally from the diet until recovery. During recovery, protein is increased gradually as tolerated to 40-60 grams per day. Use of IV or oral branched-chain amino acid supplements in an attempt to correct the amino acid imbalance that is common among encephalopathic patients is advocated by some, but their effectiveness is not well documented. Research in this area is ongoing.

5. **Pharmacotherapy**
   - *Corticosteroids:* May be helpful in individuals whose liver biopsy documents the presence of chronic active hepatitis. They are not helpful with cirrhosis and increase the risk of infection and gastric erosion if used.
   - *Sedatives:* Avoided if at all possible because they can precipitate or contribute to encephalopathy. If sedative use is necessary, oxazepam (Serax) is the best choice because it can be eliminated safely by patients with hepatic disease.
   - *Histamine H_2-receptor antagonists:* Prophylactic cimetidine (Tagamet) and ranitidine (Zantac) are prescribed to prevent gastric erosions, which are common in patients with chronic or severe hepatic failure.
   - *Dextrose:* Moderate to severe hypoglycemia can occur owing to impaired gluconeogenesis and other metabolic alterations. Checks of blood sugar q8-12h are necessary to detect hypoglycemia. In the event of hypoglycemia, a bolus of 50% dextrose or continual infusion of a 10% solution is indicated.
   - *Thiamine:* Given to patients with alcoholic cirrhosis who are likely to be deficient in this vitamin and are at risk for developing neuropathies due to B-vitamin deficiencies.

< N O T E : See Table 6-2 for a list of drugs that are hepatotoxic.

6. **Protection of health-care personnel:** Health-care workers must protect themselves from potential infection by frequent handwashings and implementation

T A B L E 6 - 2

Drugs with the potential for hepatotoxicity

Acetaminophen	Clindamycin	Oral contraceptives
Acetylsalicylic acid	Dantrolene	Oxacillin
Ampicillin	Diazepam	Penicillin
Carbamazepine	Ethanol	Phenytoin
Carbenicillin	Halothane	Prophylthiouracil
Chloramphenicol	Hydrochlorothiazide	Rifampin
Chlorpropamide	Isoniazid	Sulfonamides
Chlorpromazine	Methyldopa	Tetracyclines (especially parenteral)

of appropriate barrier precautions. Gloves must be worn when contact with blood, mucous membranes, or body secretions is likely. Masks, gowns, and eye coverings (goggles or glasses) should be used if splashes are likely. Care must be taken in the disposal of needles and sharp instruments. High-risk health-care workers such as critical care, emergency, hemodialysis, and IV therapy personnel should be vaccinated against HBV.

7. **Management of bleeding complications:** Fresh frozen plasma and platelets are administered to correct defects in clotting factors and thrombocytopenia. Vitamin K may be prescribed to help correct bleeding tendencies. Serious coagulopathies requiring specialized component therapy may develop (see "Disseminated Intravascular Coagulation," p. 418).

8. **Management of respiratory failure:** Intubation or mechanical ventilation may be indicated in the following instances: impaired gag reflex due to encephalopathy, aspiration of gastric contents, or impairment of ventilation secondary to ascites.

9. **Management of ascites**
   - *Sodium:* If ascites is severe, it is limited to <500 mg/day.
   - *Diuretics:* If more conservative measures are ineffective in controlling ascites, spironolactone (Aldactone), an aldosterone antagonist with weak diuretic action and potassium conservation, may be used. Another potassium-sparing diuretic, amiloride, may be used as well. If ineffective, more potent diuretics such as furosemide or thiazides are added. For severe ascites, mannitol may be added to the regimen. The goal with diuresis is 1 L/day, as estimated by a 0.5 kg weight loss/day.
   - *Paracentesis:* Repeated daily removal of 4-6 L/day of ascitic fluid may be attempted for refractory ascites. Concurrent administration of salt-poor albumin aids in maintaining intravascular volume.
   - *Ultrafiltration:* An automated ultrafiltration device is used to remove and filter ascitic fluid *via* a peritoneal dialysis catheter. The concentrated fluid is returned to the patient intravenously. Complications of this technique include clogging of the membrane, infection, transient pyrexia, pulmonary edema, and intraperitoneal hemorrhage.
   - *Peritoneal-venous shunt:* A shunt system (e.g., LeVeen) may be placed surgically in patients with refractory or life-threatening ascites. The peritoneal cavity is drained by a long, perforated catheter, which is connected to a

pressure-sensitive valve. The valve attaches to a subcutaneous catheter that drains into the intrathoracic superior vena cava. The many complications include fluid overload, infection, disseminated intravascular coagulation (DIC), peritonitis, and shunt occlusion. A rapid increase in intravascular volume may precipitate variceal hemorrhage in susceptible individuals.

10. **Management of hepatorenal syndrome:** The syndrome is characterized by renal failure with normal tubular function in a patient with severe hepatic failure. Often, it is initiated by over-aggressive diuretic therapy, paracentesis, hemorrhage, diarrhea, or other source of dehydration. Because it is exceedingly difficult to manage, prevention, when possible, is essential. Alleviation of precipitants and conservative measures such as fluid restriction, electrolyte correction, and withdrawal of potentially nephrotoxic drugs (e.g., aminoglycosides) are employed. Ascites is mobilized slowly and hepatic failure, which is the causative factor, is treated. Generally, sodium-containing solutions are avoided, even in the presence of significant hyponatremia. Renal dialysis is seldom employed because it does not improve survival and can lead to complications such as GI hemorrhage and shock.

11. **Management of encephalopathy**
   - Elimination or correction of precipitating factors (e.g., variceal or other hemorrhage, infection, electrolyte imbalance, sedative use, dietary protein intake, constipation).
   - Elimination of dietary protein, which is reintroduced gradually when symptoms improve.
   - Early and thorough catharsis by magnesium citrate or enemas (usually tap water), which remove intestinal contents and are exceedingly helpful in reducing encephalopathy.
   - Administration of neomycin, a nonabsorbable antibiotic, to reduce intestinal bacteria that produce ammonia. It may be given orally, by NG tube, or per rectal enema. Owing to its nephrotoxic and ototoxic effects, neomycin is used only in acute situations.
   - Administration of lactulose, which creates an environment unfavorable to ammonia-forming intestinal bacteria and causes osmotic diarrhea. The dose is adjusted to produce two semi-formed stools per day.

12. **Management of esophageal varices:** See section "Bleeding Esophageal Varices," p. 357.

13. **Hepatic transplantation:** Indicated only for patients with irreversible, progressive liver disease for whom there is no alternative therapy. Hepatic transplantation requires a highly-skilled team of specialists and is offered only at a few centers.

NURSING DIAGNOSES AND INTERVENTIONS

Fluid volume deficit related to decreased intake secondary to medically-prescribed restrictions; and decreased circulating volume secondary to hypoalbuminemia, altered hemodynamics, fluid sequestration, and diuretic therapy

---

Desired outcome: Patient's circulating plasma volume is restored and maintained as evidenced by MAP ≥ 70 mm Hg; HR 60-100 bpm; brisk capillary refill (<3 seconds); distal pulses $>2+$ on a 0-4+ scale; CVP 2-6 mm Hg; PAP 20-30/8-15

mm Hg; PAWP 6-12 mm Hg; CI $\geq$2.5 L/min/m^2; SVR 900-1200 dynes/sec/cm^{-5}; urinary output $\geq$30 ml/hr; and patient oriented to person, place, and time.

1. Monitor and document BP hourly, or q15min in the presence of unstable VS. Be alert to MAP decreases of $\geq$10 mm Hg from previous measurement.
2. Monitor and document HR, EKG, and cardiovascular status hourly, or more frequently in the presence of unstable VS. Be alert to increases in HR suggestive of hypovolemia or circulatory decompensation. Be aware that HR increases also may be due to fever.
3. Measure central pressures and thermodilution CO q1-4h. Be alert to low or decreasing CVP, PAWP, and CO. Calculate SVR q4-8h, or more frequently in unstable patients. An elevated HR, decreased PAWP, CO less than baseline, or CI <2.5 along with decreased urinary output suggest hypovolemia. Because of altered vascular responsiveness, the SVR may not be increased in hypovolemic hepatic failure patients. Be aware that a "normal" CO actually may be decreased for these patients.
4. Measure and record urinary output hourly. Be alert to output <30 ml/hr for two consecutive hours. Estimate volume status and adequacy of cardiovascular function by evaluating BP, HR, CVP, PAP, PAWP, urinary output, amplitude of distal pulses, capillary refill, and LOC. Consider cautious increase in fluid intake (e.g., 50-100 ml/hr) and then reevaluate volume status as described above. Use extreme caution in administering potent diuretics as they may precipitate encephalopathy or renal disease by causing rapid diuresis and electrolyte changes. If potent diuretics are necessary, the initial dose should be small in order to evaluate the patient's response.
5. Estimate ongoing fluid losses. Measure all drainage from peritoneal or other catheters q2-4h. Weigh patient daily, using the same scale and method. Compare 24-hour intake to output and record the difference. Weight loss should not exceed 0.5 kg/day, as more rapid diuresis can lead to intravascular volume depletion and impair renal function.
6. Monitor serum albumin and notify MD if levels are reduced. Administer albumin replacements as prescribed.
7. < N O T E : If fluid volume deficit is related to variceal hemorrhage, see same nursing diagnosis in "Bleeding Esophageal Varices," p. 360.

Fluid volume excess: Intravascular, related to retention secondary to sodium and electrolyte disturbances, functional renal failure, and medical therapy (peritoneal-venous shunt insertion and hemofiltration therapy for ascites); extravascular related to edema and ascites secondary to sequestration of fluid

Desired outcomes: Patient is normovolemic as evidenced by CVP $\leq$6 mm Hg, PAWP $\leq$12 mm Hg, HR $\leq$100 bpm, RR 12-20 breaths/min with normal depth and pattern (eupnea), decreasing or stable abdominal girth, and absence of crackles, edema, and other clinical indicators of fluid volume excess. Serum sodium is 137-147 mEq/L and serum potassium is 3.5-5.5 mEq/L.

1. Monitor VS, hemodynamic parameters, and cardiovascular status q1-2h, more frequently if patient is undergoing ultrafiltration therapy, and immediately after

LeVeen valve or similar peritoneal-venous shunt surgery. Be alert to CVP values >6 mm Hg or PAWP >12 mm Hg. Notify MD of elevated values.

2. Monitor patient for evidence of pulmonary edema related to fluid overload. Note presence of dyspnea, orthopnea, basilar crackles (rales) that do not clear with coughing, and tachypnea. Notify MD if these signs develop.

3. Use minimal amounts of fluids necessary to administer IV medications and maintain IV catheter patency.

4. If fluids are restricted, offer mouth care, ice chips (included as part of oral fluid measurement), gum, or hard candy.

5. Measure and record abdominal girth daily. Be aware that abdominal girth measurements are subject to error and great care is necessary to ensure accurate measurements. Measure at the widest point and mark this level for subsequent measurement. Always position the patient supine when making abdominal girth measurements.

6. Be aware that rapid increases in intravascular volume may precipitate variceal hemorrhage in susceptible patients. Notify MD promptly for evidence of hemorrhage (see "Bleeding Esophageal Varices," p. 357).

7. Monitor serum electrolytes, especially sodium and potassium, and notify MD of significant deviations from normal.

8. Ensure proper functioning of peritoneal-venous shunt in postoperative patients
   - Anticipate rapid fluid mobilization, as evidenced by increased CVP and increased urinary output from preoperative values.
   - Anticipate prescription for IV furosemide during the first 24h after surgery. Furosemide frequently causes potassium depletion; monitor potassium levels closely and supplement as prescribed.
   - Teach patient to use incentive spirometer or similar device that creates inspiratory resistance. Use of such devices promotes negative inspiratory pressure and facilitates flow of ascitic fluid.
   - Apply elastic abdominal binder to increase pressure gradient and facilitate flow of ascitic fluid.
   - Monitor for evidence of variceal bleeding: sudden decrease in hematocrit, unexplained nausea, light-headedness, dark stools, or hematemesis.

Alteration in nutrition: Less than body requirements related to decreased intake secondary to anorexia, nausea, and medically-prescribed dietary restrictions; and decreased metabolism of nutrients secondary to decreased intestinal motility, altered portal blood flow, decreased intestinal absorption of vitamins and minerals, and altered protein metabolism

---

Desired outcomes: Patient has adequate nutrition as evidenced by a state of nitrogen balance found on nitrogen balance studies, thyroxine-binding prealbumin 200-300 μg/ml, and retinol-binding protein 40-50 μg/ml. Blood glucose levels remain within normal range (65-110 mg/dl).

---

1. Confer with MD, dietician, and pharmacist (if parenteral feedings are necessary) to estimate patient's current nutritional and metabolic needs, based on the presence of encephalopathy, chronic hepatic disease, infection, and nutritional status prior to hospitalization. For general information, see section "Providing Nutritional Support," p. 490.

2. Provide enteral feedings if possible. In the absence of adequate bowel functioning or with poor oral intake, confer with MD regarding administration of parenteral supplements.

3. Note and carefully record oral intake. Note all sources of food (including meals not prepared in the hospital), paying particular attention to foods containing sodium and significant amounts of protein.

4. Administer vitamin supplements as prescribed.

5. Encourage supplements brought from home if desired by patient and appropriate for the patient's diet.

6. Encourage bed rest to reduce metabolic demands on the liver and encourage hepatic regeneration. Increase patient's activity levels gradually as condition improves and to patient tolerance.

7. Monitor blood glucose levels q8h or as prescribed. Notify MD of levels <65 mg/dl.

8. Monitor patient for clinical indicators of hypoglycemia: altered mentation, irritability, diaphoresis, anxiety, weakness, tachycardia.

< N O T E :   Clinical signs of hypoglycemia can be confused with hepatic encephalopathy. Be sure to validate clinical signs with blood glucose levels.

9. Be aware that mild elevations in blood sugar are anticipated in some patients with chronic liver disease.

Impaired gas exchange related to shallow breathing with decreased diffusion of oxygen secondary to diaphragmatic limitation with ascites, hydrothorax, or central respiratory depression occurring with encephalopathy

---

Desired outcome: Patient has adequate gas exchange as evidenced by $Pao_2 \geq 80$ mm Hg; $Paco_2 <45$ mm Hg; RR 12-20 breaths/min with normal depth and pattern (eupnea); oxygen saturation >90%; and orientation to person, place, and time.

< N O T E :   LOC is difficult to evaluate in the presence of moderate to severe hepatic encephalopathy.

1. Monitor and document respiratory rate q1-4h. Note pattern, excursion depth, and effort.

2. Administer supplemental oxygen as prescribed to enhance cerebral and hepatic oxygenation.

3. Maintain body positions that optimize ventilation. Elevate HOB 30 degrees or higher, depending on patient comfort and hemodynamic status.

4. Monitor Pao_2, $Paco_2$, and oxygen saturations; notify MD of abnormalities.

5. Assess patient q4-8h for indicators of atelectasis (e.g., diminished breath sounds, basilar crackles); hydrothorax (e.g., diminished breath sounds, dullness to percussion); and pulmonary infection (e.g., yellow, greenish, or thick sputum; rhonchi; fever). Notify MD if physical assessment findings are suggestive of respiratory complications.

6. Evaluate obtunded patient for presence of the gag reflex. Confer with MD regarding need for endotracheal intubation if the gag reflex is depressed.

Sensory-perceptual alterations related to impaired mentation secondary to accumulation of ammonia or other CNS toxins occurring with hepatic dysfunction

---

Desired outcomes: Patient exhibits stable personality pattern, age-appropriate behavior, intact intellect appropriate for level of education, distinct speech, and coordinated gross and fine motor movements. Handwriting remains legible and psychometric test scores are within the normal range.

---

1. Avoid or minimize the precipitating factors:
   - Check NG secretions, vomitus, and stools for occult blood. Notify MD promptly if tests are positive for blood or if GI bleeding is obvious.
   - Evaluate Hct and Hgb for evidence of bleeding. Notify MD for very low values or values deviating from baseline. Anticipate mild to moderate anemia.
   - Notify MD promptly for indicators of infection (for detail, see **Potential for infection**, p. 376).
   - Evaluate serum ammonia levels. Report significant elevations from baseline.

< N O T E : Ammonia values vary greatly and do not always correlate directly with encephalopathy. To help ensure accurate results, place specimens for ammonia analysis on ice and transport immediately to laboratory.

   - Be alert to potential sources of electrolyte imbalance (e.g., diarrhea, gastric aspiration).
   - Avoid use of sedative or tranquilizing agents. If sedatives are necessary, oxazepam (Serax) and antihistamines (e..g, Benadryl) are the safest.
   - Avoid use of hepatotoxic drugs (see Table 6-2).
   - Correct hypoxemia (see **Impaired gas exchange**, p. 374).

2. Evaluate patient for CNS effects such as personality changes, childish behavior, intellectual impairment, slurred speech, ataxia, and asterixis.

3. Administer daily handwriting or psychometric tests (if appropriate for patient's LOC) to evaluate mild or subclinical encephalopathy. Report significant deterioration in handwriting or in test scores.

4. Notify MD of abnormal EEG reports.

5. Eliminate dietary protein in severely encephalopathic patients. As prescribed, reintroduce protein gradually as tolerated after patient's clinical symptoms improve (i.e., patient becomes more alert and neuromuscular coordination improves). Limit protein to 40-60 grams/day in recently or chronically encephalopathic patients.

6. Administer enemas as prescribed to clear the colon of intestinal contents that contribute to encephalopathy. Repeat enemas as necessary to ensure thorough cleansing of the colon.

7. Administer neomycin as prescribed to reduce intestinal bacteria, which produces ammonia. Monitor patient for evidence of ototoxic (i.e., decreased hearing) and nephrotoxic (e.g., urinary output <30 ml/hr, increased creatinine levels) effects caused by neomycin. Avoid neomycin administration in patients with renal insufficiency.

8. Administer lactulose as prescribed to reduce ammonia formation in the intestine. Consult with MD to adjust dose to produce two semi-formed stools daily. Avoid

lactulose-related diarrhea, as it may cause dangerous dehydration and electrolyte imbalance.

9. Protect confused or unconscious patient from injury.
   - Leave siderails up; consider padding them if patient is active.
   - Tape all catheters and tubes securely to prevent dislodgement.
   - Consider possibility of seizures in the severely encephalopathic patient; have airway management equipment readily available.

Potential for infection related to susceptibility secondary to anemia, leukopenia, impaired immunity, decreased serum globulins, and multiple invasive diagnostic tests and medical therapies

---

Desired outcome: Patient is free of infection as evidenced by normothermia, HR $\leq$100 bpm, RR $\leq$20 breaths/min, negative cultures, WBC count $\leq$11,000 μl, clear urine, and clear and thin sputum.

---

1. Monitor VS for evidence of infection (e.g., increases in heart and respiratory rates). Check rectal or core temperature q4h for increases.
2. If temperature elevation is sudden, culture blood, sputum, urine, or other sites as prescribed. Report positive culture reports promptly.
3. Monitor CBC and report significant increases in WBC. Be aware that a normal or mildly elevated leukocyte count may signify infection in patients with hepatic failure, since patients with chronic liver disease often are leukopenic with WBCs as low as 1500-3000/mm^3.
4. Evaluate secretions and drainage for evidence of infection (e.g., sputum changes, cloudy urine).
5. Evaluate IV, central line, and paracentesis site(s) for evidence of infection (erythema, warmth, unusual drainage). It is normal for paracentesis puncture site to have a small amount of drainage immediately after the procedure. Prolonged or foul-smelling drainage can signal infection.
6. Prevent transmission of infectious agents by washing hands well before and after caring for patient and by wearing gloves when contact with blood or other body substances is likely. Dispose of all needles and other sharp instruments in puncture-resistant, rigid containers. Keep containers in each patient room and in other convenient locations. Avoid recapping and manipulating needles prior to disposal.
7. Administer antibiotics as prescribed. Use caution in administering antibiotics (especially aminoglycosides) to patients with low urinary output or renal insufficiency.

Potential for injury related to risk of bleeding secondary to altered clotting factors and thrombocytopenia

---

Desired outcomes: Clots form and bleeding is not prolonged. Patient's PT is 11-15 seconds, PTT is 30-40 seconds, and platelet count is $\geq$100,000 μl.

---

1. Avoid giving IM injections. If they are necessary, use small-gauge needles and maintain firm pressure over injection sites for several minutes. Avoid massaging IM injection sites.

2. Maintain pressure for several minutes over venipuncture sites. Inform lab personnel of patient's bleeding tendencies.

3. Avoid arterial punctures. If ABGs are necessary, confer with MD regarding use of an in-dwelling arterial line. If this is not possible, be certain to maintain pressure for at least 10 minutes over the arterial puncture site.

4. Monitor PT levels and platelet counts daily. Inform MD of significant prolongation of the PT or of significant reduction in the platelet count.

5. Assess patient for signs of bleeding. Note oral and nasal mucosal bleeding and ecchymotic areas and test stools and emesis for occult blood. Notify MD of positive findings.

6. Use electric rather than straight razor for patient shaving. Provide soft-bristled toothbrush or toothettes and mouthwash for oral hygiene.

7. Avoid in-dwelling NG drainage tubes as they may irritate gastric mucosa or varices, causing bleeding to occur.

8. Administer fresh frozen plasma and platelets as prescribed. Monitor carefully for fluid volume overload (see **Fluid volume excess**, p. 372).

9. Administer vitamin K as prescribed.

10. A post shunt coagulopathy may develop in some patients after peritoneal-venous shunt surgery. Monitor these patients closely and notify surgeon at once if bleeding complications are suspected.

11. If fibrin split products are present in the blood and there is significant thrombocytopenia, DIC may be present. See "Disseminated intravascular coagulation," p. 418, for further detail.

Potential alteration in tissue perfusion: Renal, related to risk of reduced renal cortical blood flow and consequent functional renal failure secondary to hepatic failure

< N O T E : This condition can be precipitated by dehydration, hemorrhage, paracentesis, or diarrhea.

Desired outcome: Patient has optimal renal function/perfusion as evidenced by urinary output $\geq$30 ml/hr, serum creatinine 0.7-1.5 mg/dl, serum potassium 3.5-5.5 mEq/L, serum sodium 137-147mEq/L, and urine sodium >10 mEq/L.

---

1. Monitor CVP and PAWP q1-4h to ensure optimal filling pressures (see **Fluid volume deficit**, p. 371). Monitor filling pressures qh immediately following paracentesis or if patient is dehydrated or hemorrhaging.

2. Monitor serum and urine sodium levels. Serum sodium <120 mEq/L and urine sodium <10 mEq/L are associated with the development of hepatorenal syndrome. Notify MD of significant alterations in serum and urine sodium.

3. Monitor creatinine and potassium values and report significant increases. Be aware that BUN is not an accurate indicator of renal function, especially in the patient with hepatic failure, since alterations in hepatic function can cause decreased levels and GI bleeding results in increased values.

4. Minimize infusion of sodium-containing fluids as they contribute to ascites and peripheral edema and may potentiate functional renal failure.
5. For additional information, see nursing diagnoses and interventions in "Acute Renal Failure," p. 176-184.

Impairment of skin and tissue integrity related to pruritus, tissue edema, or impaired tissue healing

---

Desired outcome: Patient's skin and tissue remain intact.

---

1. Restrict use of soap to baths only. Follow baths with lotion, which should be applied while the skin is still moist.
2. Use eggcrate or other low-pressure mattress to minimize pressure on fragile tissues.
3. Turn and reposition patient at least q2h.
4. If patient is confused or obtunded, place his or her hands in soft gloves or mitts to minimize scratching.
5. Administer cholestyramine (e.g., Cuemid, Questran) as prescribed to reduce bile acids in the serum and skin and thereby relieve itching. Avoid administration of other oral medications within two hours of cholestyramine administration, as they may bind with them in the intestine and reduce their absorption.

As appropriate, see the following for additional nursing diagnoses and interventions: "Management of the Adult on Mechanical Ventilation," pp. 66-70; "Providing Nutritional Support," pp. 490-505; "Caring for the Critically Ill on Prolonged Bed Rest," pp. 506-511; "Caring for the Critically Ill with Life-Threatening Disorders," pp. 511-522; and "Caring for the Family of the Critically Ill," pp. 522-526.

REHABILITATION AND PATIENT-FAMILY TEACHING CONCEPTS

Give patient and significant others verbal and written instructions for the following:
1. Importance of sufficient rest and adherence to prescribed diet.
2. Infection control: If hepatic failure is related to HBV infection, HBV prophylaxis for sexual partners and household contacts with possible blood exposure to HBV (i.e., those who share toothbrushes or razors) should be considered. Prescreening for the presence of HB antibodies is encouraged if it does not delay treatment for more than 14 days after last exposure. A single dose of hepatitis B immune globulin (HBIG) is recommended for sexual contacts and household contacts with possible blood exposure. The HB vaccine series should be initiated for exposures among homosexual men but is optional for heterosexual exposure.
3. Availability of alcohol and drug treatment programs for patients with alcohol- and drug-related hepatic failures.
4. Availability of support groups (i.e., Alcoholics Anonymous, Alanon) for patients and family members when hepatic failure is related to chronic alcohol ingestion.

5. Importance of avoiding OTC medications without first consulting MD. Confer with MD regarding use of acetaminophen after hospital discharge for minor aches and pains.

6. Medications, including drug name, dose, purpose, schedule, precautions, and potential side effects.

7. Signs and symptoms of infection: fever, unusual drainage from paracentesis or other invasive procedure sites, warmth and erythema surrounding the invasive sites, or abdominal pain. Have patient demonstrate technique for measurement of oral temperature using glass thermometer or type of thermometer used at home.

8. Signs and symptoms of unusual bleeding, including prolonged mucosal bleeding, very large or painful bruises, and dark stools. If possible, major dental procedures should be postponed until bleeding times normalize.

9. Sodium restriction if patient developed ascites during the course of the illness.

10. Protein restriction if the patient has residual or chronic encephalopathy. Instruct patient to avoid constipation by increasing bulk in the diet or using agents prescribed by MD.

11. Alcohol cessation for at least several months after complete recovery from the acute episode. After full recovery, one or two glasses of beer or wine a day usually are usually allowed if hepatic failure was not related to alcohol ingestion.

12. Daily weights: Instruct patient to report significant loss or gain to MD.

Acute pancreatitis

Pancreatitis is an autodigestive process of pancreatic tissue by its own enzymes. In chronic pancreatitis, the gland is abnormal before the onset of symptoms and remains abnormal. Acute pancreatitis is distinguished by a normal gland before and after the onset of symptoms. Initially, pancreatic ductal flow becomes obstructed, injuring the adjacent acinar cell where pancreatic enzymes are stored in their inactive form (zymogens). Once acinar cell damage has occurred, zymogens are released and autodigestion of the organ begins. Reflux of duodenal or bile content into the ductal system due to structural weaknesses or stone impaction can activate the autodigestive cascade. In addition, diseases that overstimulate enzyme secretion or activate the complement system can transform the zymogens. Edema and vascular insult frequently lead to rupture of the pancreatic ducts and spillage of pancreatic enzymes into the peritoneum, resulting in a chemical peritonitis. Necrosis and hemorrhage are precursors of complete pancreatic dysfunction. Mortality from acute pancreatitis is high and is estimated by some to be as high as 80% in patients with widespread necrosis and hemorrhage.

Complications: If hypovolemia is not detected and treated promptly, acute renal failure becomes likely. Marked depletion of intravascular plasma volume is the result of fluid sequestration into the interstitium and retroperitoneum. Massive, life-threatening hemorrhage from gastroduodenal ulceration or rupture of necrotic tissue results in blood volume depletion. Hypoalbuminemia frequently is present and contributes to hypovolemia. Cardiovascular failure persists in some patients despite volume repletion. In these patients, CVP and PAP are low and the CO is high. It is believed that activation of bradykinin peptides produces these cardiovascular changes. Edema and increased vascular permeability are additional consequences of bradykinin formation. Mild to severe respiratory failure is common with acute pancreatitis and is attributed to the release of phospholipase A. This enzyme is believed to destroy alveolar surfactant, decreasing lung compliance and impairing ventilatory capacity. Some patients develop an intravascular coagulopathy that can lead to life-threatening complications such as pulmonary emboli. Hypocalcemia is common and is attributed to calcium binding in areas of fat necrosis within the pancreas. Hypoalbuminemia contributes to hypocalcemia as about 40% of calcium is bound to serum protein under normal circumstances. Glucagon release also is believed to lower serum calcium levels in acute pancreatitis. The formation of pancreatic pseudocysts or abscesses as a result of necrosis and the collection of purulent material within the tissue can lead to rupture, which in turn can cause sepsis. The ensuing circulatory and respiratory failure often leads to death.

ASSESSMENT

Signs and symptoms: Sudden onset of pain (often following excessive food or alcohol ingestion) lasting 12-48 hours, described as mild discomfort to severe distress, and located from the mid-epigastrum to the RUQ. The pain may radiate to the back. Nausea and vomiting typically accompany the pain; diarrhea, melena, and hematemesis also may be present. Dyspnea and cyanosis, which are signs of adult respiratory distress syndrome (ARDS, see p. 18), may occur as serious complications of acute pancreatitis. With biliary tract disease, jaundice may be present. Turner's sign, a gray-green discoloration of the flanks, is present in about 1% of patients. Hypocalcemia manifests as numbness or tingling in the extremities that can progress to tetany if calcium is severely depleted.

Physical assessment: Restlessness due to patient's furtively seeking a comfortable position, jaundice if patient has biliary tract disease, and diminished or absent bowel sounds reflective of GI dysfunction and ileus. Palpation will reveal localized tenderness in the RUQ or diffuse discomfort over the upper abdomen. Mild to moderate ascites is present and contributes to moderate abdominal distention. Diminished or absent bowel sounds reflect GI dysfunction and possible ileus. Breath sounds may be decreased or absent, suggesting focal atelectasis or pleural effusion. Effusions usually are left-sided but can be bilateral. Auscultation of crackles (rales) may reflect hypoventilation due to pain, early ARDS, or microemboli. In the presence of hemorrhage or severe hypovolemia, the hands will be cool and sweaty, capillary refill will be delayed, and peripheral pulses will be diminished. Urine output will decrease as the body attempts to conserve intravascular volume.

Vital signs and hemodynamic measurements: Increased temperature associated with tachycardia and increased BP. Tachycardia, decreased BP, decreased PAP, and decreased CO are present with hemorrhage, shock, or dehydration. Increase in PVR suggests the presence of ARDS or pulmonary emboli. If septic complications occur, CO may be elevated and SVR decreased.

History and risk factors: Excessive alcohol ingestion; biliary tract disease; high cholesterol levels; use of drugs such as steroids, furosemide, thiazides, and azathioprine; viral infections (especially mumps and hepatitis); open heart surgery; penetrating and blunt injuries to the pancreas. Pregnancy, primary hyperparathyroidism, uremia, and renal transplantation have been implicated as causes because they can lead to ductal stone formation and, as a result, pancreatitis.

DIAGNOSTIC TESTS

1. *Hematologic studies:* Leukocytosis with a WBC count of 11,000-20,000 cells/mm^3 is reflective of the inflammatory process. Hematocrit and hemoglobin lev-

els vary, depending on the presence of hemorrhage (decreased) or dehydration (increased).

2. *Chemistry studies:* Serum amylase usually is elevated 3-5 times normal for the first several days. As damage subsides, the level decreases. A rapid decrease in amylase occurs either with rapid remission or total pancreatic necrosis (Berck, 1985). If available, serum lipase levels parallel amylase levels and are more specific for pancreatitis. Generally, urine amylase is elevated for 1-2 weeks. The creatinine/amylase index usually is elevated with obvious pancreatitis. Hypocalcemia is a frequent finding and values <8 mg/dl are not uncommon. Since part of the calcium is protein bound, serum levels are dependent upon albumin levels. As serum albumin levels decrease, reductions in serum calcium levels are anticipated. Hyperglycemia and glycosuria are a consequence of glucagon release. Blood glucose values are commonly greater than 200 mg/dl. Persistent elevation of liver enzymes suggests alcoholic pancreatitis. Increased serum bicarbonate and hypokalemia are reflections of metabolic alkalosis, usually due to vomiting or gastric suctioning.

3. *Coagulation studies:* Decreases in platelets and fibrinogen will be present. Elevations in circulating levels of fibrin are associated with microthrombi in the pancreas and other tissues.

4. *ABG values:* Decreased arterial oxygen tension is a common finding and may be present without other symptoms of pulmonary insufficiency. Early hypoxia produces a mild respiratory alkalosis.

5. *EKG:* ST-segment depression and T-wave inversion may be seen, owing to the shock state, severe pain that causes coronary artery spasm, or the effect of trypsin and bradykinins on the myocardium. Hypocalcemia results in widening of the ST segment.

6. *Radiologic procedures:* Abdominal x-ray may show dilation of the bowel and ileus. Chest x-rays are helpful in distinguishing effusions from atelectasis and in diagnosing ARDS. Endoscopic retrograde cholangiopancreatography (ERCP) may be helpful after the acute episode in identifying stones or stenosis. Barium studies may reveal displacement of the stomach or duodenum due to edema or pseudocysts.

7. *Ultrasonography and CT scan:* Identify pseudocysts, visualize biliary tract abnormalities, and monitor inflammatory swelling of the pancreas.

8. *Endoscopy:* Visualizes gastroduodenal ulcers and other abnormalities when GI bleeding complicates the disease course.

MEDICAL MANAGEMENT AND SURGICAL INTERVENTIONS

Treatment is more palliative than curative. Efforts are directed at pain relief and resting the pancreas until the autodigestive process subsides.

1. **Analgesia:** Meperidine (Demerol) is used rather than morphine. Morphine is associated with spasms of the smooth muscle of the pancreatic and biliary ducts and the ampulla of Vater, where the ducts enter the duodenum. Administration of morphine could impede ductal flow further. Epidural blockage may be employed for severe pain.

2. **Fluid and electrolyte management:** The inflammatory process results in fluid sequestration and extensive intravascular volume loss. Nausea, vomiting, NG suctioning, and hemorrhage contribute to the hypovolemic state. Colloids, albumin, fresh frozen plasma, and packed cells are administered to replace vol-

ume losses and minimize interstitial edema. Fluid sequestration in the peritoneum and interstitium continues until the acute phase is arrested, therefore
continual volume replacement is essential. If serum potassium and calcium levels are decreased, replacement therapy may be necessary. Because hypercalcemia has been implicated in the genesis of pancreatitis, calcium replacement
is prescribed cautiously.

3. **Suppression of pancreatic secretions:** Accomplished by withholding oral feedings, including water; aspirating gastric secretions *via* NG suction; reducing
gastric acidity by administering anticholinergics, cimetidine, glucagon, and antacids; and reducing physical activity. NG suction has the additional benefit of
relieving abdominal distention and vomiting.

4. **Respiratory support:** Pulmonary congestion, pleural effusion, and atelectasis
result in respiratory insufficiency. Abdominal distention and retroperitoneal fluid
sequestration cause diaphragmatic elevation and ventilatory restriction. Early
respiratory failure is detected by a decrease in oxygen tension (<60-70 mm
Hg). Serial ABG tests are performed during the first 2-3 days of therapy to
detect early hypoxemia. Oxygen is initiated if hypoxemia is present. Patients
who develop severe pulmonary insufficiency require endotracheal intubation and
positive end expiratory pressure (PEEP) ventilation. If there is evidence of progressive respiratory failure, IV fluids are given cautiously to prevent cardiopulmonary compromise.

5. **Management of infection:** Triple antibiotic coverage by a penicillin, cephalosporin, and aminoglycoside may be employed to minimize septic complications.

6. **Nutritional support:** Parenteral feedings that provide nutrients necessary for
tissue healing are initiated for patients with severe pancreatitis. Oral feedings
are not indicated during the acute episode as they result in pancreatic inflammation by stimulating glandular secretions. A feeding jejunostomy tube may be
inserted to provide enteral feedings for some patients. Low-fat oral feedings are
begun after the initial episode subsides and bowel function returns.

7. **Peritoneal lavage:** Removes toxic factors present in peritoneal exudate and can
result in immediate clinical improvement in many patients with severe pancreatitis. The procedure is similar to peritoneal dialysis. A soft lavage catheter is
positioned in the peritoneum, and continual lavage is instituted for 2-7 days,
depending upon the patient's clinical response. Generally, 2 liters of an isotonic, balanced electrolyte solution are infused into the peritoneum over a 15-
minute period. The solution dwells in the peritoneum for 20-30 minutes and
then is drained into a bedside collection container for 15-20 minutes. The cycle
is repeated hourly. Common lavage additives include potassium, heparin, and a
broad-spectrum antibiotic.

8. **Surgical management:** In general, nonsurgical management of acute pancreatitis is most effective. Surgical intervention does not improve the patient's condition and increases respiratory complications. Because acute pancreatitis is easily confused with acute abdominal emergencies requiring urgent surgery,
exploratory laparotomy is necessary for some patients. More aggressive surgical
procedures such as early pancreatic drainage or resection remain controversial.

NURSING DIAGNOSES AND INTERVENTIONS

Fluid volume deficit related to inadequate intake or decreased circulating volume
secondary to fluid sequestration or active bleeding

Desired outcome: Circulating plasma volume is restored as evidenced by MAP >70 mm Hg, HR 60-100 bpm, normal sinus rhythm on EKG, CVP 2-6 mm Hg, PAWP 6-12 mm Hg, CI ≥2.5 L/min/m², CO 4-7 L/min, SVR 900-1200 dynes/sec/cm⁻⁵, PVR 60-100 dynes/sec/cm⁻⁵, brisk capillary refill (<3 seconds), peripheral pulses >2+ on a 0-4+ scale, urinary output ≥30 ml/hr, and stable weights and abdominal girth measurements.

1. Monitor BP q1-4h if losses are due to fluid sequestration, inadequate intake, or slow bleeding. Monitor BP q15min if patient has active blood loss or unstable VS. Be alert to MAP decreases of ≥10 mm Hg from previous BP.
2. Monitor HR, EKG, and cardiovascular status qh. Monitor these parameters q15min or more frequently in the presence of active bleeding or unstable VS. Be alert to increases in HR, which suggest hypovolemia.

< N O T E : Increases in HR also may be due to fever.

3. Measure hemodynamic parameters (i.e., CVP, PAWP, and CO) and thermodilution CO q1-4h. Be alert to low or decreasing CVP, PAWP, and CO. Calculate SVR and PVR q4-8, or more frequently in unstable patients. An elevated HR, decreased PAWP, decreased CO (CI<2.5 L/min/m²), and increased SVR suggest hypovolemia. Pulmonary hypertension is anticipated in patients with ARDS. Assess for signs of overaggressive fluid resuscitation (see **Potential fluid volume excess,** below). Elevate PAWP to minimally acceptable level to maintain CO and tissue perfusion for patients with pulmonary insufficiency (see **Potential for impaired gas exchange,** p. 385).
4. Measure urinary output qh. Be alert to output <30 ml/hr for two consecutive hours. Evaluate intravascular volume and cardiovascular function and increase fluid intake promptly if decreased urinary output is due to hypovolemia and hypoperfusion.
5. Monitor for physical indicators of hypovolemia, including cool extremities, delayed capillary refill (>4 seconds), and decreased amplitude of or absent distal pulses.
6. Estimate ongoing fluid losses. Measure all drainage from tubes, catheters, and drains. Note the frequency of dressing changes due to saturation with fluid or blood. Weigh patient daily, using the same scales and method. Compare 24-hour urine output to 24-hour fluid intake and record the difference.
7. Evaluate character of all fluid losses (see Table 6-6, p. 411). Note color and odor. Be alert to the presence of particulate matter, fibrin, and clots. Test GI aspirate, drainage, and excretions (including stool) for the presence of occult blood.
8. Evaluate abdominal girth q8h. Measure and record girth daily or more often if there is evidence of distention or ascites. Be aware that abdominal girth measurements are subject to wide measurement errors and great care is necessary in ensuring accurate measurements. Measure at the widest point and mark this level for subsequent measurement. Always position the patient supine when performing girth measurements.

Potential fluid volume excess related to retention secondary to overaggressive fluid resuscitation and peritoneal lavage

Desired outcome: Patient is normovolemic as evidenced by MAP 70-105 mm Hg, HR 60-100 bpm, RR 12-20 breaths/min with normal pattern and depth (eupnea), CVP 2-6 mm Hg, PAWP 6-12 mm Hg, CI 2.5-4 L/min/m^2, and absence of adventitious breath sounds and S$_3$ gallop.

1. Evaluate patient q1-4h for clinical indicators of fluid volume excess: dyspnea, orthopnea, increased respiratory rate and effort, S$_3$ gallop, or crackles (rales). Document and report changes and new findings.
2. Measure hemodynamic parameters (BP, HR, CVP, PAWP) qh in patients undergoing peritoneal lavage or in patients with evidence of hypervolemia (i.e., CVP or PAWP increased from baseline or above normal or presence of clinical indicators of fluid volume excess).
3. As prescribed, administer inotropic agents such as dopamine to augment myocardial contractility. Evaluate effectiveness by measuring CO and calculating CI q1-2h and by measuring urine output q1-2h. Document and report CI <2.5 L/min/m^2 and urine output <30 ml for two consecutive hours.
4. Administer furosemide (Lasix) or other diuretic as prescribed to promote diuresis. Document response to diuretic therapy by noting onset and amount of diuresis.
5. Carefully implement peritoneal lavage as prescribed (see Table 6-3, below).

Alteration in comfort: Pain related to peritoneal inflammation and tissue destruction by pancreatic enzyme release

---

TABLE 6-3

Nursing interventions for the patient undergoing peritoneal lavage for acute pancreatitis

- Ensure sterile technique throughout all phases of lavage to prevent serious complications caused by infection.
- Warm lavage fluid to patient's body temperature to prevent cramping, hypothermia, and discomfort.
- Measure lavage infusion fluid loss/retention. Document input and output throughout entire procedure. Document and report daily fluid balance, either excess or deficit.
- Turn patient gently from side to side as needed to promote drainage.
- Monitor patient carefully for decrease in ventilatory excursion due to pressure from lavage fluid. Drain fluid and notify MD promptly if patient develops signs and symptoms of respiratory distress.
- Maintain HOB at 30 degrees or greater.
- Check urine for glucose and monitor blood glucose levels. Glucose in the lavage fluids can contribute to the glucose intolerance that occurs frequently in patients with pancreatitis. Insulin administration may be required in some instances.
- Note and document characteristics (color, odor, clarity, amount) of lavage return. Document and report changes.

Desired outcomes: Patient states that a reduction in discomfort has occurred. Ventilation and hemodynamic status are uncompromised as evidenced by MAP 70-105 mm Hg, HR 60-100 bpm, RR 12-20 breaths/min with normal depth and pattern (eupnea), CVP 2-6 mm Hg, and PAWP 6-12 mm Hg.

1. As prescribed, administer meperidine or other analgesia before pain becomes severe. If route is IM, rotate injection sites and inspect sites carefully for hematoma in patients with hemorrhagic complications. Patients with serious coagulation problems or those receiving heparin therapy for problems with intravascular coagulation usually require IV analgesia.

< C A U T I O N :   Narcotic analgesics decrease GI motility and may delay return to normal bowel functioning.

2. Avoid administration of morphine as it may cause ductal spasm.
3. Pancreatitis can be very painful. Prepare significant others for personality changes and behavioral alterations associated with extreme pain and narcotic analgesia. Family members sometimes misinterpret patient's lethargy or unpleasant disposition and may even blame themselves. Reassure them that these are normal responses.
4. Supplement analgesics with nonpharmacologic maneuvers to aid in pain reduction. Modify patient's body position to optimize comfort. Many patients with abdominal pain find a dorsal recumbent or lateral decubitus bent-knee position most comfortable.
5. Because reducing anxiety contributes to pain relief, ensure consistency and promptness in delivering analgesia to relieve patient's anticipation anxiety.
6. Patients and family members sometimes are distressed at the health team members' inability to relieve pain. Provide continual reassurance that all possible measures are being implemented.
7. Monitor respiratory pattern and LOC closely, since both may be depressed by the large amounts of narcotics usually required to control pain.
8. Monitor HR and BP q1-4h. Monitor CVP and PAWP q4h or more frequently in unstable patients. Report significant deviations from baseline to MD. Be aware that narcotics cause vasodilatation and can result in serious hypotension, especially in volume depleted patients.
9. Evaluate effectiveness of medication and discuss dose and drug manipulation with the MD. If medications are not effective, prepare patient for splanchnic block or other pain-relieving procedure planned by the MD.

Potential for impaired gas exchange related to decreased diffusion of oxygen secondary to microatelectasis and fluid accumulation in the alveoli

Desired outcome: Patient has adequate gas exchange as evidenced by Pao_2 ≥80 mm Hg; $Paco_2$ 35-45 mm Hg; RR 12-20 breaths/min with normal depth and pattern (eupnea); patient oriented to person, place, and time; and clear and audible breath sounds.

1. Monitor and document respiratory rate q1-4h as indicated. Note pattern, degree of excursion, and whether or not patient uses accessory muscles of respiration. Report significant deviations from baseline.
2. Auscultate both lung fields q4-8h. Note presence of abnormal (crackles, rhonchi, wheezes) or diminished sounds.
3. Be alert to early signs of hypoxia, such as restlessness, agitation, and alterations in mentation.
4. Monitor ABG values q12h during the first 48 hours and more often in the unstable patient. Many patients with pancreatitis do not have obvious clinical symptoms of respiratory failure and a decreased arterial oxygen tension may be the first sign of failure. Alert the MD if PaO_2 is <60-70 mm Hg or if oxygen saturation falls below 90%.
5. Administer oxygen as prescribed. Check oxygen delivery system at frequent intervals to ensure proper delivery, as oxygen is critical to these patients.
6. Maintain body position that optimizes ventilation and oxygenation. Elevate HOB 30 degrees or higher, depending on patient comfort. If pleural effusion or other defect is present on one side, position patient with the unaffected lung dependent to maximize the ventilation-perfusion relationship.
7. Avoid overaggressive fluid resuscitation (see **Fluid volume excess**, p. 383).
8. See "Adult Respiratory Distress Syndrome," p. 18, for additional information. tion.

Potential for infection related to susceptibility secondary to formation and possible rupture of abscess or pseudocyst

---

Desired outcome: Patient remains free from infection as evidenced by core or rectal temperature ≤100° F (≤37.8° C); negative cultures; HR 60-100 bpm; RR 12-20 breaths/min; BP within patient's normal range; CI ≤4 L/min/m^2; SVR 900-1200 dynes/sec/cm^{-5}; and orientation to person, place, and time.

---

1. Check rectal or core temperature q4h for increases. Be aware that hypothermia may precede hyperthermia in some patients.
2. If there is a sudden increase in temperature elevation, culture blood, sputum, urine, and other sites as prescribed. Monitor culture reports and report positive cultures promptly.
3. Evaluate orientation and LOC q2-4h. Document and report significant deviations from baseline.
4. Monitor BP, HR, RR, CO, and SVR q1-4h. Be alert to increases in HR and RR associated with temperature elevations. An elevated CO (CI >4.0 L/min/m^2) and decreased SVR (<900 dynes/sec/cm^{-5}) are suggestive of sepsis.
5. Administer parenteral antibiotics in a timely fashion. Reschedule antibiotics if a dose is delayed for more than one hour. Recognize that failure to administer antibiotics on schedule can result in inadequate blood levels and treatment failure. Aminoglycosides are used frequently; therefore, monitor patient for hearing loss. Older adults are especially susceptible to the ototoxic and nephrotoxic effects of aminoglycosides. Monitor BUN, creatinine, and urinary output, which are indicators of renal function.

6. Prevent transmission of potentially infectious agents by using good handwashing before and after caring for patient and by isolating dressings and drainage.

Impaired tissue integrity: GI tract, related to irritation secondary to release of chemical irritants into the pancreatic parenchyma and surrounding tissue, including the peritoneum

---

Desired outcomes: Patient exhibits no further GI tissue destruction as evidenced by reduction in pain; GI aspirate, stools, drainage, and vomitus negative for blood; and return of bowel sounds and bowel functioning. Gastric pH remains >5.

---

1. Withhold oral feedings to avoid stimulation of pancreatic enzymes.
2. Ensure patency of NG sump tube to provide continual gastric drainage and prevent pancreatic stimulation. Do not occlude the air vent of double-lumen tube as this may result in vacuum occlusion. Check placement of NG tube at least q8h and reposition as necessary.
3. Administer anticholinergics, cimetidine, and glucagon as prescribed to decrease gastric and pancreatic secretions and reduce gastric pH. Monitor gastric pH and administer antacids to maintain pH >5.
4. Because increased activity can stimulate gastric secretions, limit patient's physical activity during the acute phase.
5. Test GI aspirate, drainage, and excretions for the presence of occult blood q12-24h.
6. Initiate peritoneal lavage as prescribed (see Table 6-3, p. 384).

Alteration in nutrition: Less than body requirements related to decreased oral intake secondary to nausea, vomiting, and NPO status; and increased need secondary to tissue destruction or infection

---

Desired outcome: Patient maintains baseline body weight and demonstrates a state of nitrogen balance on nitrogen studies.

---

1. Collaborate with MD, dietician, and pharmacist to estimate patient's individual metabolic needs, based on activity level, presence of infection or other stressor, and nutritional status prior to hospitalization. Develop a plan of care accordingly.
2. As prescribed, provide parenteral nutrition during acute phase of pancreatitis.
3. Administer enteral feedings *via* feeding jejunostomy as prescribed for patients with intestinal peristalsis.
4. Monitor bowel sounds q4h. Document and report deviations from baseline. "Hold" oral or jejunostomy feedings if bowel sounds are absent.
5. Monitor blood or urine glucose levels q4-8h or as prescribed. Notify MD of blood levels >200 mg/dl.
6. Begin low-fat oral feedings when acute episode has subsided and bowel function has returned. This may take several weeks in some patients.
7. For more detail, see "Providing Nutritional Support," p. 490.

As appropriate, see nursing diagnoses and interventions in the following: "Adult Respiratory Distress Syndrome," pp. 20-21; "Acute Renal Failure," pp. 176-184; "Disseminated Intravascular Coagulation," p. 418; "Caring for the Critically Ill on Prolonged Bed Rest," pp. 505-511; "Caring for the Critically Ill with Life-Threatening Disorders," pp. 511-522; and "Caring for the Family of the Critically Ill," pp. 522-526.

REHABILITATION AND PATIENT-FAMILY TEACHING CONCEPTS

Give patient and significant others verbal and written instructions for the following:
1. Alcohol rehabilitation programs, as indicated for patients whose pancreatitis is caused by excessive alcohol intake.
2. Medications, including drug name, dosage, purpose, schedule, precautions, and side effects such as dry mouth with anticholinergics and drowsiness with narcotics.
3. Importance of adhering to a low-fat diet if prescribed.
4. Indicators of actual or impending GI hemorrhage: nausea, vomiting of blood, dark stools, light-headedness, passage of frank blood in stools.
5. Indicators of infection: fever, unusual drainage from surgical incisions or peritoneal lavage site, warmth or erythema surrounding surgical sites, and abdominal pain. Have patient demonstrate oral temperature-taking technique using glass thermometer or type of thermometer that will be used at home.
6. Importance of seeking medical attention promptly if signs of recurrent pancreatitis (i.e., pain, change in bowel habits, passing of blood in the stools, or vomiting blood) or infection (see #5 above) appear.

Peritonitis

Peritonitis is an inflammation of all or part of the peritoneal cavity caused by diffuse microbial proliferation or chemical irritation from leakage of corrosive gastric or intestinal contents into the peritoneum. Ruptured appendix, perforated peptic ulcer, pancreatitis, abdominal trauma, and ruptured abdominal abscesses are among the many etiologic factors associated with peritonitis. In-dwelling tubes and catheters such as those used for postoperative drainage and continuous ambulatory peritoneal dialysis (CAPD) are foreign bodies that compromise peritoneal integrity and permit the entry of infective organisms that can trigger peritonitis.

Regardless of the initiating factor, the inflammatory process is similar in every case. The initial reactions, which usually are triggered by histamine release, include hyperemia, edema, and vascular congestion. Fluid shifts from intravascular to interstitial spaces as a result of increased vascular permeability. The circulating blood volume is depleted and hypovolemic shock may ensue. The transudated fluid contains high levels of fibrinogen and thromboplastin. The fibrinogen is converted to fibrin by the thromboplastin. Under normal conditions, the peritoneum has fibrinolytic abilities to stop the fibrin formation. However, when weakened or injured, this ability is hampered and fibrin adhesions form around the damaged area. The fibrin deposits form a barrier that harbors and protects bacteria from the body's defenses, resulting in multiple pockets of infection, which can lead to recurrent infection or septicemia. In most cases the fibrin deposits dissolve, but prolonged or severe inflammation can result in the continuing presence of fibrin, leading to adhesions and potential bowel obstruction.

ASSESSMENT

Signs and symptoms: The primary symptom is pain, which may be quite severe, causing the patient to maintain a fetal position and resist any movement that aggravates the pain. Its onset can be sudden or insidious, with the location varying according to the underlying pathology. Fever and restlessness are common findings in many patients. Nausea, vomiting, anorexia, and changes in bowel habits also may be present and are reflective of GI dysfunction.

Physical assessment: Auscultation of all four quadrants usually reveals diminished or absent bowel sounds. The complete absence of bowel sounds suggests an ileus, a frequent complication of peritonitis. Palpation of the abdomen elicits tenderness that can be generalized or localized, depending on the nature and extent of infection. Rebound tenderness, guarding, and involuntary rigidity also may be present. Occasionally, mild to moderate ascites is observed, depending on the cause of peritonitis. Respiratory rate is rapid, and the patient usually has a shallow ventilatory pattern to minimize abdominal movement and pain; as a consequence, breath sounds may be diminished. Fluid shifts and hypovolemia can cause restlessness and confusion due to impaired cerebral perfusion.

Vital signs and hemodynamic measurements: Usually, fever is present, accompanied by tachypnea and tachycardia due to increased metabolic demands. During the acute phase, the cardiovascular system may be compromised by large fluid shifts from the intravascular space into the abdominal interstitium and peritoneum. This disruption of intravascular volume can lead to hypovolemia with marked tachycardia, hypotension, low CO, decreased PA pressures, and decreased urine output. Depending on disease progression, the patient may exhibit signs of septic shock. Endotoxemic vasodilatation is manifested by a low SVR, with an initial increase in HR and CO. This state complicates the initial hypovolemia and may result in a dangerously low MAP, thus impairing renal and cerebral perfusion.

History and risk factors: Inflammatory processes such as diverticulitis, appendicitis, or Crohn's disease; obstructive events in the small bowel and colon; vascular events such as ischemic colitis, mesenteric thrombosis, or embolic phenomena; blunt or penetrating trauma, especially to hollow viscera; severe hepatobiliary disease; and CAPD. General risk factors include those related to poor tissue healing and infection, for example, old age, diabetes, vascular disease, advanced liver disease, malignancy, and malnutrition.

DIAGNOSTIC TESTS

1. *Hematologic studies:* Leukocytosis will be present, with the WBC count usually >20,000 mm^3. Initially, the hemoglobin and hematocrit may be increased due to hemoconcentration, but will decrease to baseline levels as normal intravascular volume is restored.

2. *Blood chemistry studies:* Depending on the severity of the patient's condition, blood electrolytes may be abnormal. If nausea and vomiting are persistent, metabolic alkalosis is expected. This state is reflected by high CO_2 and low Cl^- values. Serum albumin levels often are decreased, especially with bacterial peritonitis. The underlying disease process affects chemistry studies; for example, patients with pancreatitis usually have elevated amylase levels.

3. *Radiologic procedures:* The abdominal x-ray usually reveals dilation of the large and small bowel, with edema of the small bowel wall. Free air in the abdomen suggests visceral perforation. Although radionuclide scanning of the peritoneum can be done, a more useful procedure is the CT scan. With CT

scanning, abscesses can be visualized and even drained during the procedure, thus avoiding surgery.

4. *Ultrasonography:* Useful in locating small amounts of loculated fluid, as well as differentiating fluid collections in the abdomen.

5. *Diagnostic paracentesis:* Abdominal paracentesis involves the insertion of a catheter or trocar into the abdomen to obtain specimens. Sterile saline is infused through the catheter and the return fluid is analyzed for RBC, WBC, amylase, and bacteria content. If ascites is present, it may not be necessary to infuse saline because fluid can be removed directly for analysis.

MEDICAL MANAGEMENT AND SURGICAL INTERVENTIONS

Because peritonitis usually is a complication of another condition, the aim of therapy is to treat the underlying disease process. The following are some of the general therapies that apply to the management of peritonitis.

1. **Antimicrobial therapy:** Both aerobic and anerobic organisms are found within the abdomen. An aminoglycoside is used for aerobic organisms; while clindamycin, chloramphenicol, cefoxitin, or metronidazole is used for anaerobic bacteria.

2. **Pain management:** The degree of discomfort caused by peritonitis varies greatly. Narcotic analgesics are used to ensure patient comfort but are given cautiously to avoid compromise of abdominal and respiratory function. These analgesics usually require frequent administration, with the dose titrated for each individual. Initiation of narcotic analgesia is delayed until the patient has been fully evaluated by a surgeon, as important diagnostic clues can be masked.

3. **Fluid and electrolyte management:** With bacterial peritonitis, a significant intravascular volume depletion may occur. In most cases crystalloids are used initially, unless there is evidence of decreased intravascular proteins, in which event colloids such as albumin or plasma protein fraction are indicated. If peritonitis is complicated by hemorrhage, packed red blood cells may be given. Electrolyte replacement, typically potassium, is implemented according to laboratory findings.

4. **Nutritional therapy:** Because of the inflammatory process, GI function is compromised and motility is minimal. An enteric tube is inserted to reduce or prevent distention and promote function. Initially, the patient is NPO until some GI function is regained. When the resumption of bowel sounds or passing of flatus signals the return of GI motility, enteral nutrition is begun. If the return of gastric motility is delayed for several days, parenteral nutrition may be necessary.

5. **Surgical management:** Is often necessary, depending on the cause of peritonitis. All intra-abdominal foreign material is removed and nonviable tissue is debrided. Leaky anastomoses are identified and repaired. If present, bowel perforations and obstructions are corrected, and abscesses are drained.

NURSING DIAGNOSES AND INTERVENTIONS

Fluid volume deficit related to decreased circulating volume secondary to fluid sequestration, decreased oral intake, and possibly active loss due to bleeding

---

Desired outcome: Circulating intravascular volume is restored and maintained as evidenced by the following parameters: MAP 70-105 mm Hg; HR 60-100 bpm;

normal sinus rhythm on EKG; CVP 2-6 mm Hg; PAWP 6-12 mm Hg; CI 2.5-4 L/min/m^2; urinary output $\geq$30 ml/hr; warm extremities; peripheral pulses >2+ on a 0-4+ scale; brisk capillary refill (<3 seconds); patient oriented to person, place, and time; and stable weights.

1. Monitor BP q1-4h, depending on patient stability. Be alert to MAP decreases of $\geq$10 mm Hg from previous BP reading.
2. Monitor HR and EKG q1-4h, or more often if VS are unstable. Be alert to increases in HR, which are suggestive of hypovolemia. Usually the EKG will show sinus tachycardia. In the presence of hypokalemia due to prolonged vomiting or gastric suction, EKG may show ventricular ectopy, prominent U wave, and depression of the ST segment.

< N O T E :   HR increases also may be due to fever.

3. Measure CVP, PAWP, thermodilution CO q1-4h, depending on patient stability. Be alert to low or decreasing CVP, PAWP, and CO. Calculate SVR q4-8h or more frequently in unstable patients. A decreased CVP and PAWP, decreased CO (CI <2.5 L/min/m^2), and increased SVR (>1200 dynes/sec/cm^{-5}) suggest hypovolemia.
4. Measure urinary output qh. Be alert to output <30 ml/hr for two consecutive hours, which may signal intravascular volume depletion. Consult with MD and increase fluid intake promptly if decreased urinary output is due to hypovolemia and hypoperfusion.
5. Monitor patient for physical indicators of hypovolemia, including cool extremities, capillary refill >4 seconds, decreased amplitude of peripheral pulses, and neurologic changes such as restlessness and confusion.
6. .Estimate ongoing fluid losses. Measure all drainage from tubes, catheters, and drains. Note the frequency of dressing changes due to saturation with fluid or blood. Weigh the patient daily, using the same scales and method. Compare 24-hour urine output to 24-hour fluid intake and record the difference.

Alteration in comfort: Pain related to peritoneal inflammation

Desired outcome: Patient states that a reduction or absence in pain has occurred and does not exhibit nonverbal indicators of discomfort such as restlessness and facial grimacing. Ventilation and hemodynamic status are uncompromised as evidenced by MAP 70-105 mm Hg, HR 60-100 bpm, RR 12-20 breaths/min with normal depth and pattern (eupnea), PAWP 6-12 mm Hg, and CVP 2-6 mm Hg.

1. Monitor patient for the presence of discomfort; administer analgesics promptly, before pain becomes severe. Consistency and promptness in delivering analgesia also may help to decrease patient's anxiety, which can contribute to the severity of the pain.

< N O T E :   Narcotic analgesics decrease GI motility and may delay the return of normal bowel functioning.

2. Modify patient's body position to optimize comfort. Many patients with severe

abdominal pain find a dorsal recumbent or lateral decubitus bent-knee position more comfortable than other positions.

3. Monitor respiratory pattern and LOC qh, since both may be depressed if large amounts of narcotics are required to control the pain.
4. Monitor HR and BP q1-4h. Monitor CVP and PAWP q4h or more frequently in unstable patients. Report significant deviations to MD. Be aware that narcotics cause vasodilatation and can result in serious hypotension, especially in volume-depleted patients.
5. Evaluate effectiveness of the medication on an ongoing basis. Based on patient's clinical response, discuss dose and drug manipulation with the MD.
6. Avoid administration of narcotics to newly admitted patients until they have been fully evaluated by a surgeon, as narcotic analgesics can mask important diagnostic clues.

Alteration in nutrition: Less than body requirements related to decreased intake secondary to impaired GI function

---

Desired outcome: Patient maintains baseline body weight and demonstrates state of nitrogen balance on nitrogen studies.

---

1. Monitor bowel sounds q1-8h; report significant changes (i.e., sudden absence or return).
2. Maintain NPO status during the acute phase of peritonitis. Gradually increase oral or enteral intake when gastric motility returns.
3. If patient has abdominal distention, measure and document abdominal girth q8h. Distention can signal complications such as ileus or ascites.
4. Administer antacids and histamine H_2 antagonists as prescribed to reduce corrosiveness of gastric acid and prevent complications such as stress ulcers.
5. Administer prescribed antiemetic medications as indicated.
6. Ensure that gastric, intestinal, and other GI drainage tubes are functioning properly. Evaluate character of the drainage (see Table 6-6, p. 411). Irrigate or reposition tubes as necessary. Patency and proper position of decompression tubes such as the Miller-Abbott are essential for proper functioning.
7. For more information, see section "Providing Nutritional Support," p. 490.

Potential for infection related to likelihood of septicemia in patients with intra-abdominal infection

---

Desired outcome: Patient does not develop septicemia as evidenced by HR 60-100 bpm; RR 12-20 breaths/min; SVR 900-1200 dynes/sec/cm^{-5}; CI 2.5-4 L/min/m^2; normothermia; negative cultures; and orientation to person, place, and time.

---

1. Monitor VS and hemodynamic measurements for evidence of septicemia: increases in HR, RR, and CO (CI >4.0 L/min/m^2) and a decrease in SVR (<900 dynes/sec/cm^{-5}). Check rectal or core temperature q4h for increases. Be aware that hypothermia may precede hyperthermia in some patients.
2. If the patient has a sudden temperature elevation, culture blood, sputum, urine,

and other sites as prescribed. Monitor culture reports and report positive cultures promptly.

3. Administer antibiotics as prescribed. Aminoglycosides are used frequently; therefore, monitor patient for hearing loss. Older adults are especially susceptible to the ototoxic effects of aminoglycosides. Check BUN and creatinine and monitor urinary output to ensure that patient has adequate renal function as aminoglycosides are potentially nephrotoxic.

4. In order to minimize microbial growth, facilitate drainage of pus, GI secretions, old blood, necrotic tissue, foreign material such as feces, and other bodily fluids from wounds.
   - Evaluate and maintain patency of wound drains by suction or sterile irrigation as prescribed. Notify MD in the event of loss of patency or other malfunction of drainage tubes.
   - Document and report unusual characteristics or changes in wound drainage (see Table 6-6, p. 411).
   - Change saturated dressings, using aseptic technique.
   - Pack open wounds as prescribed, using aseptic technique.
   - Irrigate wounds as prescribed, using aseptic technique.
   - Document and report presence of nonviable tissue.
   - Turn patient frequently to encourage gravity drainage of secretions.

5. Evaluate wounds for evidence of infection (e.g., erythema, warmth, swelling, unusual drainage). Culture any unusual drainage (see Table 6-6, p. 411, for a description of normal drainage).

6. Evaluate patient's orientation to person, place, and time and LOC q2-4h. Document and report significant deviations from baseline.

Hyperthermia related to infectious process occurring with peritonitis

Desired outcome: Patient's temperature returns to normal limits within an acceptable timeframe.

1. Monitor rectal or core temperature q2-4h.
2. If a hypothermia blanket is required, perform the following interventions:
   - Protect the skin that is in contact with the blanket by placing a sheet between the blanket and patient.
   - Inspect patient's skin q2h for evidence of tissue damage due to local vasoconstriction. Massage patient's skin q2h to promote circulation and minimize tissue damage.
   - Check patient's temperature at frequent intervals to ensure that sudden decreases (along with shivering) do not occur, which could increase metabolic demand.
3. If patient has a very high fever (i.e., >38.9° C [102° F]), administer tepid baths, which may be helpful in reducing the fever.
4. Administer antipyretics as prescribed.

For other nursing diagnoses and interventions, see the following as appropriate: "Management of the Adult with Hemodynamic Monitoring," pp. 168-170; "Caring for the Critically Ill on Prolonged Bed Rest," pp. 506-511; "Caring for the Critically Ill with Life-Threatening Disorders," pp. 511-522; and "Caring for the Family of the Critically Ill," pp. 522-526.

REHABILITATION AND PATIENT-FAMILY TEACHING CONCEPTS

Give patient and significant others verbal and written instructions for the following:
1. Medications, including drug name, purpose, dosage, schedule, precautions, and potential side effects.
2. Signs and symptoms of infection: fever, unusual drainage from surgical incision or diagnostic pericentesis site, unusual warmth or redness surrounding surgical sites, and abdominal pain. Have patient demonstrate technique for measurement of oral temperature, using glass thermometer or type of thermometer that will be used at home.
3. Importance of seeking medical attention promptly for signs and symptoms of complications such as adhesions (e.g., pain, persistent vomiting, fecal vomiting, abdominal distention, sudden change in bowel habits), or infection (see #2, above).

Acute gastrointestinal bleeding

Bleeding can occur at any point along the alimentary tract. The following is a brief overview of common GI bleeding sites or occurrences.

Esophagus: Esophageal varices (see p. 357) are the most common cause of massive esophageal hemorrhage. Esophagitis and esophageal ulcers and tumors also can cause acute bleeding but they occur less frequently. Maneuvers that increase intra-abdominal pressure (i.e., retching, vomiting, straining, coughing) can lead to Mallory-Weiss syndrome, a laceration or tear of the mucosa and submucosa of the cardia or lower esophagus, resulting in massive bleeding.

Stomach and duodenum: The most common causes of hematemesis and melena are duodenal and gastric ulcers, accounting for half of massive upper GI bleeding disorders. Stress ulcers are common phenomena in critically ill patients. Groups likely to develop stress ulcers include patients with burn injuries, head injuries, ventilator dependency, and shock states. Gastritis, another common cause of GI bleeding, usually presents as slow, diffuse oozing that is difficult to control. Benign or malignant gastric tumors may initiate severe bleeding episodes, especially tumors located in the vascular system that supplies the GI tract.

Small intestine: This area of the alimentary tract accounts for only 3% of GI bleeding episodes. Diverticular disease, intussusception of the small bowel, acute superior mesenteric artery occlusion, and Crohn's disease are some of the possible causes for bleeding.

Large intestine: Arteriovenous malformation of the ascending colon and the cecum is the usual cause of massive colonic bleeding. Inflammatory bowel diseases such as ulcerative colitis and Crohn's disease result in friable intestinal mucosa, which can lead to massive hemorrhage and other serious complications including bowel obstruction and perforation. In addition, diverticular disease can cause serious, intermittent bleeding episodes. Other causes include benign or malignant neoplasms and congenital malformation such as hemangioma or telangiectasia.

Neighboring organs: Acute pancreatitis (see p. 379) and pancreatic pseudocyst are disorders associated with hemorrhage.

Systemic organ diseases: Hypoperfusion associated with severe cardiac disease can lead to GI ischemia, resulting in tissue damage that may lead to necrosis and hemorrhage. Uremia has a high incidence of bleeding due to platelet dysfunction. Collagen diseases can result in thrombosis of small vessels in the small intestine, eventually leading to ulceration. Many blood dyscrasias (e.g., disseminated intravascular coagulation [DIC], thrombocytopenia) are associated with hematemesis and melena due to a decreased ability to form clots.

Medications: Long-standing use of aspirin, steroids, or anticoagulants sometimes is associated with serious GI bleeding.

Other trauma: In addition to major abdominal trauma (see p. 401), foreign bodies (e.g., razors, screws, nails) may lacerate gastric or intestinal mucosa, causing bleeding to occur.

Postoperative hemorrhage: Postoperative hemorrhage can occur immediately or as long as 10-20 days after surgery. Bleeding in the postoperative period may be due to residual or stress-related ulcers, vascular disruption along the suture line, or blood dyscrasias. A sudden massive loss of circulating volume (>20%) results in decreased venous return and diminished cardiac output. Reflex peripheral vasoconstriction shunts blood to vital cerebral and cardiopulmonary systems. In turn, renal and mesenteric blood flow diminish, resulting in organ ischemia. If bleeding continues, cerebral and coronary flow become compromised, eventually resulting in multisystem organ failure. Renal ischemia results in acute tubular necrosis (see "Acute Renal Failure," p. 173), hepatic dysfunction results in metabolic derangements (see "Hepatic Failure," p. 364), and pulmonary dysfunction leads to adult respiratory distress syndrome (see p. 18).

ASSESSMENT

Signs and symptoms: Vary, depending on the amount of blood lost, rate of bleeding, and its effects on cardiovascular and other body systems. Adults can lose up to 500 ml of blood in 15 minutes and remain asymptomatic. A loss of 1000 ml in 15 minutes usually produces tachycardia, hypotension, nausea, weakness, and diaphoresis. Syncope associated with hypotension also may occur. Hematemesis, melena (passage of black, shiny, fetid stools containing blood), and hematochezia (passage of bloody stools) usually are present. Blood can irritate the bowels, thereby increasing transit time and causing diarrhea. Mild to severe pain usually is associated with ulcerative or erosive disease. As blood covers and protects the eroded tissue, pain may disappear. Severe hypovolemic shock and decreased cardiac output can lead to ischemia of various organs, especially the lungs, brain, and kidneys.

Physical assessment: With profuse, active bleeding, a fast assessment can determine if a shock state is present: the presence of tachycardia, hypotension, cool and diaphoretic extremities, decreased peripheral pulses, delayed capillary refill (>4 seconds), pallor or cyanosis, restlessness, confusion, decreased urine output, and obvious bleeding. Initially, auscultation of the abdomen may reveal hyperactive bowel sounds due to mucosal irritation by blood, or a silent abdomen, which suggests serious complications such as ileus, perforation, or vascular occlusion. Palpation may reveal epigastric tenderness, which is expected in peptic ulceration; or an epigastric mass or enlarged lymph nodes, which are indicative of gastric malignant disease. Jaundice, spider veins, ascites, and hepatosplenomegaly suggest liver disease. A careful digital rectal examination should be performed along with the testing of vomitus and stool for occult blood. With upper GI bleeding, emesis or NG aspirate contains obvious whole blood or coffee-ground appearing old blood. Stools usually are black and tarry (melena), with a distinctive fetid odor. With lower GI bleeding, stools may be dark or contain fresh blood. Massive lower GI bleeding is associated with dark red "currant jelly" stools or passing of fresh blood with clots (hematochezia). Bleeding below the level of the duodenum is not associated with hematemesis.

Vital signs and hemodynamic measurements: HR and BP are quick indicators of a hypovolemic state. Systolic BP <100 mm Hg with a HR >100 bpm in a previously normotensive individual signal a 20% or greater reduction in blood volume. Postural VS should be measured, as well. A decrease in systolic BP >10 mm Hg or an increase in HR of 10 bpm is indicative of a recent blood loss of at least 1000 ml in the adult. Hemodynamic measurements usually reveal a decreased PAP and CO and an increased SVR. After abdominal surgery, a hyperdynamic state may exist, with an increased CO and decreased SVR. The mechanism of this phenomenon is not completely understood. RR will be mildly elevated as a response to the diminished oxygen-carrying capacity of the blood. If abdominal pain is present, ventilatory excursion may be limited.

History and risk factors: Excessive alcohol, salicylate, or steroid ingestion; foreign body ingestion; hiatal hernia; hepatic, pancreatic, or biliary tract disease; blood dyscrasias; penetrating or blunt trauma; familial cancer; recent abdominal surgery.

DIAGNOSTIC TESTS

1. *Hematologic tests:* Serial hemoglobin and hematocrit values will reflect the amount of blood lost. Because the ratio of blood cells to plasma remains unchanged initially, the first hematocrit value may be near normal. However, the hematocrit is expected to fall dramatically as volume is restored and extravascular fluid mobilizes into the vascular space. Platelet count rises within an hour of hemorrhage and leukocytosis follows.

2. *Chemistry studies:* Electrolyte imbalance is not commonly seen in GI bleeding, although excessive vomiting or gastric suction may cause a hypochloremic, hypokalemic state accompanied by a rise in the serum bicarbonate level. Increases in BUN without corresponding creatinine increases occur owing to excess intestinal protein from the digestion of RBCs. BUN increases are not seen with colonic or lower small intestinal bleeding as protein digestion occurs higher in the upper small intestine. Dehydration and renal insufficiency contribute to an elevated BUN in affected patients. Plasma protein levels may rise in response to increased hepatic production. Mild hyperglycemia is the result of the body's compensatory response to a stressful stimulus. Hyperbilirubinemia is caused by the breakdown of reabsorbed blood and its pigments. Ammonia levels usually are elevated in patients with liver disease.

3. *ABG values:* If the shock state is severe, lactic acidosis occurs, reflected by low pH and serum bicarbonate levels. With a low perfusion state, hypoxemia may be present.

4. *Coagulation studies:* Depending on preexisting disease, hypocoagulability may be present. Elevation of fibrinogen levels, fibrin split products (FSP), and prothrombin and partial prothrombin times may be seen.

5. *12-lead EKG:* May reflect severe cardiac ischemia as a result of hypoperfusion. Ischemic changes include T-wave depression or inversion.

6. *Esophagogastroduodenoscopy (panendoscopy):* The esophagus, stomach, and duodenum are visualized directly with a fiberoptic endoscope, which is passed through the mouth. Lesions in these areas are noted and attempts are made to

identify the exact source of bleeding. The study usually is performed within the first 12 hours after admission. It may be necessary to clear the stomach of blood and clots by lavage prior to the procedure. Antacids should be held until after the procedure because they alter the appearance of the lesions. Electrocautery, laser, and other therapeutic techniques may be employed during this procedure.

7. *Proctosigmoidoscopy:* The rectum and sigmoid colon are visualized directly through an endoscope, which is passed through the anus into the lower GI tract. Mucosal bleeding, polyps, hemorrhoids, and other lesions may be seen. Biopsies may be taken during this procedure.

8. *Radiologic procedures:* Flat plate abdominal x-ray may reveal free air under the diaphragm, which suggests perforation. A chest x-ray is taken to establish baseline pulmonary status. Barium studies usually are reserved for nonemergent situations to verify the presence of tumors or other large gastrointestinal lesions.

9. *Angiography:* If the bleeding is rapid and suspected of being vascular in origin, selective angiography of various GI arterial systems may aid in the visualization of bleeding site(s). If the bleeding site is vascular, therapeutic embolization may be attempted during angiography. See precautions under this topic in ''Bleeding Esophageal Varices,'' p. 358.

MEDICAL MANAGEMENT AND SURGICAL INTERVENTIONS

1. **Fluid and electrolyte management:** Volume replacement in acute GI bleeding must be performed as quickly as possible. In addition to GI blood loss, sequestration of fluid into the peritoneum and interstitium depletes intravascular volume. With severe hypovolemia, a combination of crystalloids and colloids is used for volume expansion. Packed cells and fresh frozen plasma should be balanced to provide replacement of cells and clotting components. Large transfusions will cause Ca^{++} to bind with the citrate in the blood and deplete free Ca^{++} levels. In addition, large volume blood transfusions can lead to coagulopathy disorders. If bleeding is massive, lactated Ringer's solution is the preferred crystalloid volume expander because electrolyte disturbances are minimized. Vasopressors and inotropes should be used *only* if tissue perfusion remains compromised despite adequate intravascular volume replacement. Hemodynamic monitoring is essential for continuous evaluation of the patient's volume status, especially in patients over age 50 or those with chronic illnesses such as cardiovascular, pulmonary, renal, or hepatic disease. Over-aggressive volume resuscitation results in overhydration with complications of cardiac failure and pulmonary edema. Electrolytes are closely monitored, especially in patients with renal or hepatic disease.

2. **Respiratory support:** Because of a decrease in the oxygen-carrying capacity of the RBCs in massive blood loss, oxygen therapy by nasal cannula or face mask usually is initiated. More aggressive ventilatory support may be required for patients with persistent hypoxemia and other evidence of early respiratory failure or impending adult respiratory distress syndrome (see p. 18).

3. **Nutritional support:** As soon as the patient's hemodynamic status stabilizes, nutritional support must be considered. Total parenteral nutrition is started for patients who are likely to remain NPO for days to weeks. Enteral or oral feedings are started when there is no further evidence of GI hemorrhage and bowel function has returned.

4. **Gastric lavage:** Gastric intubation often is necessary, especially with upper GI

bleeding. Lavage with room-temperature or iced saline or with water is performed to clear blood and clots from the stomach and allow for estimation of ongoing blood loss. Intragastric cooling with iced saline lavage is a commonly performed procedure, but its effectiveness in controlling upper GI bleeding has not been well established.

5. **Analgesia:** Caution is exercised if pain medications are used, as many analgesics have a vasodilatation effect and can decrease preload, afterload, and BP significantly.

6. **Pharmacotherapy:** Antacids raise the gastric pH and may decrease the corrosiveness of gastric acid. However, a major goal of antacid therapy is pain control, as antacids are helpful in relieving pain associated with peptic ulcer disease. Histamine H_2 receptor antagonists such as cimetidine and ranitidine block gastric acid and pepsin secretion and are employed in the treatment of erosive and ulcerative disease. Oral sucralfate may be prescribed for patients with gastric erosions. The sucralfate combines with gastric acid and forms an adhesive protective coating over damaged mucosa. Vasopressin is sometimes used for uncontrolled massive bleeding. For additional information on vasopressin, see "Bleeding Esophageal Varices," p. 359.

7. **Surgical management:** Many surgical techniques are used, depending on the location and severity of the lesion. Ulcerative disease requires surgery if the lesions continue to bleed despite aggressive medical therapy or if complications such as perforation or obstruction develop. Vagotomy, pyloroplasty, antrectomy, and partial or total resection of the affected area are some of the many surgical procedures employed. A common procedure for duodenal ulcers is gastrojejunostomy (Billroth II procedure). Massive lower GI bleeding is difficult to control and may require aggressive surgical procedures such as a colectomy, with the creation of a permanent ileostomy or internal ileal pouch. If GI bleeding is due to gastroesophageal varices, see "Bleeding Esophageal Varices," p. 357.

NURSING DIAGNOSES AND INTERVENTIONS

Fluid volume deficit related to decreased circulating volume secondary to inadequate intake, active bleeding, or fluid sequestration

---

Desired outcome: Circulating plasma volume is restored, as evidenced by MAP $\geq$70 mm Hg, HR 60-100 bpm, CVP 2-6 mm Hg, PAWP 6-12 mm Hg, CI $\geq$2.5 L/min/m^2, normal sinus rhythm on EKG, and urinary output $\geq$30 ml/hr.

---

1. Monitor BP q15min during episodes of rapid active blood loss or unstable VS. Be alert to MAP decreases of >10 mm Hg from previous reading.
2. Monitor postural VS on admission, q4-8h, and more frequently if recurrence of active bleeding is suspected: measure BP and HR with patient in a supine position, followed immediately by measurement of BP and HR with patient in a sitting position (as tolerated). A decrease in systolic BP >10 mm Hg or an increase in HR of 10 bpm with patient in a sitting position suggests a significant intravascular volume deficit, with approximately 15-20% loss of volume.
3. Monitor HR, EKG, and cardiovascular status qh or more frequently in the

presence of active bleeding or unstable VS. Be alert to a sudden increase in HR, which is suggestive of hypovolemia.

< N O T E : Increases in HR may be due to other factors such as pain and anxiety.

4. Measure central pressures and thermodilution CO q1-4h. Be alert to low or decreasing CVP, PAWP, and CO. Calculate SVR q4-8h, or more frequently in unstable patients. An elevated HR, decreased PAWP, decreased CO (CI <2.5 L/min/m^2), and increased SVR suggest hypovolemia and the need for volume restoration.

5. Replace volume with prescribed fluids (usually a combination of crystalloid and blood products) *via* large bore IV (18 gauge or larger).

6. Measure urinary output qh. Be alert to output <30 ml/hr for two consecutive hours. Increase fluid intake if decreased output is due to hypovolemia and hypoperfusion.

7. Monitor hematocrit; immediately report values <28-$30/100$ ml.

8. Measure and record all GI blood losses from hematemesis, hematochezia, melena.

9. Check all stools and gastric contents for occult blood.

10. Ensure proper function and patency of NG tubes. Do not occlude the air vent of double-lumen tubes as this may result in vacuum occlusion. Confirm placement of NG tube at least q8h and reposition as necessary.

11. Administer histamine H$_2$ receptor antagonists, antacids, and sucralfate as prescribed to minimize tissue damage and bleeding due to corrosive gastric acid.

Alteration in cardiac output: Decreased, related to diminished venous return and decreased preload secondary to acute blood loss

---

Desired outcome: CO returns to or approaches normal limits as evidenced by CI ≥ 2.5 L/min/m^2, urinary output ≥ 30 ml/hr, normal sinus rhythm on EKG, distal pulses $>2+$ on a 0-4+ scale, and brisk capillary refill (<3 seconds).

---

1. Administer oxygen as prescribed to facilitate maximal oxygen delivery to the tissues.

2. Monitor ABG values for hypoxemia. Alert MD if arterial Pa$_{O_2}$ value is <80 mm Hg or if oxygen saturation falls below 90%.

3. Monitor EKG for evidence of myocardial ischemia (i.e., T-wave depression, QT prolongation, ventricular dysrhythmias).

4. Monitor for physical indicators of diminished cardiac output including pallor, cool extremities, capillary refill delayed for >4 seconds, and decreased or absent amplitude of distal pulses.

5. Monitor thermodilution CO (see intervention #4 under **Fluid volume deficit**, above).

6. Monitor urine output qh; document and report urine output <30 ml/hr for two consecutive hours.

Alteration in comfort: Pain related to GI mucosal irritation, inflammation, or surgical procedure

Desired outcomes: Patient states that a reduction in discomfort has occurred. Ventilation and hemodynamic status are uncompromised as evidenced by RR 12-20 breaths/min with normal depth and pattern (eupnea), and MAP 70-105 mm Hg.

1. Administer antacids as prescribed to relieve pain due to upper GI disorders.
2. Monitor and document presence of abdominal pain or discomfort. Be aware that pain may disappear concomitant with a bleeding episode as blood covers and protects eroded tissue.
3. If narcotic analgesics are prescribed for postoperative or severe pain, administer with caution. Many narcotic analgesics cause vasodilatation, thereby decreasing preload and afterload. For patients with GI bleeding and markedly reduced preload, narcotic administration can result in dramatic hypotension.
4. Monitor respiratory rate and depth to avoid narcotic-induced respiratory depression.
5. Supplement analgesics with nonpharmacologic maneuvers to aid in pain reduction. Modify patient's body position to optimize comfort. Patients who have pain associated with gastric reflux may be more comfortable with HOB elevated, if this position does not compromise hemodynamic status.
6. Because reducing anxiety contributes to pain relief, ensure consistency and promptness in delivering analgesia.

Alteration in nutrition: Less than body requirements related to decreased oral intake secondary to nausea, vomiting, and NPO status; and increased need secondary to tissue destruction or infection

Desired outcome: Patient has adequate nutrition as evidenced by stable weights, thyroxine-binding prealbumin 200-300 µg/ml, and a state of nitrogen balance on nitrogen studies.

1. Collaborate with MD, dietician, and pharmacist to estimate patient's individual metabolic needs, based on activity level, underlying disease process, and nutritional status prior to hospitalization.
2. Provide parenteral nutrition during acute phase of the bleeding, as prescribed.
3. Begin enteral therapy when acute hemorrhagic episode has subsided and bowel function has returned. This may take several weeks in some patients.
4. Monitor thyroxine-binding prealbumin and report decreasing levels.
5. Weigh patient daily at the same time of day, using the same scales. Weight can be a practical indicator of nutritional status if patient's weight changes are interpreted based on the following factors: fluid shifts (edema, diuresis, third-spacing), surgical resection, and weight of dressings and equipment.
6. For more information, see "Providing Nutritional Support," p. 490.

Alteration in bowel elimination: Diarrhea related to increased motility secondary to irritation by the presence of blood in the GI tract or disease process

Desired outcome: Stools are normal in consistency and frequency and negative for occult blood. Serum sodium is 137-147 mEq/L, serum potassium is 3.5-5.5 mEq/L, and serum calcium is 8.5-10.5 mg/dl.

1. Monitor and record the amount, frequency, and character of patient's stools.
2. Provide or have bedpan or bedside commode (only for hemodynamically stable patients) readily available.
3. Minimize embarrassing odor by removing stool promptly and using room deodorizers.
4. Use matter-of-fact approach when assisting patient with frequent bowel elimination. Reassure patient that frequent elimination is a common problem for most patients with GI bleeding.
5. Evaluate bowel sounds q4-8h. Anticipate normal to hyperdynamic bowel sounds. Absence of bowel sounds (especially in association with severe pain or abdominal distention) may signal serious complications such as ileus or perforation.
6. Monitor serum electrolytes and notify MD of abnormalities.
7. Keep patient NPO until diarrhea episodes have subsided.

See other nursing diagnoses and interventions in the following, as appropriate: "Management of the Adult on Hemodynamic Monitoring," pp. 171-174; "Caring for the Critically Ill on Prolonged Bed Rest," pp. 506-511; "Caring for the Critically Ill with Life-Threatening Disorders," pp. 511-522; and "Caring for the Family of the Critically Ill," pp. 522-526.

REHABILITATION AND PATIENT-FAMILY TEACHING CONCEPTS

Give patient and significant others verbal and written instructions for the following:
1. Medications, including drug name, dosage, purpose, schedule, precautions, and potential side effects.
2. Signs and symptoms of actual or impending GI hemorrhage: nausea, vomiting of blood, dark stools, light-headedness, passage of frank blood in stools.
3. Importance of seeking medical attention promptly if signs of recurrent bleeding (i.e., pain, change in bowel habits, passing of blood in the stools, or vomiting blood) appear.

Abdominal trauma

The degree of injury to abdominal contents is related to the nature of the force applied and the consistency of the affected structures. Forces involved are classified as penetrating (e.g., stab, gunshot wounds) or blunt (e.g., those caused by falls, physical assault, motor vehicle accidents, crush injury). Organs are categorized as solid (e.g., liver, spleen, pancreas) or hollow (e.g., stomach, intestine). Usually, injury inflicted by stab wounds follows a more predictable pattern and involves less tissue destruction than injury from gunshot wounds, although stab wounds to major vascular structures and organs can be fatal. Removing penetrating objects can result in additional injury, so attempts at removal should be made only under controlled situations with a surgeon and operating room immediately available. High-velocity weapons (e.g., rifles) not only cause injury to tissue in the direct path of the missile but to adjacent organs as well because of energy shock waves that surround the missile path. Tissue destruction is not as great with low-velocity pistols. Blunt abdominal trauma typically results in injury to solid viscera because hollow viscera tend to be more compressible. However, hollow organs may rupture, especially when full, if there is a sudden increase in intraluminal pressure. The rate of complications and death increases greatly if injury to multiple abdominal organs is sustained.

Abdominal trauma results in direct injury to organs, blood vessels, and supporting structures. Other pathophysiologic changes associated with abdominal trauma include: (1) massive fluid shifts related to tissue damage, blood loss, and shock; (2) metabolic changes associated with stress and catecholamine release; (3) coagulation problems associated with massive hemorrhage and multiple transfusions; (4) inflammation, infection, and abscess formation due to release of GI secretions and bacteria into the peritoneum; and (5) nutritional and electrolyte alterations that develop as a consequence of disruption of GI tract integrity. The following is a brief overview of common injuries:

Spleen: The organ most frequently injured following blunt trauma. Massive hemorrhage from splenic injury is common. Splenic injury often is associated with hepatic or pancreatic injury. All efforts are made to repair the spleen since total splenectomy increases the long-term risk of sepsis, especially in children and young adults.

Liver: Because of its size and location, it is the organ most frequently involved in penetrating trauma and often is affected with blunt injury, as well. Control of bleeding and bile drainage are major concerns with hepatic injury.

Lower esophagus and stomach: Occasionally, the lower esophagus is involved in penetrating trauma. Because the stomach is flexible and readily displaced, it is usually not injured with blunt trauma, but may be injured by direct penetration. Injury to the lower esophagus and stomach results in the escape of irritating gastric fluids and the release of free air below the level of the diaphragm. Esophageal injuries often are associated with thoracic injuries.

Pancreas and duodenum: Although traumatic pancreatic or duodenal injury occurs relatively infrequently, it is associated with high morbidity and mortality rates because of the difficulty of detecting these injuries and the likelihood of massive injury to nearby organs. These organs are retroperitoneal and clinical indicators of injury often are not obvious for several hours.

Small intestine and mesentery: These injuries are common and may be caused by penetrating or nonpenetrating forces. Compromised intestinal blood flow with eventual infarction is the consequence of undetected mesenteric damage. Perforations or contusions can result in release of bacteria and intestinal contents into the abdominal cavity, causing serious infection.

Colon: Injury most frequently caused by penetrating forces, although lap belts, direct blows, and other blunt forces cause a small percentage of colonic injuries. Because of the high bacterial content, infection is even more a concern than with small bowel injury. Many patients with colon injuries require temporary colostomy.

Pelvis: See "Lower Urinary Tract Trauma," p. 184, and "Renal Trauma," p. 189.

Major vessels: Injuries to the abdominal aorta and inferior vena cava are most often caused by penetrating trauma but also occur with deceleration injury. Hepatic vein injuries frequently are associated with juxtahepatic vena caval injury and result in rapid hemorrhage. Blood loss after major vascular injury is massive and survival depends on rapid prehospital transport and immediate surgical intervention.

Retroperitoneal: Tears in retroperitoneal vessels associated with pelvic fractures or damage to retroperitoneal organs (pancreas, duodenum, kidney) can cause bleeding into the retroperitoneum. Even though the retroperitoneal space can accommodate up to 4 L of blood, detection of retroperitoneal hematomas is difficult and sophisticated diagnostic techniques may be required.

ASSESSMENT

Signs and symptoms: A wide variation can occur. Mild tenderness to severe abdominal pain may be present, with the pain either localized to the site of injury or diffuse. Blood or fluid collection within the peritoneum causes irritation resulting in involuntary guarding, rigidity, and rebound tenderness. Fluid or air under the diaphragm may cause referred shoulder pain. Kehr's sign (left shoulder pain caused by splenic bleeding) also may be noted, especially when the patient is recumbent. Nausea and vomiting may be present, and the conscious patient who has sustained blood loss often complains of thirst, an early sign of hemorrhagic shock. Symptoms of abdominal injury may be minimal or absent in the patient who is intoxicated or has sustained head or spinal cord injury.

< N O T E :   The absence of signs and symptoms does not exclude the presence of major abdominal injury.

Physical assessment: Abdominal assessment is highly subjective and serial evaluations by the same examiner are strongly recommended in order to detect subtle changes.

- *Inspection:* Abrasions and ecchymoses may be indicative of underlying injury. For example, ecchymosis over LUQ suggests splenic rupture; ecchymotic areas on the flank are suggestive of retroperitoneal bleeding; and erythema and ecchymosis across the lower abdomen suggest intestinal injury due to lap belts. Ecchymoses may take hours to days to develop, depending on the rate of blood loss. Absence of ecchymosis does not exclude major abdominal trauma and massive internal bleeding. In the event of gunshot wounds, entrance and exit (if present) wounds should be identified.
- *Auscultation:* It is important to auscultate before palpation and percussion, as these maneuvers can stimulate the bowel and confound assessment findings. Bowel sounds are likely to be decreased or absent with abdominal organ injury or intraperitoneal bleeding. However, the presence of bowel sounds does not exclude significant abdominal injury. Immediately after injury, bowel sounds may be present, even with major organ injury. Bowel sounds should be auscultated in each quadrant q1-2h in patients with suspected abdominal injury. Absence of bowel sounds is expected immediately after surgery. Failure to auscultate bowel sounds within 24-48 hours after surgery is suggestive of ileus, possibly caused by continued bleeding, peritonitis, or bowel infarction.
- *Palpation:* Tenderness to light palpation suggests pain from superficial or abdominal wall lesions, such as that occurring with seatbelt contusions. Deep palpation may reveal a mass in the area of hematoma. See Table 6-4, p. 404, for signs and symptoms suggestive of peritoneal irritation. Subcutaneous em-

T A B L E 6 - 4
Signs and symptoms suggestive of peritoneal irritation

- Generalized abdominal pain or tenderness.
- Involuntary guarding of the abdomen.
- Abdominal wall rigidity.
- Rebound tenderness.
- Abdominal pain with movement or coughing.
- Decreased or absent bowel sounds.

physema of the abdominal wall usually is caused by thoracic injury, but also may be produced by bowel rupture. Measurements of abdominal girth may be helpful in identifying increases in girth attributable to gas, blood, or fluid. Visual evaluation of abdominal distention is a late and unreliable sign of bleeding.

- *Percussion:* Unusually large areas of dullness may be percussed over ruptured blood-filled organs. For example, a fixed area of dullness in the LUQ suggests a ruptured spleen. An absence (or decrease in the size) of liver dullness may be caused by free air below the diaphragm, a consequence of hollow viscus perforation, or in unusual cases, displacement of the liver through a ruptured diaphragm. The presence of tympany suggests gas; dullness suggests the enlargement is caused by blood or fluid.

Vital signs and hemodynamic measurements: Ventilatory excursion often is diminished because of pain, thoracic injury, or diaphragmatic elevation due to abdominal distention. Initial compensatory tachycardia and vasoconstriction secondary to blood loss usually maintain a normal BP until blood loss becomes major. At that point, BP deteriorates to an MAP <70 mm Hg. Vascular resistance remains high. A diminished CVP and PAP reflect hypovolemic shock; CO decreases because of hypovolemia but will normalize with correction. Initial hypothermia is common.

History: Details regarding circumstances of the accident and mechanism of injury are invaluable in detecting the possibility of specific injuries. In addition, ascertain time of patient's last meal, previous abdominal surgeries, and use of safety restraints (if appropriate). If possible, determine current medications and allergies, particularly to contrast material, antibiotics, and tetanus toxoid. The history may be difficult to obtain due to alcohol or drug intoxication, head injury, breathing difficulties, or impaired cerebral perfusion. In such cases, family members and emergency personnel may be valuable sources of information.

DIAGNOSTIC TESTS

1. *Hematocrit:* Serial levels reflect the amount of blood lost. If drawn immediately after the injury hematocrit may be normal, but serial levels will reveal dramatic decreases during resuscitation and as extravascular fluid mobilizes during the recovery phase.

2. *WBC count:* Leukocytosis is expected immediately after injury. Splenic injuries in particular result in the rapid development of a moderate to high WBC count. A later increase in WBCs or a shift to the left reflects an increase in the number of neutrophils, which signals an inflammatory response and pos-

sible intra-abdominal infection. In the patient with abdominal trauma, ruptured abdominal viscera must be considered as a potential source of infection.

3. *Platelet count:* Mild thrombocytosis is seen immediately following traumatic injury. Spontaneous bleeding and a very low platelet count (<20,000-30,000 per mm^3) are signals of the need for transfusion of fresh platelets.

4. *Glucose:* Initially elevated due to catecholamine release and insulin resistance associated with major trauma. Glucose metabolism is abnormal following major hepatic resection and patients should be monitored at frequent intervals in order to prevent severe hypoglycemic episodes.

5. *Amylase:* Elevated serum levels are associated with pancreatic or upper small bowel injury, but values may be normal even with severe injury to these organs.

6. *SGOT, SGPT, LDH:* Elevations of these enzymes reflect hepatic dysfunction due to liver ischemia during prolonged hypotensive episodes or direct traumatic damage. Fluctuations in these enzymes during the postoperative period can be used to detect evidence of liver necrosis.

7. *X-rays:* Flat and upright chest x-rays exclude chest injuries (frequently associated with abdominal trauma) and establish a baseline, since surgery is likely. In addition, chest, abdominal, and pelvic x-rays may reveal fractures, missiles, free intraperitoneal air, hematoma, or hemorrhage. All patients in motor vehicle accidents, falls, or similar accidents require cervical spine x-rays to exclude the possibility of cervical spine injury (see ''Acute Spinal Cord Injury,'' p. 293).

8. *Occult blood:* Gastric contents and stool should be tested for blood in the initial and recovery periods because GI bleeding can occur both as a result of direct injury and later complications.

9. *Diagnostic peritoneal lavage (DPL):* Involves insertion of a peritoneal dialysis catheter into the peritoneum to check for intra-abdominal bleeding. DPL is indicated for confirmed or suspected blunt abdominal trauma for the following patients: (1) those in whom signs and symptoms of abdominal injury are obscured by intoxication, head or spinal cord trauma, narcotic administration, or unconsciousness; (2) those about to undergo general anesthesia for repair of other injuries (e.g., orthopedic, facial); and (3) any patient with equivocal assessment findings. DPL is unnecessary for patients who have obvious intraabdominal bleeding or other indications for immediate laparotomy (see ''Surgical Considerations,'' p. 408).

If gross blood is recovered when the catheter is inserted, immediate laparotomy is indicated. If blood is not recovered, a liter of normal saline or Ringer's lactate is infused rapidly through the catheter and then drained into a sterile bedside drainage device. If possible, the patient is moved from side to side after fluid instillation in order to distribute the lavage fluid evenly. If the drained lavage is grossly bloody, intraperitoneal bleeding is confirmed. Other indicators of a positive lavage are >100,000 RBC/μl, >500 WBC μl, amylase >175 units/dl, presence of bile or bacteria, or obvious intestinal contents in the drainage.

< N O T E : An in-dwelling urinary catheter is inserted before DPL to prevent inadvertent puncture of a full bladder. The stomach is decompressed with a gastric tube in order to check for bleeding and avoid pressure on a full stomach, vomiting, and aspiration.

10. *CT scan:* Can detect intraperitoneal and retroperitoneal bleeding and free air (associated with rupture of hollow viscera). It is most useful in assessing injury to solid abdominal organs.

< C A U T I O N :   Because of the risk of rapid deterioration, patient should be accompanied by emergency or critical care nurse during the 30-minute period it takes to perform CT scan. Appropriate monitoring and resuscitation equipment must be readily available.

11. *Angiography:* Performed selectively with blunt trauma to evaluate injury to spleen, liver, pancreas, duodenum, and retroperitoneal vessels when other diagnostic findings are equivocal.

< C A U T I O N :   Because of the large amount of contrast material used during this procedure, monitor urine output closely for several hours for a decrease and ensure adequate hydration.

12. Abdominal injuries often are associated with multi-system trauma. Also see diagnostic test discussions in "Chest Trauma," p. 33, "Cardiac Trauma," p. 103, "Urinary Tract Trauma," p. 185, "Renal Trauma," p. 190, "Head Injury," p. 274, and "Acute Spinal Cord Injury," p. 295.

MEDICAL MANAGEMENT AND SURGICAL INTERVENTIONS

1. **Oxygen:** Individuals sustaining abdominal trauma are likely to be tachypnic with the potential for poor ventilatory effort. Supplemental oxygen is delivered until patient's ABG values while breathing room air are acceptable.
2. **Fluid management:** Since massive blood loss is associated with most abdominal injuries, immediate volume resuscitation is critical. Initially, Ringer's lactate or similar balanced salt solution is given. Colloid solutions such as albumin are helpful in the postoperative period if the patient is hypoalbuminemic due to hepatic injury or ischemia, or if there are low filling pressures and evidence of decreased plasma oncotic pressure. Typed and cross-matched fresh blood is the optimal fluid for replacement of large blood losses. However, since fresh whole blood is rarely available, a combination of packed cells and fresh frozen plasma is often used.

< C A U T I O N :   Large volumes of fluid given rapidly must be warmed in order to prevent complications of hypothermia and coagulopathy.

3. **Pneumatic anti-shock garment (PASG, MAST):** Can be used as a temporary means to elevate BP in patients with severe abdominal trauma and marked hypovolemia. The inflatable garment consists of a pair of trousers with an abdominal extension. When inflated with air, the garment's external pressure compresses the legs and abdomen, resulting in direct tamponade of bleeding and possibly other effects, including increased preload from autotransfusion of blood from the legs and abdomen and a direct increase in afterload from vascular compression.

< N O T E :   Use of PASG is controversial. The critical care nurse working with PASG must be certain the patient is volume resuscitated and that each section is deflated slowly before removal. Fluid and blood should be kept readily available during the deflation in case of hemodynamic instability.

4. **Gastric intubation:** Gastric tube permits gastric decompression, aids in removal of gastric contents, and prevents accumulation of gas or air in the GI tract. Aspirated contents can be checked for blood to aid in the diagnosis of lower esophageal, gastric, or duodenal injury. The tube usually remains in place until bowel function returns.

5. **Urinary drainage:** An in-dwelling catheter is inserted soon after admission to obtain a specimen for urinalysis and monitor hourly urine output and aid in the diagnosis of genito-urinary trauma. See "Urinary Tract Trauma," p. 185, for precautions.

6. **Pharmacotherapy**
   - *Antibiotics:* Abdominal trauma is associated with a high incidence of intra-abdominal abscess, sepsis, and wound infection, particularly injury to the terminal ileum and colon. Individuals with penetrating or blunt trauma and suspected intestinal injury are started on parenteral antibiotic therapy immediately. Broad-spectrum antibiotics are continued postoperatively and stopped after several days unless there is evidence of infection.
   - *Analgesics:* Because narcotics alter the sensorium, making evaluation of the patient's condition difficult, they are seldom used in the early stages of trauma. Analgesics are used in the immediate postoperative period to relieve pain and promote ventilatory excursion.
   - *Tetanus prophylaxis:* Tetanus immune globulin and tetanus toxoid are considered, based on CDC recommendations (see Table 6-5).

7. **Nutrition:** Patients with abdominal trauma have complex nutritional needs owing to the hypermetabolic state associated with major trauma and traumatic or surgical disruption of normal GI function. Often, infection and sepsis contribute to negative nitrogen state and increased metabolic needs. Prompt initiation of parenteral feedings in patients unable to accept enteric feedings and the administration of supplemental calories, proteins, vitamins, and minerals are essential for healing. For more information, see "Providing Nutritional Support," p. 490.

TABLE 6-5

Tetanus prophylaxis in routine wound management—United States, 1985*

History of adsorbed tetanus toxoid (doses)	Clean, minor wounds		All other wounds[1]	
	Td[2]	TIG	Td[2]	TIG
Unknown or < three	Yes	No	Yes	Yes
≥three[3]	No[4]	No	No[5]	No

*From Centers for Disease Control: Morbidity Mortality Weekly Report **34**(27):422, 1985.

[1]Such as, but not limited to, wounds resulting from missiles, crushing, burns, and frostbite.

[2]For children under 7 years old; DPT (DT, if pertussis vaccine is contraindicated) is preferred to tetanus toxoid alone. For persons 7 years old and older, Td is preferred to tetanus toxoid alone.

[3]If only three doses of *fluid* toxoid have been received, a fourth dose of toxoid, preferably an absorbed toxoid, should be given.

[4]Yes, if more than 10 years since last dose.

[5]Yes, if more than 5 years since last dose. (More frequent boosters are not needed and can accentuate side effects).

8. **Surgical considerations for penetrating abdominal injuries:** The issue of mandatory surgical exploration versus observation and selective surgery, especially with stab wounds, remains controversial. There is a trend toward observation of patients without obvious injury or peritoneal signs. Indications for laparotomy include one or more of the following: (1) penetrating injury suspected of invading the peritoneum; (2) positive peritoneal signs (e.g., tenderness, rebound tenderness, and involuntary guarding); (3) shock; (4) GI hemorrhage; (5) free air in the peritoneal cavity as seen on x-ray; (6) evisceration; (7) massive hematuria; or (8) positive diagnostic peritoneal lavage.

< N O T E : The patient should be evaluated for peritoneal signs at least hourly by the same professional. Notify surgeon immediately if the patient develops peritoneal signs, evidence of shock, gastric or rectal bleeding, or gross hematuria.

9. **Surgical considerations for nonpenetrating abdominal injuries:** Physical examination usually is reliable in determining the necessity for surgery in alert, cooperative, unintoxicated patients. Additional diagnostic tests such as DPL or CT scan are necessary to evaluate the need for surgery in the patient who is intoxicated, unconscious, or who has sustained head or spinal cord trauma. Immediate laparotomy for blunt abdominal trauma is indicated under the following circumstances: (1) clear signs of peritoneal irritation (see Table 6-4); (2) free air in the peritoneum; (3) hypotension due to suspected abdominal injury or persistent and unexplained hypotension; (4) positive DPL; (5) GI aspirate or rectal smear positive for blood; or (6) other positive diagnostic tests such as CT scan or arteriogram. Carefully evaluated, stable patients with blunt abdominal trauma may be admitted to critical care for observation. These patients should be evaluated in the same manner as that described above in "penetrating trauma." It is important to note that damage to retroperitoneal organs such as the pancreas and duodenum may not cause significant signs and symptoms for 6-12 hours or longer. Relatively slow bleeding from abdominal viscera may not be clinically apparent for 12 hours or longer after the initial injury. In addition, the nurse should be aware that complications such as bowel obstruction due to adhesions or narrowing of the bowel wall from localized ischemia, inflammation, or hematoma may develop days or weeks after the traumatic event. The need for vigilant observation in the care of these patients can not be overemphasized.

NURSING DIAGNOSES AND INTERVENTIONS

Fluid volume deficit related to decreased circulating volume secondary to active bleeding; GI drainage through gastric, intestinal, or drainage tubes; diarrhea; or fistulas

---

Desired outcomes: Circulating volume is restored as evidenced by MAP ≥70 mm Hg, HR 60-100 bpm, normal sinus rhythm on EKG, CVP 2-6 mm Hg, PAWP 6-12 mm Hg, CI ≥2.5 L/min/m^2, SVR 900-1200 dynes/sec/cm^{-5}, urinary output ≥30 ml/hr, warm extremities, brisk capillary refill (<3 seconds), and distal pulses >2+ on a 0-4+ scale.

---

1. Monitor BP q15min, or more frequently in the presence of obvious bleeding or unstable VS. Be alert to changes in the MAP of >10 mm Hg. Even a small but sudden decrease in BP signals the need to notify MD, especially with the trauma patient in whom the extent of injury is unknown. Most trauma patients are young and excellent neurovascular compensation results in a near normal BP until there is a large intravascular volume depletion. Routine VS assessment (q1-4h in most critical care units) is indicated in the stable postoperative patient.

2. Monitor HR, EKG, and cardiovascular status q15 min until volume is restored and VS are stable. Check EKG to note HR elevations and myocardial ischemic changes (i.e., ventricular dysrhythmias and ST-segment changes).

3. In the patient with evidence of volume depletion or active blood loss, administer pressurized fluids rapidly through several large caliber (16 gauge or larger) catheters. Use short, large-bore IV tubing in order to maximize flow rate. Avoid use of stopcocks, as these slow the infusion rate.

< C A U T I O N : Evaluate patency of IV catheters continuously during rapid volume resuscitation.

4. Measure central pressures and thermodilution CO q1-2h or more frequently if there is ongoing blood loss. Calculate SVR and PVR q4-8h or more often in unstable patients. Be alert to low or decreasing CVP and PAWP. An elevated HR, along with a decreased PAWP, decreased CO (CI <2.5 L/min/m^2), and increased SVR suggest hypovolemia. Anticipate slightly elevated HR and CO due to hyperdynamic cardiovascular state in some volume resuscitated patients. Also, anticipate mild to moderate pulmonary hypertension, especially in patients with concurrent thoracic damage such as pulmonary contusion, smoke inhalation, or early ARDS. ARDS is a concern in patients who have sustained major abdominal injury, as there are many potential sources of infection and sepsis that make the development of ARDS more likely. For more information, see ''Adult Respiratory Distress Syndrome,'' p. 18.

5. Measure urinary ouput q1-2h. Be alert to output <30 ml/hr for two consecutive hours. Low urine output usually reflects inadequate intravascular volume in the abdominal trauma patient. Before administering diuretics, be certain that patient does not exhibit evidence of hypovolemia.

6. Monitor for physical indicators of hypovolemia, including cool extremities, capillary refill >4 seconds, and absent or decreased amplitude of distal pulses.

7. Estimate ongoing blood loss. Measure all bloody drainage from tubes or catheters, noting drainage color (e.g., coffee ground, burgundy, bright red). Note the frequency of dressing changes due to saturation with blood to estimate amount of blood loss *via* wound site.

Alteration in comfort: Pain related to irritation from intraperitoneal blood or secretions, actual trauma or surgical incision, and manipulation of organs

---

Desired outcome: Patient states that a reduction in pain has occurred and does not exhibit nonverbal indicators (i.e., grimacing, guarding) of discomfort.

---

1. Evaluate patient for presence of preoperative and postoperative pain. Preoperative pain is anticipated and is a vital diagnostic aid. The nature of postoperative pain also can be important. Incisional and some visceral pain can be anticipated, but intense pain or prolonged pain, especially when accompanied by other peritoneal signs, can signal bleeding, bowel infarction, infection, or other complications.

2. Administer narcotics and other analgesics as prescribed. Avoid administering analgesics preoperatively until the patient has been evaluated thoroughly by a trauma surgeon. Postoperatively, administer prescribed analgesics promptly before the pain becomes severe. Analgesics are helpful in relieving pain as well as aiding in the recovery process by promoting greater ventilatory excursion. Be aware that substance abuse often is involved in traumatic events; victims, therefore, may be drug or alcohol users, with a higher-than-average tolerance to narcotics. These same individuals may suffer symptoms of alcohol or narcotic withdrawal that need recognition and treatment. In addition, recognize that narcotic analgesics can decrease GI motility and may delay return to normal bowel functioning.

3. Supplement analgesics with nonpharmacologic maneuvers (e.g., positioning, backrubs, distraction) to aid in pain reduction.

Potential for infection related to vulnerability secondary to disruption of the GI tract, particularly of the terminal ileum and colon; traumatically inflicted open wound; multiple in-dwelling catheters and tubes; and compromised immune state due to stress of trauma and massive blood loss

---

Desired outcome: Patient is free of infection as evidenced by core or rectal temperature <37.8° C (100° F); HR ≤100 bpm; CI ≤4.0 L/min/m^2; SVR ≥900 dynes/sec/cm^{-5}; orientation to person, place, and time; and absence of unusual redness, warmth, or drainage at surgical incisions.

---

1. Monitor VS for evidence of infection, noting temperature increases and associated increases in heart and respiratory rates. An elevated CO and decreased SVR are suggestive of sepsis. Notify surgeon if these are new findings.

2. Evaluate orientation and LOC q2-4h.

3. Ensure patency of all surgically placed tubes or drains. Irrigate or attach to low-pressure suction as prescribed. Promptly report unrelieved loss of tube patency.

4. Evaluate incisions and wound sites for evidence of infection: unusual redness, warmth, delayed healing, and purulent or unusual drainage.

5. Note color, character, and odor of all drainage. Report the presence of foul-smelling or abnormal drainage. See Table 6-6, on the next page, for a description of the *usual* character of GI drainage.

6. Administer parenteral antibiotics in a timely fashion. Reschedule antibiotics if a dose is delayed for more than one hour. Recognize that failure to administer antibiotics on schedule may result in inadequate blood levels and treatment failure.

7. As prescribed, administer pneumococcal vaccine in patients with total splenectomy to minimize the risk of postsplenectomy sepsis.

TABLE 6-6

Characteristics of GI drainage

Source	Composition and usual character
Mouth and oropharynx	Saliva; thin, clear, watery; pH 7.0
Stomach	Hydrochloric, gastrin, pepsin, mucus; thin, brownish to greenish; acidic
Pancreas	Enzymes and bicarbonate; thin, watery, yellowish brown; alkaline
Biliary tract	Bile, including bile salts and electrolytes; bright yellow to brownish green
Duodenum	Digestive enzymes, mucus, products of digestion; thin, bright yellow to light brown, may be greenish; alkaline
Jejunum	Enzymes, mucus, products of digestion; brown, watery with particles
Ileum	Enzymes, mucus, digestive products, greater amounts of bacteria; brown, liquid, feculant
Colon	Digestive products, mucus, large amounts of bacteria; brown to dark brown, semi-formed to firm stool
Postoperative (GI surgery)	Initially, drainage expected to contain fresh blood; later, drainage mixed with old blood and then approaches normal composition
Infection present	Drainage cloudy, may be thicker than usual; strong or unusual odor, drain site often erythematous and warm

8. Administer tetanus immune globulin and tetanus toxoid as prescribed (see Table 6-5, p. 407).
9. Change dressings as prescribed, using aseptic technique. Prevent cross-contamination from various wounds by changing one dressing at a time.
10. If patient presents with or develops evisceration, do not reinsert tissue or organs. Place a sterilely saline-soaked gauze over the evisceration and cover with a sterile towel until the evisceration can be evaluated by the surgeon.

Potential alteration in tissue perfusion: GI tract, related to risk of interruption of blood flow to abdominal viscera from vascular disruption or occlusion or moderate to severe hypovolemia caused by hemorrhage

Desired outcomes: Patient does not develop bowel or organ ischemia as evidenced by normoactive bowel sounds; soft, nondistended abdomen; and return of bowel elimination. Hematocrit remains >30%; SGOT is 5-40 IU/L; SGPT is 5-35 IU/L; LDH is 90-200 ImU/ml; and gastric secretions, drainage, and excretions are negative for occult blood.

1. Auscultate for bowel sounds hourly during the acute phase of abdominal trauma and q4-8h during the recovery phase. Report prolonged or sudden absence of bowel sounds during the postoperative period as these signs may signal bowel ischemia or infarction.
2. Evaluate patient for peritoneal signs (see Table 6-4, p. 404), which may present

acutely secondary to injury or may not develop until days or weeks later if complications due to slow bleeding or other mechanisms occur.

3. Ensure adequate intravascular volume (see discussion in **Fluid volume deficit,** p. 408).
4. Evaluate laboratory data for evidence of bleeding (e.g., serial hematocrit) or organ ischemia (e.g., SGPT, SGOT, LDH).
5. Document amount and character of GI secretions, drainage, and excretions. Note changes suggestive of bleeding (presence of frank or occult blood), infection (e.g., increased or purulent drainage), or obstruction (e.g., failure to eliminate flatus or stool within 72 hours of surgery).

Impairment of skin and tissue integrity related to direct trauma and surgery; hypermetabolic, catabolic posttraumatic state; impaired tissue perfusion; or exposure to irritating GI drainage

---

Desired outcomes: Patient exhibits wound healing within an acceptable timeframe and there is no evidence of skin breakdown due to GI drainage. Nitrogen studies show a balanced nitrogen state.

---

1. Promptly change all dressings that become soiled with drainage or blood.
2. Protect the skin surrounding tubes, drains, or fistulas, keeping the areas clean and free from drainage. Gastric and intestinal secretions and drainage are irritating and can lead to skin excoriation. If necessary, apply ointments, skin barriers, or drainage bags to protect the surrounding skin. If available, consult ostomy nurse for complex or involved cases.
3. Inspect wounds, fistulas, and drain sites for signs of irritation, infection, and ischemia.
4. Identify infected and devitalized tissue. Aid in their removal by irrigation, wound packing, or preparing patient for surgical debridement.
5. Ensure adequate protein and calorie intake for tissue healing (see **Alteration in nutrition**, p. 413).

Hypothermia related to exposure at the scene of injury, temporary loss of temperature regulatory mechanisms due to shock or CNS ischemia, evisceration injury, surgical exposure of abdominal viscera, and administration of large volumes of unwarmed fluid or blood

---

Desired outcomes: Patient's temperature remains or returns to normal. Complications of hypothermia are avoided, as evidenced by normal sinus rhythm on EKG; patient oriented to person, place, and time; $Pao_2 \geq 80$ mm Hg; and absence of prolonged bleeding from wounds, incisions, and venipuncture sites.

---

1. Warm all fluids administered during the initial resuscitation phase and until the postoperative patient approaches normothermia. Prewarm crystalloids so that they are ready for immediate use. Because standard blood warmers are ineffective in rapid warming of large volumes of blood, avoid their use if blood loss is massive as the patient may become seriously hypotensive due to the

delay caused by the slow passage of blood through the warmer. Recently, rapid volume-infusors have become available and are invaluable in the immediate warming of large volumes (i.e., 800-1200 ml/min) of blood and fluids as they are infused.

2. Keep ambient room temperature in trauma receiving, surgical, and critical-care areas as warm as possible.

3. Avoid unnecessary exposure of the patient. Keep patient covered with warmed blankets whenever possible.

4. Because standard glass thermometers usually do not register below 94° F, electric thermometers may be necessary. If patient has severe hypothermia, monitor core temperature *via* rectal or esophageal probe or PA catheter until normothermia is attained.

5. Be aware that vasodilatation during rewarming can result in an intravascular fluid volume deficit (see **Fluid volume deficit**, p. 408).

6. Be aware that vasodilatation during rewarming necessitates evaluation and frequent titration of vasoactive infusions.

7. Monitor for and promptly report serious dysrhythmias (i.e., atrial fibrillation with rapid ventricular response, ventricular dysrhythmias, and A-V conduction block), which are associated with severe or prolonged hypothermia.

8. Be aware that hypothermia compromises cortical functioning and the patient may be confused, disoriented, somnolent, or have other neurologic derangements. These symptoms may make it difficult to evaluate concurrent head injury.

9. Monitor ABGs at frequent intervals for evidence of hypoxemia. Hypothermia causes a shift to the left in the oxyhemoglobin dissociation curve and may impair oxygen unloading to peripheral tissue.

10. Because DIC may develop several days after a hypothermic episode, monitor for excessive bleeding from wounds, surgical incisions, and venipuncture sites and promptly report the presence of serious or progressive thrombocytopenia. For more information, see "Disseminated Intravascular Coagulation," p. 418.

Alteration in nutrition: Less than body requirements related to decreased intake secondary to disruption of GI tract integrity (traumatic or surgical) and increased need secondary to hypermetabolic posttrauma state

---

Desired outcome: Patient has adequate nutrition as evidenced by maintenance of baseline body weight and state of nitrogen balance on nitrogen studies.

---

1. Collaborate with MD, dietician, and pharmacist to estimate patient's metabolic needs, based on type of injury, activity level, and nutritional status prior to injury.

2. Consider patient's specific injuries when planning nutrition. For example, expect patients with hepatic or pancreatic injury to have difficulty with blood sugar regulation. Patients with trauma to the upper GI tract may be fed enterally, but feeding tube must be placed distal to the injury. Disruption of the GI tract may require feeding gastrostomy or jejunostomy. Patients with major hepatic trauma may have difficulty with protein tolerance.

3. Ensure patency of gastric or intestinal tubes in order to maintain decompression

and encourage healing and return of bowel function. Avoid occlusion of the vent side of sump suction tubes, as this may result in vacuum occlusion of the tube. Use caution when irrigating NG or other tubes that have been placed in or near recently sutured organs.

4. Do not start enteral feeding until bowel function returns (i.e., bowel sounds are present, patient experiences hunger).
5. Recognize that narcotics decrease GI motility and may cause nausea and vomiting.
6. Weigh patient daily to evaluate trend. Be alert to steady decreases in weight and evaluate loss by assessing and comparing to volume status and fluid shifts.
7. Collect 24-hour urine for urea nitrogen, as prescribed, to evaluate nitrogen balance.
8. For more information, see section "Providing Nutritional Support," p. 490.

Posttrauma response related to stress reaction secondary to life-threatening accident or event resulting in trauma

---

Desired outcome: Patient verbalizes that the psychosocial impact of the event has decreased; cooperates with treatment plan; and does not exhibit signs of severe stress reaction such as display of inconsistent affect, suicidal or homicidal behavior or extreme agitation or depression.

< N O T E :   Many victims of major abdominal trauma sustain life-threatening injury. The patient is often aware of the situation and fears death. Even after the physical condition stabilizes, the patient may have a prolonged or severe reaction triggered by the trauma.

1. Evaluate mental status at systematic intervals during the acute and recovery periods. Be alert to indicators of severe stress reaction such as display of affect inconsistent with statements or behavior, suicidal or homicidal statements or actions, extreme agitation or depression, and failure to cooperate with instructions related to care.
2. Consult with specialist such as psychologist, psychiatric nurse clinician, or pastoral counselor if patient displays signs of severe stress reaction as described above.
3. Consider organic causes that may contribute to posttraumatic response stress (e.g., severe pain, alcohol intoxication or withdrawal, electrolyte imbalance, metabolic encephalopathy, or impaired cerebral perfusion).
4. For other pyschosocial interventions, see section "Caring for the Critically Ill with Life-Threatening Disorders," p. 511.

Alteration in bowel elimination related to disruption of normal function secondary to fecal diversion in patients with colonic injury and colostomy

---

Desired outcome: Patient has bowel sounds and eliminates gas and stool *via* stoma.

1. Auscultate abdomen for bowel sounds q4-8h. Document presence or absence of bowel sounds. Notify surgeon in the event of diminished or absent bowel sounds after the first 36-72 hours postcolostomy.

2. Empty stool from the bottom opening of the ostomy appliance. Note quality and quantity of stool. The presence of blood in the stool is abnormal after the initial postoperative period and should be reported to the surgeon.

3. Evaluate stoma q8h for viability and document its appearance. Paleness or a dark purple or black color are signals of circulatory impairment and should be reported at once.

4. If constipation is suspected by absence of stool elimination in the presence of bowel sounds, colostomy irrigation may be indicated. Confer with MD accordingly.

5. Consult with ostomy nurse as needed.

Disturbance in self-concept related to alteration in body image secondary to fecal diversion in patients with colonic injury and colostomy

---

Desired outcome: Patient acknowledges body changes, views stoma, and demonstrates movement toward incorporating changes into self-concept.

---

1. Offer patient opportunity to view stoma. Use mirrors if necessary.

2. Encourage patient and significant others to verbalize feelings regarding the colostomy.

3. Anticipate feelings of shock and disbelief initially. Be aware that trauma patients do not receive the emotional preparation that elective surgical patients receive.

4. Anticipate and acknowledge normalcy of feelings of rejection, isolation, and uncleanliness.

5. Encourage acceptance of colostomy by enabling patient to participate in care.

6. Confer with surgeon regarding advisability of a visit by another ostomate.

7. Be aware that most colostomies are temporary in patients with colonic trauma. This fact can be reassuring to the patient, but it is important to validate the type of colostomy with the surgeon before explaining this to the patient.

For more information, see nursing diagnoses and interventions in the following as appropriate: "Management of the Adult with Hemodynamic Monitoring," pp. 171-174; "Caring for the Critically Ill on Prolonged Bed Rest," pp. 506-511; "Caring for the Critically Ill with Life-Threatening Disorders," pp. 511-522; and "Caring for the Family of the Critically Ill," pp. 522-526.

REHABILITATION AND PATIENT-FAMILY TEACHING CONCEPTS

Anticipate extended physical and emotional rehabilitation for the patient and significant others. Provide them with verbal and written information for the following:

1. Probable need for emotional care, even for patients who have not required extensive physical rehabilitation. Provide referrals to support groups for trauma patients and family members.

2. Availability of rehabilitation programs for substance abuse, as indicated. Immediately following the traumatic event, the patient and family members are very impressionable, making this period an ideal time for the substance abuser to begin to resolve the problem.

3. Medications, including drug name, purpose, dosage, schedule, precautions, and potential side effects. Encourage patients on antibiotics to take the medications for the prescribed length of time, even though they may be asymptomatic. If patient received tetanus immunization, ensure that he or she receives a wallet-sized card documenting the immunization.

4. Wound and catheter care. Have patient or caregiver describe and demonstrate proper technique prior to hospital discharge.

5. Importance of seeking medical attention if indicators of infection or bowel obstruction occur (e.g., fever, severe or unusual abdominal pain, nausea and vomiting, unusual drainage from wounds or incisions, or a change in bowel habits).

6. Injury prevention. Immediately following a traumatic injury, the patient is especially likely to respond to injury prevention education. Provide instructions on proper seatbelt applications (across the pelvic girdle rather than across soft tissue of the lower abdomen), safety for infants and children, and other factors suitable for the individuals involved.

SELECTED REFERENCES

ACIP: Recommendations for protection against viral hepatitis. *MMWR* 1985; 34(22): 313-335.

American College of Surgeons Committee on Pre and Postoperative Care, Gann, DS (chairperson): *Manual of Preoperative and Postoperative Care,* 3rd ed. Saunders, 1983.

Berk JE (ed): *Gastroenterology,* 4th ed. Saunders, 1985.

Cameron JL (ed): *Current Surgical Therapy 1984-1985.* Decker, 1984.

Center for Infectious Diseases, Centers for Disease Control: Guideline for Prevention of Surgical Wound Infections. US Department of Health and Human Services, 1985.

Galambos JT: *Cirrhosis.* Saunders, 1979.

Harmon AR: *Nursing Care of the Adult Trauma Patient.* Wiley, 1985

Lebrec, et al: Propranolol for prevention of recurrent gastrointestinal bleeding in patients with cirrhosis: A controlled study. *New Engl J Med,* 1981; 305(12): 1371.

Martin DM, Galambos JT: Fulminant hepatic failure. *Crit Car Qu* 1982; 5(2): 9.

Millikan WJ, et al: The Emory prospective randomized trial: Selective versus nonselective shunt to control variceal bleeding. *Ann Surg* 1985; 201(6): 712.

Moss G, et al: Colloid or crystalloid in the resuscitation of hemorrhagic shock: A controlled clinical trial. *Surg* 1981; 89: 434.

Petersdorf R, et al (ed): *Harrison's Principles of Internal Medicine,* 10th ed. McGraw-Hill, 1983.

Sherlock S: *Diseases of the Liver and Biliary System,* 7th ed. Blackwell, 1985.

Trunkey D, Lewis FR (ed): *Current Therapy of Trauma, Vol 2.* Decker, 1986.

Warren WD, et al: Distal splenorenal shunt versus endoscopic sclerotherapy for long-term management of variceal bleeding. *Ann Surg* 1986; 202(4): 454.

7
HEMATOLOGIC
DYSFUNCTIONS

Disseminated intravascular coagulation

Hemolytic crisis

Idiopathic thrombocytopenia purpura

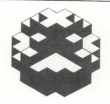

Disseminated intravascular coagulation

Disseminated intravascular coagulation (DIC) is a syndrome characterized by a disruption of the normal coagulation process. A predisposing event occurs that activates either the extrinsic or intrinsic coagulation pathway, resulting in an abnormal acceleration of the clotting process and a rapid consumption of prothrombin, platelets, factor V, and factor VIII. In conjunction with this accelerated coagulation process, fibrinolysis occurs *via* the conversion of plasminogen to plasmin (a proteolytic enzyme). This enzyme digests both fibrinogen and fibrin and produces fibrin degradation products (FDPs), which have an anticoagulant effect. Circulating FDPs combine with fibrinogen and sometimes form insoluble clots that are deposited in the microvasculature of such organs as the brain, liver, heart, lungs, or kidneys. The presence of these microthrombi can lead to ischemia, hypoxia, or necrosis. The combination of the processes of coagulation, anticoagulation, and fibrinolysis leads to a depletion of clotting factors, and ultimately, to hemorrhage. DIC always occurs secondary to an underlying pathology that triggers this cycle of disequilibrium between clot formation and clot lysis. See Table 7-1 for a list of conditions that can activate DIC.

ASSESSMENT

Signs and symptoms: Abrupt onset of bleeding or oozing of blood from venipuncture sites, mucosal surfaces (e.g., oral, nasal, tracheal, gastric, urethral, vaginal, rectal), and surgical or trauma wounds. In addition, the patient may have hematuria, guaiac-positive stools or nasogastric aspirate, bruising, pallor, dyspnea, acidosis, tachycardia, vertigo, hypotension, ecchymoses (e.g., on palate, gums, skin, conjunctiva), petechiae, lethargy, irritability, confusion, abnormal behavior, fatigue, muscle weakness, oliguria, ST-T wave changes, acrocyanosis (cyanotic extremities), mottled skin, and mottled skin lesions.

Physical assessment: Focus of assessment will relate to underlying disease (see Table 7-1); however, some general findings for DIC will include oozing of blood from mucosal surfaces, petechiae, ecchymoses, acrocyanosis, and mottling.

Risk factors: Any clinical state or pharmacologic therapy (e.g., chemotherapy) that inhibits the reticuloendothelial removal of activated clotting factors, fibrin split products (FSPs, also called fibrin degradation products), and thromboplastin. See Table 7-1 for a list of clinical states in which this can occur.

DIAGNOSTIC TESTS

1. *Fibrinogen levels:* Decreased (<200 mg/dl) because fibrinogen is consumed in the formation of fibrin clots.
2. *Fibrin split products (FSPs):* Increased (>8 μg/ml) because activation of fibrinolytic system produces FSPs as an end product of clot dissolution.
3. *Platelet count:* Decreased (<150,000/μl) because platelets are removed from active circulation to form clots.
4. *Prothrombin time (PT):* Prolonged (>15 seconds) because of depletion of coagulation factors.
5. *Partial thromboplastin time (PTT):* Prolonged (>40 seconds) because of consumption of coagulation factors.
6. *Protamine sulfate test:* Protomine sulfate is added to plasma. In the presence of fibrin monomers (material resulting from the action of thrombin on fibrinogen) or early FDPs, fibrin strands are formed. Because the test is insensitive to fi-

TABLE 7-1

Clinical conditions that can activate DIC

Obstetric	Liver disease	Tissue damage	Infections
Abruptio placentae	Cirrhosis	Surgery	Viral
Toxemia	Hepatic necrosis	Trauma	Bacterial
Amniotic fluid embolism		Burns	Rickettsial
Septic abortion		Prolonged extracorporeal	Protozoal
Retained dead fetus		circulation	
		Rejection transplant	
		Heat stroke	
Hemolytic processes	**Vascular disorders**	**Miscellaneous**	
Transfusion reaction	Shock	Fat or pulmonary embolism	
Acute hemolysis secondary to	Aneurysm	Snake bite	
infection or immunologic	Giant hemangioma	Neoplastic disorder	
disorder		Acute anoxia	
		Necrotizing enterocolitis	

brinogen or FDPs, the construction of these fibrin strands reflects the formation of excessive amounts of thrombin. This test is strongly positive in the presence of DIC.

7. *Clotting factor assay:* Reduction in factors V and VIII, which implicates DIC as a causative factor.

8. *Euglobulin lysis time:* To differentiate primary fibrinolysis (short euglobulin time) from DIC, which usually presents a normal or slightly prolonged euglobulin time.

9. *Peripheral blood smear:* For visualization *via* microscopic exam of schistocytes and burr cells, which are indicative of the deposition of fibrin in the small blood vessels.

MEDICAL MANAGEMENT

Treatment of the underlying disorder often corrects the secondary coagulopathy. However, there are three controversial treatment modalities available: (a) heparin therapy; (b) blood factor replacement; and (c) epsilon-aminocaproic acid therapy. The latter alternative is used *only* in those rare cases of *primary* fibrinolysis, when the disadvantages versus benefits issues have been resolved clinically. In most settings, the first two alternatives are the therapies that are utilized most often. In addition, the risk of intracranial bleeding secondary to hypertension must be considered before anticoagulant therapy is initiated.

1. **Treatment of the primary pathology**

2. **Continuous IV heparin therapy:** Although its use is controversial, it is administered because heparin interferes with the coagulation cascade at several sites. It blocks the clotting cascade by neutralizing the freely circulating thrombin and prevents the deposition of microvascular thrombi by its anticoagulant effect, thus allowing for the accumulation of clotting factors. In addition, it deactivates the fibrinolytic system.

3. **Blood component replacement:** Replacement of clotting factors in the form of fresh frozen plasma, cryoprecipitate, packed red blood cells, and platelets in an attempt to supplant the deficiencies caused by the consumptive process. Blood replacement also supports volume and maintains blood pressure.

4. Epsilon-aminocaproic acid therapy: Stops bleeding by disrupting the fibrinolytic process. It inhibits plasmin, which normally digests both fibrinogen and fibrin, and thus allows clots to form.

NURSING DIAGNOSES AND INTERVENTIONS

Alteration in tissue perfusion: Peripheral, renal, pulmonary, and cerebral, related to impaired circulation secondary to presence of microthrombi occurring with coagulation phase of DIC

Desired outcomes: Patient has adequate perfusion as evidenced by BP within patient's normal limit, HR ≤100 bpm, RR ≤20 breaths/min, peripheral pulses >2+ on a scale of 0-4+, urinary output ≥30 ml/hr, and capillary refill <3 seconds. Patient is asymptomatic of emboli and has fibrinogen levels 200-400 mg/dl and platelet count 150,000-400,000/μl.

---

1. Monitor VS for evidence of coagulation, including a decrease in BP, increases in HR and RR, and decreased amplitude of peripheral pulses.
2. Monitor I&O for a decrease in urinary output (in the presence of adequate intake), which can signal the onset of coagulation.
3. Monitor laboratory tests for evidence of clotting, including decreased fibrinogen levels and platelet count.
4. Assess for the presence of microemboli by noting an increase in petechiae, cyanosis, ecchymosis, and acrocyanosis, or decrease in amplitude of distal pulses.
5. Monitor patient for signs of pulmonary embolism: tachypnea, tachycardia, cyanosis, sudden onset of dyspnea, diaphoresis, diffuse chest pain, hemoptysis, anxiety, restlessness, and apprehension. If patient exhibits evidence of pulmonary embolism, institute oxygen therapy and notify MD immediately.
6. Monitor ABG values for respiratory alkalosis, which can occur owing to hyperventilation and hypoxemia. Assess the alveolar-arterial oxygen (A-a) gradient for an increase (>30 mm Hg), which can be indicative of a pulmonary embolus.
7. Assess patient's neurologic status at least q2h during the acute phase, using the Glasgow coma scale.
8. Turn patient q2h while awake and q4h during the night. Institute coughing and deep-breathing exercises with each turning procedure.

Potential fluid volume deficit related to risk of blood loss secondary to hemorrhagic phase of DIC or heparin therapy

---

Desired outcome: Patient is asymptomatic of bleeding as evidenced by partial thromboplastin time (PTT) 30-40 seconds; abdominal girth measurement within patient's normal range; secretions and excretions negative for blood; and patient oriented to person, place, and time.

---

1. Monitor coagulation tests. Be alert to a partial thromboplastin time (PTT) >40 seconds.
2. Assess for internal bleeding by measuring abdominal girth q8h and testing tra-

cheal aspirate, urine, stool, emesis, NG drainage, and sputum for the presence of blood.

3. Monitor gastric pH q2h and keep pH >4.5 by administering antacids or hydrogen blocker therapy as prescribed to prevent gastric ulceration.

4. Monitor neurologic status by assessing LOC, orientation, pupillary reaction, and movement and strength of extremities. Changes in status can be indicative of intracranial bleeding.

5. Encourage patient to use mouthwash and cotton swabs for oral care to minimize the risk of bleeding from gum injury. Also teach patient to use electric rather than straight razor for shaving.

6. Avoid giving IM injections, as they can precipitate bleeding.

7. If patient undergoes an invasive procedure, maintain pressure over the insertion site until bleeding ceases.

8. As appropriate, teach patient the importance of avoiding platelet aggregation inhibitors, such as aspirin, which can prolong episodes of bleeding.

Potential alteration in cardiac output: Decreased, related to risk of dysrhythmias secondary to acidosis or electrolyte disturbance caused by massive blood loss

---

Desired outcomes: Patient has adequate cardiac output as evidenced by HR 60-100 bpm; SVR 900-1200 dynes/sec/cm^{-5}; cardiac output (CO) 4-7 L/min; PAWP 6-12 mm Hg; CI 2.5-4 L/min/m^2; and normal sinus rhythm on EKG. Serum sodium is 137-147 mEq/L; serum potassium is 3.5-5.5 m/Eq/L; serum chloride is 95-108 mEq/L; and pH is 7.35-7.45.

---

1. Monitor cardiac rhythm continuously for evidence of dysrhythmias, which can decrease cardiac output.

2. Monitor for increased HR, which can result in a decreased ventricular filling time.

3. If a pulmonary artery catheter is present, calculate SVR and be alert to an abnormally high reading, which is indicative of peripheral vasoconstriction that occurs with hypovolemia. Also assess for a decreased CO, decreased PAWP, or decreased CI, which may signal hypovolemia with resultant hypoperfusion.

4. Assess for other signs of vasoconstriction, including cold and clammy skin, decreased urinary output (<30 ml/hr for two consecutive hours), increased capillary refill time (>3 seconds), and restlessness.

5. Monitor serum sodium, potassium, and chloride levels, which may decrease with blood loss. Also monitor pH for decrease secondary to carbon dioxide retention, which can produce dysrhythmias.

6. During periods of decreased cardiac output, support the patient hemodynamically *via* prescribed vasopressors such as dopamine or dobutamine hydrochloride.

7. Replace blood loss as appropriate to patient's clinical condition.

8. Promptly report significant findings to MD.

Impaired gas exchange related to decreased diffusion of oxygen secondary to increased pulmonary alveolar-capillary permeability or embolus formation

Desired outcome: Patient's gas exchange is adequate as evidenced by Pao_2 80-100 mm Hg; $Paco_2$ 35-45 mm Hg; pH 7.35-7.45; RR 12-20 breaths/min with normal depth and pattern (eupnea); HR 60-100 bpm; and orientation to person, place, and time.

1. Assess respiratory status, noting rate, rhythm, depth, and regularity of respirations.
2. Monitor ABG values, being alert to an increase in $Paco_2$ and decrease in pH, which can signal hypoventilation.
3. If patient is able, encourage deep-breathing exercises as often as tolerated.
4. Place patient in high-Fowler's position to promote lung expansion.
5. Monitor sputum and tracheal secretions for evidence of blood.
6. Assess the lungs for the presence of bibasilar crackles (rales), which can occur with fluid accumulation.
7. Assess patient for changes in sensorium, which can be indicative of the need for oxygen. Notify MD accordingly.
8. Ensure that patient is wearing antiembolic hose to prevent venous stasis and possible embolus formation.
9. Monitor for the presence of a pulmonary embolus. Be alert to sharp, stabbing chest pain; dyspnea; cyanosis; pupillary dilation; rapid, irregular pulse; profuse diaphoresis; and anxiety. If patient exhibits signs and symptoms of a pulmonary embolus, administer oxygen and notify MD immediately.

REHABILITATION AND PATIENT-FAMILY TEACHING CONCEPTS

Refer to patient's primary diagnosis.

Hemolytic crisis

Hemolytic crisis is an acute disorder that frequently accompanies hemolytic anemias. It is characterized by premature pathologic destruction (hemolysis) of red blood cells (erythrocytes). As erythrocyte destruction accelerates, there is a decrease in the oxygen-carrying capacity of the blood, which results in a reduction in the amount of oxygen delivered to the tissues. This hypoxic state produces tissue ischemia and can progress to tissue infarction. Hemolytic episodes can be triggered both by emotional and physiologic states, including stress, trauma, surgery, acute infectious processes, and abnormal immune responses.

ASSESSMENT

Acute indicators: Fever; abdominal, chest, and back pain; jaundice; headache; dizziness; palpitations; SOB; hemoglobinuria; lymphadenopathy; splenomegaly; and signs of peripheral nerve damage, including paresthesias, paralysis, chills, and vomiting.

Chronic indicators: Anemia, pallor, fatigue, dyspnea on exertion, icterus, bone infarctions, monoarticular and polyarticular arthritis, hematuria, renal failure, increased gallstone formation, and skin ulcers.

Physical assessment: Depending on severity and duration of the anemia, the patient may exhibit impaired growth and development. Inspection may reveal the presence of jaundice, SOB, monoarticular or polyarticular arthritis, retinal detachment and associated vitreous hemorrhage, and hemiplegia. Palpation may reveal splenomegaly, lymphadenopathy, hepatomegaly, or abdominal guarding. Chronic skin ulcers may be seen, particularly in the ankle area.

Risk factors: Any patient with a clinical state that promotes premature destruction of RBCs, whether the cause is genetic (e.g., sickle cell or thalassemia) or acquired (e.g., drug-induced or autoimmune), is at risk for hemolytic crisis.

DIAGNOSTIC TESTS

1. *Sickle cell test:* Screens for the presence of sickle cell anemia, particularly in Blacks.
2. *Erythrocyte sedimentation rate (ESR):* Decreased as a result of sickle cell interference with normal rouleau formation.
3. *Sodium metabisulfite slide test:* Screens for sickle cell anemia. When this reagent is added to blood containing red cells with sickle hemoglobin (HbS), it induces sickling by decreasing oxygen tension.
4. *Hemoglobin (Hg) and hematocrit (Hct):* Decreased because of the premature destruction of RBCs and increased number of premature RBCs.
5. *Unconjugated bilirubin:* Elevated because of the liver's inability to process the large quantity of bilirubin released during hemolysis.
6. *Serum lactic dehydrogenase isoenzymes (LDH_1 and LDH_2):* Levels will be elevated because of the release of these enzymes when the RBC is destroyed.
7. *Reticulocyte count and index:* Elevated because of the rapid destruction of RBCs.
8. *Haptoglobin level:* Decreased because of the binding of haptoglobin (a plasma protein) to vast quantities of hemoglobin in an attempt to remove the hemoglobin from plasma.
9. *Hemoglobin electrophoresis:* Used as a screening tool for identifying the sickle cell trait (HbA).
10 *Peripheral blood smear:* Will reveal presence of abnormally shaped erythrocytes (poikilocytes and anisocytes).
11. *Bone marrow aspiration:* Will reveal presence of enlarged erythrocytes (erythroid hyperplasia).
12. *Coombs test:* Positive in the presence of antibody-mediated hemolysis.

MEDICAL MANAGEMENT AND SURGICAL INTERVENTIONS

1. **Volume replacement:** If patient is hypovolemic, aggressive replacement of fluids is mandatory to prevent hypovolemic shock and deposition of hemolyzed RBCs in the microvasculature of the major organs.
2. **Transfusions:** RBCs are given if circulatory failure or hypoxia occurs. Blood replacement supports volume and provides additional hemoglobin for transport of oxygen.
3. **Oxygen therapy:** For patients who are hypoxic.
4. **Corticosteroids:** Produce clinical remission in approximately 85% of patients.
5. **Splenectomy:** Surgical removal of the spleen destroys the site at which RBC destruction occurs.
6. **Elimination of causative factor:** If possible, precipitating cause (e.g., drug, chemical, stress state) is eradicated to prevent prolongation of the crisis.
7. **Folic acid supplementation:** Folic acid is necessary for hematopoiesis (production of blood cells). Supplementation of 1 mg/day is recommended to prevent hemolytic crisis in individuals with chronic hemolytic diseases.

NURSING DIAGNOSES AND INTERVENTIONS

Potential for injury related to risk of hemolytic crisis secondary to stress, trauma, surgery, acute infectious process, or abnormal immune response

---

Desired outcomes: Patient is asymptomatic of hemolytic crisis as evidenced by presence of patient's normal visual acuity, motor strength, and coordination; normothermia; HR 60-100 bpm; and absence of abdominal pain, headache, palpitations, and dizziness. Patient and significant others verbalize the importance of keeping patient's emotional and physiologic stress to a minimum.

---

1. Instruct patient to report changes in vision, which can signal an impending crisis.
2. For patient who does suffer temporary vision loss, ensure that side rails are up and that patient's call light is within easy reach.
3. Use Glasgow coma scale to assess motor strength and coordination with special attention to identifying paresthesias and paralysis, which occur with peripheral nerve damage secondary to hypoxia. These signs, along with fever, abdominal pain, headache, dizziness, and palpitations can signal the onset of hemolytic crisis.
4. Protect patient from extremes of temperature, which can precipitate a crisis. Caution patient about the importance of keeping emotional and physiologic stress to a minimum.

Alteration in tissue perfusion: Peripheral, renal, cardiopulmonary, and cerebral, related to impaired circulation with cellular hypoxia secondary to microthrombi (resulting from destruction of RBCs) and a decrease in circulating RBCs

---

Desired outcome: Patient has adequate perfusion as evidenced by BP within patient's normal range; HR 60-100 bpm; RR 12-20 breaths/min with a normal depth and pattern (eupnea); urinary output ≥30 ml/hr; amplitude of peripheral pulses >2+ on a scale of 0-4+; capillary refill <3 seconds; warm skin; Pao_2 ≥80 mm Hg; urinary creatinine clearance levels 107-141 ml/min (male) or 87-132 ml/min (female); and patient oriented to person, place, and time.

---

1. Monitor for decreased Pao_2, an indicator of cellular hypoxia.
2. Monitor VS and urine output for evidence of decreased perfusion. Be alert to a decrease in BP, increase in HR, increase in RR, dyspnea, or a decrease in urinary output.
3. Assess amplitude of peripheral pulses as an indicator of peripheral perfusion. Use Doppler if unable to palpate pulses.
4. Assess extremities for coolness, pallor, and prolonged capillary refill, which are signals of decreased peripheral perfusion.
5. Keep lower extremities elevated to promote venous blood flow.
6. Administer IV fluids as prescribed to prevent deposition of hemolyzed RBCs in the microvasculature.
7. Monitor neurologic status, using Glasgow coma scale.

8. Monitor urinary creatinine clearance for decreased levels, which may be a signal of decreased renal blood flow or renal obstruction.

Fluid volume deficit related to loss secondary to excretion of urine of abnormally low molecular concentration (hyposthenuria) caused by damage to the renal concentrating mechanism

---

Desired outcome: Patient is normovolemic as evidenced by urinary output ≥30 ml/hr, stable weights, BP within patient's normal range, HR 60-100 bpm, good skin turgor, moist mucous membranes, urine osmolality 300-1090 mOsm/kg, serum osmolality 275-300 mOsm/kg, PAWP 6-12 mm Hg, CO 4-7 L/min, and SVR 900-1200 dynes/sec/cm^{-5}.

---

1. Monitor I&O q8h, being alert to a decreased urinary output in the presence of adequate intake.
2. Weigh patient daily, noting losses >0.5 kg/day, which may signal excessive volume loss.
3. Assess patient for indicators of volume depletion, including poor skin turgor; dry mucous membranes; hypotension; tachycardia; and decreasing urine output, urinary and serum osmolality, PAWP, CO, and SVR.
4. If patient is able, encourage an increase in normal oral intake to compensate for excessive fluid loss; or, adjust IV fluids accordingly.

Impairment of skin and tissue integrity related to tissue hypoxia secondary to vasocclusive process

---

Desired outcome: Patient's skin and tissue remain intact.

---

1. Keep extremities warm to promote circulation and help prevent tissue hypoxia.
2. Eliminate or reduce tissue pressure points by changing patient's position at least q2h, using sheepskin under elbows and heels and a bed cradle to reduce pressure of covers on extremities. If available, use "air" beds for these patients.
3. Maintain patient in a well-hydrated state to promote circulation.
4. Monitor skin changes over bony prominences, noting the following signs that are indicative of skin integrity disruption: elevated skin temperature, erythema, prolonged blanching in response to digital pressure, and blister formation. Teach these signs to patient and significant others.
5. Apply sterile dressing or skin barriers (e.g., Tegaderm, Duoderm, Op-Site) to areas of breakdown to prevent extension of the ulcer or infection.
6. Monitor visceral protein status and nitrogen studies. A negative nitrogen state puts the patient at higher risk for skin and tissue impairment. Encourage patient to eat a diet that is high in protein and carbohydrates to promote a balanced nitrogen state. See "Providing Nutritional Support," pp. 490-505, for more information.

Alteration in comfort: Pain related to vessel occlusion and hemarthrosis

---

Desired outcome: Patient relates a reduction in pain and does not exhibit evidence of discomfort such as guarded positioning.

---

1. Monitor patient for signs of discomfort, including guarded positioning, muscle spasm, rubbing or pulling of body part, tense body posture, and increases in HR, BP, and RR.
2. Medicate for pain and assess effectiveness of medication. Confer with MD regarding efficacy of antiinflammatory agents.
3. Apply warm compresses to joints to increase circulation and thereby improve oxygenation to the tissues.
4. Apply elastic stockings to promote venous return and enhance circulation.
5. Encourage patient to perform isotonic or ROM exercises of the lower extremities to promote circulation.
6. Help allay fears by reassuring patient that pain will decrease as the crisis subsides.
7. Provide emotional support to patient during the crisis episode.

REHABILITATION AND PATIENT-FAMILY TEACHING CONCEPTS

Give patient and significant others verbal and written instructions for the following:
1. Importance of assessing extremities daily for evidence of injury (e.g., tissue breakdown or blood sequestration in joints or tissues).
2. Comfort measures for hemarthrosis (see **Alteration in Comfort**, p. 425).
3. Importance of avoiding physically and psychologically stressful situations, which can precipitate hemolytic crisis.
4. Medications, including drug name, purpose, dosage, frequency, and side effects, particularly of steroids: increased appetite, weight gain, headache, moonface, "buffalo hump," increased predisposition to infection, and fluctuating glucose levels.
5. Signs of sensorimotor impairment, including unsteady gait, paresthesias, blurring of vision, and paralysis.
6. Importance of having pneumococcal vaccine and wearing an ID bracelet if splenectomy has been performed.
7. Care of recurrent skin ulcers.
8. Indicators of impending *hemolytic crisis:* fever, abdominal pain, headache, dizziness, palpitation; and signs of *peripheral nerve damage:* paresthesias and paralysis.
9. Addresses and phone numbers of support groups for sickle cell anemia or thalassemia.
10. Importance of smoking cessation due to the vasoconstrictive effects of nicotine.

Idiopathic thrombocytopenia purpura

Idiopathic thrombocytopenia purpura (ITP) is a coagulation disorder characterized by a premature destruction of platelets, which causes the platelet count to fall below 100,000/mm^3. The survival time of platelets decreases from the normal time of 1-3 weeks to 1-3 days due to the presence of antiplatelet IgG antibodies, which destroy platelets in the reticuloendothelial system of the spleen. The coagulopathy is believed to be an autoimmune response that occurs in both an acute and chronic form. Primarily, the acute form of ITP is a childhood disease (reaching its peak incidence in children aged 2-6 years old) that is related immunologically to an antecedent viral infection. The chronic form is seen most often in the 18-50 year range, occurring 3 times more frequently in women. The cause of the adult form is unknown.

ASSESSMENT

Signs and symptoms: Petechiae, purpura, and bleeding often are the only clinical signs, but gingival bleeding, epistaxis, gastrointestinal bleeding, and an increase in menstrual flow can occur as well. The most serious complication is intracranial (subarachnoid) hemorrhage, occurring in <1% of patients. Other signs and symptoms such as fever, splenomegaly, or lymphadenopathy mandate that other diagnoses be considered.

Physical assessment: Presence of petechiae, purpura, bruising, and bleeding from mucosal surfaces or wounds.

Risk factors: In the acute form there is usually a history of antecedent viral infection occurring about 3 weeks prior to the hemorrhagic episode. The chronic form usually is insidious and the patient has a long history of hemorrhagic symptoms.

DIAGNOSTIC TESTS

1. *Peripheral blood smear:* Will reveal megathrombocytes (large platelets), which are present during premature destruction of platelets.
2. *Platelet count:* Decreased to <100,000/mm^3 because of premature destruction.
3. *Bleeding time:* Usually prolonged because of a decrease in platelet count.
4. *Platelet antibody screen:* Positive because of the presence of IgG antiplatelet antibodies.
5. *CBC:* Hemoglobin and hematocrit may be decreased because of insidious blood loss; WBC count will be normal.
6. *Bone marrow:* Increased number of megakaryocytes (platelet precursors).
7. *Screening coagulation tests* (prothrombin time, partial thromboplastin time, thrombin time): Normal because these tests measure clotting factors other than platelets.

MEDICAL MANAGEMENT AND SURGICAL INTERVENTIONS

1. **Glucocorticoid therapy:** Adrenocorticosteroids (e.g., prednisone 1-2 mg/kg/day) are effective in increasing the platelet count in approximately 85% of patients because they suppress the phagocytic activity of the reticuloendothelial system (RES).
2. **Platelet transfusions:** Platelets are replaced only in cases of life-threatening hemorrhage because of the rapid destruction of the platelets by the RES.
3. **Splenectomy:** Treatment of choice in cases that are refractory to glucocorticoid therapy. The effectiveness of the splenectomy is believed to be related to the removal of the site of destruction of the antibody sensitized platelets.
4. **Plasma exchange *via* apheresis:** Short-term therapy utilized until glucocorticoid therapy takes effect. Currently under investigation, this procedure removes the mediating plasma factor. It involves the removal of 2-3 liters of plasma, with replacement by a suitable solution such as albumin, crystalloids, or fresh frozen plasma.

NURSING DIAGNOSES AND INTERVENTIONS

Potential for injury related to the increased risk of bleeding secondary to decreased levels of platelets

---

Desired outcomes: Patient exhibits no new evidence of bleeding or bruising episodes. Platelet count is 150,000-400,000/μl; secretions and excretions are negative for blood; BP is within patient's normal range; HR is 60-100 bpm; and RR is 12-20 breaths/min with a normal depth and pattern (eupnea). Patient verbalizes knowledge of techniques that will help decrease the risk of bleeding.

---

1. During the acute phase of ITP, teach patient to perform oral hygiene using mouthwash and oral swabs or toothettes to help prevent gum bleeding. Once the crisis has been resolved, teach patient to use an electric razor and soft-bristled toothbrush to prevent mechanical injury that would promote bleeding.
2. Avoid giving IM injections, which may result in continuous oozing of blood from the injection site.
3. Avoid administering aspirin products, which increase the risk of bleeding by decreasing platelet adhesiveness.
4. Monitor platelet count daily for significant changes. Be alert to values that continue to be low.
5. Monitor patient for signs of bleeding including hematuria, melena, hematemesis, or bleeding from mucosal membranes. Test secretions, including nasogastric aspirate, for blood q2h.
6. Assess heart rate and rhythm, respiratory rate and rhythm, and BP for evidence of active bleeding. Be alert to increased heart and respiratory rates and a decrease in BP.
7. If severe menorrhagia is present, confer with MD regarding the need for progestational hormones (e.g., norethindrone acetate, 5-10 mg PO, qd) for suppression of menses.

Potential fluid volume excess: Cerebral, related to risk of intracranial hemorrhage secondary to platelet destruction (occurs in <1% of patients)

Desired outcomes: Patient is asymptomatic of intracranial hemorrhage as evidenced by orientation to person, place, and time; normoreactive pupils and reflexes; patient's normal visual acuity, motor strength, and coordination; and absence of headache and other clinical indicators of increased intracranial pressure (IICP). Patient verbalizes the importance of avoiding the Valsalva maneuver.

---

1. Assess patient for signs of IICP, including changes in LOC, pupillary responses, and reflexes. Patient may have diplopia or blurred vision. Pupils will range from sluggish to fixed and dilated. Loss of motor function can take the form of paresis, paralysis, or abnormal extension posturing (decerebration).
2. Monitor patient for the presence of headaches, visual disturbances, or motor dysfunction, which are symptoms of IICP.
3. Position patient with HOB slightly elevated (30-40 degrees) to decrease intracranial pressure.

4. Maintain neck in neutral position at all times *via* use of a collar or neck roll, if necessary, to prevent increases in ICP, which occur with neck flexion.

5. Teach patient to avoid Valsalva maneuver (e.g., straining at stool or forceful blowing of nose), which could cause intracranial bleeding.

6. Confer with MD regarding use of stool softeners or cough suppressants, as necessary.

Impairment of tissue integrity related to vulnerability secondary to intradermal bleeding

---

Desired outcome: Patient is asymptomatic of further tissue injury (i.e., bruising, petechiae, or purpura).

---

1. Apply ice bag or manual pressure over sites of intradermal bleeding to promote vasoconstriction and thus decrease the bleeding.

2. Handle patient gently to minimize the risk of tissue trauma.

3. Avoid use of IM injections, which would promote intradermal bleeding. If IM injections are necessary, use the smallest gauge needle possible and maintain pressure on the injected site for 5-10 minutes to prevent bleeding into the tissues.

4. Inspect and document condition of patient's skin on a daily basis, noting evidence of new or worsening petechiae, purpura, or bruising.

Alteration in comfort: Pain related to hemarthrosis

Desired outcome: Patient relates a reduction in pain and does not exhibit signs of uncontrollable discomfort.

---

1. Monitor patient for signs of fatigue and malaise. As appropriate, instruct patient to decrease or eliminate those activities that cause fatigue and malaise.

2. Elevate patient's legs to decrease joint pain in the lower extremities.

3. Decrease stress on joints by supporting extremities with pillows, making sure bed is not gatched at the knee.

4. Use a bed cradle and lightweight blankets and bed clothing to decrease pressure on tissues.

Potential fluid volume deficit related to loss secondary to postsplenectomy or intra-abdominal bleeding

---

Desired outcomes: Patient is normovolemic as evidenced by BP within patient's normal range, HR 60-100 bpm, RR 12-20 breaths/min with normal depth and pattern (eupnea), and urinary output ≥30 ml/hr. Patient is free of abdominal pain or tenderness and frank bleeding from the operative site and exhibits the following: hematocrit 37%-47% (female) or 40%-54% (male), hemoglobin 12-16 g/dl (female) or 14-18 g/dl (male), and abdominal girth measurements within patient's normal range.

---

1. Monitor patient for signs of hypovolemia, including increases in HR and RR, decreases in BP and urinary output, and restlessness.
2. Monitor hematocrit and hemoglobin values for a decrease, which can signal active bleeding.
3. Inspect operative site for evidence of frank bleeding.
4. Measure abdominal girth q8h and assess for abdominal pain or tenderness, which can signal intra-abdominal bleeding.

REHABILITATION AND PATIENT-FAMILY TEACHING CONCEPTS

Give patient and significant others verbal and written instructions for the following:
1. Assessment for bleeding (e.g., presence of petechiae, purpura, melena, hematuria, hematemesis, oozing from oral mucous membranes).
2. Importance of avoiding activities that can cause trauma, and hence, promote bleeding. These activites range from shaving with razor blades and brushing the teeth with a hard-bristled toothbrush, to engaging in contact sports. Teach patient the necessity of using a soft-bristled toothbrush and shaving with an electric razor.
3. Importance of follow-up care and continuing medical therapy (e.g., glucocorticoid drugs) for prescribed amount of time, which can be short-term, long-term, or lifelong. Teach patient the side effects of these drugs, including GI effects, such as nausea, vomiting, epigastric pain, ulceration of GI tract; Cushingoid features; fluid and electrolyte imbalances, including hypernatremia, hypokalemia, and hypocalcemia; and increased susceptibility to infection. In addition, mental and emotional effects, such as depression, euphoria, insomnia, nervousness, and psychoses can occur, as well as metabolic effects, including hyperglycemia, diabetes mellitus, myopathy, and osteoporosis.
4. Indicators of intracranial bleeding, such as change in LOC, pupil abnormalities, visual disturbances, motor dysfunction, and headaches.
5. Importance of abstaining from cigarettes, which can impair arterial circulation *via* the vasoconstrictive effects of nicotine and the resultant inability of platelets to pass through the smaller vessels.
6. Necessity for having pneumococcal vaccine and wearing an ID bracelet if splenectomy has been performed.

SELECTED REFERENCES

Abels L: *Critical Care Nursing: A Physiologic Approach.* Mosby, 1986.

Carpenito LJ: *Nursing Diagnosis: Application to Clinical Practice.* Lippincott, 1983.

Champion LAA: Platelet disorders. In *Guide to Hematologic Disorders.* Hartman PM (ed). Grune & Stratton, 1980.

Davoric G: Disseminated intravascular coagulation. *Crit Care Nurse* 1982; 2(6): 36-46.

Eastman RD: *Clinical Hematology.* John Wright & Sons, 1984.

Erslev AJ, Gabuzda TG: *Pathophysiology of Blood,* 3rd edition. Saunders, 1985.

Hamilton GC. Hemostasis out of order. *Emerg Med* 1985; 15: 83-116.

Kenner CV, Guzzetta CE, Dossey BM: *Critical Care Nursing: Body-Mind-Spirit.* Little, Brown, 1985.

Luby CK, Wood PW: Thrombotic thrombocytopenia purpura. *Dim Crit Care Nurs* 1985; 4(4): 209-214.

MacKinney AA: *Pathophysiology of Blood.* Wiley, 1984.

Newland JR: Coagulation and the tests for DIC. *Consultant* 1985; 25(3): 112-120.

Pagana KD, Pagana TJ: *Pocket Nurse Guide to*

Laboratory and Diagnostic Tests. Mosby, 1986.

Porth CM: *Pathophysiology.* Lippincott, 1986.

Reich PR: Hematology: *Physiopathologic Basis for Clinical Practice.* Little, Brown, 1978.

Rooney A, Haviley C: Nursing management in disseminated intravascular coagulation. *Onc Nurs Forum* 1985; 12(1): 15-22.

Rosove MH: Approach to the diagnosis of quantitative and qualitative disorders of platelets. In *Hematology.* Figueroa WG (ed). Wiley, 1981.

Rosove MH: Bleeding disorders. In *Practical*

Hematology. Hocking WG (ed). Wiley, 1983.

Shoemaker WC, Thompson WL, Holbrook PR: Textbook of Critical Care. Saunders, 1984.

Thompson JM, et al: *Clinical Nursing.* Mosby, 1986.

Tueller BL: Hematologic Disorders. In: *Manual of Nursing Therapeutics: Applying Nursing Diagnoses to Medical Disorders.* Swearingen, PL (ed). Addison-Wesley, 1986.

Vogelpohl RA: Disseminated intravascular coagulation. *Crit Care Nurse* 1981; 1(3): 38-43.

Zschoche DA: *Mosby's Comprehensive Review of Critical Care.* Mosby, 1986.

8
MULTI-SYSTEM
S T R E S S O R S

Sepsis

Anaphylaxis

Toxic shock syndrome

Burns

Compartment syndrome

Organ rejection

Acquired immune deficiency syndrome

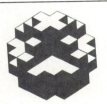

Sepsis

Sepsis is a pathologic state caused by bacteria, viruses, or fungi in the blood. It can be described as a continuum from bacteremia to profound septic shock. During the initial stages of sepsis the sympathetic nervous system is stimulated and cate-cholamines are released. This results in increased cardiac contractility and a hyper-dynamic cardiac state. The subsequent changes that occur are mediated by cellular release of enzymes and chemical substances. Although it is not precisely clear what stimulates release of these chemical substances, possible stimuli include offending microorganisms, the phagocytic process, or immunocompetent cells (T- and B-cell lymphocytes). Complement is the primary chemical mediator in sepsis.

A major systemic response to sepsis is vasodilatation, which occurs secondary to activation of the complement system, along with kinin release. Complement proteins have the ability to release vasoactive and chemotactic substances. Kinins, such as bradykinin and serotonin, cause vasodilatation and increase capillary permeability, thereby decreasing systemic vascular resistance and facilitating fluid shifts from intravascular to interstitial spaces. Another response is increased capil-lary permeability secondary to histamine release, which results in vascular fluid shifts to interstitial spaces. In addition, there is selective blood vessel constriction

TABLE 8-1

Assessment guidelines for the patient with sepsis in the early (warm) stage

Clinical indicator	Cause
Cardiovascular	
Increased HR ($\geq$100 bpm)	Sympathetic nervous system stimulation
Decreased BP (<90 mm Hg systolic)	Vasodilatation
CO >7 L/min; CI >4.0 L/min/m^2	Hyperdynamic state
SVO$_2$ >80%	Decreased utilization of oxygen by cells
PAWP usually <6 mm Hg	Venous dilatation; decreased preload
SVR <900 dynes/sec/cm^{-5}	Vasodilatation
Strong, bounding peripheral pulses	Hyperdynamic cardiovascular system
Respiratory	
Tachypnea (>20 breaths/min) and hyperventilation	Decreases in cerebrospinal fluid pH stimulate the central respiratory center
Crackles (rales)	Interstitial edema occurring with increased vascular permeability
Pa$_{CO_2}$ <35 mm Hg	Tachypnea and hyperventilation
Renal	
Decreased urine output (<30 ml/hr)	Decreased renal perfusion
Cutaneous	
Flushed and warm skin	Vasodilatation
Metabolic	
Increasing body temperature	Increased metabolic activity; release of pyrogens secondary to invading microorganisms
Neurologic	
Changes in LOC	Decreased cerebral perfusion and brain hypoxia

(e.g., renal, pulmonary, and splanchnic vessels) and vascular occlusion with subsequent sluggish blood flow and tissue ischemia. This stage often is referred to as "warm shock." As the septic state progresses, the hemodynamics change from vasodilatation to a classic shock presentation, with vasoconstriction and decreased cardiac output. These changes are stimulated by the powerful catecholamines and prostaglandins that are released from ischemic tissues. The stage during which tissue perfusion becomes severely compromised and ischemic cellular damage occurs is termed "cold shock." Additionally, fever occurs when the invading microorganisms release pyrogens (e.g., prostaglandins), which affect the thermoregulatory center in the hypothalamus.

The patient with sepsis is at high risk for development of disseminated intravascular coagulation (DIC, see p. 418) and adult respiratory distress syndrome (ARDS, see p. 18). Endotoxins, which are released from gram-negative bacilli, damage the vascular endothelium of pulmonary vessels, and along with the increased capillary permeability cause interstitial edema, increased vascular resistance, and decreased surfactant production. These changes precipitate ARDS. DIC is caused by a widespread, inappropriate activation of the coagulation cascade, a process that may be stimulated by chemical mediators in sepsis. See Figure 8-1 for a depiction of the pathologic process of sepsis.

ASSESSMENT

Physical assessment: See Table 8-1, p. 433, and Table 8-2, p. 436.

History and risk factors: Malnutrition, immunosuppression, chronic health problems (e.g., liver or renal disease), or recent traumatic injuries or surgical or invasive procedures; infection due to the following organisms: *E. coli, Klebsiella, Enterobacter, Serratia, Pseudomonas aeruginosa, Streptococcus pneumoniae, Staphylococcus aureus,* and *Pneumococcus,* as well as viruses and fungi.

DIAGNOSTIC TESTS

1. *WBC count:* Early in septicemia, WBCs will be decreased because of the binding of endotoxins to WBCs. These WBCs then are removed from the circulation. Later in the process after the immune system becomes active, leukocytosis will occur.
2. *WBC differential:* An increase in the number of immature neutrophils occurs because the cells are released into the bloodstream as the body attempts to fight the infection. These cells are called band neutrophils or nonsegmented neutrophils.
3. *Serum glucose:* Elevated because of catecholamine-induced hepatic gluconeogenesis and glycogenolysis.
4. *Blood cultures and antibiotic sensitivity testing of isolates:* Identify causative organism(s).
5. *Culture and antibiotic sensitivity testing of suspect infection sites:* Correlate with blood cultures to identify source(s) of the sepsis.
6. *Abdominal x-ray* (flat plate): To rule out perforated viscus as the cause of the sepsis.
7. *ABGs:* Will reflect metabolic acidosis (low HCO_3^-). Early in septicemia a low $PaCO_2$ may be reflective of hyperventilation. As shock progresses, however, respiratory acidosis (retention of CO_2) will occur and hypoxemia will be present because of respiratory failure.
8. *BUN and creatinine:* Increases are reflective of decreasing renal perfusion.
9. *Clotting studies:* Will demonstrate an increased PT, increased PTT, increased

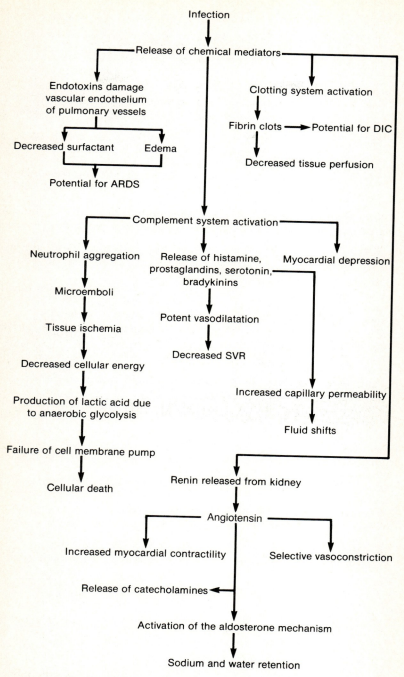

FIG. 8-1. The pathophysiologic process of sepsis.

TABLE 8-2
Assessment guidelines for the patient with sepsis in the late (cold) stage

Clinical indicator	Cause
Cardiovascular	
Extreme tachycardia with S_3 sound	Compensatory attempt by sympathetic autonomic nervous system to maintain cardiac output
Profound hypotension	Decreased stroke volume. Diastolic BP may remain high due to vasoconstriction.
CO <4.0 L/min; CI <2.5 L/min/m^2	Failure of compensatory mechanisms
PAWP usually >12 mm Hg	Increased left ventricular end diastolic pressure (LVEDP) due to increased residual volume from decreased stroke volume
SVR >1200 dynes/sec/cm^{-5}	Vasoconstriction
Weak or absent peripheral pulses	Decreased peripheral perfusion due to decreased cardiac output
SVO$_2$ ≤60%	Decreased oxygen binding to hemoglobin due to acidosis
Respiratory	
Decreased respiratory rate (<12 breaths/min) and depth	Failure of compensatory mechanisms (central respiratory center depression)
Crackles, rhonchi, wheezes	Accumulation of lung secretions
Increased FIO$_2$ required to maintain PaO$_2$ (may signal development of ARDS)	Ventilation/perfusion mismatch and decreased lung compliance
Increased PaCO$_2$ (>45 mm Hg)	Respiratory failure
Renal	
Decreased urine output progressing to anuria	Decreased renal perfusion and tubular ischemia
Decreased fractional excretion of sodium	Activation of the aldosterone mechanism and release of antidiuretic hormone, which stimulate retention of sodium and water
Cutaneous	
Cool, pale skin or cyanosis	Sustained vasoconstriction
Metabolic	
Decreasing body temperature	Decreased metabolic activity
Neurologic	
Decreased LOC (e.g., no response to verbal stimuli; deteriorating response to painful stimuli)	Severe hypoxia
Hematologic	
Oozing from previous venipuncture sites	Development of DIC due to stimulation of coagulation process, followed by fibrinolysis

bleeding time, thrombocytopenia, and increased fibrin split products. These results all reflect activation of the clotting cascade and may signal development of DIC.

10. *Liver studies:* SGOT, SGPT, and LDH will be elevated secondary to liver ischemia.

MEDICAL MANAGEMENT

1. Antibiotic therapy specific to the causative organism. Therapy usually is begun immediately after cultures are obtained and before sensitivity studies are completed (usually 24-48 hours).
   - *For gram-positive organisms* (e.g., *Streptococcus pneumoniae, Staphylococcus aureus, Pneumococcus):* Crystalline penicillin G or ampicillin; nafcillin plus ampicillin or vancomycin.

< C A U T I O N : Be alert to hypersensitivity reactions to penicillin-type drugs (see "Anaphylaxis," p. 443).

   - *For gram-negative organisms* (e.g., *E. coli, Klebsiella, Enterobacter, Serratia, Pseudomonas aeruginosa):* Tobramycin, amikacin, or an aminoglycoside (e.g., tobramycin or amikacin) plus cefotaxime or other cephalosporin.

< C A U T I O N : Aminoglycosides are nephrotoxic and can be dangerous in oliguric patients because they may cause further damage to renal tubules. When used in combination with cephalosporins, aminoglycosides significantly increase the risk of nephrotoxicity. If renal function is compromised, drug dosage should be adjusted accordingly. Because aminoglycosides are ototoxic as well, the drug should be used with extreme caution in hearing-impaired individuals.

   - *For anaerobes:* Clindamycin, chloramphenicol, or metronidazole (Flagyl, mainly used for fungal infections).
2. **Nutritional support:** Short- and medium-chain fatty acids and branched-chain amino acids are administed to stop protein catabolism. The short- and medium-chain fatty acids are absorbed more readily and metabolized more easily than long-chain fatty acids. They may be given orally, such as MCT (brand name meaning medium chain triglyceride) oil, or given IV (e.g., intralipid solutions). Branched-chain amino acid solutions are used in sepsis because they are metabolized by muscle rather than the liver, and therefore can be used in the presence of organ failure.
3. **Fluid administration:** To maintain adequate ventricular filling pressures and volume, which become compromised with increased capillary permeability and vasodilatation. Lactated Ringer's solution, normal saline, plasma protein fraction (Plasmanate), albumin, and fresh frozen plasma are used.
4. **Steroids** (e.g., dexamethasone 3-6 mg/kg or methylprednisone sodium 30 mg/kg): Although their use is controversial, steroids may be used to decrease capillary permeability, decrease leukocyte aggregation, decrease formation of microemboli, decrease histamine release, and decrease coagulopathy.
5. **Antipyretic agents, cooled IV fluid, or cooling blanket:** To normalize temperature.
6. **Intubation and mechanical ventilation:** To maintain adequate oxygenation. Positive end expiratory pressure (PEEP) may be necessary if the patient is developing ARDS.
7. **Vasopressors,** such as dopamine hydrochloride, norepinephrine, and metaraminol: May be administered to reverse vasodilatation and maintain perfusion.

< N O T E : Dopamine hydrochloride dosages >10 μg/kg/min will stimulate the alpha (vasoconstrictor) effects. Norepinephrine often is administered along with

phentolamine, which counteracts the tissue damaging effects of norepinephrine. Vasopressors are contraindicated in hypovolemic states.

8. **Positive inotropic drugs** such as dopamine and dobutamine: May be given to augment cardiac contractility and cardiac output. In the late stages of sepsis, positive inotropic drugs may be given along with **vasodilators**, such as nitroprusside and nitroglycerine, which decrease preload and afterload by dilating veins and arteries.

9. **Sodium bicarbonate:** Administered judiciously to correct metabolic acidosis. Dosage is guided by ABG findings so that metabolic alkalosis does not occur.

10. **Naloxone hydrochloride (Narcan):** May be used to reverse some of the vasodilatation effects of sepsis.

11. **Glucose-Potassium-Insulin (GKI):** This combination may be given to increase cardiac performance during sepsis.

NURSING DIAGNOSES AND INTERVENTIONS

Fluid volume deficit related to decreased circulating volume secondary to increased capillary permeability and loss of intravascular volume into interstitial spaces

---

Desired outcomes: Patient is normovolemic as evidenced by peripheral pulses >2+ on a 0-4+ scale, stable body weight, urine output ≥30 ml/hr, systolic BP >90 mm Hg or within patient's normal range, specific gravity 1.010-1.030, and absence of edema and adventitious lung sounds. PAWP is 6-12 mm Hg, CO is 4-7 L/min, and SVR is 900-1200 dynes/sec/cm^{-5}.

---

1. Assess fluid volume by monitoring BP and peripheral pulses hourly. Report systolic BP ≤90 mm Hg (or 20-30 mm Hg less than presepsis level) and decreasing amplitude of peripheral pulses.

2. Weigh patient daily; monitor I&O q shift, noting 24-hour trends. Report urine output <30 ml/hr.

< N O T E :   In sepsis, the patient's weight may increase with fluid volume deficit due to loss of intravascular volume into interstitial spaces.

5. Monitor specific gravity hourly, being alert to increases >1.030, which are indicative of a dehydration state, or a fixed specific gravity of 1.010, which may signal inadequate glomerular filtration.

4. Assess for interstitial edema as evidenced by pretibial, sacral, ankle, and hand edema, as well as crackles (rales) on auscultation of lung fields.

5. Monitor hemodynamic pressures, particularly PAWP, CO, and SVR. During the early (warm) stage of sepsis, PAWP usually is decreased to <6 mm Hg but will be increased to >12 mm Hg in the late (cold) stage. CO usually is >7 L/min in the early stage and decreased to <4 L/min in the late stage. SVR can be <900 dynes/sec/cm^{-5} in the early stage but increased to >1200 dynes/sec cm^{-5} in the late stage.

6. Administer crystalloid and colloid fluid replacement as prescribed. Often, fluid replacement therapy will be given to maintain a PAWP of 6-12 mm Hg. Assess PAWP and lung sounds at frequent intervals during fluid replacement to detect evidence of fluid overload: crackles (rales) and increasing PAWP.

7. As prescribed, administer vasopressor agents to help maintain perfusion, and steroids to decrease capillary permeability.
8. Administer positive inotropic agents as prescribed to maintain adequate CO in the presence of massive vasodilatation.
9. Position patient supine with legs elevated to increase venous return and preload.

Alteration in cardiac output: Decreased, related to relative hypovolemia (early stage) secondary to effects of endotoxins; or decreased contractility (late stage) secondary to effects of tissue hypoxia

---

Desired outcome: Patient has adequate cardiac output as evidenced by systolic BP ≥90 mm Hg (or within patient's normal range), HR ≤100 bpm, peripheral pulses >2+ on a scale of 0-4+, urine output ≥30 ml/hr, PAWP ≤12 mm Hg, CO ≥4 L/min, and CI ≥2.5 L/min/m^2.

---

1. Assess patient for signs of decreased cardiac output: decreasing BP, increasing HR, decreasing amplitude of peripheral pulses, restlessness, decreasing urinary output, and increasing PAWP.
2. Administer positive inotropic agents as prescribed to augment cardiac contractility.
3. Position patient supine with legs elevated to optimize preload and enhance stroke volume.
4. Assess CO at least q4h. Optimally, CO will be ≥4 L/min and CI will be ≥2.5 L/min/m^2.
5. Monitor cardiac rhythm per monitor at frequent intervals. Observe for development of dysrhythmias, such as PVCs, which may occur with hypoxia, and extreme tachycardia, both of which will potentiate a decreased cardiac output.
6. Minimize myocardial oxygen demand by assisting patient with ADLs and ensuring uninterrupted periods of rest.

Alteration in tissue perfusion: Cerebral, renal, and splanchnic, related to decreased circulating volume secondary to vasodilatation (early stage) or vasoconstriction and thrombus obstruction (late stage)

Desired outcomes: Patient has adequate perfusion as evidenced by orientation to person, place, and time; peripheral pulses >2+ (on a scale of 0-4+); urine output ≥30 ml/hr; BUN ≤20 mg/dl; serum creatinine ≤1.5 mg/dl; serum potassium ≤5.5 mEq/L; serum amylase ≤180 Somogyi units/dl; and platelet count ≥150,000/μl. BP is 110-120/70-80 mm Hg (or within patient's normal range); SVO$_2$ is ≤80%; SVR is 900-1200 dynes/sec/$^{-5}$; CO is 4-7 L/min; and CI is 2.5-4 L/min/m^2.

---

1. Assess for changes in LOC as an indicator of decreasing cerebral perfusion.
2. Assess for the following signs of decreasing renal perfusion: urine output <30 ml/hr and increased BUN, serum creatinine, and serum potassium.
3. Assess for evidence of decreasing splanchnic (visceral) circulation, including elevated serum amylase and decreased platelet count.
4. Monitor arterial BP continuously. Be alert to decreased systolic BP, normal or

increased diastolic BP, and decreased pulse pressures, which occur in the presence of decreasing perfusion.

< N O T E : Systolic BP will be decreased because of decreased cardiac output and the diastolic BP may be high secondary to compensatory vasoconstriction.

5. Assess peripheral pulses, temperature, and color of skin. With hypoperfusion, pulse amplitude decreases, extremities become cool due to vasoconstriction, and skin color becomes pale or mottled because of decreased perfusion.
6. Monitor cellular oxygen consumption (SVO_2) as an indicator of tissue perfusion. With sepsis, cellular oxygen delivery is decreased (precapillary vasoconstriction) and thus, cellular oxygen utilization is decreased. Therefore, the mixed venous blood oxygen saturation (SVO_2) will be abnormally high.
7. Administer vasoactive drugs as prescribed and assess SVR and CO during administration to determine effect of these drugs. Optimally, SVR will increase to ≥ 900 dynes/sec/cm^{-5}, CO will be 4-7 L/min, and CI will be 2.5-4 L/min/m^2.

< N O T E : Vasoactive drugs probably will include vasopressors (e.g., norepinephrine) early in sepsis and vasodilators (e.g., nitroprusside) late in sepsis. Vasopressors are always accompanied by fluid resuscitation as needed.

8. Administer steroids as prescribed to decrease capillary permeability; monitor for increasing renal perfusion (urinary output ≥ 30 ml/hr), which may occur with the decreased loss of circulating volume.

Impaired gas exchange related to decreased diffusion of oxygen secondary to interstitial edema, alveolar destruction, and eventual (late) respiratory depression

---

Desired outcome: Patient's PaO_2 is ≥ 80 mm Hg; $PaCO_2$ is ≤ 45 mm Hg; and pH is 7.35-7.45.

---

1. Assess for and maintain a patent airway by assisting patient with coughing and suctioning trachea as necessary. Ensure that patient demonstrates adequate air movement by noting presence of breath sounds over all lung fields.
2. Assist patient into position of comfort for breathing. Depending on stability of hemodynamics, the optimal position may be a 15°-30° HOB elevation.
3. Assess rate and depth of respirations and ABG values at frequent intervals. Be alert to dyspnea, SOB, restlessness, decreased air movement, change in rate and depth of respirations (e.g., increased rate/decreased depth or decreased rate/decreased depth) as well as the following ABG findings: decreasing PaO_2, increasing $PaCO_2$, and acidosis (decreasing pH).
4. If patient exhibits evidence of inadequate gas exchange, prepare for the probability of endotracheal intubation.
5. If patient is being ventilated mechanically, monitor inspiratory peak pressures for increasing trends, which may signal decreasing compliance and development of ARDS. Also, assess for and document mode of ventilation, tidal volume, FIO_2, rate of respirations, and level of PEEP. Typically, as ARDS develops, an increasing FIO_2 ($>.50$) and increasing levels of PEEP are required to maintain adequate PaO_2 (>60 mm Hg). Notify MD if inspiratory peak pressures increase with each breath or if the following signs of hypoxia occur at the prescribed

FIo_2 and level of PEEP: increased HR ($\geq$100 bpm), anxiety, cool extremities, change in mentation, or skin color changes (pallor or cyanosis). See section "Management of the Adult on Mechanical Ventilation," p. 61, for more information.

6. Turn patient q2h to maintain optimal ventilation/perfusion ratios and prevent atelectasis.

7. Administer sodium bicarbonate as prescribed to buffer metabolic acidosis. Dosages are determined by level of pH in ABG findings.

< N O T E :   Administration of sodium bicarbonate may worsen respiratory acidosis.

Ineffective thermoregulation related to fluctuations secondary to alterations in metabolic rate due to endotoxin effect on hypothalamic temperature regulating center

---

Desired outcome: Patient is in a state of normothermia.

---

1. Monitor patient's temperature continuously or at frequent intervals. Use temperature probe (rectal or tympanic) for continuous monitoring of core temperature. Body temperature can range from 38.3° C-40.6° C (101° F-105° F) in the early stage of sepsis and can be <35.6° C (96° F) in the late stage. Be alert to shaking chills early in sepsis as temperature increases and profuse diaphoresis as temperature decreases late in sepsis. The following are weighed for each patient to determine the extent of treatment (e.g., aspirin) that should be employed to decrease fever:
   • Good results from a fever: Decreased viral and bacterial replication.
   • Bad results from a fever: Increased cardiac workload and increased oxygen consumption.

2. Administer antibiotics as prescribed.

< N O T E :   Observe for untoward effects of antibiotics including renal toxicity, ototoxicity, allergic reactions, anaphylaxis, pseudomembranous colitis, overgrowth of normal flora, and superimposed infectious processes of the skin, urinary tract, or respiratory tract. Large doses of antibiotics may cause the release of endotoxins from dying bacteria, which may potentiate the progression of the deleterious effects of sepsis.

3. Administer antipyretic agents as prescribed.

4. If the patient is hyperthermic, a cooling blanket may be prescribed to decrease the metabolic rate, thereby decreasing myocardial oxygen demand. Avoid "chilling," which will cause shivering and thus increase myocardial oxygen demand and cardiac workload.

5. For hyperthermic patients, employ tepid baths, which decrease body temperature by releasing internal heat. Cooled IV fluids may decrease core temperature, as well.

6. In the presence of hypothermia, use warm blankets to increase body temperature. Heating devices can damage ischemic cells in peripheral tissues and usually are avoided.

Alteration in nutrition: Less than body requirements related to increased need for nutritional substrates secondary to increased metabolic rate

---

Desired outcome: Patient has adequate nutrition as evidenced by stable weights, serum albumin 3.5 gm/dl, thyroxine-binding prealbumin 200-300 μg/ml, retinol-binding protein 40-50 μg/ml, urine urea nitrogen 10-20 mg/dl, and a state of nitrogen balance as determined by nitrogen studies.

---

1. Assess and record weight and nutritional intake daily. Have a calorie count done by nutritional services.
2. If patient is receiving oral feedings, assess for the presence of bowel sounds at least q2h. Paralytic ileus can occur secondary to an ischemic bowel.
3. If the patient is on continuous NG tube feedings, assess for residual feeding q2h. Assess for residual prior to intermittent tube feedings. If residual is ≥100 ml, hold feeding and consult with MD.
4. To meet patient's tremendous metabolic demands, provide foods that are high in calories.
5. Encourage intake of foods high in protein and carbohydrates.
6. Administer nutritional supplements as prescribed.

< N O T E :   Standard hyperalimentation solutions are not metabolized well in the septic state. Branched-chain amino acid solutions and short- to medium-chain fatty acid solutions are best, for example MCT oil or Freamine HBC.

7. Observe for and document areas of tissue breakdown, which can be indicative of a negative nitrogen state.
8. Monitor lab value results for serum albumin, thyroxine-binding prealbumin, retinol-binding protein, and nitrogen studies.
9. For more information, see section "Providing Nutritional Support," p. 490.

See nursing diagnoses and interventions in "Management of the Adult with Hemodynamic Monitoring," p. 171. See "Renal Transplant" for the following: **Knowledge deficit:** Immunosuppressive medications and their side effects, p. 195; **Impaired skin integrity** secondary to immunosuppression with corticosteroids, p. 198; and **Potential for infection** secondary to immunosuppression, p. 197. See "Disseminated Intravascular Coagulation" for the following: **Alteration in tissue perfusion**: Microthrombi occurring with coagulation phase of DIC, p. 420; and **Potential fluid volume deficit** secondary to hemorrhagic phase of DIC, p. 420. Also see the following: "Caring for the Critically Ill with Life-Threatening Disorders," pp. 511-522, and "Caring for the Family of the Critically Ill," pp. 522-526.

REHABILITATION AND PATIENT-FAMILY TEACHING CONCEPTS

Because sepsis is a condition that usually occurs secondary to another disorder, patient-family teaching most likely will be directed toward the primary illness. In addition, provide patient and significant others with verbal and written information that is specific to sepsis:

1. Risk factors for sepsis specific to the event that caused patient's disorder, for example, a chemotherapeutic agent.

2. Measures for minimizing risk of sepsis, such as maintaining optimal nutritional state and avoiding obvious sources of infection such as crowds.
3. Indicators of systemic infection.
4. Importance of consultation with a health professional if indicators of systemic infection occur.

Anaphylaxis

Systemic anaphylactic shock (anaphylaxis) is a medical emergency stimulated or caused by an exaggerated response to an allergen. It occurs in a sensitized person (i.e., someone who has been exposed previously to the same allergen), usually 1-20 minutes following introduction of the antigenic substance.

In the immediate phase, the hypersensitivity response occurs on the surface of the mast cells, which are located primarily in connective tissue. There, the antigen combines with sensitized antibodies from previous exposure (usually IgE type). The antigen also attaches to basophils circulating in the blood. This triggers release of substances from the granules within the cells, including histamine, serotonin, and eosinophil and neutrophil chemotactic factors. In addition, the antigen-antibody complex activates a cellular process that produces prostaglandins and leukotrienes (called SRS-A). These chemical mediators produce systemic effects that can have deleterious results, including profound shock.

Histamine causes increased capillary permeability, increased lung secretions, bronchoconstriction, and systemic vasodilatation. The leukotrienes produce bronchoconstriction that is even more severe than that caused by histamine. The prostaglandins exaggerate the bronchoconstriction and potentiate the effects of histamine on vascular permeability and lung secretions. The combined effects of these substances cause respiratory distress and obstruction, which can lead to respiratory arrest and fluid loss from the vascular space, with possible vasogenic shock and end-organ dysfunction due to tissue hypoxia.

ASSESSMENT

Early indicators: Uneasiness, light-headedness, itching of palms.

Late indicators: Rapid progression from light-headedness to syncope; urticaria that involves large surface areas of the skin. In addition, patient may have angioedema (tissue swelling), especially of the eyes, lips, tongue, hands, feet, and genitalia; dyspnea and respiratory distress; and abdominal cramps, diarrhea, and vomiting.

Physical assessment: See Table 8-3, p. 445.

Hemodynamic measurements: Decreased arterial BP and MAP due to vasodilatation; decreased CO (<4.0 L/min) if shock ensues; decreased CI (<2.5 L/min); decreased SVR (<900 dynes/sec/cm^{-5}) because of vasodilatation; and low PAWP (<6 mm Hg) because of vasodilatation, decreased venous return, and loss of intravascular fluid.

History and risk factors: Recent exposure to pharmacologic agents, such as the penicillins; anesthetic agents; contrast medium; blood transfusions; and insect bites or stings.

DIAGNOSTIC TESTS

The diagnosis of anaphylaxis is based on presenting signs and symptoms. IgE levels may confirm allergic origin and ABG values may be assessed to evaluate respiratory status.

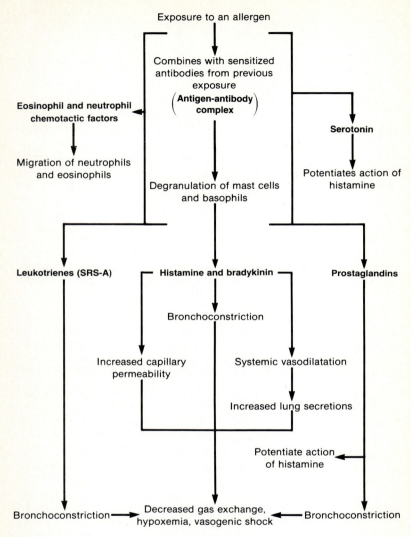

FIG. 8-2. The pathophysiologic process of anaphylaxis. Major chemical mediators are in bold faced print.

MEDICAL MANAGEMENT

1. **Airway maintenance:** May require endotracheal intubation. If laryngeal edema is severe and causes obstruction, a tracheostomy may be necessary.

2. **Epinephrine:** Counteracts the effects of anaphylaxis by increasing myocardial contractility, dilating bronchioles, constricting blood vessels, inhibiting histamine release, and counteracting histamine that already is circulating. Standard dosage is 0.3-0.5 mg (0.3-0.5 ml of a 1:1000 solution) IV or SC, although

TABLE 8-3

Systemic effects of anaphylaxis

System	Effects	Cause
Neurologic	Decreased LOC progressing to coma	Brain hypoxia or cerebral edema occurring with interstitial fluid shifts
Respiratory	Dyspnea progressing to air hunger and complete respiratory obstruction; impaired phonation; noisy breating; high-pitched "barking" cough; and wheezes, crackles, rhonchi, decreased breath sounds	Laryngeal edema; bronchoconstriction; increased lung secretions
Cardiovascular	Decreased BP leading to profound hypotension; increased heart rate; decreased amplitude of peripheral pulses; palpitations (atrial tachycardias, premature atrial beats, premature ventricular beats progressing to ventricular tachycardia or ventricular fibrillation); lymphadenopathy	Systemic vasodilation; vasogenic shock; decreased cardiac output with decreased circulating volume
Renal	Decreased urine output; incontinence	Decreased renal perfusion; smooth muscle contraction of urinary tract
Gastrointestinal	Nausea; vomiting; diarrhea; abdominal cramping	Smooth muscle contraction of GI tract
Cutaneous	Urticaria; angioedema (hands, lips, face, feet, genitalia); cyanosis	Histamine-induced disruption of cutaneous vasculature; increased capillary permeability; decreased oxygen saturation of hemoglobin

some researchers recommend 0.1 mg (0.1 ml of a 1:1000 solution). If given IV, the route preferred in the presence of shock, it usually is diluted in 10 ml of normal saline. This initial dosage is followed by IV infusion of 1 μg/min, which is increased to 4 μg/min in the absence of a positive response.

3. **Supplemental oxygen:** May be administered to support oxygen delivery to the tissues. The amount and method of administration are guided by ABG results.

4. **Fluid resuscitation:** Crystalloids (e.g., lactated Ringer's solution) or colloids (e.g., albumin and plasma protein fraction {Plasmanate}) to increase colloid osmotic pressure and pull fluids back into the vascular spaces, thus attaining adequate vascular volume. This may require a rapid infusion of 2-3 liters.

5. **Vasopressors:** Necessary if fluid replacement does not reverse or prevent shock. Drugs such as dopamine hydrochloride and norepinephrine are titrated for the desired response. Usual dosages: dopamine hydrochloride 5-20 μg/kg/min and norepinephrine 2-8 μg/kg/min.

6. **Antihistamines:** For example, diphenhydramine may be given IV to relieve urticaria and abdominal cramping. Usual dosage is 20-50 mg.

7. **Theophylline (Aminophylline):** May be given IV drip to stimulate bronchodilatation and relieve bronchospasm. Usual dosage is 2-4 mg/min (0.5 mg/kg).

8. **Corticosteroids:** May be given to decrease both capillary permeability and release of chemical mediators. The effect is not immediate.

9. **Military anti-shock trousers (MAST):** Advocated by some to increase systemic vascular resistance and maintain BP.

NURSING DIAGNOSES AND INTERVENTIONS

Impaired gas exchange related to decreased diffusion of oxygen secondary to dyspnea and airway obstruction occurring with laryngeal edema and bronchoconstriction

---

Desired outcome: Patient has adequate gas exchange as evidenced by auscultation of air movement over lung fields and $Pao_2 \geq 80$ mm Hg.

---

1. Assess patency of airway on a continuing basis. Be alert to decreasing air movement heard on auscultation of the lungs, expiratory wheezing, SOB, and dyspnea, which can progress to "air hunger." Notify MD if assessment reveals signs of impaired gas exchange or airway compromise; prepare for endotracheal intubation if signs are present. Keep suction equipment readily available.

2. Administer epinephrine IV or SC, as prescribed. Dosage and route vary. Generally, the following guidelines are used:
   - IV route if patient is in shock.
   - Initially, a dose of 0.1 mg (0.1 ml of a 1:1000 solution) diluted in 10 ml normal saline is infused over 5-10 minutes. The dose may be increased to 0.3-0.5 mg.
   - After initial dosage, an IV drip of 1 mg of 1:1000 epinephrine in 250 ml 5% dextrose in water is established. Initial infusion usually is 1 μg/min. If given SC, the dose is 0.3-0.5 mg (0.3-0.5 ml of a 1:1000 solution) and it is repeated q15-20min as needed.

< N O T E : Patients on beta-blocking drugs, such as propranolol, may not respond to epinephrine.

3. Administer oxygen as prescribed.

4. Auscultate lung fields for presence of wheezes and air movement.

< N O T E : With further bronchoconstriction and obstruction, wheezes may decrease; therefore, it is important to listen for air movement as well.

5. Prepare for endotracheal intubation if SOB and respiratory distress continue.

< C A U T I O N : An oral airway provides airway support only as far as the posterior pharynx. If laryngeal edema is present, the oral airway will be ineffective because the obstruction is lower.

6. If laryngeal edema prevents intubation, prepare for the possibility of a tracheostomy.

7. Antihistamines, such as diphenhydramine, may be given IV or IM to compete

with histamine at receptor sites and control edema and itching. Usual dose is 20-50 mg.

8. If prescribed, administer IV bronchodilators, such as theophylline (Aminophylline), to induce bronchodilatation. Usual dosage is 2-4 mg/min. Monitor for side effects such as dysrhythmias.

9. Keep "crash cart" nearby in the event of respiratory arrest.

10. As prescribed, administer glucocorticoids (e.g., hydrocortisone) for their anti-inflammatory effects and potential ability to decrease capillary permeability. Be aware that the effects of glucocorticoids will not be noticed immediately.

11. Monitor ABG values for evidence of in improving or worsening condition. Be alert to increasing $Paco_2$ (>50 mm Hg) and decreasing Pao_2 (<60 mm Hg).

12. If BP is stable, assist patient to sitting position to enhance gas exchange.

13. Remain with patient; encourage slow, deep breathing if possible. Help alleviate patient's anxiety by responding calmly and explaining all procedures before performing them.

Alteration in cardiac output: Decreased, related to dysrhythmias or risk of cardiac arrest secondary to decreased circulating volume occurring with vasodilatation and increased capillary permeability

---

Desired outcomes: Patient has adequate cardiac output as evidenced by BP >90/60, peripheral pulses >2+ on a scale of 0-4+, CO ≥4.0 L/min, CI ≥2.5 L/min/m^2, and SVR ≥900 dynes/sec/cm^{-5}. EKG reveals normal sinus rhythm.

---

1. Assess for physical and hemodynamic indicators of decreased cardiac output:
   - Check apical pulse for irregularity.
   - Palpate peripheral pulses for decreasing amplitude.
   - Assess arterial BP for decrease, an indicator of failed compensatory mechanisms.
   - Calculate SVR. A decrease (<900 dynes/sec/cm^{-5}) is associated with decreased afterload (vasodilatation) and may precipitate decreased CO.
   - Measure CO if a thermodilution catheter is present.
   - Calculate CI for a more precise measurement of adequacy of CO. A finding of <2.5 L/min/m^2 usually is associated with hypoperfusion.

2. Assess electrical rhythm *via* EKG monitor for dysrhythmias, such as atrial tachycardias, premature ventricular beats, ventricular tachycardia, and ventricular fibrillation.

3. Inspect face, lips, hands, feet, and genitalia for edema as an indicator of fluid loss to interstitial spaces. Document edema on a scale of 1+ to 4+.
   - 1+: A slight depression that disappears quickly.
   - 4+: A deep depression that disappears slowly.

4. As prescribed, administer epinephrine to decrease capillary permeability, stimulate vasoconstriction, increase systemic vascular resistance, and increase myocardial contractility. Observe for therapeutic effects as evidenced by increased calculated SVR, increased CO/CI, increased arterial BP and MAP, stronger peripheral pulses, warming of extremities, and increased urine output (indicator of increased renal perfusion).

5. Administer fluid replacement therapy as prescribed. Be aware that it may take as much as 2-3 liters to attain adequate vascular volume.

< N O T E : During fluid resuscitation, assess patient for indicators of fluid volume excess, including crackles with chest auscultation, presence of S_3 heart sounds, and jugular venous distention. If hemodynamic monitoring lines are present, be alert to increasing PAP, PAWP, and RAP.

6. Prepare for possible vasopressor infusion to reverse shock state. Possible pharmacologic agents include:
   • *Dopamine hydrochloride:* To increase cardiac contractility and systemic vascular resistance *via* its alpha and beta properties. Usual dose is 5-20 µg/kg/min.
   • *Norepinephrine:* Alpha adrenergic stimulator. Initial dose is 2-8 µg/min and can be increased to achieve the necessary BP.
   • *Metaraminol* (rarely used): Potent sympathomimetic drug that increases strength of cardiac contractions and stimulates vasoconstriction. It is given by IV drip and titrated to achieve the desired hemodynamics.
   • *Methoxamine hydrochloride:* Alpha adrenergic drug that stimulates intense vasoconstriction.

7. If prescribed, apply MAST suit to increase systemic vascular resistance.

< C A U T I O N : MAST suit must be released gradually to prevent hypovolemia.

Alteration in tissue perfusion: Peripheral, renal, and cerebral, related to decreased circulation of blood to the tissues secondary to edema and loss of vascular volume

---

Desired outcome: Patient has adequate perfusion as evidenced by peripheral pulses >2+ (on a scale of 0-4+); brisk capillary refill (<3 seconds); urinary output ≥30 ml/hr; warm and dry skin; and orientation to person, place, and time.

---

1. Palpate peripheral pulses in arms and legs (radial, brachial, dosalis pedis, posterior tibial) and rate them according to a 0-4+ scale. Report decreased amplitude of pulses.
2. Assess capillary refill. Note whether it is brisk (<3 seconds) or delayed (>4 seconds), which is likely with edema and decreased vascular volume.
3. Assess degree of peripheral edema, rating it on a scale of 1+ to 4+.
4. Assess color and warmth of extremities; report presence of coolness and pallor.
5. Monitor BP at frequent intervals. Be alert to readings >20 mm Hg below patient's normal and other indicators of hypotension, including dizziness, restlessness, altered mentation, and decreased urinary output.
6. Observe for indicators of decreased cerebral perfusion, such as restlessness, confusion, and decreased LOC.

< N O T E : Changes in LOC may signal either decreased cerebral perfusion (tissue hypoxia) or increasing ICP caused by interstitial swelling from capillary permeability.

7. Administer fluid and pharmacologic agents as prescribed (see previous nursing diagnosis).

Impaired skin integrity related to urticaria and angioedema secondary to allergic response

---

Desired outcomes: Patient states that urticaria is controlled. Skin remains intact.

---

1. Assess patient for the presence of urticaria (hives) and itching of hands, feet, neck, and genitalia, which are characteristic of anaphylaxis.
2. Administer antihistamines as prescribed to relieve itching.
3. Administer epinephrine as prescribed to counteract most of the effects of the hypersensitivity response.
4. Discourage patient from scratching the skin. If scratching is unavoidable, teach patient to use pads of fingertips rather than nails.
5. Apply cool washcloths or covered ice as a soothing measure to irritated and edematous areas.

REHABILITATION AND PATIENT-FAMILY TEACHING CONCEPTS

Give patient and significant others verbal and written instructions for the following:
1. Information about the antigenic agent that caused the anaphylaxis, including ways to avoid it in the future. For example, if the anaphylaxis was caused by penicillin, the patient needs to avoid all penicillin-related drugs and possibly molds, since penicillin is made from mold.
2. Importance of describing allergies to all health professionals.
3. Purpose of the Medic-Alert tag or bracelet to identify the allergy.
4. Necessity of anaphylaxis emergency treatment kits. Teach patient self-administration technique and the importance of prompt treatment.
5. Importance of reporting immediately the symptoms of allergy, such as flushing, warmth, itching, anxiety, and hives.

Toxic shock syndrome

Research suggests that toxic shock syndrome (TSS) is caused by a bacterial toxin or poison. Toxins, low-molecular-weight proteins, produced by a strain of *Staphylococcus aureus,* enter the blood from the site of infection by diffusing across the mucous membranes and are then distributed throughout the body. The toxins cause massive peripheral vasodilatation, rapid movement of serum proteins and fluid from the intravascular space to interstitial space, and fever. They contribute further to the shock state by suppressing myocardial functioning. TSS affects many body systems (see Table 8-4 for more information).

ASSESSMENT

Early indicators: Fever, rash, hypotension, vomiting, diarrhea, disorientation, petechiae, joint pain, muscular tenderness.

Late indicators: Full thickness desquamation of the hands and feet, dyspnea, cyanosis.

TABLE 8-4

Multi-system involvement in toxic shock syndrome

Organ system	Symptoms	Possible pathophysiology due to toxins
Cardiovascular	Hypotension and edema	Fluid and protein loss into soft tissue caused by increased capillary permeability.
Cutaneous	Hyperemia of mucous membranes	Mucous membranes become inflamed as toxins bind to cells.
	Erythroderma	Toxins and antibody bind to the skin and cause rash, followed by desquamation (shedding of epithelial cells in scales or sheets) of hands and feet.
	Alopecia and nail loss	Binding of toxins and antibody causes cellular destruction of hair and nails.
Gastrointestinal	Rebound tenderness	Inflamed mucous membranes caused by toxin binding.
	Vomiting and diarrhea	Acute gastroenteritis caused by toxins.
Hemopoietic	Thrombocytopenia with oozing from punctures	Platelet destruction, bone marrow suppression, and DIC caused by toxins.
Renal	Oliguria	Prerenal acute renal failure results from pump failure (myocarditis) and hypovolemia; intrarenal acute renal failure results from injury to renal tubule epithelium caused by toxins.
Central Nervous	Disorientation, confusion, restlessness	Changes in cerebrovascular capillary permeability, cerebral vasculitis, and cerebritis caused by toxins.
Musculoskeletal	Total body and joint pain	Systemic absorption of the toxins causes joint and muscular discomfort.
Respiratory	Pulmonary congestion, dyspnea, cyanosis	Increased vascular permeability in the lungs causes pulmonary infiltrates, alveolar collapse, and adult respiratory distress syndrome (ARDS).

Physical assessment: Gallop rhythms, abdominal rebound tenderness, hyperemia of mucous membranes (strawberry tongue, conjunctivitis, pharyngitis, vaginitis), diffuse erythroderma (sunburn-like rash), pulmonary congestion, oozing from puncture sites, pyrexia (rectal or core temperature will be elevated markedly), edema, photophobia.

Monitoring parameters

1. *Pulmonary artery catheters:* Low PAWP and RAP.
2. *Arterial blood pressure:* Profoundly decreased.
3. *Cardiac monitor:* Sinus tachycardia, supraventricular tachycardia.

   History and risk factors: Tampon use during first five days of menstrual period, recent childbirth or abortion, surgical wound infection, soft tissue wound (subcutaneous and cutaneous lesion, abscess, ulcer, cellulitis, insect bite, burn, abrasion).

DIAGNOSTIC TESTS

1. *Culture and sensitivities* (blood, urine, sputum, vagina, cervix, anterior nose, stool, CSF, soft tissue wounds): Generally, blood cultures will be negative, but cultures of some body sites may be positive for *Staphylococcus aureus.*
2. *Chest x-ray:* May show interstitial and alveolar infiltrates due to pulmonary congestion.
3. *Serum albumin, calcium, and phosphate studies:* Hypocalcemia and hypoalbuminemia result from rapid movement of intravascular fluid and protein into the extravascular space. Hypophosphatemia results from decreased intake, absorption, excretion, or transcellular movement of phosphate.
4. *BUN and serum creatinine:* Elevated. Dehydration and hypoperfusion cause prerenal acute renal failure; toxins cause intrarenal acute renal failure.
5. *Platelet count:* May show evidence of thrombocytopenia due to platelet destruction and bone marrow suppression by toxins.
6. *Bilirubin:* Elevated due to liver dysfunction.
7. *ABGs:* Hypoxemia may be present if patient experiences pulmonary congestion; metabolic acidosis may be present due to circulatory shock.
8. *Clotting studies:* May reflect disseminated intravascular coagulation (i.e., increased fibrin split products, PT, PTT, and bleeding time).

MEDICAL MANAGEMENT

1. **Fluid resuscitation** (colloids or crystalloids) **and pressor agents:** To correct hypovolemia. Pressor therapy always must be accompanied by fluid resuscitation.
2. **Pharmacotherapy**
   - *Antistaphylococcal antibiotics* that are beta-lactamase resistant: For example, nafcillin, oxacillin, cephalothin, vancomycin, gentamycin, clindamycin, methicillin.
   - *Parenteral high-dose corticosteroids:* Controversial. Reliable data on the efficacy of steroids in TSS is not available. Steroids may stabilize the cell membrane, blocking the effects of the toxin.
   - *Analgesia:* Acetaminophen, morphine sulfate.
   - *Antipyretics:* Acetaminophen.

   < N O T E : Aspirin should be avoided because of its tendency to aggravate bleeding disorders.

   - *Calcium supplements* (e.g., calcium chloride): To correct hypocalcemia.
   - *Antiemetics and antidiarrheal agents.*
3. **Acetaminophen and cooling blanket:** To correct pyrexia.
4. **Oxygen, intubation, and mechanical ventilation**, if necessary: To correct hypoxia.

NURSING DIAGNOSES AND INTERVENTIONS

Fluid volume deficit related to decreased circulating volume secondary to fluid shifts, fever, vomiting, and diarrhea caused by bacterial toxins

Desired outcomes: Patient is normovolemic as evidenced by urine output ≥30 ml/hr, urine specific gravity ≤1.030, BP within patient's normal range, PAWP ≥6 mm Hg, moist mucous membranes, good skin turgor, and absence of thirst. Serum albumin is ≥3.5 g/dl, serum calcium is ≥8.5 mg/dl, and serum phosphate is ≥2.5 mg/dl.

1. Maintain aggressive fluid resuscitation with colloids or crystalloids through a large-bore IV catheter, as prescribed by MD.
2. Monitor fluid replacement *via* pulmonary artery catheter readings q2h or as needed. Maintain wedge pressure in the high-normal range (10-15 mm Hg) to augment heart filling pressure.
3. Monitor I&O hourly. Maintain in-dwelling urinary catheter to gravity drainage; notify MD if urine output is <30 ml/hr.
4. Assess for indicators of dehydration: dry mucous membranes, poor skin turgor, increased urine specific gravity.
5. Monitor BP continuously *via* arterial catheter. Notify MD if mean BP becomes <70 mmHg.
6. Monitor serum electrolytes q6h (see information under "Diagnostic Tests," p. 451). Supplement electrolytes as prescribed.
7. Administer antiemetics and antidiarrheal agents as needed for vomiting and diarrhea. Avoid use of NG tube, which can aggravate emesis.

Alteration in cardiac output: Decreased: Risk of pump failure related to myocardial suppression secondary to bacterial toxins and hypocalcemia

Desired outcomes: Patient has adequate cardiac output as evidenced by sinus rhythm 60-100 bpm on cardiac monitor, peripheral pulses >2+ (on a 0-4+ scale), and brisk capillary refill (<3 seconds). Serum calcium levels are within normal range (8.5-10.5 mg/dl).

1. Assess cardiovascular status q4h, evaluating heart sounds, capillary refill, and peripheral pulses. Notify MD of new murmurs, rubs, gallops; document whether capillary refill is brisk (<3 seconds) or delayed (>4 seconds). Palpate peripheral pulses bilaterally in upper and lower extremities (radial, brachial, dorsalis pedis, and posterior tibial) and rate on a scale of 0-4+. Notify MD of absent pulses.
2. Maintain continuous heart monitoring. Notify MD of changes in rhythm or changes in rate >20 bpm.
3. Assess for indicators of hypocalcemia: hyperreflexia, tetany, prolonged QT interval on EKG, muscle cramping, abdominal cramping, nervous system excitability, numbness, tingling of fingers, seizures, altered mental status, laryngeal stridor, laryngospasm. Also be alert to positive *Chvostek's sign:* twitching of facial muscles on the same side that facial nerve is tapped; and to positive *Trousseau's sign:* contraction of the muscles of the hands and arms when circulation is interrupted with a blood pressure cuff inflated above systolic pressure

for 3 minutes. The metacarpophalangeal joints become flexed, fingers extended, thumb drawn to the palm, and wrist and elbows flexed.

4. As prescribed, supplement calcium intravenously *via* infusion device, optimally through central access.

Hyperthermia related to increased metabolic rate and dehydration secondary to bacterial infection and response to toxins

Desired outcome: Patient's body temperature is within normal limits.

1. Monitor rectal or core temperature q4h if <38.3° C (101° F), or qh if >38.3° C (101° F).
2. Administer acetaminophen q4h as needed for temperatures >38.3° C (101° F).
3. If patient is unresponsive to acetaminophen, provide hypothermia blanket for temperature >38.9° C (102° F). Pad blanket with one thickness bath blanket to prevent skin breakdown; assess skin hourly. To allow for heat diffusion, limit the number of blankets covering patient to a single sheet and a bath blanket.
4. Ensure optimal hydration. See interventions in **Fluid volume deficit**, p. 451.

Alteration in comfort: Pain related to myalgias and arthralgias

Desired outcome: Patient relates a reduction in discomfort and does not exhibit signs of uncontrolled pain.

1. Recognize the severity of diffuse myalgias (muscular pain) and arthralgias (joint pain) in TSS. Muscular tenderness, particularly in the back, abdomen, and extremities, makes even gentle touch painful for the TSS patient. Explain the cause of the pain (bacterial toxins) to the patient.
2. Medicate patient with IV morphine sulfate or comparable narcotic analgesia up to qh, as prescribed by MD. However, in the presence of hypotension or respiratory suppression (if the patient is not intubated), refrain from giving the analgesia.
3. Assist patient into a position of comfort. Often, knee flexion will relax lower abominal muscles and help reduce discomfort.
4. Turn patient only when necessary for maintaining skin integrity and maximizing pulmonary functioning. Avoid unnecessary moving. Keep obstacles away from bedside to avoid jostling bed.
5. Avoid use of aspirin for pain (aggravates bleeding disorders) or heating pads (aggravates erythroderma and pyrexia).

Sensory-perceptual alterations related to confusion and agitation secondary to bacterial toxins, hypotension, dehydration, febrile state, and hospitalization in critical care area

Desired outcome: Patient verbalizes orientation to person, place, and time.

1. Perform a complete neurologic assessment q4h, including strength and movement of the extremities, pupillary exam, best verbal response, and patient's ability to open eyes.
2. Provide rest by darkening the room and limiting interruptions.
3. Allow liberal visiting hours for patient's family if their presence decreases patient's agitation.
4. Ensure safety precautions as needed, e.g., bed in lowest position, side rails up, and soft restraints.
5. Orient patient to person, place, and time, as needed. Explain all procedures, using terms patient can understand. Keep clocks and calendars visible to patient.

Impaired skin integrity related to erythroderma secondary to bacterial toxins

---

Desired outcome: Patient's skin remains intact.

---

1. Moisturize skin with emollient lotion q2h. Patient may be more comfortable if the hospital gown is removed.
2. Use bath oil rather than soap for bathing patient.
3. Explain to patient that rash will heal similarly to sunburn.
4. Turn and position patient at least q2h.
5. Elevate HOB to 45 degrees if patient has facial edema.
6. If alopecia (loss of hair) occurs, explain to patient that it usually is a temporary condition. Patient also may lose nails, which grow back after several weeks.
7. Refer patient to dermatology service for unusual problems.

Knowledge deficit: Disease process and treatment

Desired outcome: Patient verbalizes knowledge of TSS, including the disease process, treatment, and measures that promote wellness.

---

1. Assess patient's and significant others' knowledge of the disease process and treatment of TSS when the critical phase of the illness is over or as soon as questions arise. Respond to the patient's and significant others' questions first, and then teach other information the patient needs for full understanding of the disease.
2. Discuss the purpose of the antistaphylococcal antibiotics.
   - *Critical phase:* Antibiotics probably do not alter the course of critical illness (the disease process results from the bacterial toxins, not the bacteria) but are used to decrease incidences of relapse. Antibiotics will be administered IV during the critical phase.
   - *Rehabilitative phase:* Following recovery, if *Staphylococcus aureus* is present on vaginal cultures, oral antibiotics are given one week prior to and during menstruation.
3. Teach patient the importance of taking all antibiotics until the prescription is finished.

4. Discuss the association of TSS with tampon use (see Rehabilitation and Patient-Family Teaching, below). Encourage patient to adopt the following practices:
  - Do not use superabsorbent tampons.
  - Change tampons at least q4h.
  - Use pads or napkins at night.
  - Wash hands before inserting or removing tampons.
  - Bathe or shower daily, with tampons removed if during menstruation.
  - Do not leave vaginal diaphragms in place for longer than 12 hours.

5. Teach patient to check for signs of suprainfection during antibiotic administration: fever, black or white-coated tongue, nausea, vomiting, diarrhea, vaginal itching, vaginal discharge. Advise patient to notify MD if signs of suprainfection occur.

6. Advise patient to check with MD regarding routine vaginal cultures to detect the presence of *Staphylococcus aureus* after hospital discharge.

7. Explain that restrictions on vaginal intercourse are not necessary.

REHABILITATION AND PATIENT-FAMILY TEACHING CONCEPTS

Give patient and significant others written and verbal instructions for the following:

1. Medications, including drug name, purpose, dosage, schedule, precautions, and potential side effects, particularly of the antibiotics.

2. If TSS was caused by vaginal infection, the importance of avoiding tampon and vaginal diaphragm use for at least 3-4 menstrual periods. If tampons are to be used in the future, patient should change them q4h and use a pad at night.

3. Possibility of recurrence, which is considerable. Tampons should not be used if vaginal cultures show *Staphylococcus aureus*.

4. Importance of removing the tampon and seeing MD immediately if patient has a fever >38.9° C (102° F).

5. Regeneration of nails and hair, which usually occurs after 4 weeks.

Burns

The skin is complex and is the largest organ of the body. It protects against infection, prevents loss of body fluids, controls body temperature, functions as an excretory and sensory organ, aids in activating vitamin D, and influences body image. Burns, the most dramatic injury that can occur to skin, are classified according to the causative agent: thermal (scald, contact, flame), electrical, chemical, and radiation. Extent and depth of the burn injury depend on the *intensity* and *duration of exposure* to the offending agent. The American Burn Association (ABA) has developed an injury severity grading system that categorizes burns as minor, moderate, and major (see Table 8-5). The ABA advocates that major burns be treated in a burn center or facility with expertise in burn care. Moderate burns usually require hospitalization, though not necessarily in a burn unit, and minor burns are often treated in the emergency room or on an out-patient basis.

Damage to the skin frequently is defined in terms of partial-thickness and full-thickness injury, which correspond to the various layers of the skin. Partial-thickness injuries are further differentiated into superficial and deep partial-thickness categories. *Superficial partial-thickness injury,* commonly referred to as "first-degree" burn, for example, sunburn, damages the epidermis, which is composed

TABLE 8-5
ABA classification system

Magnitude of burn injury	Second-degree		Third-degree adults and children %BSA	Special location	Complications, poor risk, fractures, other trauma
	Adult %BSA*	Children %BSA			
Major	>25%	>20%	>10%	+	+
Moderate	15-25%	10-20%	<10%	−	−
Minor	<15%	<10%	<2%	−	−

*BSA: body surface area

of keratinized fiber that is replenished continuously from underlying desquamated cells migrating to the superficial layer; forms a protective barrier between host and environment; and heals within 24-72 hours. *Deep partial-thickness injury,* called a "second-degree" burn, involves varying levels of the dermis, which contains structures essential to skin function (e.g., sweat and sebaceous glands, hair follicles, sensory and motor nerves, and capillary network); and heals within 3-35 days, depending on depth, because epidermal elements germinate and migrate until the epidermal surface is restored. *Full-thickness injury,* a "third-degree" burn, exposes the poorly vascularized fat layer, which contains adipose tissue, roots of sweat glands, and hair follicles; and destroys all epidermal elements. Wounds <4 cm in diameter are allowed to heal by granulation and migration of healthy epithelium from wound margins; larger wounds are closed *via* skin grafting.

ASSESSMENT

The extent of the burn wound is estimated quickly by use of the "rule of nines." For adults, each body area is assigned a percentage of surface area to establish the degree of involvement: head and neck 9%, each upper extremity 9%, anterior chest 18%, posterior chest 18%, each lower extremity 18%, and the genitalia 1%. For odd-shaped burns, the surface area of the victim's palm usually equals 1% of the total BSA. A chart that accounts for changes in the size of body parts occurring with growth is recommended for children and is the most accurate method of determining the extent of the burn.

Respiratory system: Singed nasal hairs; burns in perioral area or neck; burns of oral or pharyngeal mucous membranes; change in voice or coughing up of soot; inelastic, constricting, tight eschar of neck or chest; swelling of membranes of naso-oropharyngeal passage.

- *Clinical indicators:* Crackles (rales), rhonchi, stridor, severe hoarseness, hacking cough, labored breathing, dyspnea, tachypnea, and possible altered LOC, depending on degree of hypoxia.

< N O T E : Physical evidence of respiratory compromise may be absent in spite of marked pulmonary injury.

- *Risk factors:* History of having been burned in a confined area. Patients with preexisting cardiac or respiratory condition and those who are heavy smokers are most susceptible to respiratory complications associated with smoke inhalation.

TABLE 8-6
Factors determining burn severity

Extent	Severity dependent on intensity and duration of exposure.
Depth	Severity dependent on intensity and duration of exposure.
Age	Patients <2 years old and >60 years of age.
Medical history	Preexisting conditions such as heart disease, chronic renal failure.
Body part	Special burn areas: hands, face, eyes, ears, feet, and genitalia.
Complications	Burns with concomitant trauma (i.e., fractures).

Cutaneous system: Increased evaporative water loss and hypothermia caused by impaired skin integrity. To determine burn wound severity, see Table 8-6.
  • Clinical indicators: See Table 8-7, Characteristics of Burn Wound Depth.

< N O T E :   True depth of the burn may not manifest for several hours or up to several days post-burn injury.

Cardiovascular system: There will be third spacing of fluids with decreased circulatory volume proportional to extent and depth of injury caused by increased capillary permeability, decreased vascular colloid osmotic pressure, and a deranged capillary hydrostatic pressure. Patient may have complaints of tingling or numbness in extremities, dry mucous membranes, and thirst. In response to the burn insult, there is an increase in catecholamine, cortisol, renin-angiotensin, antidiuretic hormone, and aldosterone production as the body struggles to retain sodium and water.
  • *Clinical indicators:* Edema formation; skin temperature and color changes; decreased or absent peripheral pulses and delayed capillary refill caused by compromised blood flow occurring with circumferential burns of extremities;

TABLE 8-7
Characteristics of burn wound depth

	Partial-thickness	**Full-thickness**
Cause	Flash, flame, ultraviolet (sunburn), hot liquid or solid, chemicals, radiation.	Flame, hot liquid or solid, chemical, electrical, radiation.
Surface appearance	*Superficial:* Dry, no blisters or edema. *Deep:* Moist blebs, blisters, edema, oozing of plasma-like fluid.	Dry, leathery, eschar. Thombosed blood vessels may be visible.
Color	Cherry red to mottled white; will blanch and refill.	Ranges in color from red to khaki-colored; waxy; charred; does not blanch.
Sensation	*Superficial:* Very painful to the touch. *Deep:* Extremely sensitive to touch, temperature, and air currents.	Anesthetic to touch and temperature because of destruction of sensory nerve endings.
Healing	3-35 days.	Wounds ≥4 cm must be grafted.

elevated serum potassium (first 24-36 hours post burn) secondary to hemolysis of cells; hemoconcentration; decreased hemoglobin; tachycardia; hypotension; and decreased filling pressures (CVP, PAP, PAWP). Hair may be sparse and brittle; the eyes sunken and dull; lips cracked and dry; buccal cavity sore and inflamed; mucous membranes and conjunctiva pale; muscle tone poor. Hypoproteinuria may be present due to escape of proteins into the interstitial space. In addition, patient will have dramatically elevated basal metabolic rate with protein catabolism and increased fat mobilization from fatty acids and triglycerides, resulting in decreased body weight.

- *Risk factors:* Patients with renal disease, diabetes, or preexisting cardiac or respiratory conditions may have complications associated with fluid resuscitation therapy.

Gastrointestinal system: Paralytic ileus associated with or resulting in decreased or absent peristalsis (usually resolves within 72 hours post burn); development of Curling's ulcer (acute ulceration of stomach or duodenum), a common life-threatening complication in burn patients, which is associated with a gastric ph <5 and a positive guaiac stain.

- *Clinical indicators:* Absence of bowel sounds, stools, flatus; nausea and vomiting in the presence of alcohol intoxication.
- *Risk factors:* History of peptic ulcer or duodenal ulcer disease, steroid use, hypokalemia, or alcohol abuse.

Renal system: As early intravascular dehydration causes hemoconcentration and oliguria, a high myoglobin or hemoglobin load may be reflected by a dark brown "sludgy" urine. Inadequate fluid resuscitation may lead to acute tubular necrosis and acute renal failure.

- *Clinical indicators:* Urine output <30 ml/hr; dark, amber, "thick" urine; high urine specific gravity; glycosuria secondary to a decreased glucose tolerance and decreased insulin effectiveness.

In addition, assess for the following:

Wound sepsis: Evaluate for increased rapidity of eschar separation, increased amount of exudate, and isolated pockets containing purulent material, which are all suggestive of burn wound sepsis.

- *Clinical indicators:* Disappearance of well-defined burn margins; presence of edema, discoloration, superficial ulceration of burned skin at wound margin/ skin interface. Granulation tissue may become pale and boggy; focal black, dark brown, or violet areas of discoloration in the wound; partial-thickness burn may change from pink or mottled red to full-thickness necrosis (i.e., sloughing of subcutaneous fat layer); vesicular lesions may appear in healing or healed partial-thickness injury; and there may be erythematous, nodular lesions in unburned skin. In addition, there may be hemorrhagic discoloration of subeschar fat, with remaining eschar spongy and poorly demarcated; cellulitis of unburned skin (common with gram-positive invasion); turquoise-colored, sweet-smelling exudate (with *Pseudomonas* infection); changes in LOC (confusion, disorientation, agitation); labile temperature ranging from 35°-40.5° C (95°-105° F), gastric distention, and paralytic ileus.
- *Risk factors:* Concommittant injuries (e.g., fractures), long-term steroid therapy, immunosuppression, diabetes mellitus, history of cardiopulmonary disease.

DIAGNOSTIC TESTS

1. *Serial ABG's:* Will demonstrate hypoxemia and acid-base abnormalities.
2. *Carboxyhemoglobin level:* Determines presence of carbon monoxide in the blood secondary to smoke inhalation.
3. *Serial chest x-rays:* Usually normal upon admission, but changes 24-48 hours after the burn injury has occurred may be reflective of atelectasis, pulmonary edema, or acute respiratory distress.
4. *Culture and sensitivity studies:* To evaluate sputum, blood, urine, and wound tissue for evidence of infection. Burn wound sepsis is defined as microorganisms 10^5 per gram burn wound tissue with active invasion of adjacent, viable, unburned skin. Examples of gram-negative organisms that may be found include: *Pseudomonas aeruginosa, Klebsiella, Serratia, E. coli, Enterobacter cloacae.* Less frequently, gram-positive organisms (*Staphylococcus* and *Streptococcus*) and fungal organisms *(Candida* and *Aspergillus)* may be present.

< N O T E : If a burn wound culture is positive for Group A *Streptococcus,* this may signal the need for an epidemiologic investigation. Contact your facility's infection control nurse or epidemiology department for assistance in evaluating such a culture, especially if more than one patient has a positive culture at approximately the same time.

5. *Laryngoscopy and bronchoscopy:* Although not routine, may be helpful in determining presence of extramucosal carbonaceous material and the state of the mucosa (e.g., edema, denudation, erythema, blistering) in inhalation injuries.
6. *Vital capacity, tidal volume, and inspiratory force:* Performed q2-4h to evaluate respiratory status. They will demonstrate falling values with inhalation injury associated with the development of respiratory distress or failure.
7. *Urine specimen:* For urinalysis and culture and sensitivity studies. Nitrogen is measured with the return of capillary integrity (3-5 days after the burn injury) and mobilization of third-spaced fluids *via* 24-hour urine collection for total nitrogen, urea nitrogen, and amino acid nitrogen. Large amounts of nitrogen are excreted in the urine secondary to long periods of catabolism during the healing of a burn wound.
8. *Baseline bloodwork*
   * *Hematocrit:* Increased secondary to fluid shifts from intravascular space.
   * *Hemoglobin:* Decreased secondary to hemolysis.
   * *Serum sodium:* Decreased secondary to massive fluid shifts into interstitial spaces.
   * *Serum potassium:* Elevated due to cell lysis and fluid shifts into interstitial spaces.
   * *BUN:* Elevated secondary to hypovolemic status.
   * *Total protein:* Decreased secondary to leakage of plasma proteins into interstitial spaces.
   * *Creatine phosphokinase (CPK):* Evaluated as an index of muscle damage, so it is particularly important in electrical injuries. The higher the CPK, the more extensive the muscle damage.
9. *EKG:* For baseline evaluation of patient's cardiac status and for comparison should changes occur.

MEDICAL MANAGEMENT

1. **Humidified oxygen therapy:** Treats hypoxemia and prevents drying and sloughing of the mucosal lining of the tracheobronchial tree.
2. **Intubation and mechanical ventilation:** As indicated for respiratory distress. Because laryngeal edema resolves in 3-5 days, tracheostomy is avoided for upper airway distress.
3. **Bronchodilators and mucolytic agents:** Aid in the removal of secretions.
4. **Escharotomy** (surgical incision through the eschar or fascia): Relieves respiratory distress secondary to circumferential, full-thickness burns of neck and trunk, or in extremities to lessen pressure from underlying edema and restore adequate perfusion. It may be done at the bedside or in the emergency room. Indications for escharotomy include cyanosis of distal unburned skin, delayed capillary filling, progressive neurologic changes (may mimic compartment syndrome), burns of thorax that restrict respiratory motion, and weak or absent peripheral pulses.
5. **Fluid resuscitation therapy:** IV fluids (usually lactated Ringer's solution or normal saline) are delivered *via* a large-bore catheter at a high rate of flow to maintain urine output at a minimum of 30-50 ml/hour. Colloids are avoided during the first 24 hours post burn because they can increase edema formation during this period of increased capillary permeability.
6. **In-dwelling urinary catheter:** Enables accurate measurement of urine output.
7. **Nasogastric suction:** Allows aspiration of gastric contents secondary to paralytic ileus in patients with a ≥30% BSA burn or for those who present with alcohol intoxication.
8. **Tetanus-toxoid prophylaxis:** Given IM to combat *Clostridium tetani,* an anaerobic infection.
9. **Morphine sulphate:** Small doses are given IV for comfort.

< N O T E :   All medications, except for tetanus-toxoid, are administered IV to avoid sequestration of medication, which would then "flood" the vascular system with the return of capillary integrity and the diuresis of third-spaced fluids.

10. **Antacid administration:** Maintains gastric pH >5.0 and prevents development of Curling's ulcer.
11. **High-protein/high-calorie diet:** Achieves nitrogen balance for optimal wound healing. Many formulas are available to determine nutritional requirements and are based on preburn body weight in kilograms, total body surface area burned (TBSA), age, sex, and basal metabolic rate. Patients unable to meet nutritional requirements for healing *via* the enteral route are started on total parenteral nutrition (TPN) by a central line.

< N O T E :   Nutritional deficiencies generally are not apparent initially unless the patient was malnourished preinjury.

12. **Multivitamin and mineral supplements:** Vitamins A and C and zinc are especially important for promoting wound healing.
13. **IV antibiotics:** As indicated for specific culture and sensitivity findings.
14. **Wound care:** Cleansing, debridement (manual or surgical), and antimicrobial therapy (i.e., topical agents: silvadene, povidone iodine, mafenide, silver nitrate, proteolytic enzymes) control bacterial proliferation and provide a wound capable of producing granulation tissue and a capillary network.

15. Split-thickness skin grafting: Provides closure for full-thickness injuries. Biologic dressings such as cadaver skin or porcine or amniotic membranes may be utilized for temporary closure prior to autografting.

NURSING DIAGNOSES AND INTERVENTIONS

Impaired gas exchange related to hypoventilation and decreased diffusion of oxygen secondary to circumferential burns to neck and thorax or swelling of the membranes of the naso-oropharyngeal passage due to smoke inhalation

Desired outcome: Patient exhibits adequate gas exchange as evidenced by PaO_2 ≥80 mm Hg; oxygen saturation ≥95%; RR 12-20 breaths/min with a normal pattern and depth (eupnea); absence of adventitious breath sounds and other clinical indicators of respiratory dysfunction; and orientation to person, place, and time.

1. Assess and document respiratory status qh, noting rate and depth, breath sounds, and LOC. Be alert to a declining respiratory status as evidenced by crackles (rales), rhonchi, stridor, severe hoarseness, hacking cough, labored breathing, dyspnea, tachypnea, restlessness, and decreasing LOC. Notify MD promptly of all significant findings.
2. Monitor serial ABGs for decreasing PaO_2 and oxygen saturation as evidence of worsening hypoxemia. Also be alert to gradually declining values in vital capacity, tidal volume, and inspiratory force.
3. Place patient in high-Fowler's position to enhance respiratory excursion. Reposition patient from side to side q1-2h to help mobilize secretions and prevent atelectasis.
4. Teach patient the necessity of coughing and deep-breathing exercises q2h, including incentive spirometry.
5. Monitor for indicators of upper airway distress (e.g., severe hoarseness, stridor, dyspnea, and less frequently, CNS depression) and lower airway distress (e.g., crackles, rhonchi, hacking cough, and labored or rapid breathing). Report significant findings promptly.
6. Administer oxygen therapy, mechanical ventilation, or bronchodilator treatment (i.e., theophylline, sympathomimetics) as prescribed.
7. As prescribed, administer percussion and postural drainage to facilitate airway clearance (this is contraindicated with fresh skin grafts).
8. Perform oropharyngeal or endotracheal suctioning as indicated by the presence of adventitious breath sounds.

Fluid volume deficit related to decreased circulating volume secondary to leakage of fluid, plasma proteins, and other cellular elements into the interstitial space and loss through the burn wound

Desired outcomes: Patient's circulating volume is restored without signs of fluid overload or excessive edema formation as evidenced by BP 110-120/70-80 mm Hg (or within patient's normal range), peripheral pulses >2+ (on a 0-4+ scale), urine output 30-50 ml/hr, and urine specific gravity 1.010-1.030. Hematocrit is 40%-

54% (male) or 37%-47% (female); hemoglobin is 14-18 g/dl (male) or 12-16 g/dl (female); serum sodium is 137-147 mEq/L; and serum potassium is 3.5-5.5 mEq/L.

1. Monitor patient for evidence of fluid volume deficit, including tachycardia, decreased BP, decreased amplitude of peripheral pulses, urine output <30 ml/hr, thirst, and dry mucous membranes.
2. Monitor I&O; administer fluid therapy as prescribed, titrating hourly infusion to maintain urine output at a minimum of 30-50 ml/hour.
3. Monitor weight daily; report significant gains or losses. For example, 2 kg acute weight loss may signal a 2 L fluid loss. However, weight loss also may be due to catabolism and an increased metabolic rate as the body attempts to heal itself.
4. Monitor urine specific gravity. As fluid resuscitation occurs, urine specific gravity will become normal, reflecting a normovolemic status; conversely, an elevated value occurs with a dehyrated state and a decreased value reflects an overhydrated state.
5. Monitor serial hematocrit, hemoglobin, serum sodium, and serum potassium values. As the circulating volume is restored, the hematocrit decreases to within normal limits. Hemoglobin values may decrease secondary to hemolysis within the first 1-2 hours post burn. Transfusions with packed red blood cells generally are required by day five post burn. Usually, potassium is elevated during the first 24-36 hours post burn due to hemolysis and the lysis of cells. After 72-96 hours, hypokalemia may be seen as cell membranes regain their integrity and the patient experiences diuresis. At this point, it may be necessary to add potassium to the IV solutions. Notify MD of significant findings.
6. Monitor patient for evidence of fluid volume excess secondary to rapid fluid resuscitation, especially in patients with preexisting respiratory or cardiac disease. Be alert to urine output >50 ml/hr, crackles (rales), SOB, and tachypnea.
7. Confer with MD regarding use of mannitol in the presence of myoglobinuria to "flush" the kidney tubules. All other diuretics are avoided because they further deplete an already compromised intravascular volume, aggravating the shock state.
8. With the onset of spontaneous diuresis, decrease infusion rates by 25% for one hour if the urine output is 30-50 ml/hr for two consecutive hours. Repeat the reduction, or as prescribed.

Alteration in bowel elimination related to decreased peristalsis secondary to paralytic ileus

---

Desired outcomes: Bowel sounds are auscultated within 48-72 hours postburn and patient demonstrates bowel elimination within patient's normal pattern.

---

1. Monitor bowel sounds q2h. Be alert to an absence of bowel sounds, which occurs with paralytic ileus.
2. During period of absent bowel sounds maintain NG tube to intermittent low suction as prescribed.
3. Maintain NPO status until return of bowel sounds. Provide mouth care at frequent intervals.

Potential for injury related to risk of development of gastric (Curling's) ulcer secondary to gastric pH <5

Desired outcome: Patient's gastric pH tests >5 and gastric aspirate is negative for blood.

< N O T E :   After return of bowel sounds, any major trauma victim is at high risk for development of gastric ulcers. In the burn patient acute ulceration of the stomach and duodenum is called Curling's ulcer.

1. Monitor gastric pH q2h. Administer antacids as prescribed to maintain pH >5.0.
2. Administer oral or IV H_2 receptor blocking agents q2-4h or as prescribed to prevent formation of gastric acids.
3. Test gastric aspirate for blood q8h. Promptly report presence of blood to MD.

Impaired tissue and skin integrity related to damage to epidermal elements secondary to burn injury

---

Desired outcomes: Patient's wound exhibits evidence of granulation and healing by primary intention or split-thickness skin grafting within an acceptable time frame. Tissue perfusion in burned extremities is adequate as evidenced by peripheral pulses >2+ (on a scale of 0-4+), brisk capillary refill (<3 seconds), and skin temperature warm to the touch.

---

1. Assess and document time and circumstances of burn injury, as well as extent and depth of burn wound. See Tables 8-6 and 8-7, p. 457.
2. In burned extremities, evaluate tissue perfusion by monitoring capillary refill, temperature, and peripheral pulses qh. Be alert to signs of decreased peripheral perfusion, including coolness of the extremity, weak or absent peripheral pulses (≤2+), and delayed capillary refill (>4 seconds). Report significant findings to MD.
3. Cleanse and debride wound as prescribed. Control ambient temperature carefully to prevent hypothermia.
4. Apply topical antimicrobial treatments as prescribed, using aseptic technique.
5. Elevate burned extremities above heart level to promote venous return and prevent excessive dependent edema formation.
6. To prevent pooling of fluid or seroma formation, which contribute to graft loss, express fluid between graft and recipient bed as prescribed by using a rolling motion with sterile applicators. Always roll the applicator in the same direction over the graft to prevent disruption of graft "take." If prescribed, aspirate hematomas or seromas with a tuberculin syringe and 26-gauge needle. This also is done to prevent pooling of fluids.
7. Monitor type and amount of drainage from wounds. Promptly report the presence of bright red bleeding, which would inhibit graft "take," and purulent exudate, which is indicative of infection.
8. Maintain immobility of grafted site for 3 days or as prescribed. This is

achieved with a combination of positioning, splinting, or light pressure and sedation. In some instances, restraints, stents, bulky dressings, or occlusive dressings may be required to maintain immobilization and promote hemostasis of graft.

9. Elevate grafted extremity above heart level to promote venous return and decrease pooling of blood and plasma.
10. Apply elastic wraps to grafted legs to promote venous return.
11. Utilize bed cradle to prevent bedding from coming into contact with open grafted area.
12. Provide donor site care as prescribed and be alert to signs of donor site infection.

Potential impairment of physical mobility related to risk of contracture formation secondary to immobilization from pain, splints, or scar formation

---

Desired outcome: Patient displays complete range of motion without verbal or nonverbal indicators of discomfort.

---

1. Provide ROM exercises q4h. When possible, combine with hydrotherapy in a Hubbard tank.
2. Apply splints as recommended by physical therapy to maintain body parts in functional positions and prevent contracture formation.
3. For graft patient, institute ROM exercises and ambulation on tenth day post-graft, or as prescribed.

Potential for infection related to vulnerability secondary to bacterial proliferation in burn wounds, presence of invasive lines or urinary catheter, and immunocompromised status

---

Desired outcome: Patient is free of infection as evidenced by normothermia, WBC count <11,000 µl, negative cultures, well defined burn wound margin, and absence of pockets containing purulent matter and other clinical indicators of burn wound infection.

---

1. Except for eyebrows, shave all hair within 2 inches of wound margin to prevent contamination of wound.
2. Monitor temperature q2h. Report temperatures >38.9° C (102° F).
3. Assess burn wound daily for status of eschar separation and granulation tissue formation, color, vascularity, sensation, and odor. Be alert to signs of infection, including fever, elevated WBC count, rapid eschar separation, increased amount of exudate, pockets containing purulent material, disappearance of a well-defined burn margin with edema formation, wound discoloration (e.g., black or dark brown), change in color of partial-thickness burn from pink or mottled red to full-thickness necrosis, superficial ulceration of burned skin at wound margins, pale and boggy granulation tissue, hemorrhagic discoloration of subeschar fat, spongy and poorly demarcated eschar. Report significant findings promptly.

4. Assess appearance of grafted site, including adherence to recipient bed, appearance, and color. Be alert to erythema, hyperthermia, increasing tenderness, purulent drainage, and swelling around the grafted site.
5. Observe for clinical indicators of sepsis: tachypnea, hypothermia, hyperthermia, ileus, subtle disorientation, unexplained metabolic acidosis, and glucose intolerance, as evidenced by glycosuria and elevated blood sugar levels. For more information, see "Sepsis," p. 433.
6. As prescribed, obtain wound, blood, sputum, and urine cultures in the presence of a temperature >38.9° C (102° F).
7. Administer systemic antibiotics and antipyretics as prescribed.
8. Ensure aseptic technique when administering care to burned areas and performing invasive techniques.
9. Place patients with burns >30% BSA in protective isolation.
10. For patients with skin grafts, monitor donor site for evidence of infection.

Alteration in nutrition: Less than body requirements of protein, vitamins, and calories related to hypermetabolic state secondary to burn wound healing

---

Desired outcome: Patient has adequate nutrition as evidenced by stable weights, balanced nitrogen state per nitrogen studies, serum albumin ≥3.5 g/dl, thyroxine-binding prealbumin 200-300 μg/ml, retinol-binding protein 40-50 μg/ml, and evidence of burn wound healing and graft "take" within an acceptable time frame.

---

1. Record all intake for daily calorie counts. Measure weight daily and evaluate based on patient's preburn weight.
2. Monitor serum albumin, thyroxine-binding prealbumin, retinol-binding protein, and urine nitrogen measurements. Burn victims undergo long periods of catabolism, with large amounts of nitrogen excreted in the urine. Serum values will be decreased from normal. Be alert to continuing deficiencies, weight loss, and poor graft "take," all of which are signals that nutritional needs are not being met.
3. Provide high-protein, high-calorie diet. When patient can take foods orally, promote supplemental feedings of milkshakes, ice cream, etc. between meals.
4. Confer with MD regarding need for enteral feedings in patients with burns >10% BSA, preinjury illness, or associated injuries, as they have calorie requirements that cannot be met orally. Patients with ileus that persists for more than 4 days or those unable to meet caloric needs enterally will require TPN as prescribed by MD.

Alteration in comfort: Pain related to exposed sensory nerve endings secondary to burn injury

---

Desired outcome: Patient expresses relief of or decrease in degree of pain and does not exhibit signs of uncontrolled discomfort.

---

1. Assess patient's level of discomfort at frequent intervals. Patients with partial-thickness burns may experience severe pain because of exposure of sensory

nerve endings. Be aware that pain tolerance decreases with prolonged hospitalization and sleep deprivation.

2. Monitor patient for clinical indicators of pain: increased BP, tachypnea, dilated pupils (unless patient has received narcotic analgesia), shivering, rigid muscle tone, or guarded position.

3. Administer narcotic analgesia or tranquilizers as prescribed and at least 20-30 minutes before painful procedures.

4. Provide a full explanation of procedures and honest feedback, using a calm, organized, and firm manner.

5. Employ nonpharmacologic interventions as indicated: relaxation breathing, guided imagery, soft music.

6. Ensure that patient receives periods of uninterrupted sleep (optimally 90 minutes at a time) by grouping care procedures when possible and limiting visitors.

Sensory-perceptual alterations related to tactile and visual deficits, medications, sleep-pattern disturbance, or pain secondary to severe burn injury

---

Desired outcomes: Patient verbalizes orientation to person, place, and time and describes rationale for necessary treatments.

---

1. Assess patient's orientation to person, place, and time.

2. Answer patient's questions simply and succinctly, providing information regarding immediate surroundings, procedures, and treatments. During the emergent phase of the burn injury, anticipate the necessity of having to repeat information at frequent intervals.

3. For patient with full-thickness injury, explain why tactile sensation is decreased or absent and that it will return with eschar separation and debridement.

4. If patient's eyelids are swollen shut due to facial edema, reassure patient that he or she is not blind and that swelling will resolve within 4-5 days.

5. Touch patient often on unburned skin to provide nonpainful tactile stimulation.

6. For more information, see the same nursing diagnosis in ''Caring for the Critically Ill with Life-Threatening Disorders,'' p. 513.

For other nursing diagnoses and interventions, see the following, as appropriate: ''Management of the Adult on Mechanical Ventilation,'' pp. 66-70; ''Providing Nutritional Support,'' pp. 490-505; ''Caring for the Critically Ill on Prolonged Bed Rest,'' pp. 506-511; ''Caring for the Critically Ill with Life-Threatening Disorders,'' pp. 511-522; and ''Caring for the Family of the Critically Ill,'' pp. 522-526.

REHABILITATION AND PATIENT-FAMILY TEACHING CONCEPTS

Burn patients admitted to the intensive care unit usually are hospitalized for a prolonged period of time. Patient and family teaching efforts are directed toward the rehabilitative phases. Give patient and significant others verbal and written instructions for the following:

1. Splinting and exercise program for contracture prevention, as directed by physical therapist. Teach patient and significant others to monitor for pain or pressure

due to improperly applied splint and to assess splinted extremity for coolness, pallor, cyanosis, decreased pulses, and impaired function.

2. Skin care
   - Explain that a lubricating cream without alcohol (e.g., Nivea) should be applied several times a day and after bathing to promote soft and pliant skin and assist with control of pruritus.
   - Explain that dressings or padding should be applied to areas that may be traumatized by pressure.
   - Teach patient to avoid exposure to sun, as healed skin is highly sensitive to ultraviolet rays for up to a year.
   - Explain to black patient that permanent pigmentation changes are likely due to destruction of melanocytes and that burned areas usually will stay pink.
   - Wound care: Provide simplified dressing change procedure; explain indicators of infection and importance of notifying MD should they appear.
   - Teach patient the importance of wearing pressure garment as prescribed to prevent excessive or hypertrophic scarring.
3. Nutrition: Explain the importance of maintaining an adequate intake of protein and calories for optimal wound healing.
4. Medications, including drug name, purpose, dosage, schedule, precautions, and potential side effects.
5. Home care and the importance of counseling to provide support for adjustment to life outside the hospital environment following disfiguring injury.
6. Importance of follow-up care; confirm date and time of first appointment if it has been established.

Compartment syndrome (ischemic myositis)

Compartment syndrome is defined as increased pressure within an anatomic compartment, which compromises function and circulation to the tissues within the compartment. It is a surgical emergency that requires rapid intervention to prevent permanent cosmetic or functional deformity or loss of limb. Although compartment syndrome most commonly follows fractures, especially those of the tibia and fibula, it can occur from a variety of conditions (see Table 8-8).

As compartmental tissue pressure increases, it compromises capillary blood flow. Unremitting pressure results in tissue injury, which causes the release of histamine, producing vasodilatation and increased capillary permeability. Dilated blood vessels and loss of fluids and proteins through the more permeable capillaries contribute to higher tissue pressures. These higher pressures eventually exceed capillary pressure, and ultimately, exceed venous pressure, which in turn promotes further tissue ischemia. Tissue ischemia results in the release of more histamine, which exacerbates the problem. As a result of impaired venous return, anaerobic metabolism creates more lactic acid, which stimulates vasodilatation, increases BP, and elevates tissue pressure even further. As this cycle continues, ischemic tissue begins to necrose, resulting in permanent tissue changes.

The average onset between the initial injury to the compartment and the beginning symptoms of compartment syndrome is two hours. Compartmental tissue ischemia exceeding 6 hours results in tissue necrosis and irreversible tissue changes. Neurologic injury begins within 30 minutes of inadequate blood supply and becomes irreversible after 12-24 hours.

TABLE 8-8
Etiology of compartment syndrome

Localized compartmental trauma	Tissue reaction/edema formation
Fractures	Prolonged use of operative tourniquets
Surgery	Arterial or venous obstruction
Hematoma	Limb reimplantation
Venomous bites (snake, spider)	Thermal injury (especially when circumferential)
Vascular injury	Excessive exercise (e.g., March gangrene)
Coagulation defects	**Other**
Hemophilia	Compression during obtundness (anesthesia,
Anticoagulant therapy	drug overdose)
	Infiltrated IV therapy
	Muscle hypertrophy (e.g., shin splints)

< S O U R C E : Callahan (1985)

ASSESSMENT

Early indicators: Excruciating pain is the cardinal finding. Passive motion of the involved muscle group (*via* passive extension of the digits) increases the pain significantly. Tissue pressures >8 mm Hg are considered significantly elevated above the normal 0-4 mm Hg.

Late indicators: If compartment syndrome is left untreated, the necrosed muscle becomes fibrosed and contracted, resulting in a functionally useless compartment (e.g., Volkmann's ischemic contracture), which drastically effects function of the involved limb.

Physical assessment

- *Muscle involvement:* Inability to control pain with normal amounts of narcotics in any patient at risk of compartment syndrome requires closer physical assessment. Pain on passive extension of the digits is an early finding indicative of muscle tissue involvement.
- *Neurovascular involvement:* Increasing extremity circumference, sluggish capillary refill, and tautness over tissue compartments are signs of early neurovascular involvement. Eventually, all neurovascular structures traversing the involved compartment will show deficit, although noncompartmental neurovascular structures remain uninvolved until the majority of the compartment has been affected. Late findings include the **six P's** mnemonic: pain (increased with pressure applied over the compartment and passive movement of the digits), pallor, polar (coolness), pulselessness, paresthesia, and paralysis.

History and risk factors: Any patient with a peripheral injury listed in Table 8-8 is at risk. Patients undergoing IV therapy and those with circumferential casts or dressings are at risk for iatrogenic compartment syndrome.

DIAGNOSTIC TESTS

1. *Intracompartmental pressure monitoring:* Although simple needle manometers may be used to measure compartment tissue pressures, they are subject to obstruction from muscle tissue and are inappropriate for continuous monitoring. Wick or slit catheters allow continuous pressure monitoring *via* fluid-filled catheters, pressure transducers, and arterial pressure monitors. Compartmental pressures exceeding continuous readings of 30 mm Hg or intermittent readings ≥40

mm Hg require immediate surgical intervention, regardless of distal pulses.

2. *Arteriorgrams and venograms:* Radiologic examination of blood vessels may be done when embolus, thrombus, or other vascular injury is suspected.

MEDICAL MANAGEMENT

1. **Release of external pressure:** Loosening or removing circumferential casts or dressings; escharotomy for circumferential burns or frostbite.
2. **Analgesia, elevation to improve venous return, and ice for vasoconstriction:** Early interventions for initial indicators of compartment syndrome.
3. **Fasciotomy of myofascial compartment:** Imperative for strongly suspected compartment syndrome to permit unrestricted swelling. After a few days, the fasciotomy is closed primarily; skin grafting may be needed to ensure complete covering of the exposed compartment.
4. **Compartment syndrome caused by vascular injury:** Requires exploration of the involved vessel to facilitate application of papavarine, injection of a bolus of fluid to regain normal internal artery dynamics, and repair of lacerations or resection of involved vessels.

NURSING DIAGNOSES AND INTERVENTIONS

Potential alteration in tissue perfusion: Compartment tissues, related to impaired circulation secondary to developing or recurring compartment syndrome

---

Desired outcomes: Patient has adequate perfusion to compartment tissues as evidenced by brisk (<3 seconds) capillary refill; peripheral pulses >2+ on a 0-4+ scale; normal tissue pressures (0-4 mm Hg); and absence of edema, tautness, and the mnemonic six P's over the compartment. Patient verbalizes understanding of the importance of reporting symptoms indicative of impaired neurovascular status.

---

1. Monitor neurovascular status of injured extremity with each VS check (at least q2h). Monitor for the mnemonic **six P's:** pain (especially on passive digital movement and with pressure over the compartment), paresthesia, paralysis, polar, pallor, and pulselessness. Also assess for sluggish capillary refill, increasing limb edema, and tautness over individual compartments.
2. Report deficits in neurovascular status promptly. Elevate the extremity, apply ice, and loosen circumferential dressings as appropriate.
3. Teach patient the symptoms that necessitate prompt reporting: increasing pain, paresthesia (diminished sensation, hyperesthesia, or anesthesia), paralysis, and coolness.
4. Monitor tissue pressures on a continuous basis if an intracompartmental pressure device is present. Alert MD to pressures higher than normal. Be aware that pressures >8 mm Hg are considered significantly elevated above normal.

Alteration in comfort: Pain related to tissue ischemia secondary to compartment syndrome

---

Desired outcomes: Patient verbalizes that pain has been controlled and does not exhibit signs of uncontrolled discomfort. Patient verbalizes understanding of the need to report uncontrolled or increasing pain.

---

1. Assess the patient's complaints of pain for onset, duration, progression, and intensity, rating the pain as ''1'' for minor to ''10'' for unbearable.
2. Determine if passive stretching of digits and pressure over limb compartments increase the pain, as both are likely with compartment syndrome.
3. Adjust the medication regimen to the patient's needs; document medication effectiveness.
4. Elevate patient's extremity; prevent pressure on involved compartment and neurovascular structures.
5. If patient has had a fasciotomy, be aware that if the pain does not subside following this procedure, it could be indicative of an incomplete fasciotomy. Pain that increases several days following a fasciotomy may signal compartmental infection.
6. Continue to monitor neurovascular function with each VS check to assess for recurring compartment syndrome or infection.

Potential for infection related to vulnerability secondary to necrotic tissue, wide compartmental fasciotomy, and open wound

---

Desired outcome: Patient is free of infection as evidenced by normothermia, WBC count ≤11,000 μl, erythrocyte sedimentation rate (ESR) ≤20 mm/h (women) or ≤15 mm/h (men), and absence of wound erythema and other clinical indicators of infection.

---

1. Monitor patient for fever, increasing pain, and laboratory data indicative of infection (e.g., increased WBC count, increased ESR).
2. Assess exposed wounds and dressings for erythema, increasing wound drainage, purulent wound drainage, increasing wound circumference, edema, and localized tenderness.
3. Assess neurovascular structures for deficit, which can signal infection or pressure from adjacent inflamed tissues.
4. After primary closure or grafting of wound, continue to assess wound for signs of infection (see #2).
5. Be aware of and assess for chronic infection and osteomyelitis as potential complications following compartment syndrome.
6. Notify MD promptly of significant findings.

Disturbance in self-concept related to altered body image secondary to large, irregular fasciotomy wound and skin grafted scar; loss of function and cosmesis of an extremity; or amputation

---

Desired outcomes: Patient acknowledges body changes and demonstrates movement toward incorporating changes into self-concept. Patient does not exhibit maladaptive response (e.g., severe depression) to wound or functional loss.

---

1. Encourage questions about compartment syndrome, therapeutic interventions, and long-term effects.

1. Assess the patient's complaints of pain for onset, duration, progression, and intensity, rating the pain as ''1'' for minor to ''10'' for unbearable.
2. Determine if passive stretching of digits and pressure over limb compartments increase the pain, as both are likely with compartment syndrome.
3. Adjust the medication regimen to the patient's needs; document medication effectiveness.
4. Elevate patient's extremity; prevent pressure on involved compartment and neurovascular structures.
5. If patient has had a fasciotomy, be aware that if the pain does not subside following this procedure, it could be indicative of an incomplete fasciotomy. Pain that increases several days following a fasciotomy may signal compartmental infection.
6. Continue to monitor neurovascular function with each VS check to assess for recurring compartment syndrome or infection.

Potential for infection related to vulnerability secondary to necrotic tissue, wide compartmental fasciotomy, and open wound

---

Desired outcome: Patient is free of infection as evidenced by normothermia, WBC count ≤11,000 µl, erythrocyte sedimentation rate (ESR) ≤20 mm/h (women) or ≤15 mm/h (men), and absence of wound erythema and other clinical indicators of infection.

---

1. Monitor patient for fever, increasing pain, and laboratory data indicative of infection (e.g., increased WBC count, increased ESR).
2. Assess exposed wounds and dressings for erythema, increasing wound drainage, purulent wound drainage, increasing wound circumference, edema, and localized tenderness.
3. Assess neurovascular structures for deficit, which can signal infection or pressure from adjacent inflamed tissues.
4. After primary closure or grafting of wound, continue to assess wound for signs of infection (see #2).
5. Be aware of and assess for chronic infection and osteomyelitis as potential complications following compartment syndrome.
6. Notify MD promptly of significant findings.

Disturbance in self-concept related to altered body image secondary to large, irregular fasciotomy wound and skin grafted scar; loss of function and cosmesis of an extremity; or amputation

---

Desired outcomes: Patient acknowledges body changes and demonstrates movement toward incorporating changes into self-concept. Patient does not exhibit maladaptive response (e.g., severe depression) to wound or functional loss.

---

1. Encourage questions about compartment syndrome, therapeutic interventions, and long-term effects.

3. Identify and emphasize patient's strengths to facilitate adaptation to cosmetic and functional loss.

or discuss the injury.

6. If the extremity will be amputated, collaborate with MD regarding visitation by a successfully adapted amputee, who may serve as patient's role model.
7. Encourage maximum self care. Provide necessary adjunctive aids (e.g., built-up utensils, button hooks, orthotics) to facilitate independence.
8. For other interventions, see the same nursing diagnoses in the appendicized section, "Caring for the Critically Ill with Life-Threatening Disorders," pp. 511-522.

REHABILITATION AND PATIENT-FAMILY TEACHING CONCEPTS

Give patient and significant others verbal and written instructions for the following:
1. Information about compartment syndrome and ways to prevent it from occurring or recurring. Elaborate on description of patient's pain, as discussed under **Alteration in comfort:** Pain, p. 469.
2. For patients who have undergone fasciotomy, skin grafting

promptly: fever, localized warmth, increasing pain, increasing wound drainage (especially purulent drainage), swelling, and redness.
3. For patients who have undergone vessel exploration, the importance of reporting the following signs and symptoms promptly: change in the color of the extremity (i.e., paleness, duskiness, cyanosis); coolness; sluggish capillary refill; and pulselessness.
4. For patients with functional loss or amputation, the use of orthotics and adjunctive devices to facilitate self care.

Organ rejection

The major, universal problem with all types of organ transplantation is graft rejection. When the body detects the presence of a foreign substance, it mounts the defense of nonspecific inflammation and phagocytosis. The next level of immune response involves antibody-mediated (humoral immunity) and cell-mediated immunity. Both responses occur in a parallel fashion after exposure to an antigen. *Antibody-mediated immune response* is related to B-lymphocyte activity. When an antigen is encountered, the B lymphocyte enlarges, divides, and differentiates into a plasma cell that produces and secretes antigen-specific immunoglobulins, or antibodies. The formation of this antigen-antibody complex triggers off events that augment the nonspecific responses of inflammation and phagocytosis. *Cell-mediated immune response* involves T lymphocytes. A T lymphocyte recognizes a foreign antigen on the surface of the macrophage, binds to the antigen, and enlarges and produces a sensitized clone, which migrates through the body to the site of the antigen. When the sensitized T cell combines with the antigen, chemicals are released that kill foreign cells directly and act to facilitate phagocytosis and the inflammatory response. See Figure 8-3 for a flow chart that outlines this process.

TABLE 8-9
Types of acute rejection

Organ	Clinical presentation	Treatment options
Heart	Usually seen 10-14 days after transplant. Indicators include fever, anxiety, lethargy, low back pain, atrial or ventricular dysrhythmias, gallop, pericardial friction rub, jugular venous distention, hypotension, and decreased cardiac output late in rejection.	Methylprednisolone sodium succinate (500 mg-1 g) daily for 2-4 days. Antilymphocyte sera (rabbit, horse, or goat) IV for 6-14 days. Monoclonal antibody for 10-14 days. Retransplant necessary for intractable acute rejection.
Liver	Initially seen 4-10 days after transplant. Indicators include malaise; fever; abdominal discomfort; swollen, hard, tender graft; tachycardia; RUQ or flank pain; cessation of bile flow; change in color of bile from golden to a colorless fluid; jaundice; elevated PT, bilirubin, transaminase, and alkaline phosphatase.	Methylprednisolone sodium succinate (500 mg-1 g) daily for 2-4 days. Antilymphocyte sera (rabbit, horse, or goat) IV for 6-14 days. Retransplant necessary for recurrent, unresponsive rejection.
Pancreas	Time of rejection occurrence varies. Difficult to diagnose; patient may have hyperglycemia, pancreatitis, pain over graft. Open biopsy may be necessary to diagnose rejection.	Methylprednisolone sodium succinate (250 mg-1 g) daily for 2-4 days. Antilymphocyte sera (rabbit, horse, goat) IV for 6-14 days. Monoclonal antibody for 10-14 days. Retransplant for unresponsive rejection.

- *CBC:* Will show increased total lymphocyte count.
- *VS and heart sounds:* May reveal decreased stroke volume, cardiac output, cardiac tones, and BP; and presence of S_3 and S_4 sounds, pericardial friction rub, extrasystole, and crackles (rales).

2. **Liver**
   - *Serum bilirubin:* Total bilirubin will rise in relation to baseline postoperative level.
   - *Transaminase:* Will increase from baseline; may be markedly elevated early in rejection.
   - *Alkaline phosphatase:* Will increase from baseline.
   - *Prothrombin time:* Will be prolonged.
   - *CBC:* May reveal decreased platelet count and increased total lymphocyte count.

3. **Pancreas:** Open biopsy is the only means by which a definitive diagnosis can be made.
   - *Fasting and 2-hour postprandial plasma glucose:* Levels will be increased above normal ranges.
   - *Serum amylase:* Levels may be elevated, indicating presence of pancreatitis, an inconsistent marker of rejection.
   - *C-peptide (serum and urine):* Levels may be decreased.

4. **Renal:** See ''Renal Transplant,'' pp. 192-199, in the chapter ''Renal-Urinary Dysfunctions.''

MECHANISMS OF IMMUNOSUPPRESSIVE AGENTS

The following drugs may be used in various combinations for additive effect in preventing or modifying the rejection response. The goal of therapy is to achieve enough immunosuppression to prevent graft rejection, but not so much as to leave the patient in a defenseless state.

1. **Azathioprine:** Interferes with DNA synthesis and inhibits mitosis of immunologically competent cells. Cell division and proliferation occur in response to antigenic stimulation. Azathioprine affects rapidly replicating cells at an early stage of lymphocyte activation and is believed to block proliferation of helper T cells and cytotoxic T cells. Cytoxan may be used in place of Imuran when liver function is compromised.

2. **Corticosteroids:** Suppress the production of cytotoxic T-lymphocytes from noncytotoxic precursor cells. There is some evidence that steroids prevent the release of interleukin 1 and 2. Interleukin 1, released by the macrophages, promotes the differentiation of helper T cells. The release of interleukin 2 promotes differentiation of cytotoxic cells.

3. **Antilymphocyte sera (ALG or ATGAM):** The antilymphocyte antibodies in the sera are useful in the treatment of steroid resistant rejection and potent suppressors of cell-mediated immunity. They are directed against many different antigens on the surface of human lymphocytes and affect immunity *via* reduction of T lymphocytes.

4. **Monoclonal antibody (OKT-3 Orthoclone):** This homologus antibody reacts with and blocks the function of the chemical (T-3) complex on the surface of the T lymphocytes. The T-3 complex is responsible for the T lymphocyte identifying a transplanted organ as foreign and attempting to reject it. OKT-3 binds to the T-3 antigen on the surface of the T cells, enhancing phagocytosis and entrapment of the cells in the spleen and liver. The lymphocytes are removed from the circulation by this process in approximately 10-15 minutes.

5. **Cyclosporine:** Inhibits production and release of lymphokines and generation of cytotoxic and plasma cells by blocking the response of cytotoxic T lymphocytes to interleukin 2.

NURSING DIAGNOSES AND INTERVENTIONS

Anxiety and Fear related to threat of loss of transplanted organ due to rejection

---

Desired outcomes: Patient expresses concerns regarding possibility of organ loss and verbalizes accurate information about the signs and symptoms of organ rejection. Patient's fear and anxiety are controlled as evidenced by BP within patient's normal range, HR $\leq$100 bpm, and RR $\leq$20 breaths/min with normal depth and pattern (eupnea).

---

1. Encourage patient to discuss concerns and fears.
2. Assess patient's knowledge about the rejection process and the signs and symptoms that occur.
3. Use short, simple sentences to explain patient's current organ function and the signs and symptoms of organ rejection (see description in Table 8-9, p. 473).
4. Reassure patient that appropriate medications are being given to prevent ongoing rejection. Review medication names, dosage, and action (see above).

5. Explain to patient that rejection does not necessarily mean organ loss. Under most circumstances, rejection can be reversed.
6. Reassure patient that retransplant is a viable option if organ loss occurs.
7. For other interventions related to fear, see the same nursing diagnosis in the appendicized section, "Caring for the Critically Ill with Life-Threatening Disorders," p. 515.

Potential fluid volume excess: Edema related to retention secondary to diminished organ function during a rejection episode

Desired outcome: Patient is normovolemic as evidenced by stable weights, urine output ≥30 ml/hr, BP within patient's normal range, HR 60-100 bpm, RR 12-20 breaths/min with normal depth and pattern (eupnea), and absence of edema, crackles, and other clinical indicators of fluid overload.

1. Measure weight daily. Remember that a 1 kg weight gain can signal approximately 1 liter of fluid retention.
2. Measure I&O q1-2h; note 24-hour trends.
3. Assess BP, pulse, and respirations q1-2h. Be alert to increased BP, tachycardia, and tachypnea, which are indicators of fluid overload.
4. Auscultate for the presence of crackles (rales) and pericardial friction rub at least q8h.
5. Assess and document the presence of peripheral, sacral, and periorbital edema on a scale of 1+ to 4+.
6. Notify MD promptly of any significant findings.

Powerlessness related to actual and perceived inability to control organ rejection episodes

Desired outcome: Patient relates that he or she can control aspects of daily care as well as assume responsibility for taking medications appropriately and obtaining follow-up care.

1. Encourage patient to express feelings of frustration and powerlessness regarding organ rejection.
2. Enable and encourage patient to participate in decisions about care routines. Help patient identify areas of the care plan he or she can control, such as timing of morning care or initiating rest periods.
3. Reinforce that taking medications appropriately and keeping appointments for follow-up care *are* within patient's control and are significant in the prevention of rejection and organ destruction.
4. Solicit comments and opinions from patient. Honor patient's opinions and preferences.
5. For other interventions, see the same nursing diagnosis in the appendicized section, "Caring for the Critically Ill with Life-Threatening Disorders," p. 518.

Disturbance in self-concept related to body image changes secondary to side effects from immunosuppressive medications

---

Desired outcome: Patient verbalizes understanding of body changes that may occur with immunosuppression medications, along with interventions that can be made to minimize their effect on body image.

---

1. Identify body changes associated with steroid therapy: profuse diaphoresis, changes in fat distribution, moon facies, acne, bruising.
   - Suggest that patient try different brands of deodorants or talcs to help counteract the odor from profuse diaphoresis and to wear cotton clothing, which absorbs perspiration.
   - Suggest that to minimize the effects of facial swelling, female patient apply makeup that highlights the eyes.
   - Suggest that patient refrain from wearing prints and stripes, which may increase attention to fat distribution in the trunk area.
   - Advise patient to use facial astringents to keep skin clean and minimize acne.
   - Suggest that patient wear long sleeves and slacks to cover bruised arms and legs.
2. Teach patient body changes that are associated with cyclosporine: hirsutism, gum hyperplasia.
   - Suggest that female patient use facial depilatories.
   - Teach patient to use a soft-bristled toothbrush and mouth wash for frequent, gentle mouth care.
3. For other interventions related to disturbance in body image, see the appendicized section, "Caring for the Critically Ill with Life-Threatening Disorders," p. 520.

See "Renal Transplant" for the following: **Knowledge deficit:** Immunosuppressive medications and their side effects, p. 195; **Potential for infection** secondary to immunosuppression, p. 197; **Potential alteration in oral mucous membrane** secondary to immunosuppression, p. 198; and **Impaired skin integrity** secondary to immunosuppression with corticosteroids, p. 198. For other nursing diagnoses and interventions, see the following as appropriate: "Caring for the Critically Ill on Prolonged Bed Rest," pp. 506-511; "Caring for the Critically Ill with Life-Threatening Disorders," pp. 511-522; and "Caring for the Family of the Critically Ill," pp. 522-526.

REHABILITATION AND PATIENT-FAMILY TEACHING CONCEPTS

Give patient and significant others verbal and written instructions for the following:

1. Major indicators of organ rejection (see p. 473). Emphasize those indicators that necessitate immediate medical attention: SOB caused by fluid accumulation in the lungs, pain over transplant site, temperature >37.8° C (100° F), and hyperglycemia (for pancreatic transplant patients). Teach pancreatic transplant patient to check blood sugar levels at home and to call MD for results ≥200.
2. Medications, including name, purpose, dosage, side effects, and precautions (see p. 474).

3. Contact groups for support, for example, local Heart Association, Kidney Association, and Diabetes Association. In addition, local transplant centers have information regarding patient support groups.

Acquired immune deficiency syndrome

Acquired immune deficiency syndrome (AIDS) is characterized by a disruption of cellular mediated immunity and is manifested by opportunistic infections (e.g., *Pneumocystis carinii*) or Kaposi's sarcoma in an individual less than 60 years of age who has no other known cause for immunosuppression. Typically, there is an inverted T-helper/T-suppressor ratio. T lymphocytes, which include both T-helper and T-suppressor cells, are part of the body's cellular immune system. Helper cells stimulate the B cells to produce antibodies to foreign antigens. Suppressor cells inhibit the action of the helper cells and thereby impede antibody formation.

The three confirmed routes of transmission are the bloodstream (e.g., *via* IV drug abuse or blood transfusion), intimate sexual contact during which an exchange of body fluids occurs, and perinatally. Transmission of the virus from females to males is through vaginal secretions; however, female transmission to offspring is *via* the circulatory system (i.e., the umbilical cord). It is estimated that the average time span between exposure and infection (transmission of the HIV virus) and seroconversion (development of antibodies to the virus) is 6-8 weeks. However, the time span between exposure and symptomatic infection (clinical disease) is in the range of 5-7 years. In addition, it must be assumed that anyone who has antibodies to the virus is infectious and potentially capable of transmitting the virus.

The proportion of infected persons who are diagnosed with AIDS is quite small (probably less than 10%, see Figure 8-4), but the potential for infected individuals to become symptomatic is ever-present. The Centers for Disease Control (CDC) has projected that 20-30% of those infected with the AIDS virus will develop an

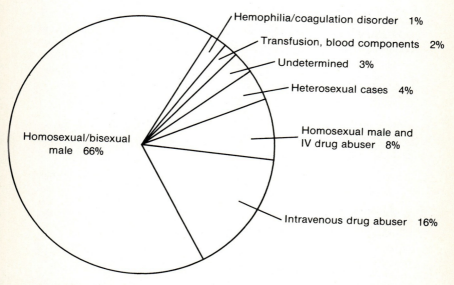

FIG. 8-4. Approximate proportions of cases within each HIV classification.

illness that fits an accepted definition of AIDS within five years. As more data become available, this projection probably will increase. It is estimated that by the end of 1991, there will have been a cumulative total of more than 270,000 cases of AIDS in the United States, with 179,000 of these cases resulting in death. The majority of persons with AIDS (66%) have been identified as homosexual or bisexual males. Other individuals at risk are listed in Table 8-10. The ultimate mortality rate for AIDS is 100%. Fewer than 14% of persons with AIDS have survived 3 years.

ASSESSMENT

Acute indicators: Rapid weight loss of >10% body weight, lymphadenopathy, persistent fevers, night sweats.

Chronic indicators: Opportunistic infections manifesting as follows: unexplained fatigue, unexplained and persistent diarrhea or bloody stools, skin rash, bruising, dysphagia, persistent dry cough, SOB, blurred vision, severe headaches, confusion, depression, progressive dementia, seizures.

Related condition: AIDS-related complex (ARC) is one of the stages of infection that is related to but not necessarily prodromal for AIDS. Its manifestations are less severe than those seen in AIDS patients and include persistent and enlarged lymph nodes, weight loss, night sweats, general malaise, aggressive lymphomas (e.g., squamous cell carcinoma of the tongue and rectum), idiopathic thrombocytopenic purpura (ITP), leukoplakia, and abnormal immune studies.

Physical assessment: Palpation may reveal enlarged, hard, sometimes painful lymph nodes; hepatomegaly; and splenomegaly. Assessment of the tongue, throat, and esophagus may reveal oral thrush. Inspection and palpation of the skin and mucous membranes may reveal rashes, plaques, or lesions that are brown, blue, or purple in color (Kaposi's lesions). Blood may be present on rectal exam. Auscultation may reveal a pericardial friction rub secondary to myocarditis. "Cotton-wool" spots, which may be seen on fundoscopic exam, are common with cytomegalovirus (CMV). Assessment of the respiratory system may reveal increased respiratory rate and inspiratory crackles (rales).

History and risk factors: Having multiple sexual partners; engaging in receptive anal intercourse (without condoms); rectal douching (because of damage to rectal mucosa); engaging in sexual practices that expose one to bodily secretions (e.g., blood, semen, feces) through mucosal abrasions; exposure to blood or viruses through shared IV needles; previous history of sexually transmitted diseases such as hepatitis, syphilis, or parasitic infections; and being a recipient of Factor

---

T A B L E 8 - 10
Groups at risk for contracting AIDS

Group	Percent
Homosexual/bisexual males who aren't IV drug abusers	66
IV drug users (males and females)	17
Homosexual males who also are IV drug abusers	8
Hemophiliacs/individuals with coagulation disorders	1
Heterosexuals	4
Individuals who have had transfusions/blood components	2
Undetermined	3

VIII concentrate, which may contain the blood from as many as 2500 donors, thereby increasing the exposure risk.

DIAGNOSTIC TESTS

1. *Human immunodeficiency virus (HIV):* Tests for presence of antibody to the virus that causes AIDS. A positive test confirms that the individual has been exposed to the AIDS virus, but it does not verify whether progression to active AIDS status has occurred.

2. *Lymphocyte count:* Will be decreased, secondary to the body's continual attempt to ward off viral and intracellular infections.

3. *WBC count:* Will be decreased because of the body's overwhelming attempt to ward off the infectious process.

4. *T-cell studies:* T-lymphocyte cells will be decreased due to the immune system's response to invading organism; T-helper/T-suppressor cell ratio will be inverted from its normal 2:1 ratio; there will be decreased number of natural T-killer lymphocytes; and skin test anergy will be present, signifying failure or delayed sensitivity of skin response to a clinically-induced antigen.

5. *B-cell studies:* B-lymphocyte cells, along with T-lymphocyte cells, are responsible for immunocompetency. With AIDS, there will be increased B-lymphocyte turnover and activity secondary to antigen-antibody response.

6. *Blood cultures:* Will reveal presence of polymicrobial infection due both to the invading organism (viral) and other opportunistic infections (viral, bacterial, fungal, and protozoal), which result from immune suppression by primary invading organism (see Table 8-11).

7. *Viral titers:* A positive result confirms exposure to such viral organisms as hepatitis A or B, herpes I or II, cytomegalovirus, and Epstein-Barr.

8. *VDRL:* Tests for exposure to syphilis.

9. *Chest x-rays:* Used initially to evaluate respiratory problems, such as pneumonia, presence of infiltrates, and pneumonitis.

10. *Gallium scan:* Increased uptake of gallium is seen in early interstitial pneumonia, even if chest x-ray is normal.

11. *Bronchoscopy:* To examine lungs and obtain lung tissue for culture.

12. *ABG values:* Usually reveal an increase in pH secondary to decrease in carbon dioxide.

TABLE 8-11
Opportunistic infections and organisms infecting AIDS patients

Viral	Fungal	Protozoal	Bacterial
Herpes (I and II)	*Candida*	*Pneumocystis carinii*	Syphilis
Cytomegalovirus	*Histoplasma capsulatum*	*Toxoplasma gondii*	*Neisseria gonorrhoeae*
Varicella	*Cryptococcus*	*Entamoeba histolytica*	*Shigella*
Epstein-Barr	*Coccidioidomycosis*	*Giardia lamblia*	*Salmonella*
		Cryptosporidium enteritis	*Mycobacterium avium-intracellulare*

13. *Total protein, albumin, thyroxine-binding prealbumin:* Will be decreased if patient is in a malnourished state.

14. *Complete neurologic workup:* Indicated for individuals in whom central neurologic complications are evident (e.g., encephalitis, meningitis, herpes zoster radiculitis, dementia).

MEDICAL MANAGEMENT AND SURGICAL INTERVENTIONS

Medical management is limited primarily to chemotherapeutic intervention in an attempt to arrest the progression of the disease. Currently, there is no single drug or combination of drugs that has restored immunocompetency to afflicted patients. Medical treatment is palliative.

Surgical interventions are limited to two specific instances: resection of tumors; and placement of central venous catheters to facilitate total parenteral nutrition, chemotherapy, or frequent blood drawings.

NURSING DIAGNOSES AND INTERVENTIONS

Potential for infection related to vulnerability secondary to immune system depression, malnutrition, fatigue, and side effects of chemotherapy

---

Desired outcome: Patient does not develop additional infections during hospitalization, as evidenced by no new positive cultures or biopsies.

---

1. Assess for indicators of opportunistic infections (e.g., oral thrush, herpes simplex, shigella, and Kaposi's lesions): persistent fatigue; night sweats; unexplained weight loss; enlarged lymph nodes; persistent diarrhea; persistent fever; and skin tumors that vary in size from a few mm to 2.5 cm, are dark blue or purple-brown in color, and may be located anywhere on the skin or mucous membranes.

2. Monitor laboratory data, including WBC count with differential, ESR, C-reactive protein, urinalysis, and cultures, to evaluate the course of infection. Be alert to leukopenia (WBC $<3500/mm^3$) and lymphopoenia (lymphocytes $<1500/mm^3$) and increased ESR and C-reactive protein. Typically, blood and urine cultures will show polymicrobial organisms. Notify MD of significant findings.

3. If patient is intubated, has a central line, or is catheterized, maintain strict asepsis for all invasive procedures to prevent introduction of new organisms.

4. Maintain meticulous body hygiene for patient to prevent spread of organisms from stool into abrasions or skin breaks. This is especially critical if patient has diarrhea.

5. Monitor temperature and VS q2h while patient is awake and q4h throughout the night for evidence of fever or sepsis. In addition to increased temperature, be alert to diaphoresis, confusion, decrease in LOC, increased HR, and decreased BP secondary to the vasodilatory effect of the increased body temperature. Perform a complete physical assessment at least q8h to identify changes from baseline assessment. Assess for changes in breath sounds, which may be indicative of an increasing level of infiltrates.

6. Promote pulmonary toilet by encouraging patient to engage in breathing or incentive spirometry exercises q2h during the day and q4h throughout the night; assist with postural drainage and chest physiotherapy as indicated.

7. Monitor sites of invasive procedures for signs of infection, including erythema, swelling, tenderness, and purulent exudate.
8. Enforce good handwashing techniques before contact with patient to minimize the risk of transmitting infectious organisms from staff and other patients.

Potential for infection related to risk of transmitting patient's infectious organisms to others

---

Desired outcomes: Needlestick injuries do not occur. Organisms causing infections or colonization in persons with AIDS are not transmitted to other patients or staff *via* the hands of personnel, as evidenced by normothermia, WBC count ≤11,000 μl, negative cultures, and absence of fatigue, diaphoresis, adventitious breath sounds, and other signs and symptoms of nosocomial infection.

---

1. Put on a gown when it is anticipated that clothing will become soiled with patient's bodily secretions.
2. Wear gloves at *any time* it is likely that there will be direct contact with patient's bodily secretions, mucous membranes, or nonintact skin. Keep a box of gloves at patient's bedside.
3. Wash hands well before leaving patient's room, using soap, water, and friction.
4. Wear a mask if patient is positive for active tuberculosis.
5. In situations during which there is risk of contact with patient's mucous membranes, such as during a bronchoscopy or wound irrigation, ensure that protective eyewear is worn.
6. Dispose of contaminated needles in a puncture-proof container. Do *not* attempt to recap needle prior to disposal.
7. To avoid the need for mouth-to-mouth resuscitation, keep disposable resuscitation equipment (manual resuscitator bag, mouth pieces) at patient's bedside.

Impaired gas exchange related to hyperventilation, increased oxygen requirements associated with sepsis, and decreased diffusion of oxygen secondary to pulmonary congestion

---

Desired outcome: Patient has adequate gas exchange as evidenced by Pao_2 ≥80 mm Hg, $Paco_2$ 35-45 mm Hg, pH 7.35-7.45, RR 12-20 breaths/min with normal depth and pattern (eupnea), and absence of adventitious sounds, nasal flaring, and other clinical indicators of respiratory dysfunction.

---

1. Assess patient's respiratory status q2h during patient's awake period, noting rate, rhythm, depth, and regularity of respiration. Observe for use of accessory muscles, flaring of nares, presence of adventitious sounds, cough, or cyanosis, which occur with respiratory dysfunction.
2. Monitor ABG results closely for decreased $Paco_2$ and increased pH, which can occur with hyperventilation.
3. Adjust oxygen therapy to attain optimal oxygenation, as determined by ABG values.
4. Instruct patient to report changes in cough, as well as dyspnea that increases with exertion.

5. To maintain adequate tidal volume, provide chest physiotherapy as prescribed; encourage use of incentive spirometry at frequent intervals.
6. Reposition patient q2h to help prevent stasis of lung fluids.
7. If patient is on ventilatory support, provide hyperinflation with 100% oxygen before and after suctioning to prevent suction-induced hypoxia. See section ''Management of the Adult on Mechanical Ventilation,'' pp. 61-70, for more information.
8. Obtain sputum for culture and sensitivity as indicated.
9. Group nursing activities to provide patient with uninterrupted periods of rest, optimally 90-120 minutes at a time.
10. When administering sulfa or experimental drugs for *Pneumocystis carinii,* monitor for evidence of respiratory depression, as well as other side effects, such as bone marrow suppression and hypotension.
11. To relieve mucous membrane irritation, which can predispose patient to coughing spells, deliver humidified air and oxygen to patient.
12. Administer sedatives and analgesics judiciously to help prevent or minimize respiratory depression.

Alteration in nutrition: Less than body requirements related to decreased intake and losses secondary to diarrhea and nausea associated with side effects of chemotherapy, malabsorption, anorexia, dysphagia, and fatigue

---

Desired outcome: Patient has adequate nutrition as evidenced by stable weights, serum albumin 3.5-5.5 g/dl, transferrin 180-260 mg/dl, thyroxine-binding prealbumin 200-300 μg/ml, retinol-binding protein 40-50 μg/ml, and a state of nitrogen balance or slightly positive nitrogen state as revealed by nitrogen studies.

---

1. Assess nutritional status daily, noting weight, caloric intake, and protein and albumin values. Be alert to progressive weight loss, wasting of muscle tissue, loss of skin tone, and decreases in both total protein and albumin, which can adversely affect wound healing as well as impair the patient's ability to withstand infection.
2. Provide small, frequent, high-caloric, high-protein meals, allowing sufficient time for patient to eat. Offer supplements between feedings. As a rule, these patients are kept in a slightly positive nitrogen state (following resolution of the critical phases of this illness) by ensuring daily caloric intake equal to 50 kilocalories/kg of ideal body weight with an additional 1.5 g of protein/kg. For example, a man weighing 70 kg should receive 3500 kilocalories, plus 105 g of protein per day.
3. Provide supplemental vitamins and minerals, as prescribed, to replace deficiencies.
4. To minimize anorexia and help treat stomatitis, which can occur as a side effect of chemotherapy, provide oral hygiene before and after meals.
5. If patient feels isolated socially, encourage significant others to visit at meal times and bring in patient's favorite high-calorie, high-protein foods from home.
6. If patient is nauseated, provide instructions for deep breathing and voluntary swallowing, which will help decrease stimulation of vomiting center.

7. If patient is dysphagic, encourage intake of fluids that are high in calories and protein; provide different flavors and textures for variation.
8. As prescribed, deliver isotonic tube feeding for patients unable to eat. Isotonic fluids will help prevent diarrhea associated with hyper- or hypotonic fluids. Check placement of NG tube before each feeding; assess absorption by evaluating amount of residual feeding q4h. Do not deliver feeding if residual is >100 ml. Keep HOB elevated 30 degrees while feeding and position patient in a right side-lying position to facilitate gastric emptying.
9. If patient's caloric intake is insufficient, discuss the potential need for total parenteral nutrition with MD.

Alterations in bowel elimination: Diarrhea, related to gastrointestinal infection, chemotherapy, or tube feeding intolerance

---

Desired outcome: Patient has formed stools and a bowel elimination pattern that is normal for him or her.

---

1. Ensure minimal use of antidiarrheal medications, which promote intestinal concentration of infectious organism.
2. Teach patient to avoid large amounts (>300 mg/day) of caffeine, which increases peristalsis and can promote diarrhea.
3. Maintain accurate I&O records to monitor for changes in fluid volume status. Be alert to signs of hypovolemia, such as cool and clammy skin, increased HR (>100 bpm), increased RR (>20 breaths/min), and decreased urinary output (<30 ml/hr). If patient is monitored hemodynamically, watch for a decrease in CO (<4 L/min), an increase in SVR (>1200 dynes/sec/cm^{-5}), and a decreased CVP (<2 mm Hg).
4. Assess stool for the presence of blood, fat, and undigested materials.
5. Monitor stool cultures for evidence of new infectious organisms.
6. Monitor patient for indicators of electrolyte imbalance, such as anxiety, confusion, muscle weakness, cramps, dysrhythmias, weak pulse, and decreased BP.
7. If patient is on tube feedings, dilute strength or decrease rate of infusion to prevent "solute drag," which may be the cause of the diarrhea.
8. Encourage foods high in potassium (see p. 228) and sodium (see p. 219) to replace any decrements of these ions.
9. Protect anorectal area by keeping it cleansed and using compounds such as zinc oxide to prevent or retard skin excoriation.

Potential impairment of skin and tissue intregity related to vulnerability secondary to cachexia and malnourishment, diarrhea, side effects of chemotherapy, Kaposi's skin lesions, negative nitrogen state, and decreased mobility due to arthralgia and fatigue

---

Desired outcome: Patient's skin and tissue remain intact.

---

1. Assess and document skin integrity, noting temperature, moisture, color, vascularity, texture, lesions, and areas of excoriation or poor wound healing. Eval-

uate Kaposi's lesions for location, dissemination, weeping, or significant changes. Note and record the presence of herpes lesions, especially those that are perirectal.

2. Avoid prolonged pressure to dependent body parts by turning and positioning patient q2h; encourage patient to change position at frequent intervals. Massage areas susceptible to breakdown (e.g., skin over bony prominences) with each position change.

3. Provide patient with an eggcrate or flotation-type mattress, as indicated.

4. Teach patient to use mild, hypoallergenic, nondrying soaps or lanolin-based products for bathing, and to pat rather than rub the skin to dry it.

5. Use soft sheets on the bed, avoiding wrinkles. If patient is incontinent, use some type of rectal device (e.g., fecal incontinence bags, rectal tube) to protect the skin and prevent perirectal excoriation and skin breakdown.

6. To enhance skin and tissue healing, assist patient toward a state of nitrogen balance by promoting adequate amounts of protein and carbohydrates (see discussion with **Alteration in nutrition**, p. 482).

7. Ensure that patient receives minimum daily requirements of vitamins and minerals; supplement them as necessary.

8. Encourage ROM and weight-bearing mobility, when possible, to increase circulation to skin and tissue.

Alteration in comfort: Pain related to prolonged immobility, side effects of chemotherapy, infections, and frequent venipunctures

---

Desired outcome: Patient verbalizes a relief in discomfort and does not exhibit signs of uncontrolled pain.

---

1. Assess and record the following: location, onset, duration, and factors that precipitate and alleviate patient's pain.

2. Provide heat or cold applications to affected areas, for example, apply heat to painful joints and cold packs to reduce swelling associated with infections or multiple venipunctures.

3. Encourage patient to engage in diversional activities as a means of increasing pain tolerance and decreasing its intensity. Examples include soothing music, quiet conversation, reading, and slow and rhythmic breathing.

4. To reduce pain intensity, teach patient techniques that decrease skeletal muscle tension, such as deep-breathing, biofeedback, and relaxation exercises (see **Knowledge deficit:** Relaxation technique effective for stress reduction and facilitation of decreased sympathetic tone, p. 99).

5. If frequent venipunctures are the cause of the patient's discomfort, discuss with MD the desirability of a capped venous catheter for long-term blood withdrawal.

6. Promote relaxation and comfort with backrubs and massage.

Activity intolerance related to weakness and fatigue secondary to fluid and electrolyte imbalance, arthralgia, myalgia, dyspnea, fever, pain, hypoxia, and effects of chemotherapy

Desired outcomes: Patient tolerates activities as evidenced by HR ≤100 bpm, RR ≤20 breaths/min, and BP within patient's normal range. Patient verbalizes the absence of fatigue and extremity weakness following activity.

1. Assess patient's tolerance to activity by assessing HR, RR, and BP prior to and immediately after activity. Be alert to increased fatigue, such as extremity weakness following periods of activity.
2. Plan adequate (90-120 minute) rest periods between patient's scheduled activities. Adjust activities, as appropriate, to reduce energy expenditures.
3. As much as possible, encourage regular periods of exercise to help prevent cardiac intolerance to activities, which can occur quickly after periods of prolonged inactivity.
4. Monitor electrolyte levels to ensure that patient's muscle weakness is not caused by hypokalemia.
5. Monitor ABG values to ensure that patient is oxygenated adequately; adjust oxygen delivery accordingly.
6. For more information, see the same nursing diagnosis in the section "Caring for the Critically Ill on Prolonged Bed Rest," p. 506.

Anxiety related to diagnosis, fear of death or social isolation, and hospitalization

Desired outcome: Patient expresses feelings and is free of harmful anxiety as evidenced by HR ≤100 bpm, RR ≤20 breaths/min with a normal depth and pattern (eupnea), and BP within patient's normal range.

1. Monitor patient for verbal or nonverbal expressions of the following: inability to cope, apprehension, guilt for past actions, uncertainty, and concerns about rejection and isolation.
2. Spend time with patient and encourage expressions of feelings and concerns.
3. Support effective coping patterns, for example, by allowing patient to cry or talk, rather than denying his or her legitimate fears and concerns.
4. Provide accurate information about AIDS and related diagnostic procedures.
5. If patient hyperventilates, teach him or her to mimic your normal respiratory pattern (eupnea).

Disturbance in self-concept related to body image changes secondary to Kaposi's lesions, side effects of chemotherapy, social stigmatization, isolation, and emaciation

Desired outcome: Patient expresses positive feelings about self to family, significant others, and primary nurse.

1. Encourage patient to express feelings, especially the way in which he or she views or feels about self.

2. Provide patient with positive feedback; help patient focus on facts, rather than myths or exaggerations about self.
3. Provide patient with access to clergy, psychiatric nurse, social worker, psychologist, or AIDS counselor as appropriate.
4. Encourage patient to join and share feelings with AIDS support group.

Knowledge deficit: Disease process, prognosis, lifestyle changes, and treatment plan

---

Desired outcome: Patient verbalizes accurate information regarding his or her disease process, prognosis, behaviors that increase the risk of transmission of the virus to others, and treatment plan.

---

1. Assess patient's knowledge about AIDS, including pathophysiologic changes that will occur, ways in which the disease is transmitted, necessary behavioral changes, and side effects of treatment. Correct misinformation and misconceptions, as necessary.
2. Inform patient of private and community agencies that are available to help with such tasks as handling legal affairs, cooking, housecleaning, and nursing care. Provide telephone numbers and addresses for AIDS support groups and self-help groups.
3. Teach patient care of long-term central venous catheter, if one will be present after hospital discharge.
4. Provide literature that explores the myths and realities of the AIDS disease process.
5. Teach patient the importance of modifying high-risk behaviors known to transmit the virus, for example, by avoiding sexual practices in which there is an exchange of bodily fluids or excretions (e.g., anal intercourse, fellatio, analingus); using condoms; exploring alternative sexual practices that eliminate direct contact with mucous membranes (e.g., masturbation, frottage); and informing sexual partners of AIDS condition.
6. Involve significant others in the teaching and learning process.
7. For more information, see "Rehabilitation and Patient-Family Teaching Concepts," p. 487.

Social isolation related to disease, societal rejection, loss of support system, fear, feelings of guilt and punishment, fatigue, and changed patterns of sexual expression

---

Desired outcome: Patient communicates and interacts with others.

---

1. Keep patient and significant others well informed of patient's status and treatment plan.
2. Provide private periods of time for patient to communicate and interact with significant others.
3. Encourage significant others to share in the care of the patient.

4. Encourage physical closeness between patient and significant others. Provide privacy, as much as possible.
5. Involve patient in unit or group activities, as appropriate.
6. Explain significance of isolation precautions to patient.

Alteration in thought processes related to mental deterioration secondary to infection or space-occupying lesion in the central nervous system (CNS)

Desired outcome: Patient verbalizes orientation to person, place, and time and correctly completes exercises in logical reasoning, memory, perception, concentration, attention, and sequencing of activities.

---

1. Assess patient for minor alterations in personality traits that cannot be attributed to other causes, such as stress or medication.
2. Assess patient for signs of dementia, which would include a slowing of all cognitive functioning: problems in attention, concentration, memory, perception, logical reasoning, and sequencing of activities.
3. Encourage patient to report persistent headaches, dizziness, or seizures, which may signal CNS involvement.
4. Note any cranial nerve involvement that differs from patient's past medical history. Most commonly, the 5th (trigeminal), 7th (facial), and 8th (acoustic) nerves are involved in infectious processes of the CNS.
5. Assess patient for signs of mental aberration, blindness, aphasia, hemiparesis, or ataxia, which may signal the presence of a demyelinating disease. Notify MD of all significant findings.

For other nursing diagnoses and interventions, see "Management of the Adult on Mechanical Ventilation," pp. 66-70; "Providing Nutritional Support," pp. 490-505; "Caring for the Critically Ill on Prolonged Bed Rest," pp. 506-511; "Caring for the Critically Ill with Life-Threatening Disorders," pp. 511-522; and "Caring for the Family of the Critically Ill," pp. 522-526.

REHABILITATION AND PATIENT-FAMILY TEACHING CONCEPTS

Give patient and significant others verbal and written instructions for the following:
1. Importance of avoiding use of recreational drugs, which are thought to potentiate the immunosuppressive process and lower resistance to infection.
2. Significance and importance of refraining from donating blood.
3. Necessity of modifying high-risk behaviors. See **Knowledge deficit**, p. 486, for specific information.
4. Principles and importance of maintaining a balanced diet; ways to supplement diet with multivitamins and other food sources, such as high-caloric substances (e.g., Isocal and Ensure).
5. Because of decreased resistance to infection, the importance of limiting contact with individuals known to have active infections.
6. Necessity of meticulous hygiene for preventing spread of any extant, or new infectious organisms.

7. Techniques for self-assessment of early signs of infection (e.g., redness, tenderness, swelling, purulent exudate) in all cuts, abrasions, lesions, or open wounds.

8. Care of central venous catheter, if appropriate; technique for self-administration of TPN or enteral tube feedings.

9. Importance of avoiding fatigue by limiting participation in social activities, getting maximum amounts of rest, and minimizing physical exertion.

10. Prescribed medications, including name, dosage, purpose, and potential side effects.

11. Importance of maintaining medical follow-up appointments.

12. Advisability of keeping anecdotal notes (perhaps in journal format) on exacerbation and remission of signs and symptoms.

13. Importance of reporting changes in neurologic status, e.g., increasing severity of headaches, blurred vision, gait disturbances, or "black-outs."

14. Advisability of sharing feelings with significant others or within a support group.

15. In addition, provide the following information regarding AIDS resources:

Public Health Service
AIDS Hotline
(800) 342-AIDS
(800) 342-2437

National Gay Task Force
AIDS Information Hotline
(800) 221-7044

Local Red Cross or
American Red Cross
AIDS Education Office
1730 D Street, N.W.
Washington, DC 20006
(202) 737-8300

National Sexually Transmitted
Diseases Hotline/American
Social Health Association
(800) 227-8922

Centers for Disease Control (CDC)
AIDS Activity
Building 6, Room 292
1600 Clifton Road
Atlanta, GA 30333
(401) 329-3479

National AIDS Network
729 Eighth St., SE
Suite 300
Washington, DC 20003
(202) 546-2424

SELECTED REFERENCES

Barach ET, et al: Epinephrine for treatment of anaphylactic shock. *JAMA* 1984; 251: 2118-2122.

Barrows JJ: Dealing with anaphylaxis STAT. *Nurs Life* May/June 1985; 33-39.

Bennett J: AIDS: What we know. *Am J Nurs* 1986; 86: 1016-1028.

Bolman RM, et al: Improved immunosuppression for heart transplantation. *Heart Transp* May 1985; 4: 315-318.

Callahan J: Compartment syndrome. *Orthop Nurs* 1985; 4(4): 11-15.

Carpenter CB, Strom TB: Transplantation: Immunogenetic and clinical aspects—Part 1. *Hosp Prac* Dec 1982: 125-134.

Centers for Disease Control: Recommendations for preventing transmission of infection with Human T-Lymphotropic Virus Type III/Lymphadenopathy Associated Virus in the workplace. *MMWR 1985* : 681-186, 691-195.

Cohen MR: Drug induced anaphylaxis. *Nursing 85* 1985; 15: 43.

Continuing Education: Burn care. *Am J Nurs* Jan 1985; 85: 30-50.

Curren JW, et al: The epidemiology of AIDS: Current status and future prospects. *Science* 1985: 1352-1357.

Cuthbert JA: Southwestern Internal Medicine Conference: Hepatic transplantation. *Am J Med Sci* April 1986; 291(4): 286-294.

Freeman JW: Nursing care of the patient with a burn injury. *Crit Car Nurs* Nov/Dec 1984: 52-68.

Gong V, Rudnick N: *AIDS. Facts and Issues.* Rutgers University Press, 1987.

Gray DWR, Morris PJ: Cyclosporine and pancreas transplantation. *World J Surg* Apr 1984; 14: 484-489.

Griffin JP: *Hematology and Immunology: Concepts for Nursing.* Appleton-Century-Crofts, 1985.

Holden CEA: Prevention of ischemic contractures. In: *The Severely Injured Limb.* Ackroyd CE, et al (eds). Churchill-Livingstone, 1983.

Holloway WA, Reinhardt J: Septic shock in the elderly. *Geriatrics* 1984; 39: 48-54.

Institute of Medicine: *Confronting AIDS.* National Academy Press, 1986.

Howard M, Puri VK, Paidipaty BB: The effects of fluid resuscitation in the critically ill patient. *Heart Lung* 1984; 13: 649-654.

Levy RM, Bredesen DE, Rosenblum ML: Neurological manifestations of acquired immune deficiency syndrome (AIDS): Experience at UCSF and review of the literature. *J Neurosurg* 1985: 475-495.

Linnemann CC: Increasing incidence of toxic shock syndrome in the 1970's. *Am J Public Health* 1986; 566-567.

Lovett JM, Karp RB: Heart transplantation. *Surg Clin N Am* June 1985; 65(3): 613-631.

Montefusco CM, Goldsmith J: Cyclosporine immunosupression in organ graft recipients: Nursing Implications. *Crit Car Nurs* March/April 1984: 117-119.

Nicolas F, Villers D, Blanloeil Y: Hemodynamic pattern in anaphylactic shock with cardiac arrest. *Crit Car Med* 1984; 12: 144-145.

Pagana KD, Pagana TJ: *Pocket Nurse Guide to Laboratory and Diagnostic Tests.* Mosby, 1986.

Painvin G, et al: Cardiac transplantation: Indications, procurement, operation, and management. *Heart Lung* Sept 1985;14: 484-489.

Porth CM: *Pathophysiology Concepts of Altered Health States,* 2nd ed. Lippincott, 1986.

Pradka L. Use of the wick catheter for diagnosing and monitoring compartment syndrome. *Orthop Nurs* 1985; 4(4): 17-18.

Price DM, Scimeca AM: The epidemic of the 80s: AIDS. *Canc Nurs* 1984; 7 (4): 283-290.

Rice V: The clinical continuum of septic shock. *Crit Car Nurs* 1984; 4: 86-109.

Rice V: Shock management, Part II: Pharmacologic intervention. *Crit Car Nurs* 1985; 5: 42-57.

Ross DG: Musculoskeletal disorders. In: *Manual of Nursing Therapeutics: Applying Nursing Diagnoses to Medical Disorders.* Swearingen PL (ed). *Addison-Wesley,* 1986.

Smith S: Liver transplantation: Implications for critical care nursing. *Heart Lung* Nov 1985;14: 617-627.

Sommers MS: Preventing complications for the toxic shock syndrome patient. *Dim Crit Care Nurs* 1985; 4: 215-225.

Stearns HC: Principles of lower extremity fracture management. In: *Assessment and Fracture Management of the Lower Extremities.* Hilt NE (ed). Monograph of the National Association of Orthopaedic Nurses, Inc, 1984.

Strom TB, Carpenter CB: Transplantation: Immunogenetic and clinical aspects—Part II. *Hosp Prac* Jan 1983: 135-150.

Sutherland DE, Goetz FC, Najarian JS: One hundred pancreas transplants at a single institution. *Ann Surg* Oct 1984: 414-440.

Thompson JM, et al: *Clinical Nursing.* Mosby, 1986.

Traiger GL, Bohachick P: Liver transplantation: Care of the patient in the acute postoperative period. *Crit Car Nurs* Sept/Oct 1983: 96-103.

Wolff SM: The treatment of gram-negative bacteremia and shock. *New Engl J Med* 1982; 307: 1267-1268.

Wooldridge-King M: Nursing considerations of the burn patient during the emergent period. *Heart Lung* 1982; 11(4): 353-361.

Wooldridge-King M, Surveyer JA: Skin-grafting for full-thickness burn injury. *Am J Nurs;* 80(11): 2000-2004.

APPENDIX

Providing
nutritional support

Many hospitalized patients are at nutritional risk or have malnutrition. Malnutrition not only increases the time of hospital stay, morbidity, and mortality, it compromises wound healing and immune function as well. Nutrition interventions minimize patient complications and the cost of health care. Nursing observations are vital to early identification of malnutrition and prevention of iatrogenic weight loss during the hospital stay. Nutritional support is especially important in critical care, as a patient's needs may be increased during this period and oral intake may not be possible. Specialized nutritional support modalities, tube feeding, or parenteral support may be required.

Screening for patients at nutritional risk

IDENTIFYING THE HIGH-RISK PATIENT

Standard criteria are used to evaluate the patient's potential for nutritional risk. These include

- Age: Infancy, childhood, advanced.
- Drug or alcohol abuse.
- History of inadequate nutrient intake.
- IV support with dextrose or saline alone for >5 days.
- Organ or system failure (e.g., ARDS, COPD, renal failure, diabetes mellitus, pancreatitis, neuromuscular dysfunction).
- Overweight status (>20% above ideal body weight).
- Pregnancy (especially in an adolescent).
- Recent, unplanned weight loss (>10 pounds).
- Serum albumin <3.5 gm/dl.
- Trauma, surgery, or disease of the oral cavity or GI tract (e.g., fractured mandible, radical head and neck resection, malabsorption syndrome).
- Underweight condition (≤80% of ideal body weight).

FORMS OF MALNUTRITION

Several varieties of malnutrition exist.

1. **Kwashiorkor:** Condition that develops when adequate calories are consumed but protein intake is inadequate. Typical signs are a low serum albumin level and edema. The patient may actually appear well-nourished, with edema masking weight loss. This type of malnutrition can occur in the patient who is maintained for a prolonged period on IV dextrose or maintenance electrolyte solutions alone.

2. **Marasmus:** Caused by chronic, inadequate intake of both calories and protein. The patient appears wasted and may have a skeleton-like appearance. Severe

depletion of lean body mass and subcutaneous fat stores is evident on physical examination. Serum albumin level may be normal, however.

3. **Protein-calorie malnutrition (PCM):** A combination of kwashiorkor and marasmus, it is the type most commonly seen in hospitalized patients in the United States. Severe wasting may be present, in conjunction with edema. Serum albumin levels may be normal or low, depending on the severity of protein inadequacy.

4. **Obesity:** State of poor nutrition associated with increased risk for a number of diseases, including diabetes mellitus, hypertension, cardiovascular disease, and some forms of cancer. Although caloric intake may exceed needs, selected nutrient deficiencies can occur because food intake may lack nutrient density. This patient, although 20% or more over ideal body weight, may have marginal stores of protein, vitamins A and C, folic acid, iron, or calcium, among other potential deficiencies.

5. **Vitamin deficiencies:** Seen most often in severe or chronic malnutrition. Some deficiencies are also associated with certain conditions or dietary patterns (e.g., thiamine and folate deficiencies in the alcholic, B_{12} deficiency in the strict vegetarian or patient with ileal resection, and vitamin C deficiency in the individual who avoids all fruits, juices, and vegetables).

6. **Mineral deficiencies:** Usually seen only after prolonged periods of inadequate intake or in certain disease states. Iron deficiency is seen more commonly in women, infants, and children. Calcium deficiency leading to rickets or osteoporosis may be seen if the diet excludes milk and milk products. Zinc deficiency, although rare, may be seen in patients with chronic diarrhea or malabsorption.

Nutritional assessment

DIETARY HISTORY

Dietary history is taken to reveal adequacy of usual and recent food intake. Excesses or deficiencies of nutrients should be noted. Unusual eating patterns may be revealed, as well (e.g., fad diets, vegetarian diet, extraordinary use of nutritional supplements). Of keen interest from a nutritional perspective is anything that impairs adequate selection, preparation, ingestion, digestion, absorption, and excretion of nutrients. Dietary history should include the following:

- Comprehensive review of usual dietary intake, including food allergies, food aversions, and use of nutritional supplements.
- Unplanned weight gain or loss.
- Chewing or swallowing difficulties.
- Nausea, vomiting, or pain with eating.
- Diarrhea, constipation, or any alteration in elimination pattern.
- Chronic disease affecting utilization of nutrients (e.g., malabsorption, pancreatitis, diabetes mellitus).
- Surgical resection or disease of the gut or accessory organs of digestion (pancreas, liver, gall bladder).
- Alcohol or drug addiction.
- Chronic use of drugs affecting appetite, digestion, utilization or excretion of nutrients (see Table A-1 for detail).

Medical, surgical, and social history also should be obtained to complete this assessment of the patient's current nutritional status.

TABLE A-1
Drugs affecting appetite, digestion, and nutrition use

Drug	Nutritional concern	Management suggestions
Aspirin	Gastric ulceration; nausea, vomiting.	Give with water or food; use buffered or enteric-coated product when possible.
Estrogen	Nausea, vomiting; sodium, water retention.	Give with meals; restrict sodium intake.
Furosemide	Increased excretion of potassium; fluid and electrolyte imbalance.	Ensure high dietary potassium intake (e.g., apricots, bananas, oranges, orange juice, most meats, peas, beans, and nuts).
Mineral oil	Malabsorption of vitamins A, D, E, K.	Avoid frequent use; avoid use at mealtime.
Methotrexate	Nausea, vomiting.	Honor food preferences; provide small meals, cold beverages.
Levodopa	Dietary protein may impair absorption.	Avoid high-protein diet.
Phenobarbital	Inactivities vitamin D; impairs folate utilization. May indirectly cause rickets or osteomalacia.	Ensure adequate dietary intake of vitamin D and folate; administer vitamin supplements as prescribed.
Phenytoin	See ''Phenobarbital,'' above. May contribute to development of megaloblastic anemia, rickets, or osteomalacia.	See ''Phenobarbital,'' above.
Tetracycline	Milk products may impair absorption.	Restrict milk and milk products.
Theophylline	Response increased with caffeine; decreased half-life with charcoal-broiled meats.	Restrict caffeine-containing beverages (coffee, tea, colas) and charcoal-broiled meats.
Warfarin	Vitamin K impairs hypoprothrombic effect.	Avoid use of vitamin-K rich foods (e.g., green leafy vegetables such as cabbage, cauliflower, and turnip greens).

PHYSICAL ASSESSMENT

Assessment may reveal important indicators of nutritional deficiencies or disorders. Examples are outlined in Table A-2.

ANTHROPOMETRICS

Measurement of the body or its parts is termed anthropometrics. Certain measurements are very useful, such as height and weight; others, such as triceps skinfold and mid-upper arm muscle circumference, are used only in special circumstances.

1. **Measuring height and weight:** Should be done on admission. If the patient's condition is too critical, reported height and weight from family or significant others should be noted on the medical record. If necessary, estimates of height and weight are made by observing body size and comparing recumbent length to known length of the mattress.

TABLE A-2
Physical assessment with nutritional implications

Abnormal appearance	Possible nutrient deficiency or disorder
Thinness, tissue wasting, poor wound healing	Protein-calorie malnutrition, marasmus
Rotundness, "moon face" appearance, presence of edema or decubiti	Obesity, kwashiorkor
Easily plucked hair	Kwashiorkor, marasmus
Nasolabial seborrhea; redness or fissures at corners of eyelids; angular lesions at corners of mouth; magenta tongue; scrotal and vulval dermatosis (skin disorder not accompanied by inflammation)	Riboflavin
Scarlet, raw tongue; swollen tongue; red, swollen pigmentation of areas exposed to sunlight	Niacin
Petechiae; bleeding, spongy gums	Vitamin C
Excessive bruising	Vitamin C or K
Xerosis (dryness of mucous membranes); follicular hyperkeratosis (epidermal hypertrophy causing horny skin formation); conjunctival xerosis	Vitamin A
Circumscribed swelling or growth of the frontal and parietal areas of the skull; knock-knees and bow legs	Vitamin D
Goiter	Iodine
Pallor, listlessness	Iron
Cyanosis, labored breathing	Respiratory distress with poor appetite and intake
Jaundice, ascites	Liver disease

- Estimates of desirable male weight can be made as follows: Allot 106 pounds for the first 5 feet of height, plus 6 pounds for each additional inch.
- Estimates of desirable female weight can be made as follows: Allot 100 pounds for the first 5 feet of height, plus 5 pounds for each additional inch.

These estimates correspond fairly well with weights for heights reported by the Metropolitan Life Insurance Company, as seen in Table A-3.

2. **Monitoring weight changes:** The patient's maintenance of body weight is one of the most readily available and practical indicators of adequacy of nutritional status and provisions. In critical care, however, weight changes may reflect the following:
   - Fluid shifts (edema, diuresis, third-spacing).
   - Surgical resections or traumatic or surgical amputations.
   - Weight of dressings or equipment.

Interpretation of weight changes must be made with these factors in mind. One liter of fluid equals approximately 2 pounds, so being "ahead" or "behind" on a patient's fluids can be reflected readily in weight changes.

TABLE A-3
Ideal weights

	Men			Women		
Height	Small frame	Medium frame	Large frame	Small frame	Medium frame	Large frame
4 ft 10 in	—	—	—	102-111	109-121	118-131
4 ft 11 in	—	—	—	103-113	111-123	120-134
5 ft	—	—	—	104-115	113-126	122-137
5 ft 1 in	—	—	—	106-118	115-129	125-140
5 ft 2 in	128-134	131-141	138-150	108-121	118-132	128-143
5 ft 3 in	130-136	133-143	140-153	111-124	121-135	131-147
5 ft 4 in	132-138	135-145	142-156	114-127	124-138	134-151
5 ft 5 in	134-140	137-148	144-160	117-130	127-141	137-155
5 ft 6 in	136-142	139-151	146-164	120-133	130-144	140-159
5 ft 7 in	138-146	142-154	148-168	123-136	133-147	143-163
5 ft 8 in	140-148	145-157	152-172	126-139	136-150	146-167
5 ft 9 in	142-151	148-160	156-176	129-142	139-153	149-170
5 ft 10 in	144-154	151-163	158-180	132-145	142-156	152-173
5 ft 11 in	146-157	154-166	161-184	135-148	145-159	155-176
6 ft	149-160	157-170	164-188	138-151	148-162	158-179
6 ft 1 in	152-164	160-174	168-192	—	—	—
6 ft 2 in	155-168	164-178	172-197	—	—	—
6 ft 3 in	158-172	167-182	176-202	—	—	—
6 ft 4 in	162-176	171-187	181-207	—	—	—

*Ages 25 through 59 for 5 lb of indoor clothing for men and 3 lb of indoor clothing for women and 1-inch heels for both. Data for 1983. Courtesy of the Metropolitan Life Insurance Company.

3. **Measurement of triceps skinfold thickness and mid-upper arm muscle circumference:** Previously was widely suggested for assessment of fat stores and lean body mass in hospitalized patients. However, for proper interpretatation of these results, the measurements must be made by a trained clinician, the patient positioned in a standard manner, and the results compared to national norms specific to age and sex. As it often is impossible to position critically ill patients appropriately to make these measurements and there is wide variability, even when specific standards are used, these measurements are not widely used at present, especially in the critical care setting. They do have value in the long-term patient who cannot be weighed. In this situation, serial measurements, using the patient as a control or standard, can be made and used as a crude indicator of adequate, inadequate, or excessive provision of nutritional support.

LABORATORY AND DIAGNOSTIC TESTING

Laboratory values pertinent to nutritional status are numerous.

1. **Visceral protein status:** Evaluated for in the following tests, with normal values in parentheses: serum albumin (3.5-5.5 g/dl), transferrin (180-260 mg/dl), thyroxine-binding prealbumin (200-300 μg/ml), and retinol binding protein (40-50 μg/ml). Normal values may vary somewhat with different laboratory proce-

dures and standards. Albumin and transferrin have relatively long half-lives of 19 and 9 days, respectively, whereas thyroxine-binding prealbumin and retinol-binding protein have very short half-lives of 24-48 hours and 10 hours, respectively. If hydration status is normal and anemia is absent, albumin and transferrin can be used as baseline indicators of adequacy of protein intake and synthesis. For evidence of response to nutritional therapy, the short turnover proteins, thyroxine-binding prealbumin and retinol-binding protein, are the most useful.

2. **Anemia:** Tested for *via* hemoglobin (Hgb), hematocrit (Hct), and RBC indices. Data from these hematologic tests are useful in nutritional assessment when hydration state is normal. The usefulness of these tests in assessing nutritional status is invalidated by massive hemorrhage. Below normal Hgb and Hct, combined with appearance of microcytic and hypochromic RBCs, may denote iron deficiency anemia. Appearance of macrocytic RBCs may signal folate deficiency; megaloblasts are associated with vitamin B_{12} deficiency.

3. **Serum levels of vitamins and minerals:** Yield little information regarding overall body stores of these nutrients; test values require cautious interpretation.

4. **Total lymphocyte count:** While previously widely used as an indicator of protein status and immune competence, it is affected by so many variables common to critical illness, such as the leukocytosis seen in sepsis, trauma, burns, or surgery, that its use is diminishing.

5. **Delayed cutaneous hypersensitivity:** Involves the application of antigens to the skin and observation of cutaneous response or lack thereof (anergy). Many iatrogenic, disease-specific, and technical factors are now known to alter this response and the use of this form of testing is no longer widely recommended or implemented.

6. **Nitrogen balance:** State of equilibrium that exists when the intake and excretion of nitrogen are equal. If more is taken in than excreted, nitrogen is said to be positive and an anabolic state exists. If more nitrogen is excreted than taken in, nitrogen balance is said to be negative and a catabolic state exists. Most nitrogen loss occurs through urinary urea nitrogen (UUN) loss, with a small, constant amount lost *via* skin and feces. Nitrogen balance is calculated as follows:

$$N_{bal} = N \text{ intake } - N \text{ excretion}$$

$$N_{bal} = \frac{\text{protein intake (gm)}}{6.25} - (24 \text{ hr UUN } + 4)$$

Nitrogen balance studies are conducted frequently in critical care settings. Accurate results rely heavily on complete 24-hour urine collections.

A positive nitrogen state is desired when anabolism is the goal, for example, following resolution of the critical phase of an illness. This is a state of "rebuilding," regaining weight and lean body mass. During critical illness the goal is nitrogen balance. In a true state of balance, needs for energy and nitrogen are being met and are adequate to provide for the following: (1) wound healing, (2) extraneous losses, (3) catabolism of stress, (4) usual synthesis of enzymes and hormones, (5) repair and replacement of worn-out cells, and (6) normal needs and physiologic functions. Although many individuals believe (erroneously) that a positive nitrogen state is needed to accomplish the above goals, nitrogen balance is adequate. In fact, anabolism in critical care may be accompanied by elevated carbon dioxide production and hepatic enzymes.

Nutritional therapy

Following completion of a comprehensive nutritional assessment, a care plan can be developed to provide optimal nutritional support for the patient. The goal for the critically ill patient is maintenance of existing lean body mass and adequate provision of energy and nutrients to sustain physiologic systems. Patients in this setting should not incur either weight loss or weight gain. Weight loss during this period of stress is likely to cause loss of protein rather than fat stores. Attempts to facilitate weight gain during critical illness may cause some of the complications of overfeeding during stress (e.g., increased CO_2 production, provision of excessive glucose and fluid load, elevation of liver enzymes, and weight gain of fluid or fat rather than repletion of lean body mass). Nutritional therapy should be provided in the most physiologic, safe, and efficacious manner possible, with cost-effectiveness considered as well.

ENERGY REQUIREMENTS

Energy expenditure is dependent on age, sex, body size, physical activity, and level of stress or catabolism. Basal energy expenditure (BEE) is defined as the energy required to support vital life functions (circulation, respirations, and other physiologic processes) in a healthy, normal, fasting individual, at rest in a neutral, thermal environment. Calculation of BEE can be made using the following equations developed by Harris and Benedict:

$$BEE \text{ (male)} = 66.5 + (13.8 \times W) + (5 \times H) - (6.8 \times A)$$
$$BEE \text{ (female)} = 655.1 + (9.6 \times W) + (1.9 \times H) - (4.7 \times A)$$
$$W = \text{weight in kg; } H = \text{height in cm; } A = \text{age in years.}$$

If the patient is being nourished, energy expenditure is increased approximately 5-10% above BEE for the specific dynamic action of nutrient utilization. This combined figure is called the resting energy expenditure (REE). As the difference in BEE and REE is often only 5%, the BEE and REE are considered relatively equal in actual clinical practice.

1. **Adjustment of BEE and REE during physical activity, illness, or injury:** The following factors are applied to the BEE and REE as suggested by Calvin Long:

$$BEE \text{ or } REE \times \text{activity factor} \times \text{injury factor} =$$
$$TEE \text{ (total energy expenditure)}$$

Activity factors	Injury factors
1.2 = bedridden patient	1.2 = surgery
1.3 = ambulatory patient	1.35 = trauma (blunt or skeletal)
	1.6 = sepsis
	2.1 = burns

Additional increases in TEE may be caused by temperature elevations, with an increase of 7% per degree of temperature elevation from normal in Fahrenheit or 13% per degree of temperature elevation from normal in Centrigrade, as reported by Kinney.

2. **Measuring energy needs directly:** Can be accomplished at the bedside by using a metabolic cart. This cart is an instrument that performs indirect calorimetry, the calculation of energy expenditure by measurement of respiratory gas exchange. This technique is based on the theory that oxygen consumption and

carbon dioxide production profile intracellular metabolism. The gas collection device can be adapted to the exhalation unit of most mechanical ventilation systems; patients not requiring mechanical ventilation can have gas exchange measured using a plastic hood or canopy. A microcomputer, which is an integral part of the metabolic cart, utilizes the data on gas exchange, urinary urea nitrogen values, as well as some basic nutritional assessment data and generates estimates of REE, protein requirements, utilization of energy substrates (carbohydrates, protein, and fat), as well as respiratory quotient (RQ). The RQ, which represents a ratio of carbon dioxide production to oxygen consumption, provides information on the adequacy of nutritional provision, that is, whether the patient is well nourished (from an energy perspective) or whether a starved or overfed state exists.

$$RQ \frac{VCO2}{VO2}$$

	Interpretation
0.7	Lipolysis or starvation; primary source of energy = fat.
0.8	Primary source of energy = protein.
0.85	Energy source = mixed substrates (carbohydrates, protein, fat)
1.0	Primary source of energy = carbohydrates.
>1.0	Overfeeding; lipogenesis (conversion of glucose to fat); increased CO_2 production.

Correct interpretation of this information on measured REE, protein needs, and substrate utilization is crucial so that proper nutritional therapy can be provided and errors in assessment avoided. For example, if measured REE represents a starved state for an individual unable to eat for several days posttrauma, the goal is not to provide support at a starvation level, but rather to adjust support to an adequate maintenance level. This may require an increase of 500 kcal per day or more over measured REE. To avoid the complications of rapid refeeding of a starved patient (e.g., cardiac failure, pulmonary compromise, or electrolyte imbalance), progression of feedings to maintenance level may have to proceed in small daily increments. The nonstarved patient, however, may require energy at levels 10-30% greater than the measured REE if they are bathed, active in bed, or undergoing pulmonary treatments or painful stimuli from other treatments (e.g., dressing changes, debridement, multiple injections). These factors must be considered in the estimate of total energy needs for each patient. In addition, reassessment is necessary at frequent intervals. For example, in closed head injury, needs are very elevated initially, and then reduced when barbiturate therapy is begun. Some intensive care therapies can elevate actual energy expenditure (Weissman, 1984). Unfortunately, metabolic cart measurements are performed over a brief period, often for only 20 minutes, and therefore cannot be expected to reveal total energy needs over a 24-hour period.

PROTEIN REQUIREMENTS AND DISTRIBUTION OF CALORIES

Once TEE has been determined, an estimate of quantities of protein, carbohydrates, and fat can be derived. Providing a relatively normal distribution of calories from these is desirable and usually adequate.

1. **Energy macronutrients and calorie:nitrogen ratio:** Percentages of total calories from carbohydrates, protein, and fat should equal approximately 50%, 15%, and 35% respectively. A nonprotein calorie per gram of nitrogen ratio of

150:1 to 100:1 usually will be achieved by providing 14-20% of total calories as protein. This will provide a range of 0.8-2.0 grams of protein/kg/day.

2. **Protein requirements in critical illness:** The usual recommendation for protein intake in critical illness is 1.2-1.5 grams of protein/kg/day.

3. **Providing glucose:** Glucose administration of 5 mg/kg/min is a suitable amount in critical care. Glucose provided in excess of this is not well utilized and may lead to hyperglycemia and excessive CO_2 production.

4. **Delivering fat:** If protein and glucose are supplied as outlined, providing the remainder of needed calories as fat will meet overall needs. Fat, particularly linoleic and linolenic acids, may be administered in minimal quantities to satisfy needs for essential fatty acids, or may be provided in larger quantities, as tolerated, to meet energy needs, especially in the patient who is glucose intolerant or being weaned from ventilator support with CO_2 retention as a complicator.

VITAMIN AND MINERAL REQUIREMENTS

It is an uncontested fact that a variety of vitamins and minerals is essential for optimal health. Even in health, quantities required vary widely, with some individuals' needs considerably higher than others'. With deficiency, several responses occur, including mobilization of stores, increased absorption, reduced excretion, and improved utilization. Some deficiencies develop more rapidly than others, but in general, vitamin and mineral deficiencies take weeks, months, or years to develop. For critically ill patients, the goals are the following:

• Provide at least minimum quantities of vitamins and minerals as outlined in standard recommendations published by American Medical Association (parenteral) and the Food and Nutrition Board of the National Research Council in the Recommended Dietary Allowances (enteral).
• Detect and treat existing deficiencies.
• Supplement specific vitamins or minerals known to be needed in increased amounts in existing disease states (e.g., zinc and vitamins A and C in burns; thiamine and folate in alcoholism).
• Observe patient for development of signs of deficiency (see Table A-2).

FLUID REQUIREMENTS

Many factors affect fluid balance. A primary goal is to achieve equilibrium between I&O. Under usual circumstances, an estimate of fluid needs can be made by providing 1 ml of free water for each calorie provided. If 1 L of 1 cal/ml tube feeding provides 75-80% free water (i.e., 750-800 ml), the patient then has a water deficit of 1000 ml minus 750-800 ml, or a deficit of 250-200 ml. Therefore, 200-250 ml of additional free water should be provided per day. Water can be administered *via* flushing of the feeding tube to maintain patency or before or after medication administration to prevent precipitation and obstruction.

An awareness is required of all sources of intake (oral, enteral, IV fluids, and medications) as well as losses (urine, stool, drains, fistulas, emesis, and expiratory and evaporative losses). Renal failure, congestive heart failure, and progression of ascites are a few conditions that necessitate careful monitoring of fluid status and may require restriction of intake. In critically ill patients, third-spacing of fluid is common and makes estimates of fluid balance and weight difficult. Fluid management must be responsive to hemodynamic variables, electrolyte balance, and optimal functioning of all bodily organs and systems.

Usual fluid requirements are 1.5 L/m². The daily loss of water includes approximately 1400 ml in urine (60 ml/hr), 350 ml *via* respiration, 350 ml as evaporative losses through skin, 100 ml in sweat, and about 200 ml in feces. If loss by any of these routes is increased, fluid needs will increase; if loss by any of these routes is impaired, fluid restriction may be necessary.

< N O T E : Urine output may be as high as 2-3 L under normal conditions. This represents a range of 80-125 ml/hr.

Nutritional support modalities

Specialized nutritional support refers to enteral and parenteral support, that is, tube feedings and intravenous delivery of nutrients. Patients in critical care frequently cannot eat enough to meet their needs. Often, several types of nutritional support are administered simultaneously when the patient is being weaned from one type of support to another. During these transition times, recording intake from all sources and obtaining calorie counts can help ensure that intake is adequate. The following are the various types of nutritional therapy.

ORAL DIET

An oral diet is based on guidelines for normal human nutrition and may be modified for consistency or for special disease states. Clear liquid and full liquid diets are nutritionally incomplete and usually are used for the purpose of testing tolerance of anything by mouth and should not be used without other nutritional supplementation for more than 5 days. For the patient with lactose intolerance, gastroenteritis (often accompanied by a lactose intolerance that can last 6-8 weeks), fat malabsorption, or pancreatitis (often accompanied by fat malabsorption), the full liquid diet is usually avoided because it contains many dairy products high in both lactose and fat. The regular hospital diet can be altered in texture to accommodate the patient with poor dentation, ill-fitting dentures, mucositis, stomatitis, oral surgery, or neuromuscular disorders. Other alterations can be made by the dietician to provide diets for patients who are diabetics, in renal failure, with hepatic disease, or with numerous other disease states and conditions requiring alterations of specific nutrients or distribution of calories.

LIQUID NUTRITIONAL SUPPLEMENTS

These are plentiful and range from complete nutritional products capable of meeting total nutritional needs if provided in adequate quantity, to others that are incomplete and intended for use as supplementation to an oral diet or as an occasional meal replacement. Caution should be exercised in selecting these aids to ensure that the patient's dietary needs are met. Most of these products are more palatable when served cold over crushed ice.

MODULAR ENTERAL COMPONENTS

These are available as individual nutrients (e.g., carbohydrates, protein, or fat; forms may vary, i.e., as long-chain triglycerides, medium-chain triglycerides, or a mixture of both) or as a carefully compounded combination of nutrients (e.g., vitamins or minerals or electrolytes). They can be used in a mix-and-match manner to produce individually tailored enteral products or to supplement other existing products. When added to foods they can enhance caloric density and protein intake, provide fat in an easy-to-absorb form, or supplement vitamins or minerals. Because deficiencies or toxicities of nutrients can occur unless requirements are carefully met and not exceeded, these products usually are used at the discretion of the clinical dietician.

ENTERAL PRODUCTS

These products are usually prepared for administration *via* a feeding tube, although some also can be taken orally. These products may be nutritionally complete or incomplete, fiber enriched or low residue, isoosmolar (300 mOsm/kg H_2O) or hyperosmolar (>300 mOsm/kg/H_2O), standard (1 cal/ml) or high calorie (1.5-2 cal/ml), restricted in protein or high in nitrogen, and containing intact or predigested nutrients. Choice of product is dependent on nutrient needs, fluid tolerance, digestive and absorptive ability, as well as route of administration (gastric, duodenal, jejunal) and lumen size of the feeding tube used. Length of the gut and function of all accessory organs of digestion are other key factors.

1. **Use of predigested products:** Currently reserved for deep jejunal feedings (in which most of the absorptive length of the gut is bypassed) and for short gut syndrome or severe malabsorption.

2. **Osmolarity and rate of administration:** Tube feeding products usually are introduced at isoosmolarity (full strength for an isoosmolar product, dilution with tap water to achieve an isoosmolar state for hyperosmolar products). Rates are often initiated at 50 ml/hr and advanced at 25 ml/hr/day until desired nutrient goals are reached. A usual maximum infusion rate is 125 ml/hr.

   - *Gastric infusions:* Increased first in concentration and then in volume as hyperosmolar solutions are better tolerated intragastrically. For example, 50 ml/hr ½ strength, 50 ml/hr full strength, 75 ml/hr full strength, then 100 ml/hr full strength.

   - *Small bowel infusions:* Advanced in volume first and concentration second. For example, 50 ml/hr ½ strength, 75 ml/hr ½ strength, 100 ml/hr ½ strength, 100 ml/hr ¾ strength, and 100 ml/hr full strength.

3. **Types of tubes used:** Temporary (oro- or nasogastric, duodenal, or jejunal) or more permanent (surgical or percutaneous endoscopically placed gastrostomy, standard jejunostomy, or needle catheter jejunostomy). The small diameter of the needle catheter jejunostomy often requires a predigested formula for lowered viscosity. It is predisposed to occlusion unless vigilant care is given to regular flushing for maintaining patency, especially if it is the only route for medication administration.

4. **Method of administration:** Gravity, syringe, or continual infusion device (pump) may be used, *via* bolus, intermittent, or continuous drip method. Of these, bolus is the most likely to cause discomfort (nausea, distention) or complications (vomiting, cramping, dumping syndrome, or diarrhea).

5. **Prevention of infection:** Hanging time should not exceed 8 hours because of the risk of bacterial proliferation at room temperature. Clean technique should be used when handling enteral products, containers, and feeding tube. Containers and tubing for enteral administration usually are changed q24h. All opened products should be dated (day, date, and time) and any unused product discarded after 24 hours.

PARENTERAL NUTRITION

Parenteral nutrition is the intravenous provision of nutrients. It may be accomplished either by peripheral or central veins.

1. **Peripheral therapy:** Used only when peripheral venous access is good and nutritional needs are low. It is used for short-term (7-10 days) delivery of nutrients or to supplement other nutritional support modalities.

2. **Central therapy:** For patients who are unable to tolerate oral or enteral feedings for a period exceeding 5-10 days.

3. **Types of parenteral solutions:** These solutions may contain dextrose, amino acids, electrolytes, vitamins, and minerals. Fat emulsions of soybean or safflower oils are available, also. The pharmacist may start with a solution of 50-70% dextrose, to which he or she adds a quantity of 8.5-10% amino acids, electrolytes, vitamins, and minerals. The final dilution of dextrose may range from 15-47%, and the quantity of amino acids may range from 2-5%, with the lower quantities provided in renal failure without dialysis, at which time only essential amino acids are provided. Amino acid solutions also may be enriched with the branched-chain amino acids or contain reduced quantities of aromatic amino acids. The former solution may be used in stress, while the latter is used in hepatic failure. IV fat emulsions are available in 10% and 20% solutions. These are used to provide essential fatty acids or for energy. In cases of glucose intolerance (e.g., diabetes, pancreatitis, sepsis, stress) or when carbon dioxide retention is a problem (e.g., COPD, weaning patient from the ventilator) carbohydrate kilocalories are replaced in part by fat.

General nursing diagnoses and interventions

Alteration in nutrition: Less than body requirements related to inadequate provision of nutrients

---

Desired outcome: Patient has adequate nutrition as evidenced by stable weights, serum albumin 3.5-5.5 g/dl, thyroxine-binding prealbumin 200-300 μg/ml, retinol-binding protein 40-50 μg/ml, and a state of nitrogen balance as determined by nitrogen studies.

For parenteral nutrition:

1. Ensure nutritional screening and assessment of patient within 72 hours of admission. For guidelines, see pp. 490-494.
2. Assist in central venous catheter placement and maintenance of sterility and patency of the line. Obtain x-ray confirmation of proper placement before commencing infusion of parenteral solutions.
3. Administer parenteral solutions as prescribed. Alert MD to
   - Indicators of sepsis.
   - Occlusion or malfunction of central line.
   - Sudden cessation of infusion in central line.
   - Factors causing impaired delivery of prescribed quantity of nutrients, for example, change in patient's status; discontinued infusion due to surgery, treatments, or therapy (OT/PT); delayed delivery due to broken bottle.
4. Test urine sugar q6h; notify MD of values ≥3.
5. Weigh patient daily at the same time of day, using the same scale. Notify MD if weight change is ≥1 kg.
6. Record I&O, noting 24-hour trends.

7. Monitor laboratory values for the following:
   - At the beginning of parenteral therapy obtain baseline serum values for:
     * Na, K, Cl, CO_2
       Platelets, PT, PTT
       CBC with differential
       Total iron-binding capacity (TIBC)
     * Glucose
     * BUN, creatinine
       Ca, Mg, PO_4
       SGPT, alkaline phosphatase, total bilirubin
       Albumin, transferrin
       Thyroxine-binding prealbumin and retinol-binding protein
   - Starred tests above often are ordered daily during initiation and progression of TPN, then as needed based on individual tolerance.
   - On a weekly basis, laboratory tests cited above are repeated.

For enteral nutrition:

1. Ensure nutritional screening and assessment of patient within 72 hours of admission. For guidelines, see pp. 490-494.
2. Insert or assist in placement of enteral tube. If patient has a small-bore feeding tube with a guide wire, obtain x-ray confirmation of proper placement before initiating infusion of tube feeding. Check placement of large-bore feeding tube by aspirating gastric contents and auscultating over epigastric area for "whoosh" of air that is noted immediately after injection of 10-20 ml of air.
3. Administer enteral product as prescribed. Alert MD to
   - Technical or mechanical complications (i.e., clogged or displaced feeding tube).
   - Signs of aspiration.
   - Metabolic complications (e.g., glycosuria, proteinuria, change in urine output or hydration status).
   - Factors causing impaired delivery of prescribed quantity of nutrients (e.g., occlusion of tube, GI distress).
4. Test urine sugar q6h; notify MD of values $\geq 3+$.
5. Weigh patient daily at the same time of day, using the same scale. Notify MD if weight change is ≥ 1 kg.
6. Record I&O, noting 24-hour trends.

For oral nutrition:

1. Ensure nutritional screening and assessment of patient within 72 hours of admission. See guidelines, pp. 490-494.
2. Position patient properly for eating; assist with eating as needed. Involve significant others in meal rituals for companionship and caring.
3. Provide small, frequent feedings of diet compatible with disease state and patient's ability to ingest foods.
4. Respect food aversions and try to maximize on food preferences.
5. Provide liquid nutritional supplements as prescribed. Serve them cold or over ice to enhance palatability.
6. Provide psychologic support.

Potential impairment of skin and tissue integrity related to vulnerability secondary to malnourished state or presence of central venous catheters or enteral tube

Desired outcome: Patient's skin remains intact, with no evidence of decubitus ulcers, skin rashes, excoriation, mucous membrane breakdown, or necrosis.

1. Ensure adequate nutrition after assessing energy, protein, fat, vitamin, mineral, and fluid needs (see pp. 496-499).
2. Alter patient's position at least q2h; check for erythematous areas.
3. Examine central catheter insertion site daily or at each dressing change, noting erythema, swelling, irritation, rash. Consider tapes or antibacterial and antifungal ointments and solutions as possible irritants. Pursue alternatives as necessary.
4. Secure feeding tube so that there is no pressure on surrounding tissues. Use transparent tape when possible for enhanced patient body image and ease of viewing patient's insertion site. Provide regular oral and nasal hygiene. Be alert to pressure areas.

Potential for infection related to vulnerability secondary to malnourished state and presence of central venous catheter or enteral tube

Desired outcome: Patient is free of infection as evidenced by normothermia, HR ≤100 bpm, RR ≤20 breaths/min, WBC count ≤11,000 μl, and absence of erythema and swelling at catheter insertion site.

1. Ensure adequate nutritional support, based on patient's needs. For guidelines, see pp. 496-499.
2. Examine catheter insertion site daily or with each dressing change for presence of erythema or swelling.
3. Assess temperature and VS q6h; report temperature >38.3° C (101° F) or temperature spike and leukocytosis. Also be alert to increased HR and RR, which are other indicators of infection.
4. Test urine for sugar q6h; report values ≥3+.
5. Use meticulous sterile technique when changing central line dressing and hanging new bottle of feeding solution.
6. Avoid using central line that is being used for nutritional support for blood drawing, pressure monitoring, or administration of medications or other fluids.
7. Hang tube feeding solution a maximum of 8 hours at a time.
8. Use clean technique in handling feeding tube and enteral products and containers.
9. Change enteral administration set q24h.
10. Report signs of GI intolerance that may be related to enteral product contamination (i.e., nausea and vomiting, abdominal distention, cramping, diarrhea).

Potential for impaired swallowing related to pain or decreased ability to ingest secondary to disease or treatment of disease (e.g., surgery, chemotherapy, radiation)

Desired outcome: Patient demonstrates adequate cough and gag reflexes and the ability to ingest foods *via* the phases of swallowing as instructed.

1. Ensure nutritional screening and assessment as well as assessment of oral motor function within 72 hours of admission or progression to oral diet.
2. Provide small, frequent meals.
3. Provide foods at temperatures acceptable to patient.
4. Respect food aversions; honor food preferences whenever possible.
5. Provide oral supplements or tube feeding supplements as prescribed. Advise patient of transition status and praise his or her progress.
6. Order extra sauces, gravies, or liquids if dryness of the oral cavity impairs patient's swallowing ability. Suggest that patient moisten each bite of food with these substances.
7. In conjunction with physical or occupational therapist, assist in retraining or facilitating patient's swallowing. Assess cough and gag reflexes before the first feeding. Initially, liquids and solids may be difficult to manage. Offer foods with thickened consistency and progress to increased texture as tolerated. Assist patient through the phases of ingesting food: opening the mouth, achieving lip closure, chewing, transferring food from side to side in the mouth and then to the back of the oral cavity, elevating the tongue to the roof of the mouth (hard palate), and swallowing between breaths.

Potential for impaired gas exchange related to risk of aspiration secondary to administration of enteral feeding

Desired outcome: Patient's proper tube position is verified by x-ray, aspiration of gastric contents, and auscultation of "whoosh" of air over epigastric area.

1. Do not initiate enteral feeding until small-bore tube position has been documented by x-ray. For large-bore feeding tube, check position *via* aspiration and auscultation (see description p. 502, under enteral nutrition, **Alteration in nutrition**).
2. Elevate HOB at least 30 degrees. Maintain this position for 45-60 minutes after feeding. If this is not possible or comfortable for the patient, turn patient into a slightly elevated right side-lying position to enhance gravity flow from the greater stomach curve to the pylorus.
3. Utilize enteral pump to facilitate infusion.
4. Aspirate gastric contents at least q4h to measure residual feeding. If residual is <100 ml, return aspirate and continue feeding. If aspirate is >100 ml, return aspirate and notify MD or follow agency policy regarding whether to hold or continue feeding.
5. Assess rate of tube feeding hourly; reset to prescribed rate as indicated. If infusion lags behind prescribed quantity significantly, do not attempt to "catch up" by increasing infusion rate greatly.

SELECTED REFERENCES

American Medical Association, Department of Foods and Nutrition: Guidelines for essential trace element preparations for parenteral use. *JAMA* 1979; 241: 2051.

American Medical Association, Department of Foods and Nutrition: Multivitamin preparations for parenteral use: a statement by the Nutrition Advisory Group. *J Parenter Enter Nutr* 1979; 3: 258.

Blackburn GL, et al: Nutritional and metabolic assessment of the hospitalized patient. *J Parenter Enter Nutr* 1977; 3: 17.

Committee on Dietary Allowances, Food and Nutrition Board, National Research Council: *Recommended Dietary Allowances*. Washington, D.C., National Academy of Sciences, 1980.

Harris JA, Benedict FG: A biometric study of basal metabolism in man. Carnegie Institute of Washington, Publication #279, 1919.

Kamath SK, et al: Hospital malnutrition: A 33-hospital screening study. *J Am Diet Assoc* 1986: 203.

Kinney JM, Roe CF: Caloric equivalent of fever: Patterns of postoperative response. *Ann Surg* 1962; 156: 610.

Lang, CE: *Nutritional Support in Critical Care*. Aspen Systems Corp., 1987.

Long CL, et al: Metabolic response to injury and illness: Estimation of energy and protein needs from indirect calorimetry and nitrogen balance. *J Parenter Enter Nutr* 1979; 3: 452.

Weissman C, et al: Effects of routine intensive care interactions on metabolic rate. *Chest* 86; 815: 1984.

2

APPENDIX

Caring for the critically ill on prolonged bed rest

TABLE A2-1
Physiologic effects of bed rest (deconditioning)

Increased HR and BP for submaximal workload.
Decrease in functional capacity.
Decrease in circulating volume.
Orthostatic hypotension.
Reflex tachycardia.
Modest decrease in pulmonary function.
Increase in thromboemboli.
Loss of muscle mass.
Loss of muscle contractile strength.
Negative protein state.
Negative nitrogen state.

Potential for activity intolerance related to deconditioning secondary to prolonged bed rest

---

Desired outcome: Patient exhibits cardiac tolerance to exercise as evidenced by HR $\leq$20 bpm over resting HR, systolic BP $\leq$20 mm Hg over or under resting systolic BP, SVO_2 $\geq$60%, RR $\leq$20 breaths/min, normal sinus rhythm on EKG, warm and dry skin, and absence of crackles, murmurs, and chest pain.

---

1. Perform ROM exercises bid to qid on each extremity. Individualize the exercise plan based on the following guidelines:
   - *Mode or type of exercise:* Begin with passive exercises, moving the joints through the motions of abduction, adduction, flexion, and extension. Progress to active assisted exercises in which you support the joints while the patient initiates muscle contraction. When the patient is able, supervise him or her in active isotonic exercises, during which the patient contracts a selected muscle group, moves the extremity at a slow pace, and then relaxes the muscle group. Have the patient repeat each exercise 5-10 times.

< CAUTION : Isometric exercises should be avoided in cardiac patients.

- *Intensity:* Begin with 3-5 repetitions as tolerated by the patient. Assess exercise tolerance by measuring HR and BP at rest, peak exercise, and 5 minutes after exercise. If HR or systolic BP increases >20 bpm or mm Hg over the resting level, decrease the number of repetitions. If HR or systolic BP decreases >10 bpm or mm Hg at peak exercise, this could be a sign of left ventricular failure, denoting that the heart cannot meet this workload. For other adverse signs and symptoms, see "Assessment," below.
- *Duration:* Begin with 5 minutes or less of exercise. Gradually increase the exercise to 15 minutes as tolerated.
- *Frequency:* Begin exercises bid-qid. As the duration increases, the frequency can be reduced.
- *Assessment of exercise tolerance:* Be alert to signs and symptoms that the cardiovascular and respiratory systems are unable to meet the demands of the low-level ROM exercises. Excessive SOB may occur if (1) transient pulmonary congestion occurs secondary to ischemia or left ventricular dysfunction; (2) lung volumes are decreased; (3) oxygen-carrying capacity of the blood is reduced; or (4) there is shunting of blood from the right to the left side of the heart without adequate oxygenation. If cardiac output does not increase to meet the body's needs during modest levels of exercise, systolic BP may fall; the skin may become cool, cyanotic, and diaphoretic; dysrhythmias may be noted; crackles (rales) may be auscultated; or a systolic murmur of mitral regurgitation may occur. If the patient tolerates the exercise, increase the intensity or number of repetitions each day.

2. As the patient's condition improves, increase activity as soon as possible to include sitting in a chair. Assess for orthostatic hypotension, which can occur as a result of decreased plasma volume and difficulty in adjusting immediately to postural change. Prepare the patient for this by increasing the amount of time spent in high-Fowler's position and moving the patient slowly and in stages. For more information about activity progression, see Table 2-1, "Activity Level Progression in Hospitalized Patients," p. 77.
3. Increase activity level by having patient perform self-care activities such as eating, mouth care, and bathing as tolerated.
4. Teach significant others the purpose and interventions for preventing deconditioning. Involve them in the patient's plan of care.
5. To help allay fears of failure, pain, or medical setbacks, provide emotional support to patient and significant others as patient's activity level is increased.

Potential for impaired physical mobility related to risk of contractures or ankylosis secondary to prolonged bed rest

---

Desired outcome: Patient displays complete range of motion (ROM) without verbal or nonverbal indicators of pain.

< N O T E : ROM exercises should be performed every day for all immobilized patients with *normal* joints. Modification may be required for patients with flaccidity (i.e., immediately following CVA or spinal cord injury) to prevent subluxation, or for patient with spasticity (i.e., during the recovery period for patients with CVA

or spinal cord injury) to prevent an increase in spasticity. Consult with physical therapist or occupational therapist for assistance with modifying the exercise plan for these patients. In addition, be aware that ROM exercises are contraindicated for patients with rheumatologic disease during the inflammatory phase and for joints that are dislocated or fractured.

1. Perform ROM routinely, as described under **Potential for activity intolerance**, p. 506. Incorporate the movement patterns into care activities such as position changes, bed baths, getting the patient on and off the bed pan, or changing the patient's gown.
2. Support patient's feet with a footboard, foam boots, or tennis shoes to prevent foot plantarflexion.
3. Encourage patient to perform dorsiflexion-plantarflexion exercises q2h.
4. Assess for footdrop by inspecting the feet for plantarflexion and evaluating patient's ability to pull the toes upward toward his or her nose. Although feet posture naturally in plantarflexion, be particularly alert to the patient's inability to pull the toes up. Document this assessment daily.
5. Post a turning schedule to ensure that position changes are performed at least q2h. Position changes not only will maintain correct body alignment, thereby reducing strain on the joints, they will also prevent contractures, minimize pressure on bony prominences, and promote maximal chest expansion as well.
   - Try to place patient in a position that achieves proper standing alignment: head neutral or slightly flexed on the neck, hips extended, knees extended or minimally flexed, and feet at right angles to the legs. Maintain this position with pillows, towels, or other positioning aids.
   - To prevent hip flexion contractures, ensure that the patient is sidelying with the hips extended for the same amount of time patient spends in the supine position.
   - When the HOB must be elevated 30 degrees, extend the patient's shoulders and arms, using pillows to support the position, and allow the fingertips to extend over the edge of the pillows to maintain normal arching of the hands.

$<$ C A U T I O N : Because elevating the HOB promotes hip flexion, ensure that patient spends equal time with the hips in extension (see intervention, above).

   - When patient is in the sidelying position, use the opportunity to extend the lower leg from the hip to help prevent hip flexion contracture.
   - When able to place patient in the prone position, move patient to the end of the bed and allow the feet to rest between the mattress and footboard. This will not only prevent plantarflexion and hip rotation, it will prevent injury to the heels and toes as well. Place thin pads under the angles of the axillae and lateral aspects of the clavicles to prevent internal rotation of the shoulders and maintain anatomic position of the shoulder girdle.

Potential for impaired skin and tissue integrity related to pressure on skin and tissue secondary to prolonged bed rest

---

Desired outcome: Patient's skin and tissue remain intact.

---

1. Identify patients at high risk for skin breakdown and tissue impairment: individuals with altered LOC, immobility, hypothermia, hyperthermia, cachexia, inability to perform ADLs, or advanced age.
2. Change patient's position at least q2h, turning from the side to the back to the side and to the front (if not contraindicated). Turn heavier patients more frequently, as there is an inverse relationship between pressure and time with decubitus ulcer formation. Use pillows to cushion bony prominences.
3. Post a position-changing schedule that is individualized to meet each patient's needs.
4. Inspect the skin during each position change, being alert to erythema. Keep patient's weight off erythematous skin as much as possible. Massage skin and tissue over susceptible areas such as bony prominences.
5. Perform backrubs q2-4h.
6. To minimize pressure on the tissues, use a protective covering over the mattress such as an eggcrate or air mattress.
7. Perform a complete assessment of the skin and tissue q8h. Document color, texture, turgor, sensation, temperature, and the presence of lesions. Be alert to skin that is erythematous and warm to the touch. Assess the ability of erythematous skin to blanch in response to digital pressure. Current research suggests that massage of erythematous skin that does not blanch in response to pressure may actually harm the tissue.
8. If skin and tissue appear to be compromised, use a low-pressure bed such as the Clinitron, Mediscus, water bed, or alternating pressure mattress.
9. Should skin breakdown occur, develop an aggressive plan of care to promote healing, including regular cleansing of the area and measures to promote circulation (i.e., ROM, ankle-circling, isometric, and deep-breathing exercises), prevent infection, and promote growth of granulation tissue, following agency protocol. Evaluate and revise the plan of care at regular intervals.
10. Help patient attain a state of nitrogen balance to prevent skin and tissue breakdown and ensure optimal tissue repair. See section "Providing Nutritional Support," p. 490, for details.
11. Unless contraindicated, ensure that patient has an intake of at least 2-3 L/day of fluid to promote optimal tissue turgor.

Potential alteration in oral mucous membrane related to self-care deficit

---

Desired outcome: Patient's oral mucosa, lips, and tongue remain intact.

---

1. Assess patient's oral mucous membrane, lips, and tongue q2h, noting presence of dryness, exudate, swelling, blisters, and ulcers.
2. If patient is alert and able to take oral fluids, offer frequent sips of water or ice chips to alleviate dryness.
3. Perform mouth care q2-4h, using a soft-bristled toothbrush to cleanse the teeth and a moistened cloth or toothette (small sponge on a stick) to moisten crusty areas or exudate on tongue and oral mucosa. If patient is intubated, suction mouth to remove fluid and debris.
4. Apply lip balm q2h and prn to prevent cracking of lips.

5. If indicated, use an artificial saliva preparation to assist in keeping mucous membrane moist. Avoid use of lemon and glycerine swabs, which can contribute to dryness.

6. As appropriate, have patient wear dentures as soon as he or she is able, to improve communication and enhance comfort.

< N O T E : If it is necessary to put fingers in patient's mouth, wear gloves on both hands. This practice will reduce the risk of acquiring herpetic Whitlow.

Self-care deficit: Inability to perform ADLs related to decreased LOC or sensorimotor deficit

Desired outcome: Patient's physical needs are met by patient, nursing staff, or significant others.

1. Assess patient's ability to perform self care, based on functional status (i.e., comatose state, hemiplegia, sensory or motor deficit, alterations in vision).

2. If patient is comatose, meet all of patient's physical needs, including bathing, oral hygiene, feeding, elimination. Involve significant others in the plan of care. Explain all procedures to patient and significant others before performing them.

3. For patient who is not comatose, collaborate with him or her on a plan of care that promotes as much self care as patient is capable of. Schedule care activities around the periods of time patient has the most energy to meet his or her needs. Use assessment criteria for activity tolerance, p. 506, to evaluate patient's tolerance of the activity.

4. If patient is alert, keep toiletries and other necessary items within his or her reach.

5. Do not rush patient; allow adequate time for performance of self-care activities.

6. Encourage patient; reinforce the value of progress that is made.

7. As appropriate, consult with occupational therapy department regarding use of assistive devices such as long-handled tools.

8. If visual impairment exists, place all objects within patient's field of vision. If diplopia is present, apply an eye patch and alternate it between patient's eyes q2-3h.

Diversional activity deficit related to monotony and boredom secondary to prolonged illness and hospitalization

Desired outcome: Patient relates that boredom is allayed.

1. Assess patient's activity tolerance as described on pp. 506-507.

2. Assess patient's prehospitalization interests and recreational activities, particularly those that are suitable to the intensive care environment.

3. Encourage significant others' involvement in patient's plan of care. Advise them of the desirability for evenly spaced visits throughout the week and encourage them to bring in diversional activities from home that are appropriate for patient's interest level and activity tolerance.

4. Provide low-level activities commensurate with patient's tolerance. Examples include books or magazines pertaining to patient's recreational or other interests, television, or writing for short intervals.

5. Initiate activities that require little concentration and proceed to more complicated tasks as patient's condition allows. For example, if reading requires more energy or concentration than patient is capable of, suggest that significant others read to patient or bring in audio tapes of books such as those that are marketed for the visually impaired.

6. Call upon volunteers or patient relation representative to visit patient.

7. Refer patient to occupational therapist for a specific, detailed plan.

8. As patient's condition improves, enable patient to sit in a chair near a window so that he or she can view outside activities.

For interventions related to prevention of atelectasis and pneumonia, see appropriate nursing diagnoses in the chapter ''Respiratory Dysfunctions,'' pp. 1-71. For **Sleep pattern disturbance** and psychosocial nursing diagnoses and interventions, see section ''Caring for the Critically Ill with Life-Threatening Disorders,'' pp. 511-522.

SELECTED REFERENCES

Stotts, N: Managing Wound Care. In *Manual of Nursing Therapeutics: Applying Nursing Diagnoses to Medical Disorders*. Ed: Swearingen, PL. Addison-Wesley, 1986.

Swearingen, PL: *Addison-Wesley Photo-Atlas of Nursing Procedures*. Addison-Wesley, 1984.

Wenger, N, Hellerstein, M: *Cardiac Rehabilitation*, 2nd ed. Lippincott, 1985.

Winslow, EH: Cardiovascular consequences of bed rest. *Heart Lung,* May 1985; 14(3): 236-246.

Caring for the critically ill with life-threatening disorders

Knowledge deficit: Current health status and therapies

Desired outcome: Patient participates in the learning process and communicates understanding of current health status and therapies.

---

1. Establish patient's current level of knowledge regarding his or her health status.

2. Assess patient's cognitive and emotional readiness to learn.

3. Recognize barriers to learning, such as ineffective communication, neurologic deficit, sensory alterations, fear, anxiety, or lack of motivation.

4. Assess patient's learning needs and establish short- and long-term goals with patient and significant others.

5. Use individualized verbal and audiovisual strategies to promote learning and enhance understanding. Give simple, direct instructions.

6. Encourage significant others to reinforce correct information regarding diagnosis and therapies to the patient.

7. As appropriate, facilitate referral of neurologically impaired patient to neurologic clinical nurse specialist, neuropsychologist.

8. Encourage patient's interest about health care information by planning care collaboratively. Explain rationale for care and therapies.
9. Interact frequently with patient to evaluate his or her comprehension of information given. Individuals in crisis often need multiple explanations before information can be understood.
10. As appropriate, assess patient's understanding of informed consent. Assist patient to use information he or she receives to make informed health care decisions (e.g., regarding surgery, resuscitation, organ donation).

Anxiety related to actual or perceived threat to biologic integrity, self concept, or role; unfamiliar people and environment; or the unknown

---

Desired outcome: Patient's anxiety is absent or reduced as evidenced by HR ≤ 100 bpm, RR ≤ 20 breaths per minute, and an absence of or decrease in irritability and restlessness.

---

1. Engage in honest communication with the patient; provide empathetic understanding. Establish an atmosphere that allows free expression.
2. Assess the patient's level of anxiety. Be alert to verbal and nonverbal cues.
   - *Mild:* Restlessness, irritability, increase in questions, focusing on the environment.
   - *Moderate:* Inattentiveness, expressions of concern, narrowed perceptions, insomnia, increased HR.
   - *Severe:* Expressions of feelings of doom, rapid speech, tremors, poor eye contact. Patient may be preoccupied with the past; unable to understand the present; and may present with tachycardia, nausea, and hyperventilation.
   - *Panic:* Inability to concentrate or communicate, distortion of reality, increased motor activity, vomiting, tachypnea.
3. For patients with severe anxiety or panic state, refer to psychiatric clinical nurse specialist or other as appropriate.
4. If patient is hyperventilating, encourage slow, deep breaths by having patient mimic your own breathing pattern.
5. Validate the nursing assessment of anxiety with the patient. ("You seem distressed; are you feeling uncomfortable now?")
6. Following an episode of anxiety, review and discuss with patient the thoughts and feelings that led to the episode.
7. Identify coping behaviors currently being used by patient, for example, denial, anger, repression, withdrawal, daydreaming, or dependence on narcotics. Review coping behaviors patient has used in the past. Assist patient with using adaptive coping to manage anxiety. ("I understand that your wife reads to you to help you relax. Would you like to spend a part of each day alone with her?")
8. Encourage patient to express fears, concerns, and questions. ("I know this room looks like a maze of wires and tubes; please let me know when you have any questions.")
9. Reduce sensory overload by providing an organized, quiet environment. See nursing diagnosis **Sensory-perceptual alterations,** pp. 513-514.

10. Introduce self and other health care members, explaining each individual's role as it relates to the patient's care.

11. Teach patient relaxation and imagery techniques. See the following: **Knowledge deficit:** Relaxation technique effective for stress reduction and facilitation of sympathetic tone, p. 99.

12. Enable support persons to be in attendance whenever possible.

Impaired verbal communication related to dysarthria secondary to neurologic deficit or physical barrier (tracheostomy, intubation)

Desired outcome: Patient communicates needs and feelings and relates decrease or absence of frustration over communication barriers.

---

1. Assess etiology of the impaired communication (e.g., endotracheal intubation, tracheostomy, cerebrovascular accident, cerebral tumor, myasthenia gravis, Guillain-Barré syndrome).

2. Along with patient and significant others, assess patient's ability to read, write, and comprehend English. If patient speaks a language other than English, collaborate with English-speaking family member or interpreter to establish effective communication.

3. When communicating with patient, use eye contact; speak in a clear, normal tone of voice; and face the patient.

4. If patient is unable to speak because of a physical barrier (e.g., intubation or tracheostomy, wired mandibles) provide reassurance and acknowledge his or her frustration. ("I know this is frustrating for you, but let's not give up. I want to understand you.")

5. Provide slate, word cards, pencil and paper, alphabet board, pictures, or other device to assist patient with communication.

6. Explain the source of the patient's communication impairment to significant others; teach them effective communication alternatives (listed above).

7. Be alert to nonverbal messages, such as facial expressions, hand movements, and nodding of the head. Validate their meaning with patient.

8. Recognize that the inability to speak may foster maladaptive behaviors. Encourage patient to communicate needs; reinforce independent behaviors.

9. Be honest with patient; do not relate understanding if you are unable to interpret patient's communication.

Sensory-perceptual alterations related to environmental overload or monotony, socially-restricted environment, psychologic stress, or pathophysiologic alterations

---

Desired outcomes: Patient verbalizes orientation to person, place, and time; relates the ability to concentrate; and expresses satisfaction with the degree and type of sensory stimulation being received.

---

1. Assess factors contributing to patient's sensory-perceptual alteration.
   - *Environmental:* Excessive noise in the environment; constant, monotonous noise; restricted environment (immobility, traction, isolation); social isolation (restricted visitors, impaired communication); therapies.
   - *Physiologic:* Decreased organ function, sleep or rest pattern disturbance, medication, previous history of altered sensory perception.
2. Determine the appropriate sensory stimulation needed for the patient and plan care accordingly.
3. Control factors that contribute to environmental overload. For example, avoid constant lighting (use blindfolds, if necessary); decrease noise whenever possible (e.g., decrease alarm volumes, avoid loud talking, close room door occasionally, provide ear plugs for patient).
4. Provide meaningful sensory stimulation.
   - Display clocks and large calendars and photographs and objects from home.
   - Provide a radio, music, reading materials, tape recordings of family and significant others.
   - Position patient toward window when possible.
   - Discuss current events, time of day, holidays, and topics of interest during patient care activities. ("Good morning, Mr. Smith. I'm Ms. Stone, your nurse for the afternoon and evening, 3 PM to 11 PM. It's sunny outside. Today is the first day of summer.")
   - As needed, orient patient to surroundings. Direct patient to reality as necessary.
   - Touch patient frequently.
   - Encourage significant others to communicate with patient frequently, using a normal tone of voice.
   - Convey concern and respect for the patient. Introduce self and call patient by name.
   - Stimulate patient's vision with mirrors, colored decorations, and pictures.
   - Stimulate patient's sense of taste with sweet, salty, and sour substances as allowed.
   - Encourage use of eyeglasses and hearing aids.
5. Explain routines, therapies, and equipment simply and directly. Critically ill individuals often cannot comprehend complex information.
6. Encourage patient to participate in health-care planning and decision making whenever possible.
7. Assess patient's sleep-rest pattern to evaluate its contribution to patient's sensory-perceptual disorder. Ensure that patient attains at least 90 minutes of uninterrupted sleep as frequently as possible. For more information, see next nursing diagnosis.

Sleep pattern disturbance related to environmental overload, therapeutic regimen, pain, immobility, or psychologic stress

---

Desired outcomes: Patient identifies factors that promote sleep, attains 90-minute periods of uninterrupted sleep, and verbalizes satisfaction with his or her ability to rest.

---

1. Assess patient's usual sleeping patterns (e.g., bedtime routine, hours of sleep per night, sleeping position, use of pillows and blankets, napping during the day, nocturia).

2. Explore relaxation techniques that promote patient's rest-sleep (e.g., imagining relaxing scenes, listening to soothing music or taped stories, using muscle relaxation exercises).

3. Identify causative factors and activities that contribute to patient's insomnia, awaken patient, or adversely affect sleep patterns. Examples include pain, anxiety, therapies, depression, hallucinations, medications, underlying illness, sleep apnea, respiratory disorder, caffeine use, fear.

4. Organize procedures and activities to allow for 90-minute periods of uninterrupted rest-sleep. Limit visiting during these periods.

5. Whenever possible, maintain a quiet environment by providing ear plugs or decreasing alarm levels. The use of "white noise" (e.g., low-pitched, monotonous sounds; electric fan; soft music) may facilitate sleep. Dim the lights for a period of time each day by drawing the drapes or providing blindfolds.

6. If appropriate, put limitations on patient's daytime sleeping. Attempt to establish regularly scheduled daytime activity (e.g., ambulation, sitting in chair, active ROM), which may promote nighttime sleep.

7. Investigate and provide comfort measures that are known to promote patient's sleep, for example, soft music, massage, reading to patient, personal hygiene (e.g., bath at bedtime), snack.

Fear related to threat to biologic integrity, potential for loss, altered body image, loss of control, or therapeutic regimen

---

Desired outcomes: Patient communicates fears and concerns, relates the attainment of increased psychologic and physical comfort, and does not exhibit ineffective coping techniques.

---

1. Assess patient's perceptions of the environment and his or her health status and determine contributing factors to patient's feelings of fear. Evaluate patient's verbal and nonverbal responses.

2. Acknowledge patient's fears. ("I understand that all this equipment frightens you, but it is necessary to help you breathe.")

3. Assess patient's history of coping behavior to determine sources of strength. ("What helps you get through stressful situations?") Identify negative coping behaviors, including severe depression, withdrawal, prolonged denial, hostility, and violence.

4. Provide opportunities for the patient to express fears and concerns. ("You seem very concerned about receiving more blood today.") Listen actively to the patient. Recognize that anger, denial, occasional withdrawal, and demanding behaviors may be coping responses.

5. Encourage patient to ask questions and gather information about the unknown. Provide ongoing information about equipment, therapies, and unit routines according to patient's ability to understand.

6. To promote an increased sense of control over self, encourage patient to participate in and plan his or her care whenever possible. Provide continuity of care by establishing a routine and arranging for consistent caregivers whenever possible.
7. Discuss with health-care team the appropriateness of medication therapy for patient's disabling fear or anxiety.
8. Explore patient's desire for spiritual or other counseling.
9. If there is a possibility of survival of the illness or surgery, collaborate with MD regarding a visit by another individual with the same disorder who has survived the surgery or disorder.

Ineffective individual coping related to threat to biologic integrity, knowledge deficit, unsatisfactory support systems, or hospitalization

---

Desired outcomes: Patient verbalizes feelings, identifies strengths and coping behaviors, and does not demonstrate ineffective coping behaviors.

---

1. Assess patient's perceptions and ability to understand his or her current health status.
2. Establish honest communication with the patient. (''Please tell me what I can do to help you.'') Assist patient with identifying strengths, stressors, inappropriate behaviors, and personal needs.
3. Support positive coping behaviors. (''I see that reading that book seems to help you relax.'')
4. Provide opportunities for the patient to express concerns; gather information from nurses and other support systems. Provide patient with explanations regarding the unit routine, therapies, and equipment. Acknowledge patient's feelings and assessment of his or her current health status and environment.
5. Identify factors that inhibit patient's ability to cope (e.g., unsatisfactory support system, knowledge deficit, grief, fear).
6. Recognize maladaptive coping behaviors (e.g., severe depression, dependence on narcotics, hostility, violence, suicidal ideations). Confront patient about these behaviors. (''You seem to be requiring more pain medication. Are you experiencing more physical pain, or does it help you to remove yourself from reality?'') Refer patient to psychiatric liaison, clinical nurse specialist, or clergy, as appropriate.
7. As patient's condition allows, assist with reducing anxiety. See **Anxiety,** pp. 512-513.
8. Help reduce patient's sensory overload by maintaining an organized, quiet environment. See **Sensory-perceptual alterations,** pp. 513-514.
9. Encourage regular visits by significant others. Encourage them to engage in conversation with patient to help minimize patient's emotional and social isolation.
10. Assess significant others' interactions with patient. Attempt to mobilize support systems by involving them in patient care whenever possible.
11. As appropriate, explain to significant others that increased dependency, anger, and denial may be adaptive coping behaviors used by patient in early stages of crisis until effective coping behaviors are learned.

Anticipatory grieving related to expected loss of body function or body part, changes in self-concept or body image, or terminal illness

Desired outcomes: Patient and significant other(s) express grief, participate in decisions regarding the future, and communicate concerns to health-care team and to one another.

1. Assess factors contributing to anticipated loss.
2. Assess and accept patient's behavioral response. Expect reactions such as disbelief, denial, guilt, ambivalence, and depression.
3. Assess religious and sociocultural expectations related to loss. ("Is religion an important part of your life? How do you and your family deal with serious health problems?") Refer to the clergy or community support groups as appropriate.
4. Encourage patient and significant others to share their concerns. ("Is there anything you'd like to talk about today?") Also, respect their desire not to speak.
5. Demonstrate empathy. ("This must be a very difficult time for you and your family.")
6. In selected circumstances, provide individuals with an explanation of the grieving process. This may assist them to better understand and acknowledge their feelings.
7. Assess grief reactions of patient and significant others and identify those individuals who may have a potential for dysfunctional grieving reactions (e.g., absence of emotion, hostility, avoidance). If the potential for dysfunctional grieving is present, refer the individual to psychiatric clinical nurse specialist, clergy, or other as appropriate.

Dysfunctional grieving related to actual or perceived loss or change in body function, body image, lifestyle, relationships, or lack of support systems

Desired outcomes: Patient and significant other(s) express grief, explain the meaning of the loss, and communicate concerns with each other. The patient completes necessary self-care activities.

1. Assess grief stage and previous coping abilities. Discuss with patient and significant others their feelings, the meaning of the loss, and their goals. ("How do you feel about your condition/illness? What do you hope to accomplish in these next few days/weeks?")
2. Acknowledge and permit anger; set limits on the expression of anger to discourage destructive behavior. ("I understand that you must feel very angry, but for the safety of others, you may not throw equipment.")
3. Identify suicidal behavior (e.g., severe depression, statements of intent, suicide plan, previous history of suicide attempt). Ensure patient safety and refer patient to psychiatric clinical nurse specialist, psychiatrist, clergy, or other support system.
4. Encourage patient and significant others to participate in daily and diversional

activities. Identify physiologic problems related to loss (e.g., eating or sleeping disorders) and intervene accordingly.

5. If there is a possibility of the patient's survival of the illness, collaborate with MD regarding a visit by another individual with the same disorder who has survived the surgery or illness.

Powerlessness related to lack of control over self-care, health care status, or outcome secondary to nature of health care environment, therapeutic regimen, or life-threatening illness

---

Desired outcomes: Patient makes decisions regarding care and therapies and relates an attitude of realistic hope and a sense of control over self.

---

1. Assess with patient his or her personal preferences, needs, values, and attitudes.
2. Before providing information, assess patient's knowledge and understanding of his or her condition and care.
3. Recognize patient's expressions of fear, lack of response to events, and lack of interest in information, any of which may signal patient's sense of powerlessness.
4. Evaluate caregiver practices and adjust them to support patient's sense of control. For example, if the patient always bathes in the evening to promote relaxation before bedtime, modify the care plan to include an evening bath rather than follow the hospital routine of giving a morning bath.
5. Assist patient to identify and demonstrate activities he or she can perform independently.
6. Whenever possible, offer alternatives related to routine hygiene, diet, diversional activities, visiting hours, or treatment times.
7. Ensure patient's privacy and preserve his or her territorial rights whenever possible. For example, when distant relatives and casual acquaintances request information about the patient's status, check with patient and family members before sharing that information.
8. Discourage patient's dependency on staff. Avoid overprotection and parenting behaviors toward patient.
9. Assess support systems; enable significant others to be involved in patient care whenever possible.
10. Offer realistic hope for the future. On occasion, encourage patient to direct thoughts beyond the present.
11. Provide referrals to clergy and other support systems as appropriate.

Spiritual distress related to altered health state, separation from religious ties, life-threatening illness, or conflict between religious beliefs and therapeutic regimens

---

Desired outcomes: Patient verbalizes his or her religious beliefs and expresses hope for the future, the attainment of spiritual well-being, and that conflicts have been resolved or diminished.

---

1. Assess patient's spiritual or religious beliefs, values, and practices. ("Do you have a religious preference? How important is it to you? Are there any religious or spiritual practices you wish to participate in while in the hospital?") If the patient expresses a desire, volunteer to read scripture or other religious literature.
2. Inform patient and significant others of the availability of spiritual aids, such as a chapel or volunteer chaplain.
3. Display a nonjudgmental attitude toward patient's religious or spiritual beliefs and values. Attempt to create an environment that is conducive to free expression.
4. Identify available support systems that may assist in meeting the patient's religious or spiritual needs (e.g., clergy, fellow church members, support groups).
5. Be alert to comments related to spiritual concerns or conflicts. ("I don't know why God is doing this to me." "I'm being punished for my sins.")
6. Use active listening and open-ended questioning to assist patient to resolve conflicts related to spiritual issues. ("I understand that you want to be baptized. We can arrange to do that here.")
7. Provide privacy and opportunities for religious practices, such as prayer and meditation.
8. If spiritual beliefs and therapeutic regimens are in conflict, provide patient with honest, concrete information to encourage informed decision making. ("I understand that your religion discourages the transfusion of blood. Do you understand that by refusing blood your risk of disability increases greatly?")

Social isolation related to hospitalization in critical care unit, altered health status, inadequate support systems, terminal illness

---

Desired outcome: Patient demonstrates interaction and communication with others.

---

1. Assess factors contributing to patient's social isolation.
   * Restricted visiting hours.
   * Absence of or inadequate support system.
   * Inability to communicate (e.g., presence of mechanical ventilation).
   * Physical changes that affect self concept.
   * Patient denial or withdrawal.
   * Critical care environment.
2. Recognize patients at high risk for social isolation: the elderly, disabled, chronically ill, economically disadvantaged.
3. Assist patient with identifying feelings associated with loneliness and isolation. ("You seem very sad when your family leaves the room. Can you tell me more about your feelings?").
4. Determine patient's need for socialization and identify available and potential support systems. Explore methods for increasing social contact (e.g., TV, radio, tapes of loved ones, intercom system, more frequent visitations, scheduled interaction with nurse or support staff).
5. Provide positive reinforcement for socialization that lessens the patient's feelings of isolation and loneliness. ("Please continue to call me when you need to

talk to someone. Talking will help both of us to better understand your feelings.'')

6. Facilitate patient's ability to communicate with others (see **Impaired verbal communication,** p. 513).

Disturbance in self concept related to alteration in body image secondary to loss or change in body parts or function, physical trauma, hospitalization

---

Desired outcomes: Patient acknowledges body changes and demonstrates movement toward incorporating changes into self-concept. Patient does not demonstrate maladaptive response, such as severe depression.

---

1. Establish open, honest communication with the patient. Promote an environment that is conducive to free expression. (''Please feel free to talk to me whenever you have any questions.'')

2. When planning patient's care, be aware of therapies that may influence patient's self concept (e.g., medications, mechanical ventilation, invasive procedures and monitoring).

3. Assess patient's knowledge of the pathophysiologic process that has occurred and his or her present health status. Clarify any misconceptions. (''You seem to believe that you will never be able to breathe without a ventilator. We expect you to be breathing well without one soon.'')

4. Discuss the loss or change with the patient and significant others. Recognize that what may seem to be a small change may be of great significance to the patient (e.g., arm immobilizer, catheter, hair loss, facial abrasions).

5. Explore with patient his or her concerns, fears, and feelings of guilt. (''I understand that you are frightened. Your face looks very different now, but you will see changes and it will improve. Gradually you will begin to look more like yourself.'')

6. Encourage patient and significant others to interact with one another. Help family to avoid reinforcement of their loved one's changed body part or function. (''I know your son looks very different to you now, but it would help if you would speak to him and touch him as you would normally.'')

7. Encourage patient to participate gradually in self-care activities, as he or she becomes physically and emotionally able. Allow for some initial withdrawal and denial behaviors. For example, when changing dressings over traumatized part, explain what you are doing but do not expect the patient to watch or participate initially.

8. Discuss opportunities for reconstruction of the loss or change (i.e., surgery, prosthesis, physical therapy, cosmetic therapies, organ transplant).

9. Recognize manifestations of severe depression (i.e., sleep disturbances, change in affect, change in communication pattern). As appropriate, refer to psychiatric clinical nurse specialist, clergy, or support group.

10. Help patient attain a sense of autonomy by offering choices and alternatives whenever possible. Emphasize patient's strengths and encourage activities that interest patient.

11. Offer realistic hope for the future.

Potential for violence related to sensory overload, rage reactions, perceived threats, or physiologic imbalance

---

Desired outcome: There is no evidence that the patient has harmed self or others.

---

1. Assess factors that may contribute to or precipitate violent behavior (e.g., medication reactions, inability to cope, suicidal behavior, confusion, hypoxia, postictal states).
2. Attempt to eliminate or treat causative factors. For example, provide patient teaching, reorient patient, ensure delivery of prescribed oxygen therapy, and reduce or prevent sensory overload (see **Sensory-perceptual alterations**, pp. 513-514).
3. Recognize that maladaptive behavior may be a response to patient's fears, grief, and feelings of powerlessness.
4. Monitor for early signs of increasing anxiety and agitation (i.e., restlessness, verbal aggressiveness, inability to concentrate). Assess for body language that is indicative of violent behavior: clenched fists, rigid posture, increased motor activity.
5. Approach patient in a positive manner and encourage verbalization of feelings and concerns. ("I understand that you are frightened. I will be here from 3 PM to 11 PM to care for you.")
6. Offer patient as much personal and environmental control as the situation allows. ("Let's discuss the care you will need today. What fluids would you like to drink? Would you prefer a bath in the morning or evening?")
7. Help patient distinguish reality from altered perceptions. Orient patient to person, place, and time. Alter the environment to promote reality-based thought processes (e.g., provide clocks, calendars, pictures of loved ones, familiar objects).
8. Initiate measures that prevent or reduce excessive agitation.
   - Reduce environmental stimuli (e.g., alarms, loud or unnecessary talking).
   - Before touching patient, explain procedures and care, using short, concise statements.
   - Speak quietly (but firmly, as necessary) and project a caring attitude toward the patient. ("We are very concerned for your comfort and safety. Can we do anything to help you feel more relaxed?")
   - Avoid crowding (i.e., of equipment, visitors, health-care personnel) in patient's personal environment.
9. Explain and discuss patient's behavior with significant others. Acknowledge frustration, concerns, fears, and questions. Review safety precautions with significant others (see next intervention).
10. In the event of violent behavior, institute safety precautions.
    - Remove harmful objects from the environment, such as heavy objects, scissors.
    - Apply padding to side rails.
    - Use restraints as necessary and prescribed.
    - Never turn back toward violent patient.
    - Do not approach violent patient without adequate assistance from others.

- Set limits on patient's behavior. ("I understand you must feel very frustrated, but you cannot continue to throw supplies or strike the siderails with your fists.")
- Explain safety precautions to patient. ("We are placing these restraints on your wrists to prevent you from harming yourself.")

Hopelessness related to prolonged hospitalization or life-threatening illness

Desired outcomes: Patient verbalizes hopeful aspects of health status and relates that feelings of despair are absent or lessened.

1. Develop open, honest communication with the patient, providing empathetic understanding of fears and doubts and promoting an environment that is conducive to free expression.
2. Assess patient's and significant others' understanding of patient's health status and prognosis; clarify any misperceptions.
3. Assess for indicators of hopelessness: unwillingness to accept help, pessimism, withdrawal, lack of interest, silence, loss of gratification in roles, previous history of hopeless behavior, hypoactivity, inability to accomplish tasks, expressions of incompetence, entrapment, irritability.
4. Provide opportunities for the patient to feel cared for, needed, and valued by others. For example, emphasize importance of relationships. ("Tell me about your grandchildren." "It seems that your family loves you very much.")
5. Support significant others who seem powerful in sparking or maintaining patient's feelings of hope. ("Your husband's mood seemed to improve after your visit to the ICU.")
6. Recognize discussions and factors that promote patient's sense of hope (i.e., discussions about family members, reminiscing about better times).
7. Explore patient's coping mechanisms; assist patient with expanding positive coping behavior (see **Ineffective individual coping**, p. 516).
8. Assess patient's spiritual state and needs (see **Spiritual distress**, pp. 518-519).
9. Promote anticipation of positive events (i.e., mealtime, grandchildren's visits, bath time, extubation, discontinuation of traction).
10. Help patient recognize that although there may be no hope for returning to original lifestyle, there *is* hope for a new, but different, life.
11. Avoid insisting that the patient assume a positive attitude. Encourage hope for the future, even if it is the hope for a peaceful death.

Caring for the family of the critically ill

Ineffective family coping: Compromised, related to anxiety, knowledge deficit, role change, exhausted support systems, or unrealistic expectations

Desired outcomes: Family members verbalize feelings, identify ineffective coping patterns, identify strengths and positive coping behaviors, and seek information and support from the nurse or other support systems outside the family.

1. Establish open, honest communication with the family. Assist the family to identify strengths, stressors, inappropriate behaviors, and personal needs. ("I understand your mother was very ill last year. How did you manage the situation?" "I know your loved one is very ill. How can I help you?")
2. Assess family members for ineffective coping (e.g., depression, chemical dependency, violence, withdrawal) and identify factors that inhibit effective coping (e.g., inadequate support system, grief, fear of disapproval by others, knowledge deficit). ("You seem to be unable to talk about your husband's illness. Is there anyone with whom you can talk about it?")
3. Assess the family's knowledge about the patient's current health status and therapies. Provide information frequently and allow sufficient time for questions. Reassess the family's understanding at frequent intervals.
4. Provide opportunites in a private setting for family to talk and share concerns with nurses.
5. Offer realistic hope. Help the family to develop realistic expectations for the future and to identify support systems that will assist them with planning for the future.
6. Assist family with reducing anxiety by encouraging diversional activities (e.g., period of time outside of critical care unit) and interaction with support systems outside the family. ("I know you want to be near your son, but if you would like to go home to rest, I will call you if *any* changes occur.")

Ineffective family coping: Disabling, related to ambivalent family relationships, unexpressed feelings, lack of communication with family, or patient dependence on family

---

Desired outcomes: Family members verbalize feelings, identify sources of support as well as ineffective coping behaviors that create ambivalence and disharmony, and do not demonstrate destructive behaviors.

---

1. Establish open, honest communication and rapport with family members. ("I am here to care for your mother and to help your family as well.")
2. Identify ineffective coping behaviors (e.g., violence, depression, substance abuse, withdrawal). ("You seem to be angry. Would you like to talk to me about your feelings?") Refer to psychiatric clinical nurse specialist, clergy, or support group as appropriate.
3. Identify perceived or actual conflicts. ("Are you able to talk freely with your family members?" "Are your brothers and sisters able to help and support you during this time?")
4. Assist family to search for healthy functioning within the family unit. For example, facilitate open communication among family members and encourage behaviors that support family cohesiveness. ("Your mother enjoyed your last visit. Would you like to see her now?")
5. Assess the family's knowledge of patient's current health status. Provide opportunities for questions; reassess family's understanding at frequent intervals.
6. Assist family with developing realistic goals, plans, and actions. Refer them to clergy, psychiatric nurse, social services, financial counseling, and family therapy as appropriate.

7. Encourage family members to spend time outside of the critical care unit and to interact with support individuals. Respect the family's need for occasional withdrawal.
8. Include the family in the patient's plan of care. Offer them opportunites to become involved in patient care, for example, ROM exercises, patient hygiene, and comfort measures (e.g., backrub).

Ineffective family coping: Potential for growth, related to use of support systems and referrals, and renewed strength of family unit

---

Desired outcomes: Family members express their intent to use support systems and resources and identify alternative behaviors that enhance family communication and strengths. Family members express realistic expectations and do not demonstrate ineffective coping behaviors.

---

1. Assess family relationships, interactions, support systems, and individual coping behaviors. Permit a period of denial; then encourage further positive coping.
2. Acknowledge family expressions of hope, future plans, and growth among family members.
3. Develop open, honest communication with the family. Provide opportunities in a private setting for family interactions, discussions, and questions. ("I know the waiting room is very crowded. Would your family like some private time together?")
4. Refer the family to community or support groups (e.g., ostomy support group, head injury rehabilitation group).
5. Encourage the family to explore outlets that foster positive feelings, for example, periods of time outside the critical care area, meaningful communication with the patient or support individuals, and relaxing activities (e.g., showering, eating, exercising).

Alteration in family processes related to inability of patient and family to cope with crisis, lack of open and honest communication among family members, or lack of support systems

---

Desired outcomes: Patient and family express feelings of conflict, demonstrate effective coping mechanisms, seek external support when necessary, and share concerns among the family unit.

---

1. Assess the family's character: social, environmental, ethnic, and cultural factors; relationships; and role patterns. Identify family developmental stage. For example, the family may be dealing with other situational or maturational crises, such as an elderly parent or teenager with a learning disability.
2. Assess previous coping behaviors. ("How does your family react in stressful situations?") Discuss observed conflicts and communication breakdown. ("I noticed that your brother would not visit your mother today. Has there been a

problem we should be aware of? Knowing about it may help us better care for your mother.'')

3. Acknowledge the family's involvement in patient care and promote strengths. (''You were able to encourage your wife to turn and cough. That is very important to her recovery.'') Encourage family to participate in patient care conferences. Promote frequent, regular patient visits by family members.

4. Provide the family with information and guidance related to critically ill patient. Discuss the stresses of hospitalization and encourage the family to discuss feelings of anger, guilt, hostility, depression, or sorrow. (''You seem to be upset since having been told that your husband is not leaving the ICU today.'') Refer to clergy, clinical nurse specialist, or social services as appropriate.

5. Evaluate patient and family responses to one another. Encourage family to reorganize roles and establish priorities as appropriate. (''I know your husband is concerned about his insurance policy and seems to expect you to investigate it. I'll call the financial counselor to come and talk with you.'')

6. Encourage the family to schedule periods of rest and activity outside the critical care unit and to seek support when necessary. (''Your neighbor volunteered to stay in the waiting room this afternoon. Would you like to rest at home? I'll call you if *anything* changes.'')

Fear: Family, related to situational crisis of patient's life-threatening condition

---

Desired outcomes: Family members communicate and discuss fears and concerns, do not demonstrate ineffective coping behaviors, and relate feelings of increased well-being and lessened fear.

---

1. Assess the family's fear and their understanding of the patient's clinical situation. Evaluate verbal and nonverbal responses.

2. Acknowledge the family's fear. (''I understand these machines must frighten you, but they are necessary to help your son breathe.'')

3. Assess the family's history of coping behavior. (''How does your family react to difficult situations?'') Determine resources and significant others available for support. (''Who usually helps your family during stressful times?'')

4. Provide opportunities for family members to express fears and concerns. Recognize that anger, denial, withdrawal, and demanding behavior may be adaptive coping responses during initial period of crisis.

5. Provide information at frequent intervals regarding patient's status and the therapies and equipment used.

6. Encourage the family to use positive coping behaviors by identifying the fear(s), developing goals, identifying supportive resources, facilitating realistic perceptions, and promoting problem-solving.

7. Recognize anxiety and encourage family members to describe their feelings. (''You seem very uncomfortable tonight. Can you describe your feelings?'')

8. Be alert to maladaptive responses to fear: potential for violence, withdrawal, severe depression, hostility, and unrealistic expectations of staff or of patient's recovery. Provide referrals to psychiatric clinical nurse specialist or other as appropriate.

9. Offer *realistic* hope, even if it is the hope for the patient's peaceful death.
10. Explore the family's desire for spiritual or other counseling.
11. Assess your own feelings about the patient's life-threatening illness. Acknowledge that your attitude and fear may be reflected to the family.
12. For other interventions, see nursing diagnoses **Alteration in family processes** and **Ineffective family coping.**

Knowledge deficit: Family: Patient's current health status or therapies

---

Desired outcome: Family members verbalize knowledge and understanding of the patient's current health status or therapies.

---

1. At frequent intervals, inform the family about the patient's current health status, therapies, and prognosis. Use individualized verbal and audiovisual strategies to enhance family's understanding.
2. Evalute the family at frequent intervals for understanding of information that has been provided. Assess factors for misunderstanding and adjust teaching as appropriate. Some individuals in crisis need multiple explanations before comprehension can be assured. ("I have explained many things to you today. Would you mind summarizing what I've told you so that I can be sure you understand your husband's status and what we are doing to care for him?")
3. Encourage family to relay correct information to the patient. This will reinforce comprehension for family and patient, as well.
4. Ask family members if their needs for information are being met. ("Do you have any questions about the care your mother is receiving or about her condition?")
5. Help family members to use the information they receive to make health-care decisions regarding family member (e.g., surgery, resuscitation, organ donation.)
6. Promote family's active participation in patient care when appropriate. Encourage family to seek information and express feelings, concerns, and questions.

SELECTED REFERENCES

Carpenito LJ: *Nursing Diagnosis: Application to Clinical Practice.* Lippincott, 1983.

Doenges M, et al: *Nurse's Pocket Guide: Nursing Diagnoses with Interventions.* FA Davis, 1984.

Swearingen, PL (ed): *Manual of Nursing Therapeutics: Applying Nursing Diagnoses to Medical Disorders.* Addison-Wesley, 1986.

3
APPENDIX
ACLS Algorithms

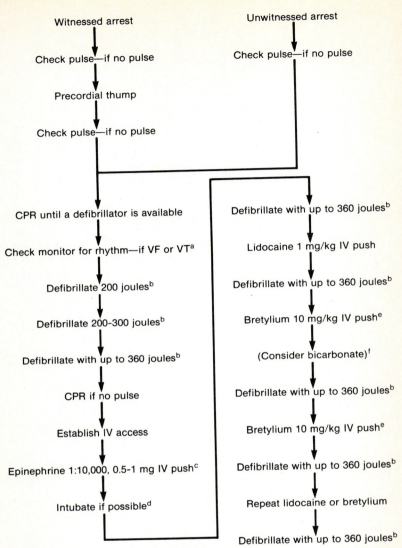

Witnessed arrest

Check pulse—if no pulse

Precordial thump

Check pulse—if no pulse

CPR until a defibrillator is available

Check monitor for rhythm—if VF or VT[a]

Defibrillate 200 joules[b]

Defibrillate 200-300 joules[b]

Defibrillate with up to 360 joules[b]

CPR if no pulse

Establish IV access

Epinephrine 1:10,000, 0.5-1 mg IV push[c]

Intubate if possible[d]

Unwitnessed arrest

Check pulse—if no pulse

Defibrillate with up to 360 joules[b]

Lidocaine 1 mg/kg IV push

Defibrillate with up to 360 joules[b]

Bretylium 10 mg/kg IV push[e]

(Consider bicarbonate)[f]

Defibrillate with up to 360 joules[b]

Bretylium 10 mg/kg IV push[e]

Defibrillate with up to 360 joules[b]

Repeat lidocaine or bretylium

Defibrillate with up to 360 joules[b]

FIG. A-1. **Ventricular fibrillation (and pulseless ventricular tachycardia).** This sequence was developed to assist in teaching how to treat a broad range of patients with ventricular tachycardia (VT). Some patients may require care not specified herein. This algorithm should not be construed as prohibiting such flexibility. Flow of algorithm presumes that VF is continuing. CPR indicates cardiopulmonary resuscitation. [a]Pulseless VT should be treated identically to VF. [b]Check pulse and rhythm after each shock. If VF recurs after transiently converting (rather than persists without ever converting), use whatever energy level has previously been successful for defibrillation. [c]Epinephrine should be repeated every 5 minutes. [d]Intubation is preferable. If it can be accomplished simultaneously with other techniques, then the earlier the better. However, defibrillation and epinephrine are more important initially if patient can be ventilated without intubation. [e]Some may prefer repeated doses of lidocaine, which may be given in 0.5 mg/kg boluses every 8 minutes to total dose of 3 mg/kg. [f]Value of sodium bicarbonate is questionable during cardiac arrest and it is not recommended for routine cardiac arrest sequence. Consideration of its use in a dose of 1 mEq/kg is appropriate at this point. Half of original dose may be repeated every 10 min if it is used.

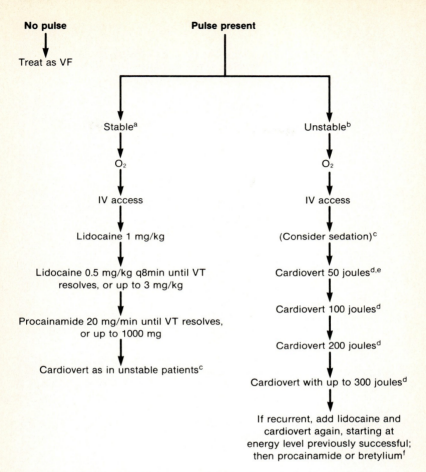

No pulse

↓

Treat as VF

Pulse present

Stable[a]	Unstable[b]
↓	↓
O₂	O₂
↓	↓
IV access	IV access
↓	↓
Lidocaine 1 mg/kg	(Consider sedation)[c]
↓	↓
Lidocaine 0.5 mg/kg q8min until VT resolves, or up to 3 mg/kg	Cardiovert 50 joules[d,e]
↓	↓
Procainamide 20 mg/min until VT resolves, or up to 1000 mg	Cardiovert 100 joules[d]
↓	↓
Cardiovert as in unstable patients[c]	Cardiovert 200 joules[d]
	↓
	Cardiovert with up to 300 joules[d]
	↓
	If recurrent, add lidocaine and cardiovert again, starting at energy level previously successful; then procainamide or bretylium[f]

FIG. A-2. **Sustained ventricular tachycardia (VT).** This sequence was developed to assist in teaching how to treat a broad range of patients with sustained VT. Some patients may require care not specified herein. This algorithm should not be construed as prohibiting such flexibility. Flow of algorithm presumes that VT is continuing. VF indicates ventricular fibrillation.

[a]If patient becomes unstable (see footnote b for definition) at any time, move to "Unstable" arm of algorithm.

[b]Unstable indicates symptoms, e.g., chest pain or dyspnea, hypotension (systolic blood pressure <90 mm Hg), congestive heart failure, ischemia, or infarction.

[c]Sedation should be considered for all patients, including those defined in footnote b as unstable, except those who are hemodynamically unstable (e.g., hypotensive, in pulmonary edema, or unconscious).

[d]If hypotension, pulmonary edema, or unconsciousness is present, unsynchronized cardioversion should be done to avoid delay associated with synchronization.

[e]In the presence of hypotension, pulmonary edema, or unconsciousness, a precordial thump may be employed prior to cardioversion.

[f]Once VT has been resolved, begin intravenous (IV) infusion of antiarrhythmic agent that has aided resolution of VT. If hypotension, pulmonary edema, or unconsciousness is present, use lidocaine if cardioversion alone is unsuccessful, followed by bretylium. In all other patients, recommended order of therapy is lidocaine, procainamide, and then bretylium.

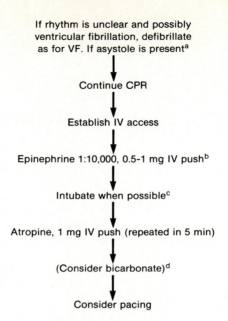

If rhythm is unclear and possibly
ventricular fibrillation, defibrillate
as for VF. If asystole is present[a]

↓

Continue CPR

↓

Establish IV access

↓

Epinephrine 1:10,000, 0.5-1 mg IV push[b]

↓

Intubate when possible[c]

↓

Atropine, 1 mg IV push (repeated in 5 min)

↓

(Consider bicarbonate)[d]

↓

Consider pacing

FIG. A-3. **Asystole (cardiac standstill).** This sequence was developed to assist in teaching how to treat a broad range of patients with asystole. Some patients may require care not specified herein. This algorithm should not be construed to prohibit such flexibility. Flow of algorithm presumes asystole is continuing. VF indicates ventricular fibrillation; IV, intravenous.

[a]Asystole should be confirmed in two leads.

[b]Epinephrine should be repeated every five minutes.

[c]Intubation is preferable; if it can be accomplished simultaneously wih other techniques, then the earlier the better. However, cardiopulmonary resuscitation (CPR) and use of epinephrine are more important initially if patient can be ventilated without intubation. (Endotracheal epinephrine may be used.)

[d]Value of sodium bicarbonate is questionable during cardiac arrest, and it is not recommended for the routine cardiac arrest sequence. Consideration of its use in a dose of 1 mEq/kg is appropriate at this point. Half of original dose may be repeated every 10 minutes if it is used.

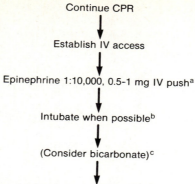

Continue CPR

Establish IV access

Epinephrine 1:10,000, 0.5-1 mg IV push[a]

Intubate when possible[b]

(Consider bicarbonate)[c]

Consider hypovolemia, cardiac tamponade, tension pneumothorax, hypoxemia, acidosis, pulmonary embolism

FIG. A-4. **Electromechanical dissociation.** This sequence was developed to assist in teaching how to treat a broad range of patients with electromechanical dissociation. Some patients may require care not specified herein. This algorithm should not be construed to prohibit such flexibility. Flow of algorithm presumes that electromechanical dissociation is continuing. CPR indicates cardiopulmonary resuscitation; IV, intravenous.

[a]Epinephrine should be repeated every 5 minutes.

[b]Intubation is preferable. If it can be accomplished simultaneously with other techniques, then the earlier the better. However, epinephrine is more important initially if the patient can be ventilated without intubation.

[c]Value of sodium bicarbonate is questionable during cardiac arrest, and it is not recommended for routine cardiac arrest sequence. Consideration of its use in a dose of 1 mEq/kg is appropriate at this point. Half of original dose may be repeated every 10 minutes if it is used.

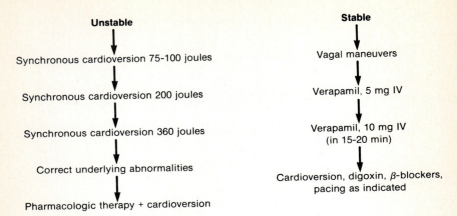

Unstable

Synchronous cardioversion 75-100 joules

Synchronous cardioversion 200 joules

Synchronous cardioversion 360 joules

Correct underlying abnormalities

Pharmacologic therapy + cardioversion

Stable

Vagal maneuvers

Verapamil, 5 mg IV

Verapamil, 10 mg IV
(in 15-20 min)

Cardioversion, digoxin, β-blockers,
pacing as indicated

If conversion occurs but PSVT recurs, repeated cardioversion is not indicated. Sedation should be used in some patients.

FIG. A-5. **Paroxysmal supraventricular tachycardia (PSVT).** This sequence was developed to assist in teaching how to treat a broad range of patients with sustained PSVT. Some patients may require care not specified herein. This algorithm should not be construed as prohibiting such flexibility. Flow of algorithm presumes PSVT is continuing.

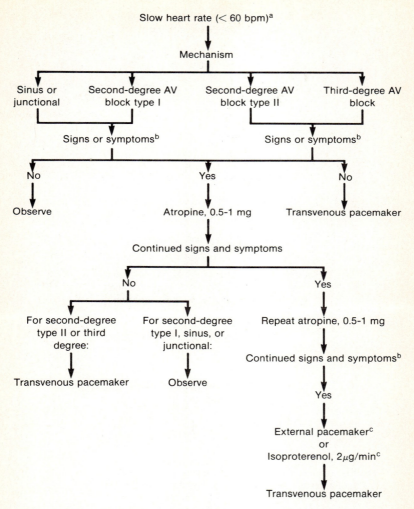

FIG. A-6. **Bradycardia.** This sequence was developed to assist in teaching how to treat a broad range of patients with bradycardia. Some patients may require care not specified herein. This algorithm should not be construed to prohibit such flexibility. AV indicates atrioventricular.

[a]A solitary chest thump or cough may stimulate cardiac electrical activity and result in improved cardiac output and may be used at this point.

[b]Hypotension (blood pressure <90 mm Hg), premature ventricular contractions, altered mental status, or symptoms (e.g., chest pain or dyspnea), ischemia, or infarction.

[c]Temporizing therapy.

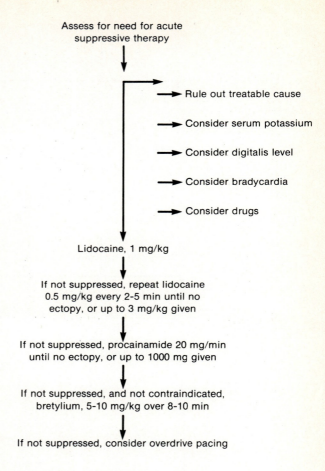

Assess for need for acute
suppressive therapy

→ Rule out treatable cause

→ Consider serum potassium

→ Consider digitalis level

→ Consider bradycardia

→ Consider drugs

Lidocaine, 1 mg/kg

If not suppressed, repeat lidocaine
0.5 mg/kg every 2-5 min until no
ectopy, or up to 3 mg/kg given

If not suppressed, procainamide 20 mg/min
until no ectopy, or up to 1000 mg given

If not suppressed, and not contraindicated,
bretylium, 5-10 mg/kg over 8-10 min

If not suppressed, consider overdrive pacing

Once ectopy resolved, maintain as follows:
    After lidocaine, 1 mg/kg . . . lidocaine drip, 2 mg/min
    After lidocaine, 1-2 mg/kg . . . lidocaine drip, 3 mg/min
    After lidocaine, 2-3 mg/kg . . . lidocaine drip, 4 mg/min
    After procainamide . . . procainamide drip, 1-4 mg/min (check blood level)
    After bretylium . . . bretylium drip, 2 mg/min

FIG. A-7. **Ventricular ectopy: Acute suppressive therapy.** This sequence was developed to assist in teaching how to treat a broad range of patients with ventricular ectopy. Some patients may require therapy not specified herein. This algorithm should not be construed as prohibiting such flexibility.

4

APPENDIX
Heart and Breath Sounds

Assessing heart sounds

Sound	Auscultation site	Timing	Pitch	Clinical occurrence	End-piece/patient position
S_1 (M_1 T_1)	Apex	Beginning of systole	High	Closing of mitral and tricuspid valves. Normal sound.	Diaphragm/patient supine
S_1 split	Apex	Beginning of systole	High	Ventricles contracting at different times due to electrical or mechanical problems. For example, a longer time span between M_1 T_1, caused by right bundle-branch heart block, or reversal (T_1 M_1) caused by mitral stenosis.	Same as S_1
S_2 (A_2 P_2)	A_2 at 2nd ICS, RSB; P_2 at 2nd ICS, LSB	End of systole	High	Closing of aortic and pulmonic valves. Normal sound.	Diaphragm/patient supine
S_2 Physiologic split	2nd ICS, LSB	End of systole	High	Accentuated by inspiration; disappears on expiration. Sound that corresponds with the respiratory cycle due to normal delay in closure of pulmonic valve during inspiration. It is accentuated during exercise or in individuals with thin chest walls; heard most often in children and young adults.	Same as S_2

Continued.

S_2 Persistent (wide) split	2nd ICS, LSB	End of systole	High	Heard throughout the respiratory cycle; caused by late closure of pulmonic valve or early closure of aortic valve. Occurs in atrial septal defect, right ventricular failure, pulmonic stenosis, hypertension, or right bundle-branch heart block.	Same as S_2
S_2 Paradoxic (reversed) split ($P_2 A_2$)	2nd ICS, LSB	End of systole	High	Because of delayed left ventricular systole, the aortic valve closes after the pulmonic valve rather than before it. (Normally during expiration the two sounds merge.) Causes may include left bundle-branch heart block, aortic stenosis, severe left ventricular failure, MI, and severe hypertension.	Same as S_2
S_2 Fixed split	2nd ICS, LSB	End of systole	High	Heard with equal intensity during inspiration and expiration due to split of pulmonic and aortic components, which are unaffected by blood volume or respiratory changes. May be heard in pulmonary stenosis or atrial septal defect.	Same as S_2

Assessing heart sounds—Continued.

Sound	Auscultation site	Timing	Pitch	Clinical occurrence	End-piece/patient position
S₃ (ventricular gallop)	Apex	Early diastole just after S₂	Dull, low	Early and rapid filling of ventricle, as in early ventricular failure, CHF; common in children, during last trimester of pregnancy, and possibly in healthy adults over age 50.	Bell/patient in left lateral or supine position
S₄ (atrial gallop)	Apex	Late in diastole just before S₁	Low	Atrium filling against increased resistance of stiff ventricle, as in CHF, coronary artery disease, cardiomyopathy, pulmonary artery hypertension, ventricular failure. May be normal in infants, children, and athletes.	Same as S₃

ICS = intercostal space; RSB = right sternal border; LSB = left sternal border.

Commonly occurring heart murmurs

Type	Timing	Pitch	Quality	Auscultation site	Radiation
Pulmonic stenosis	Systolic ejection	Medium-high	Harsh	2nd ICS, LSB	Toward left shoulder, back
Aortic stenosis	Midsystolic	Medium-high	Harsh	2nd ICS, RSB	Toward carotid arteries
Ventricular septal defect	Late systolic	High	Blowing	4th ICS, LSB	Toward right sternal border
Mitral insufficiency	Holosystolic	High	Blowing	5-6th ICS, left MCL	Toward left axilla
Tricuspid insufficiency	Holosystolic	High	Blowing	4th ICS, LSB	Toward apex
Aortic insufficiency	Early diastolic	High	Blowing	2nd ICS, RSB	Toward sternum
Pulmonary insufficiency	Early diastolic	High	Blowing	2nd ICS, LSB	Toward sternum
Mitral stenosis	Mid-late diastolic	Low	Rumbling	5th ICS, left MCL	Toward axilla
Tricuspid stenosis	Mid-late diastolic	Low	Rumbling	4th ICS, LSB	Usually none

ICS = intercostal space; RSB = right sternal border; LSB = left sternal border; MCL = mid-clavicular line.

Assessing normal breath sounds

Type	Normal site	Duration	Characteristics
Vesicular	Peripheral lung	I > E	Soft and swishing sounds. Abnormal when heard over the large airways.
Bronchial	Trachea and bronchi	E > I	Louder, coarser, and of longer duration than vesicular. Abnormal if heard over peripheral lung.
Bronchovesicular	Sternal border of the major bronchi	E = I	Moderate in pitch and intensity. Abnormal if heard over peripheral lung.

I = inspiration; E = expiration.

Assessing adventitious breath sounds

Type	Waveform	Characteristics	Possible clinical condition
Coarse crackle		Discontinuous, explosive, interrupted. Loud; low in pitch.	Pulmonary edema; pneumonia in resolution stage.
Fine crackle		Discontinuous, explosive, interrupted. Less loud than coarse crackles, lower in pitch, and of shorter duration.	Interstitial lung disease; heart failure; atelectasis.
Wheeze		Continuous, of long duration, high-pitched, musical, hissing.	Narrowing of airway; bronchial asthma; COPD.
Rhonchus		Continuous, of long duration, low-pitched, snoring.	Production of sputum (usually cleared or lessened by coughing).
Pleural friction rub		Grating, rasping noise.	Rubbing together of inflamed parietal linings; loss of normal pleural lubrication.

Assessing respiratory patterns

Type	Waveform	Characteristics	Possible clinical condition
Eupnea		Normal rate and rhythm for adults and teenagers (12-20 breaths/min).	Normal pattern while awake.
Bradypnea		Decreased rate (<12 breaths/min); regular rhythm.	Normal sleep pattern; opiate or alcohol use; tumor; metabolic disorder.
Tachypnea		Rapid rate (>20 breaths/min); hypo- or hyperventilation.	Fever; restrictive respiratory disorders; pulmonary emboli.
Hyperpnea		Depth of respirations greater than normal	Meeting increased metabolic demand (e.g., exercise).
Apnea		Cessation of breathing; may be intermittent.	Intermittent with CNS disturbances or drug intoxication; obstructed airway; respiratory arrest if it persists.
Cheyne-Stokes		Alternating patterns of apnea (10-20 seconds) with periods of deep and rapid breathing.	CHF, narcotic or hypnotic overdose, thyrotoxicosis dissecting aneurysm, subarachnoid hemorrhage, increased ICP, aortic valve disorders, may be normal in elderly during sleep.
Biot's		Irregular (can be slow and deep or rapid and shallow) followed by periods of apnea.	CNS abnormalities (e.g., meningitis, increased ICP).
Kussmaul's		Deep, rapid (>20 breaths/min), sighing, labored.	Renal failure, DKA, sepsis, shock.
Apneustic		Prolonged inspiration followed by short expirations.	Anoxia, meningitis.

INDEX OF
NURSING DIAGNOSES
USED IN THIS MANUAL

Activity intolerance related to fatigue secondary to increased work of breathing and inability to meet metabolic demands for oxygen, *"Status Asthmaticus," p. 6;* related to episodes of chest pain, *"Acute Chest Pain," p. 76;* related to weakness and fatigue secondary to decreased functioning of the myocardium, *"Congestive Heart Failure/Pulmonary Edema," p. 88;* related to weakness and fatigue secondary to decreased myocardial contractions, *"Cardiomyopathy," p. 93;* related to weakness and fatigue secondary to impaired cardiac function, ineffective breathing pattern, or deconditioning, *"Acute Pericarditis," p. 119;* related to weakness and fatigue secondary to fluid and electrolyte imbalance, arthralgia, myalgia, dyspnea, fever, pain, hypoxia, and effects of chemotherapy, *"Acquired Immune Deficiency Syndrome," p. 484;* related to deconditioning secondary to prolonged bed rest, *"Caring for the Critically Ill on Prolonged Best Rest," p. 506.*

Airway clearance, ineffective, related to presence of viscous secretions, *"Status Asthmaticus," p. 6;* related to interruption in normal respiratory mechanics secondary to intubation and mechanical ventilation, *"Management of the Adult on Mechanical Ventilation," p. 66;* related to inability to cough secondary to weakness and abnormal fatigability of diaphragmatic, intercostal, pharyngeal, and accessory muscles of respiration, *"Myasthenia Gravis," p. 244;* related to inability to cough or swallow secondary to increasing paralysis of respiratory, pharyngeal, and facial muscles and absence of gag reflex, *"Guillain-Barré Syndrome," p. 253;* related to decreased or absent cough reflex secondary to cervical or high thoracic spine injury, *"Acute Spinal Cord Injury," p. 299;* related to hypoventilation, suppression of cough reflex, and decreased diffusion of oxygen secondary to respiratory depressant effects of drugs, accumulation of pulmonary secretions, and pulmonary edema occurring with drug use or overdose, *"Drug Overdose," p. 323;* related to risk secondary to aspiration of gastric secretions, alteration in mentation (occurring with encephalopathy), or presence of balloon tamponade, *"Bleeding Esophageal Varices," p. 362.*

Anxiety related to actual or perceived threat to biologic integrity secondary to need for or presence of mechanical ventilation, *"Management of the Adult on Mechanical Ventilation," p. 69;* related to perceived threat to biologic integrity secondary to weaning process, *"Management of the Adult on Mechanical Ventilation," p. 70;* related to threat of loss of the kidney from rejection, *"Renal Transplant," p. 194;* related to threat of loss of transplanted organ due to rejection, *"Organ Rejection," p. 474;* related to diagnosis, fear of death or social isolation, and hospitalization, *"Acquired Immune Deficiency Syndrome," p. 485;* related to actual or perceived

threat to biologic integrity, self concept, or role; unfamiliar people and environment; or the unknown, *"Caring for the Critically Ill with Life-Threatening Disorders,"* p. 512.

Bowel elimination, alterations in, related to decreased intake secondary to NPO
status with hypoperistalsis or paralytic ileus, *"Guillain-Barré Syndrome,"* p. 257;
Constipation, related to prolonged immobility, decreased fluid intake, inadequate
intake of fiber, and restriction against Valsalva maneuver for straining, *"Cerebral
Aneurysm and Subarachnoid Hemorrhage,"* p. 268; Constipation or fecal impaction related to hypotonic or atonic bowel secondary to spinal shock, *"Acute Spinal
Cord Injury,"* p. 308; Constipation related to inability to defecate secondary to
lack of voluntary control of the anal sphincter and lack of sensation of a fecal mass
following return of reflex arc, *"Acute Spinal Cord Injury,"* p. 309; Diarrhea related
to increased motility secondary to irritation by the presence of blood in the GI tract
or disease process, *"Acute Gastrointestinal Bleeding,"* p. 400; related to disruption
of normal function secondary to fecal diversion in patients with colonic injury and
colostomy, *"Abdominal Trauma,"* p. 414; related to decreased peristalsis secondary to paralytic ileus, *"Burns,"* p. 462; Diarrhea, related to gastrointestinal infection, chemotherapy, or tube feeding intolerance, *"Acquired Immune Deficiency
Syndrome,"* p. 483.

Breathing pattern, ineffective, related to hyperventilation secondary to anxiety
due to use of mechanical ventilation, *"Management of the Adult on Mechanical
Ventilation,"* p. 67; related to guarding secondary to chest pain, *"Acute Pericarditis,"* p. 118; related to weakness or paralysis of respiratory muscles secondary
to severe hypokalemia (potassium <2-2.5 mEq/L), *"Fluid and Electrolyte Disturbances,"* p. 229.

Cardiac output, alterations in: Decreased, related to life-threatening dysrhythmias secondary to injury to and enhanced automaticity of the myocardium, *"Acute
Myocardial Infarction,"* p. 82; related to impaired contractility secondary to myocardial injury, *"Acute Myocardial Infarction,"* p. 82; related to impaired contractility secondary to myocardial dilatation, *"Cardiomyopathy,"* p. 92; related to dysrhythmias or impaired contractility secondary to cardiac disease, *"Dysrhythmias
and Conduction Disturbances,"* p. 96; related to cardiac arrest, *"Cardiac Arrest,"*
p. 100; related to diminished ventricular filling secondary to compression of ventricles by fluid in the pericardial sac, *"Acute Cardiac Tamponade,"* p. 107; related
to altered preload, afterload, or contractility secondary to valvular dysfunction,
"Acute Infective Endocarditis," p. 113; related to decreased or increased afterload,
increased preload, or decreased contractility secondary to loss of ≥40% of myocardial functional mass, *"Cardiogenic Shock,"* p. 134; related to risk of vessel
occlusion, myocardial infarction, coronary artery spasm, dysrhythmias, bleeding,
or cardiac tamponade secondary to complications of angioplasty, *"Percutaneous
Transluminal Coronary Angioplasty,"* p. 138; related to risk of dysrhythmias,
valve regurgitation, tamponade, or hemorrhage secondary to percutaneous balloon
valvuloplasty, *"Percutaneous Balloon Valvuloplasty,"* p. 141; related to impaired
contractility and rhythm disturbances secondary to myocardial ischemia or cardiac
injury, *"Intra-Aortic Balloon Pump,"* p. 143; related to risk of right ventricular
failure secondary to reduced right ventricular contraction occurring with left-heart-
assist device, *"Heart-Assist Device,"* p. 148; related to altered contractility sec-

ondary to intraoperative subendocardial ischemia and administration of myocardial depressant drugs, *"Coronary Artery Bypass Graft,"* *p. 150;* related to altered contractility secondary to intraoperative subendocardial ischemia and administration of myocardial depressant drugs, *"Valvular Heart Disease and Valve Surgery,"* *p. 155;* related to risk of dysrhythmias secondary to thrombolytic therapy, *"Coronary Artery Thrombolysis,"* *p. 163;* related to risk of dysrhythmias secondary to fluid and electrolyte disturbances occurring with hemofiltration, *"Continuous Arteriovenous Hemofiltration,"* *p. 210;* related to risk of ventricular dysrhythmias secondary to hypokalemia or too rapid correction of hypokalemia with resulting hyperkalemia, *"Fluid and Electrolyte Disturbances,"* *p. 227;* related to risk of ventricular dysrhythmias secondary to severe hyperkalemia or too rapid correction of hyperkalemia with resulting hypokalemia, *"Fluid and Electrolyte Disturbances,"* *p. 230;* related to decreased cardiac contractility secondary to hypocalcemia or digitalis toxicity occurring with calcium replacement therapy, *"Fluid and Electrolyte Disturbances,"* *p. 234;* related to "artificial hypovolemia" secondary to reduced peripheral vascular tone occurring with overactive sympathetic nervous system, *"Guillain-Barré Syndrome,"* *p. 256;* related to relative hypovolemia secondary to enlarged vascular space occurring with neurogenic shock, *"Acute Spinal Cord Injury,"* *p. 301;* related to risk of dysrhythmias or myocardial infarction secondary to myocardial ischemia occurring with prolonged bleeding and vasopressin-induced coronary vasoconstriction, *"Bleeding Esophageal Varices,"* *p. 361;* related to diminished venous return and decreased preload secondary to acute blood loss, *"Acute Gastrointestinal Bleeding,"* *p. 399;* related to risk of dysrhythmias secondary to acidosis or electrolyte disturbance caused by massive blood loss, *"Disseminated Intravascular Coagulation,"* *p. 421;* related to relative hypovolemia (early stage) secondary to effects of endotoxins; or decreased contractility (late stage) secondary to effects of tissue hypoxia, *"Sepsis,"* *p. 439;* related to dysrhythmias or risk of cardiac arrest secondary to decreased circulating volume occurring with vasodilatation and increased capillary permeability, *"Anaphylaxis,"* *p. 447;* Risk of pump failure related to myocardial suppression secondary to bacterial toxins and hypocalcemia, *"Toxic Shock Syndrome,"* *p. 452.*

Comfort, alteration in: Acute pain related to alteration in pleural integrity and inflammation, *"Pneumothorax,"* *p. 32;* Chest pain related to decreased oxygen supply to the myocardium, *"Acute Chest Pain,"* *p. 75;* Chest pain related to decreased oxygen supply to the myocardium, *"Acute Myocardial Infarction, p. 81;* Precordial chest pain related to myocardial damage and chest wall injuries, *"Cardiac Trauma,"* *p. 104;* Headache related to cerebral edema occurring with high perfusion pressures, *"Hypertensive Crisis,"* *p. 126;* Pain related to necrosis at the aortic media and distal tissue hypoperfusion, *"Aortic Dissection,"* *p. 130;* Chest pain related to decreased myocardial oxygen supply due to coronary artery disease, *"Percutaneous Transluminal Coronary Angioplasty,"* *p. 138;* Pain occurring with LUT structural injury, procedures for urinary diversion, or surgical incisions, *"Lower Urinary Tract Trauma,"* *p. 187;* Headache, photophobia, and fever related to meningeal irritation, *"Meningitis,"* *p. 291;* Pain related to peritoneal inflammation and tissue destruction by pancreatic enzyme release, *"Acute Pancreatitis,"* *p. 384;* Pain related to peritoneal inflammation, *"Peritonitis,"* *p. 391;* Pain related to GI mucosal irritation, inflammation, or surgical procedure, *"Acute Gastrointestinal Bleeding,"* *p. 399;* Pain related to irritation from intraperitoneal blood or secretions, actual trauma or surgical incision, and manipulation of organs, *"Abdominal*

secondary to hemorrhage, *"Valvular Heart Disease and Valve Surgery,"* p. 154; related to loss (hemorrhage) secondary to systemic lytic effects of streptokinase or urokinase, *"Coronary Artery Thrombolysis,"* p. 161; related to decreased circulating volume secondary to diuresis, vomiting, diarrhea, hemorrhage, or fluid shift to interstitial compartments, *"Acute Renal Failure,"* p. 178; related to abnormal blood loss secondary to LUT injury, *"Lower Urinary Tract Trauma,"* p. 187; related to decreased circulating volume secondary to excessive fluid removal during peritoneal dialysis or hemodialysis or bleeding associated with heparinization, *"Dialytic Therapy,"* p. 205; related to loss secondary to excessive ultrafiltration during CAVH, *"Continuous Arteriovenous Hemofiltration,"* p. 211; related to risk of blood loss secondary to line disconnection or membrane rupture, *"Continuous Arteriovenous Hemofiltration,"* p. 213; related to decreased circulating volume secondary to abnormal loss of ECF or reduced intake, *"Fluid and Electrolyte Disturbances,"* p. 217; (or excess) related to abnormal fluid loss, excessive intake of hypotonic solutions, or abnormal retention of water, *"Fluid and Electrolyte Disturbances,"* p. 224; (with concomitant risk of clotting abnormalities, electrolyte disturbances, and myasthenic or cholinergic crises) related to temporary loss of body fluids secondary to plasmapheresis, *"Myasthenia Gravis,"* p. 247; (with concomitant electrolyte imbalance) related to decreased intake secondary to decreased LOC or decreased circulating volume secondary to vomiting or diaphoresis, *"Drug Overdose,"* p. 321; (with concomitant electrolyte imbalance) related to decreased circulating volume secondary to vomiting, diaphoresis, or prolonged dehydration, *"Delirium Tremens,"* p. 326; (with concomitant electrolyte disturbance) related to decreased circulating volume secondary to hyperglycemia and osmotic diuresis, *"Diabetic Ketoacidosis,"* p. 331; related to decreased circulating volume secondary to polyuria, *"Diabetes Insipidus,"* p. 342; (with concomitant electrolyte disturbance) related to decreased circulating volume secondary to impaired secretion of aldosterone causing increased sodium excretion with resultant diuresis, *"Addisonian Crisis,"* p. 351; related to decreased circulating volume secondary to active variceal bleeding, *"Bleeding Esophageal Varices,"* p. 360; related to decreased intake secondary to medically-prescribed restrictions and decreased circulating volume secondary to hypoalbuminemia, altered hemodynamics, fluid sequestration, and diuretic therapy, *"Hepatic Failure,"* p. 371; related to inadequate intake or decreased circulating volume secondary to fluid sequestration or active bleeding, *"Acute Pancreatitis,"* p. 382; related to decreased circulating volume secondary to fluid sequestration, decreased oral intake, and possibly active loss secondary to bleeding, *"Peritonitis,"* p. 390; related to decreased circulating volume secondary to inadequate intake, active bleeding, or fluid sequestration, *"Acute Gastrointestinal Bleeding"* p. 398; related to decreased circulating volume secondary to active bleeding; GI drainage through gastric, intestinal, or drainage tubes; diarrhea; or fistulas, *"Abdominal Trauma,"* p. 408; related to risk of blood loss secondary to hemorrhagic phase of DIC or heparin therapy, *"Disseminated Intravascular Coagulation"* p. 420, related to loss secondary to excretion of urine of abnormally low molecular concentration (hyposthenuria) caused by damage to the renal concentrating mechanism, *"Hemolytic Crisis,"* p. 425; related to loss secondary to postsplenectomy or intra-abdominal bleeding, *"Idiopathic Thrombocytopenia Purpura,"* p. 429; related to decreased circulating volume secondary to increased capillary permeability and loss of intravascular volume into interstitial spaces, *"Sepsis,"* p. 438; related to decreased circulating volume secondary to fluid shifts, fever, vomiting, and diarrhea caused by bacterial toxins, *"Toxic Shock Syndrome,"* p. 451; related to decreased circulating volume secondary to leakage of fluid, plasma proteins, and other cellular elements into the interstitial space and loss through the burn wound, *"Burns,"* p. 461.

Fluid volume excess: Pulmonary and peripheral edema related to retention secondary to decreased cardiac output, *"Congestive Heart Failure/Pulmonary Edema,"* p. 86; Edema related to retention of sodium and water secondary to acute renal failure, *"Acute Renal Failure,"* p. 176; Edema related to oliguria and abnormal retention of peritoneal dialysate solution and dietary indiscretions of sodium and water, *"Dialytic Therapy,"* p. 204; Edema related to decreased ultrafiltration secondary to hypotension, clogged or clotted filter, or kinked lines, *"Continuous Arteriovenous Hemofiltration,"* p. 212; Edema (peripheral and pulmonary) related to surplus of circulating fluid secondary to expanded ECF volume, *"Fluid and Electrolyte Disturbances,"* p. 220; (or deficit) related to abnormal fluid loss, excessive intake of hypotonic solutions, or abnormal retention of water, *"Fluid and Electrolyte Disturbances,"* p. 224; Cerebral, related to risk of rebleeding from cerebral aneurysm secondary to normal hemolytic response, *"Cerebral Aneurysm and Subarachnoid Hemorrhage,"* p. 266; Cerebral, related to risk of hydrocephalus secondary to rupture of cerebral aneurysm, *"Cerebral Aneurysm and Subarachnoid Hemorrhage,"* p. 267; related to retention secondary to increased level of serum ADH with increased water reabsorption from the kidneys, *"Syndrome of Inappropriate Antidiuretic Hormone,"* p. 348; Intravascular, related to retention secondary to sodium and electrolyte disturbances, functional renal failure, and medical therapy (peritoneal-venous shunt insertion and hemofiltration therapy for ascites); extravascular, related to edema and ascites secondary to sequestration of fluid, *"Hepatic Failure,"* p. 372; related to retention secondary to overaggressive fluid resuscitation and peritoneal lavage, *"Acute Pancreatitis,"* p. 383; Cerebral, related to risk of intracranial hemorrhage secondary to platelet destruction, *"Idiopathic Thrombocytopenia Purpura,"* p. 428; Edema related to retention secondary to diminished organ function during a rejection episode, *"Organic Rejection,"* p. 475.

Gas exchange, impaired, related to decreased alveolar ventilation secondary to narrowed airways, *"Status Asthmaticus,"* p. 5; related to decreased diffusion of oxygen secondary to atelectasis and fluid accumulation in the alveoli, *"Adult Respiratory Distress Syndrome,"* p. 20; related to ventilation-perfusion mismatch secondary to pulmonary or fat emboli, *"Perfusion Disorders,"* p. 26; related to ventilation-perfusion mismatch secondary to diminished lung capacity, *"Pneumothorax,"* p. 30; related to decreased diffusion of oxygen secondary to alveolar capillary membrane changes and fluid accumulation in the lung, *"Near Drowning,"* p. 39; related to trapping of CO_2 secondary to pulmonary tissue destruction, *"Acid-Base Imbalances,"* p. 50; related to inadequate ventilation secondary to malfunction or improper setting of mechanical ventilator, *"Management of the Adult on Mechanical Ventilation,"* p. 66; related to decreased diffusion of oxygen secondary to weaning from mechanical ventilation, *"Management of the Adult on Mechanical Ventilation,"* p. 69; related to decreased diffusion of oxygen secondary to fluid accumulation in the lungs, *"Congestive Heart Failure/Pulmonary Edema,"* p. 88; related to decreased diffusion of oxygen secondary to pulmonary congestion, *"Acute Infective Endocarditis,"* p. 114; related to decreased diffusion of oxygen secondary to pulmonary congestion and acidosis occurring with anaerobic metabolism, *"Cardiogenic Shock,"* p. 136; related to hypoventilation secondary to prolonged bed rest and restricted chest excursion (HOB no higher than 30 degrees), *"Intra-Aortic Balloon Pump," p. 145;* related to decreased diffusion of oxygen secondary to postoperative atelectasis, guarding of respirations, diminished activity, retained secretions, or use of anesthesia, *"Coronary Artery Bypass Graft," p. 152;* related to decreased diffusion of oxygen secondary to pulmonary vascular congestion occurring with ECF expansion, *"Fluid and Electrolyte Disturbances," p. 221;* related to decreased availability of oxygen secondary to laryngeal spasm occurring with severe hypocalcemia, *"Fluid and Electrolyte Disturbances," p. 234;* related to decreases in chest expansion and air movement secondary to weakness and abnormal fatigability of pharyngeal, diaphragmatic, intercostal, and accessory muscles of respiration, *"Myasthenia Gravis," p. 243;* related to decreased lung expansion secondary to weakness or paralysis of intercostal and diaphragmatic muscles, *"Guillain-Barré Syndrome," p. 253;* related to risk of cerebral hypoxia secondary to aspiration pneumonia, neurogenic pulmonary edema, chest injury, imposed inactivity, or decreased ventilatory drive occurring with pressure on respiratory center, *"Head Injury," p. 277;* related to hypoventilation secondary to paresis or paralysis of the muscles of respiration (diaphragm, intercostals) occurring with high cervical spine injury or ascending cord edema, *"Acute Spinal Cord Injury," p. 298;* related to hypoventilation and bradypnea secondary to depressant effect of seizures on respiratory center and increased need for oxygen secondary to continuous seizure activity, *"Status Epilepticus," p. 314;* related to hypoventilation, suppression of cough reflex, and decreased diffusion of oxygen secondary to respiratory depressant effect of drugs, accumulation of pulmonary secretions, and pulmonary edema occurring with drug use or overdose, *"Drug Overdose," p. 323;* related to decreased diffusion of oxygen secondary to shallow breathing pattern and accumulation of pulmonary secretions occurring with chronic alcoholism (i.e., due to pneumonia or pulmonary edema) and the possibility of oversedation during treatment, *"Delirium Tremens," p. 326;* related to shallow breathing with decreased diffusion of oxygen secondary to diaphragmatic limitation with ascites, hydrothorax, or central respiratory depression occurring with encephalopathy, *"Hepatic Failure," p. 374;* related to decreased diffusion of oxygen secondary to microatelectasis and fluid accumulation in the alveoli, *"Acute Pancreatitis," p. 385;* related to decreased diffusion of oxygen secondary to increased pulmonary alveolar-capillary permeability or embolus formation, *"Disseminated Intravascular Coagulation," p. 421;* related to decreased diffusion of oxygen secondary to interstitial edema, alveolar destruction, and eventual respiratory depression, *"Sepsis," p. 440;* related to decreased diffusion of oxygen secondary to dyspnea and airway obstruction occurring with laryngeal edema and bronchoconstriction, *"Anaphylaxis," p. 446;* related to hypoventilation and decreased diffusion of oxygen secondary to circumferential burns to neck and thorax or swelling of the membranes of the naso-oropharyngeal passage due to smoke inhalation, *"Burns," p. 461;* related to hyperventilation, increased oxygen requirements associated with sepsis, and decreased diffusion of oxygen secondary to pulmonary congestion, *"Acquired Immune Deficiency Syndrome," p. 481;* related to risk of aspiration secondary to administration of enteral feeding, *"Providing Nutritional Support," p. 504.*

Grieving, anticipatory, related to expected loss of body function or body part, changes in self-concept or body image, or terminal illness, *"Caring for the Critically Ill with Life-Threatening Disorders," p. 517.*

Grieving, dysfunctional, related to actual or perceived loss or change in body function, body image, lifestyle, relationships, or lack of support systems, *"Caring for the Critically Ill with Life-Threatening Disorders,"* p. 517.

Hopelessness related to prolonged hospitalization or life-threatening illness, *"Caring for the Critically Ill with Life-Threatening Disorders,"* p. 522.

Hyperthermia related to infectious process occurring with peritonitis, *"Peritonitis,"* p. 393; related to increased metabolic rate and dehydration, *"Toxic Shock Syndrome,"* p. 453.

Hypothermia related to prolonged exposure to cold water during submersion, *"Near Drowning,"* p. 40; related to prolonged cooling of body during surgery, *"Coronary Artery Bypass Graft,"* p. 151; related to exposure at the scene of injury, temporary loss of temperature regulatory mechanisms due to shock or CNS ischemia, evisceration injury, surgical exposure of abdominal viscera, or administration of large volumes of unwarmed fluid or blood, *"Abdominal Trauma,"* p. 412.

Incontinence, reflex, related to uninhibited activity of the spinal reflex arc secondary to recovery phase from spinal shock in patients with cord lesions above T12, *"Acute Spinal Cord Injury,"* p. 306.

Infection, potential for, related to high risk secondary to recent thoracoabdominal surgery, aspiration, exposure to contaminated respiratory equipment, respiratory instrumentation, colonization of oropharynx with aerobic gram-negative bacilli, or immunosuppression, *"Acute Pneumonia,"* p. 13; related to susceptibility secondary to aspiration of water, gastric contents, and contaminants present in water, *"Near Drowning,"* p. 41; related to compromise of normal defense mechanisms secondary to intubation, contamination of respiratory equipment, or immunosuppression, *"Management of the Adult on Mechanical Ventilation,"* p. 67; related to vulnerability secondary to prolonged antibiotic use and presence of invasive catheters and lines, *"Acute Infective Endocarditis,"* p. 114; related to vulnerability secondary to presence of multiple invasive lines, cannulas, and debilitated state, *Heart-Assist Device,"* p. 149; related to vulnerability secondary to invasive procedure into thorax, *"Automatic Implantable Cardioverter-Defibrillator,"* p. 158; related to vulnerability secondary to presence of hemodynamic lines, *"Management of the Adult with Hemodynamic Monitoring,"* p. 168; related to vulnerability secondary to immunocompromised state associated with the high serum level of nitrogenous waste that occurs with renal failure, *"Acute Renal Failure,"* p. 183; related to high risk secondary to bacterial contamination of the urinary tract system occurring with penetrating trauma, rupture of the bladder into the perineum, or instrumentation, *"Lower Urinary Tract Trauma,"* p. 187; related to increased susceptibility secondary to immunosuppression, *"Renal Transplant,"* p. 197; related to vulnerability to septicemia or peritonitis secondary to peritoneal or vascular access, *"Dialytic Therapy,"* p. 203; (CNS) related to vulnerability secondary to direct access to the brain in the presence of skull fracture, penetrating wounds, craniotomy, or intracranial monitoring, *"Head Injury,"* p. 278; related to risk of cross-contamination secondary to communicable nature of bacterial and aseptic meningitis, *"Meningitis,"* p. 291; related to vulnerability secondary to presence of invasive immobilization devices, *"Acute Spinal Cord Injury,"* p. 310; related to susceptibility secondary to protein depletion and hyperglycemia, *"Diabetic Ketoacidosis,"* p. 332; related to

Mobility, impaired physical, related to precautions against movement secondary to presence of assist device or debilitated state, *"Heart-Assist Device,"* p. 148; related to movement restrictions secondary to access and equipment for hemofiltration, *"Continuous Arteriovenous Hemofiltration,"* p. 213; related to sensorimotor deficits secondary to ascending flaccid paralysis and paresthesias, *"Guillain-Barré Syndrome,"* p. 254; related to prolonged inactivity secondary to head injury, spasticity, or decreased LOC, *"Head Injury,"* p. 280; related to risk of contracture formation secondary to immobilization from pain, splints, or scar formation, *"Burns,"* p. 464; related to risk of contractures or ankylosis secondary to prolonged bed rest, *"Caring for the Critically Ill on Prolonged Bed Rest,"* p. 507.

Noncompliance with prescribed medication related to misunderstanding physician's instructions, not understanding importance of following medication schedule, running out of medication, or stopping medication intentionally owing to frustration or denial of the disease, *"Status Epilepticus,"* p. 315.

Nutrition, alteration in: *Less than body requirements* related to decreased intake secondary to oral intubation and increased need secondary to debilitated state and impaired tissue perfusion with concomitant nitrogen malabsorption, *"Heart-Assist Device,"* p. 149; related to increased catabolism or dietary restrictions secondary to acute renal failure, *"Acute Renal Failure,"* p. 179; related to dietary restrictions and protein loss occurring with peritoneal dialysis, *"Dialytic Therapy,"* p. 204; related to decreased oral intake secondary to anorexia, difficulty eating in a prone position, fear of choking and aspiration, and inability to feed self due to paralysis of upper extremities; and decreased GI motility secondary to autonomic nervous system dysfunction, *"Acute Spinal Cord Injury,"* p. 304; related to decreased intake secondary to anorexia, nausea, and medically-prescribed dietary restrictions; and decreased metabolism of nutrients secondary to decreased intestinal motility, altered portal blood flow, decreased intestinal absorption of vitamins and minerals, and altered protein metabolism, *"Hepatic Failure,"* p. 373; related to decreased oral intake secondary to nausea, vomiting, and NPO status; and increased need secondary to tissue destruction or infection, *"Acute Pancreatitis,"* p. 387; related to decreased intake secondary to impaired GI function, *"Peritonitis,"* p. 392; related to decreased oral intake secondary to nausea, vomiting, and NPO status; and increased need secondary to tissue destruction or infection, *"Acute GI Bleeding,"* p. 400; related to decreased intake secondary to disruption of GI tract integrity and increased need secondary to hypermetabolic posttraumatic state, *"Abdominal Trauma,"* p. 413; related to increased need for nutritional substrates secondary to increased metabolic rate, *"Sepsis,"* p. 442; increased requirements of protein, vitamins, and calories related to hypermetabolic state secondary to burn wound healing, *"Burns,"* p. 465; decreased intake and losses secondary to diarrhea and nausea associated with side effects of chemotherapy, malabsorption, anorexia, dysphagia, and fatigue, *"Acquired Immune Deficiency Syndrome,"* p. 482; related to inadequate provision of nutrients, *"Providing Nutritional Support,"* p. 501.

Oral mucous membrane, alteration in, related to stomatitis secondary to immunosuppression, *"Renal Transplant,"* p. 198; related to self-care deficit, *"Caring for the Critically Ill on Prolonged Bed Rest,"* p. 509.

Posttrauma response related to stress reaction secondary to life-threatening accident or event resulting in trauma, *"Abdominal Trauma,"* p. 414.

Powerlessness related to actual and perceived inability to control organ rejection episodes, *"Organ Rejection," p. 475;* related to lack of control over self-care, health care status, or outcome secondary to nature of health care environment, therapeutic regimen, or life-threatening illness, *"Caring for the Critically Ill with Life-Threatening Disorders," p. 518.*

Self-care deficit: Inability to perform ADLs related to decreased LOC or sensorimotor deficit, *"Caring for the Critically Ill on Prolonged Bed Rest," p. 510.*

Self concept, disturbance in, related to alteration in body image secondary to fecal diversion in patients with colonic injury and colostomy, *"Abdominal Trauma," p. 415;* related to altered body image secondary to large, irregular fasciotomy wound and skin grafted scar; loss of function and cosmesis of an extremity; or amputation, *"Compartment Syndrome," p. 470;* related to body image changes secondary to side effects from immunosuppression medications, *"Organ Rejection," p. 476;* related to body image changes secondary to Kaposi's lesions, side effects of chemotherapy, social stigmatization, isolation, and emaciation, *"Acquired Immune Deficiency Syndrome," p. 485;* related to alteration in body image secondary to loss or change in body parts or function, physical trauma, hospitalization, *"Caring for the Critically Ill with Life-Threatening Disorders," p. 520.*

Sensory-perceptual alterations related to decreased visual acuity secondary to retinal damage occurring with high perfusion pressures, *"Hypertensive Crisis," p. 127;* related to dialysis disequilibrium syndrome secondary to rapid removal of metabolic waste with changes in serum osmolality, *"Dialytic Therapy," p. 206;* related to diplopia or ptosis secondary to ocular involvement with myasthenia gravis, *"Myasthenia Gravis," p. 245;* related to sensorimotor dysfunction secondary to cranial nerve involvement with G-BS, *"Guillain-Barré Syndrome," p. 257;* related to visual impairment secondary to presence of immobilization device or use of therapeutic bed, *"Acute Spinal Cord Injury," p. 310;* related to disorientation, agitation, and hallucinations secondary to drug overdose and withdrawal symptoms, *"Drug Overdose," p. 322;* related to impaired mentation secondary to accumulation of ammonia or other CNS toxins occurring with hepatic dysfunction, *"Hepatic Failure," p. 375;* related to confusion and agitation secondary to bacterial toxins, hypotension, dehydration, febrile state, and hospitalization in critical care area, *"Toxic Shock Syndrome," p. 453;* related to tactile and visual deficits, medications, sleep-pattern disturbance, or pain secondary to severe burn injury, *"Burns," p. 466;* related to environmental overload or monotony, socially-restricted environment, psychologic stress, or pathophysiologic alterations, *"Caring for the Critically Ill with Life-Threatening Disorders," p. 513.*

Sexual dysfunction related to altered body image or physical limitations secondary to lower urinary tract trauma, *"Lower Urinary Tract Trauma," p. 188.*

Sexuality pattern, altered, related to fear of inducing dysrhythmias during sexual activity, *"Automatic Implantable Cardioverter-Defibrillator," p. 159;* related to loss of aspects of sexual functioning secondary to SCI, *"Acute Spinal Cord Injury," p. 310.*

Skin integrity, impaired, related to vulnerability secondary to prolonged bed rest, diminished circulation, and decreased protein intake due to NPO status, *"Intra-*

Aortic Balloon Pump,'' p. 145; related to irritation secondary to suprapubic catheter placement and maintenance, *"Lower Urinary Tract Trauma," p. 188;* related to herpetic lesions, skin fungal rashes, pruritus, and capillary fragility secondary to immunosuppression with corticosteroids, *"Renal Transplant," p. 198;* related to edema secondary to fluid volume excess, *"Fluid and Electrolyte Disturbances," p. 221;* related to prolonged immobility secondary to immobilization device or paralysis, *"Acute Spinal Cord Injury," p. 304;* related to pruritus, tissue edema, or impaired tissue healing, *"Hepatic Failure," p. 378;* related to direct trauma and surgery; hypermetabolic, catabolic posttraumatic state; impaired tissue perfusion; or exposure to irritating GI drainage, *"Abdominal Trauma," p. 412;* related to tissue hypoxia secondary to vasocclussive process, *"Hemolytic Crisis," p. 425;* related to urticaria and angioedema secondary to allergic response, *"Anaphylaxis," p. 449;* related to erythroderma secondary to bacterial toxins, *"Toxic Shock Syndrome," p. 454;* related to damage to epidermal elements secondary to burn injury, *"Burns," p. 463;* related to vulnerability secondary to cachexia and malnourishment, diarrhea, side effects of chemotherapy, Kaposi's skin lesions, negative nitrogen state, and decreased mobility due to arthralgia and fatigue, *"Acquired Immune Deficiency Syndrome," p. 483;* related to vulnerability secondary to malnourished state, or presence of central venous catheters or enteral tube, *"Providing Nutritional Support," p. 502;* related to pressure on skin and tissue secondary to prolonged bed rest, *"Caring for the Critically Ill on Prolonged Bed Rest," p. 508.*

Sleep pattern disturbance related to confusion and agitation secondary to DTs and deprivation of REM sleep secondary to alcohol ingestion, *"Delirium Tremens," p. 326;* related to environmental overload, therapeutic regimen, pain, immobility, or psychologic stress, *"Caring for the Critically Ill with Life-Threatening Disorders," p. 514.*

Social isolation related to disease, societal rejection, loss of support system, fear, feelings of guilt and punishment, fatigue, and changed patterns of sexual expression, *"Acquired Immune Deficiency Syndrome," p. 486;* related to hospitalization in critical care unit, altered health status, inadequate support systems, and terminal illness, *"Caring for the Critically Ill with Life-Threatening Disorders," p. 519.*

Spiritual distress related to altered health state, separation from religious ties, life-threatening illness, or conflict between religious beliefs and therapeutic regimens, *"Caring for the Critically Ill with Life-Threatening Disorders," p. 518.*

Swallowing, impaired, related to decreased or absent gag reflex, decreased strength or excursion of muscles involved in mastication, facial paralysis, or mechanical obstruction (tracheostomy), *"Myasthenia Gravis," p. 244;* related to lower esophageal pain or lower esophageal stricture secondary to sclerotherapy, *"Bleeding Esophageal Varices," p. 363;* related to pain or decreased ability to ingest secondary to disease or treatment of disease (e.g., surgery, chemotherapy, radiation), *"Providing Nutritional Support," p. 503.*

Thermoregulation, ineffective, related to fluctuations secondary to injury to or pressure on hypothalamus, *"Head Injury," p. 279;* related to inability of the body to adapt to environmental temperature changes secondary to poikilothermic reaction occurring with SCI, *"Acute Spinal Cord Injury," p. 307;* related to fluctuations secondary to sympathetic response occurring with cocaine overdose, *"Drug Overdose," p. 323;* related to fluctuations secondary to alterations in metabolic rate due to endotoxin effect on hypothalamic temperature regulating center, *"Sepsis," p. 441.*

Thought processes, alterations in, related to mental deterioration secondary to infection or space-occupying lesion in the CNS, *"Acquired Immune Deficiency Syndrome," p. 487.*

Tissue integrity, impaired, related to vulnerability secondary to prolonged bed rest, diminished circulation, and decreased protein intake due to NPO status, *"Intra-Aortic Balloon Pump," p. 145;* related to edema secondary to fluid volume excess, *"Fluid and Electrolyte Disturbances," p. 221;* Corneal, related to inability to blink secondary to altered LOC or cranial nerve damage, *"Head Injury," p. 280;* related to prolonged immobility secondary to immobilization device or paralysis, *"Acute Spinal Cord Injury," p. 304;* related to pruritus, tissue edema, or impaired tissue healing, *"Hepatic Failure," p. 378;* GI tract, related to irritation secondary to release of chemical irritants into the pancreatic parenchyma and surrounding tissue, including the peritoneum, *"Acute Pancreatitis," p. 387;* related to direct trauma and surgery; hypermetabolic, catabolic posttraumatic state; impaired tissue perfusion; or exposure to irritating GI drainage, *"Abdominal Trauma," p. 412;* related to tissue hypoxia secondary to vasocclusive process, *"Hemolytic Crisis," p. 425;* related to vulnerability secondary to intradermal bleeding, *"Idiopathic Thrombocytopenia Purpura," p. 429;* related to damage to epidermal elements secondary to burn injury, *"Burns," p. 463;* related to vulnerability secondary to cachexia and malnourishment, diarrhea, side effects of chemotherapy, Kaposi's skin lesions, negative nitrogen state, and decreased mobility due to arthralgia and fatigue, *"Acquired Immune Deficiency Syndrome," p. 483;* related to vulnerability secondary to malnourished state or presence of central venous catheters or enteral tube, *"Providing Nutritional Support," p. 502;* related to pressure on skin and tissue secondary to prolonged bed rest, *"Caring for the Critically Ill on Prolonged Bed Rest," p. 508.*

Tissue perfusion, alteration in: Peripheral, cardiopulmonary, renal, and cerebral, related to impaired circulation (ischemia) secondary to decreased cardiac contractility, *"Cardiac Trauma," p. 104;* Cardiovascular, peripheral, cerebral, and renal, related to impaired circulation secondary to acute cardiac tamponade, *"Acute Cardiac Tamponade," p. 107;* Renal, GI, peripheral, cerebral, and cardiopulmonary, related to impaired circulation secondary to emboli caused by vegetations, *"Acute Infective Endocarditis," p. 115;* Cardiopulmonary, cerebral, ophthalmic, and renal, related to impaired circulation secondary to vasoconstriction that occurs with interruption of the normal blood pressure control mechanism; or vasodilatation with tissue edema that occurs with loss of autoregulation, *"Hypertensive Crisis," p. 126;* Peripheral, cardiopulmonary, renal, and cerebral, related to mechanical impairment to blood flow secondary to narrowed aortic lumen, *"Aortic Dissection," p. 129;* Cerebral, renal, peripheral, and cardiopulmonary, related to impaired circulation to vital organs secondary to inadequate arterial pressure, *"Cardiogenic Shock," p. 135;* Peripheral (involved limb), related to impaired circulation secondary to presence of angioplasty sheath or risk of clot formation in vessel following sheath removal, *"Percutaneous Transluminal Coronary Angioplasty," p. 139;* Peripheral (balloon leg), related to risk of obstruction or hemorrhage of femoral artery secondary to arterial wall dissection by sheath or thrombus formation, *"Intra-Aortic*

Balloon Pump," p. 144; Cerebral, related to impaired circulation to the brain secondary to embolization resulting from cardiac surgery, "Valvular Heart Disease and Valve Surgery," p. 156; Pulmonary, related to risk of pulmonary infarction secondary to migration of pulmonary artery catheter into a wedged position, overwedging of balloon, or continuous wedge position, "Management of the Adult with Hemodynamic Monitoring," p. 169; Peripheral (hand), related to risk of impaired circulation secondary to presence of arterial catheter or thrombosis caused by catheter, "Management of the Adult with Hemodynamic Monitoring," p. 169; Access site, related to impaired circulation secondary to clots, pressure, or disconnection of shunt, "Dialytic Therapy," p. 205; Cerebral and peripheral, related to decreased circulation secondary to hypovolemia, "Fluid and Electrolyte Disturbances," p. 217; Cerebral, related to risk of cerebral vasospasm secondary to ruptured cerebral aneurysm, "Cerebral Aneurysm and Subarachnoid Hemorrhage," p. 267; Cerebral, related to impaired blood flow secondary to hypotension, intracranial hypertension, or infections that occur with secondary head injury, "Head Injury," p. 278; Peripheral and cardiopulmonary, related to risk of thromboembolism, deep-vein thrombosis (DVT), and pulmonary emboli secondary to venous stasis occurring with decreased vasomotor tone and immobility, "Acute Spinal Cord Injury, p. 302; Cerebral and cardiopulmonary, related to decreased blood flow to and increased metabolic demands on the cells secondary to continuous seizure activity, "Status Epilepticus," p. 315; Peripheral, related to risk of thromboembolism secondary to increased viscosity of the blood, increased platelet aggregation and adhesiveness, and patient immobility, "Diabetic Ketoacidosis," p. 334; Peripheral, cardiopulmonary, and renal, related to impaired circulation secondary to loss of vascular tone and decreased vascular response to catecholamines occurring with impaired secretion of glucocorticoids, "Addisonian Crisis," p. 352; Esophageal, related to risk of impaired circulation secondary to prolonged use of esophageal balloon tamponade, "Bleeding Esophageal Varices," p. 362; Renal, related to risk of reduced cortical blood flow and consequent functional renal failure secondary to hepatic failure, "Hepatic Failure," p. 377; GI tract, related to risk of interruption of blood flow to abdominal viscera from vascular disruption or occlusion or moderate to severe hypovolemia caused by hemorrhage, "Abdominal Trauma," p. 411; Peripheral, renal, pulmonary, and cerebral, related to impaired circulation secondary to presence of microthrombi occurring with coagulation phase of DIC, "Disseminated Intravascular Coagulation," p. 420; Peripheral, renal, cardiopulmonary, and cerebral, related to impaired circulation with cellular hypoxia secondary to microthrombi (resulting from destruction of RBCs) and a decrease in circulating RBCs, "Hemolytic Crisis," p. 424; Cerebral, renal, and splanchnic, related to decreased circulating volume secondary to vasodilatation (early stage) or vasoconstriction and thrombus obstruction (late stage), "Sepsis," p. 439; Peripheral, renal, and cerebral, related to decreased circulation of blood to the tissues secondary to edema and loss of vascular volume, "Anaphylaxis," p. 448; Compartment tissues, related to impaired circulation secondary to developing or recurring compartment syndrome, "Compartment Syndrome," p. 469.

Urinary elimination, alteration in pattern of, related to inadequate urinary outflow secondary to injury to LUT structures, "Lower Urinary Tract Trauma," p. 186; related to inadequate urinary outflow secondary to damaged functional renal tissue or side effects from diagnostic testing, "Renal Trauma," p. 191; Dysuria, urgency, frequency, and polyuria, secondary to administration of diuretics, calcium stone formation, or changes in renal function occurring with hypercalcemia, "Fluid and Electrolyte Disturbances," p. 237.

Urinary retention related to inhibition of the spinal reflex arc secondary to spinal shock following SCI, *"Acute Spinal Cord Injury," p. 305;* (with overflow incontinence) related to loss of reflex activity for micturition and bladder flaccidity secondary to cord lesion at or below T12, *"Acute Spinal Cord Injury," p. 307.*

Violence, potential for, related to sensory overload, rage reactions, perceived threats, or physiologic imbalance, *"Caring for the Critically Ill with Life-Threatening Disorders," p. 521.*

INDEX